SECTIONAL ANATOMY
for Imaging Professionals

THIRD EDITION

Lorrie L. Kelley, MS, RT(R)(MR)(CT)
Associate Professor, CT/MRI Program Director
Boise State University
Boise, Idaho

Connie M. Petersen, MS, RT(R)(CT)
Adjunct Instructor, Radiologic Sciences Program
Boise State University
Boise, Idaho

ELSEVIER

3251 Riverport Lane
St. Louis, Missouri 63043

SECTIONAL ANATOMY FOR IMAGING PROFESSIONALS,
THIRD EDITION

ISBN: 978-0-323-08260-0

Notice

ISBN: 978-0-323-08260-0

Senior Content Strategist: Jennifer Janson
Associate Content Development Specialist: Amy Whittier
Publishing Services Manager: Catherine Jackson
Designer: Paula Catalano

Printed in China

Last digit is the print number: 9 8 7 6 5 4 3 2 1

To *James,*
Min beste venn og evig ledsager, jeg smil hver dag på grunn av deg.
Your strength sustains me during the dark moments, your unconditional
patience and love elevates me, and your faith inspires me.

*And to **Kristina, Matt, Jennifer, John, Michael, Natalie, Angela, James,***
***Daniel, Dean, Maren, Evelyn, McKenzie,** and **Jakob,** et al, my*
greatest treasures, who bless me with their laughter and enthusiasm for
life. Thanks for reminding me to dream and never stop learning.

And to my parents,
***Bill** and **Darhl Buchanan,** for teaching me the value of hard work and sharing*
their wisdom and encouragement in ways that strengthen and inspire me.

LLK

Thank you to my family and friends whose guidance, love, and support
carried me through my most trying times.

I dedicate this book to:
*My greatest blessings, **Brady** and **Trinity,** for the countless joys you have*
graced my life with. May you never lose sight of the incredible good and
strengths within you as you reach for greatness. Always know that you
are loved and how truly honored I am to be your mom.

***Carl** and **Ellen Collins,** my parents, for the wonderful gifts of life*
and love. Thank you for your ever-present understanding, wisdom, and
encouragement. I love you both dearly.

***Grant,** my amazing gift from God, for loving me and being there*
when I needed you most.

CMP

ACKNOWLEDGMENTS

Many provided encouragement and direction as the compilation of this text commenced. Amy Whittier had the tiresome duty of encouraging us to meet deadlines, which she did with grace and humor. Jennifer Geistler had the daunting task of strategically pulling it all together. We are indebted to them for their editorial assistance in seeing this project through completion.

We wish to extend our gratitude to everyone who thought the first and second editions had value and to those who took the time to provide constructive criticism and suggestions for further improvements and increased accuracy. And to the many students who were not shy in providing feedback so that we could see the text from many different perspectives.

The following individuals and institutions deserve special acknowledgment:

- The faculty at Boise State University for their support and patience as we faced fast-approaching deadlines.

- Chris Hayden for his tremendous patience, knowledge, and time invested in helping us find and create all of the new CT images for the third edition. And St. Alphonsus Regional Medical Center for providing the CT images.
- Mary Pullin from Philips Medical Systems for providing some beautiful MR images.
- Dave Arnold and St. Luke's Regional Medical Center, as well as Kevin Bean and Intermountain Medical Imaging, for providing the majority of the MR images.

We owe a debt of gratitude to Jeanne Robertson, who provided numerous new illustrations and revised many old drawings in record time. Because of her efforts and talent, there is more consistency in the visual presentation of the artwork throughout the text.

Lorrie L. Kelley
Connie M. Petersen

Becky Britt, MSRS, RT(R)(M)
Assistant Professor
Northwestern State University
Shreveport, Louisiana

Gail Faig, BS, RT(R)(CV)(CT)
Clinical Coordinator
Shore Medical Center
School of Radiologic Technology
Somers Point, New Jersey

Lisa Fanning, MEd, RT(R)(CT)
Radiography Program Director
Massachusetts College of Pharmacy
    and Health Sciences
Boston, Massachusetts

Kelli Haynes, MSRS, RT(R)
Director of Undergraduate Studies/
    Associate Professor/Graduate
    Faculty
Radiologic Sciences Department
Northwestern State University of
    Louisiana
Shreveport, Louisiana

Marelene Johnson, MEd, RT(R)
Education Director
University of Utah
Salt Lake City, Utah

Kathleen Kienstra, MAT, RT(R)(T)
Program Director
Radiation Therapy Program
Saint Louis University
St. Louis, Missouri

Bob McGee, MEd, RT(R), CCI
Assistant Professor/Clinical
    Coordinator
South College/Asheville
Asheville, North Carolina

Marcia Moore BS, RT(R)(CT)
Instructor
St. Luke's College
Sioux City, Iowa

Roger Preston, MSRS, RT(R)(CT)
Program Director
School of Radiologic Technology
Richmond, Indiana

Theresa Roberts, MHS, RT(R)(MR)
Program Director
Radiologic Technology
Keiser University
Melbourne, Florida

Kenneth Roszel, MS, RT(R)
Program Director
Geisenger Medical Center
Danville, Pennsylvania

Rebecca Silva, MEd, MPH, RT(R)
Department Chair
South Texas College
McAllen, Texas

Karen Tillelli, RT, CT(R)
Program Instructor
University of Utah Hospital/Clinics
Salt Lake City, Utah

Diana Werderman, MSEd, RT(R)
Assistant Professor
Trinity College of Nursing and
    Health Sciences
Rock Island, Illinois

This text was written to address the needs of today's practicing health professional. As technology in diagnostic imaging advances, so does the need to competently recognize and identify cross-sectional anatomy. Our goal was to create a clear, concise text that would demonstrate in an easy-to-use yet comprehensive format the anatomy the health professional is required to understand to optimize patient care. The text was purposely designed to be used both as a clinical reference manual and as an instructional text, either in a formal classroom environment or as a self-instructional volume.

Included are close to 1000 high-quality MR and CT images for every feasible plane of anatomy most commonly imaged. An additional 350 anatomic maps and line drawings related to the MR and CT images add to the learner's understanding of the anatomy being studied. In addition, pathology boxes describe common pathologies related to the anatomy presented, assisting the reader in making connections between the images in the text and common pathologies that will be encountered in clinical practice. Tables that summarize muscle group information include points of origin and insertion, as well as functions, for the muscle structures pertinent to the images the reader is studying.

NEW TO THIS EDITION

- Nearly 150 new MR and CT images and 30 new line drawings provide more 3D and vascular images to better demonstrate anatomy seen with current technology.
- Chapter Objectives will help readers prepare for the material they will learn in each chapter.
- Addition of full labels to scans will improve usability of the images and allow readers to quickly and efficiently see the anatomy displayed on the scan.
- Addition of Test Bank to Evolve Instructor Resources will provide readers with the tools for an enhanced learning experience.

CONTENT AND ORGANIZATION

The images include identification of vital anatomic structures to assist the health professional in locating and identifying the desired anatomy during actual clinical examinations. The narrative accompanying these images clearly and concisely describes the location and function of the anatomy in a format easily understood by health professionals. The text is divided into chapters by anatomic regions. Each chapter of the text contains an outline that provides an overview of the chapter's contents, pathology boxes that briefly describe common pathologies related to the anatomy being presented, tables designed to organize and summarize the anatomy contained in the chapter, and reference illustrations that provide the correct orientation for scanning the anatomy of interest.

ANCILLARIES

A Workbook and an Evolve site complement the text. When used together, these additional tools create a virtual learning system/reference resource.

Workbook: The Workbook provides practice opportunities for the user to identify specific anatomy. The Workbook includes learning objectives that focus on the key elements of each chapter, a variety of practice items to test the reader's knowledge of key concepts, labeling exercises to test the reader's knowledge of the anatomy, and answers to exercises.

Instructor Resources on Evolve: These resources include a test bank with approximately 500 questions and an image collection with approximately 1000 images.

Lorrie L. Kelley
Connie M. Petersen

CONTENTS

1

Introduction to Sectional Anatomy

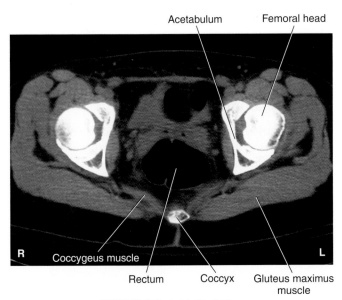

Acetabulum   Femoral head

R

Coccygeus muscle   L

Rectum   Coccyx   Gluteus maximus
muscle

FIGURE 1.1 Axial CT of hips.

Sectional anatomy has had a long history. Beginning as early as the sixteenth century, the great anatomist and artist, Leonardo da Vinci, was among the first to represent the body in anatomic sections. In the following centuries, numerous anatomists continued to provide illustrations of various body structures in sectional planes to gain greater understanding of the topographical relationships of the organs. The ability to see inside the body for medical purposes has been around since 1895, when Wilhelm Conrad Roentgen discovered x-rays. Since that time, medical imaging has evolved from the static 2-dimensional (2D) image of the first x-ray to the 2D cross-section image of computed tomography (CT), and finally to the 3-dimensional (3D) imaging techniques used today. These changes warrant the need for medical professionals to understand and identify human anatomy in both 2D and 3D images.

Sectional anatomy emphasizes the physical relationship between internal structures. Prior knowledge of anatomy from drawings or radiographs may assist in understanding the location of specific structures on a sectional image. For example, it may be difficult to recognize all the internal anatomy of the pelvis in cross-section, but by identifying the femoral head on the image, it will be easier to recognize soft tissue structures adjacent to the hip in the general location of the slice (Figure 1.1).

OBJECTIVES

- Define the four anatomic planes.
- Describe the relative position of specific structures within the body using directional and regional terminology.
- Identify commonly used external landmarks.
- Identify the location of commonly used internal landmarks.
- Describe the dorsal and ventral cavities of the body.
- List the four abdominal quadrants.
- List the nine regions of the abdomen.
- Describe the gray scale used in CT and MR imaging.
- Describe MPR, CPR, SSD, MIP and VR.

OUTLINE

1

ANATOMIC POSITIONS AND PLANES

For our purposes, sectional anatomy encompasses all the variations of viewing anatomy taken from an arbitrary angle through the body while in anatomic position.

In anatomic position, the body is standing erect, face and toes pointing forward, and arms at the side with the palms facing forward. Sectional images are acquired and displayed according to one of the four fundamental anatomic planes that pass through the body (Figure 1.2). The four anatomic planes are defined as follows:

1. **Sagittal plane:** a vertical plane that passes through the body, dividing it into right and left portions
2. **Coronal plane:** a vertical plane that passes through the body, dividing it into anterior (ventral) and posterior (dorsal) portions
3. **Axial (transverse) plane:** a horizontal plane that passes through the body, dividing it into superior and inferior portions
4. **Oblique plane:** a plane that passes diagonally between the axes of two other planes

Medical images of sectional anatomy are, by convention, displayed in a specific orientation. Images are viewed with the right side of the image corresponding to the viewer's left side (Figure 1.3).

TERMINOLOGY AND LANDMARKS

Directional and regional terminology is used to help describe the relative positions of specific structures within the body. Directional terms are defined in Table 1.1, and regional terms are defined in Table 1.2 and demonstrated in Figure 1.4.

External Landmarks

External landmarks of the body are helpful in identifying the location of many internal structures. The commonly used external landmarks are shown in Figures 1.5 and 1.6.

Internal Landmarks

Internal structures, in particular vascular structures, can be located by referencing them to other identifiable regions or locations, such as organs or the skeleton (Table 1.3).

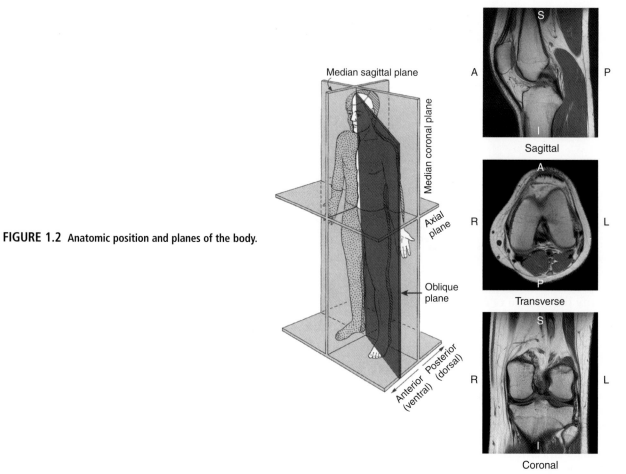

FIGURE 1.2 Anatomic position and planes of the body.

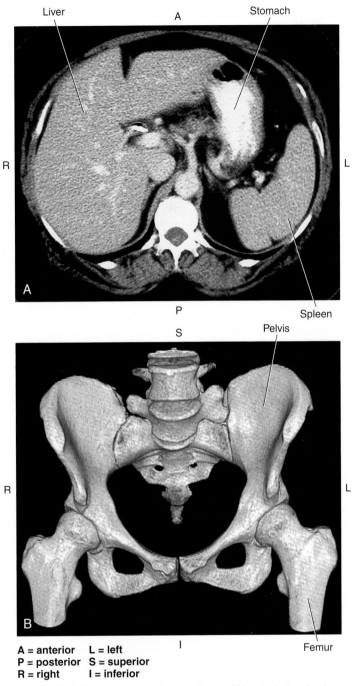

A = anterior   L = left
P = posterior S = superior
R = right   I = inferior

FIGURE 1.3 A, Axial CT of liver. B, 3D CT of hips (anterior view).

TABLE 1.1	Directional Terminology
Direction	**Definition**
Superior	Above; at a higher level
Inferior	Below; at a lower level
Anterior/ventral	Toward the front or anterior surface of the body
Posterior/dorsal	Toward the back or posterior surface of the body
Medial	Toward the midsagittal plane
Lateral	Away from the midsagittal plane
Proximal	Toward a reference point or source within the body
Distal	Away from a reference point or source within the body
Superficial	Near the body surface
Deep	Farther into the body and away from the body surface
Cranial/cephalic	Toward the head
Caudal	Toward the feet
Rostral	Toward the nose
Ipsilateral	On the same side
Contralateral	On the opposite side
Thenar	The fleshy part of the hand at the base of the thumb
Volar	Pertaining to the palm of the hand or flexor surface of wrist or the sole of the foot
Palmar	The front or palm of the hand
Plantar	The sole of the foot

TABLE 1.2	Regional Terminology		
Direction	**Definition**	**Direction**	**Definition**
Abdominal	Abdomen	Inguinal	Groin
Antebrachial	Forearm	Lumbar	Lower back between the ribs and hips
Antecubital	Front of elbow	Occipital	Back of the head
Axillary	Armpit	Ophthalmic	Eye
Brachial	Upper arm	Pectoral/mammary	Upper chest or breast
Calf	Lower posterior portion of leg	Pelvic	Pelvis
Carpal	Wrist	Perineal	Perineum
Cephalic	Head	Plantar	Sole of foot
Cervical	Neck	Popliteal	Back of knee
Costal	Ribs	Sacral	Sacrum
Cubital	Posterior surface of elbow area of the arm	Sternal	Sternum
Femoral	Thigh, upper portion of leg	Thoracic	Chest
Flank	Side of trunk adjoining the lumbar region	Umbilical	Navel
Gluteal	Buttock	Vertebral	Spine

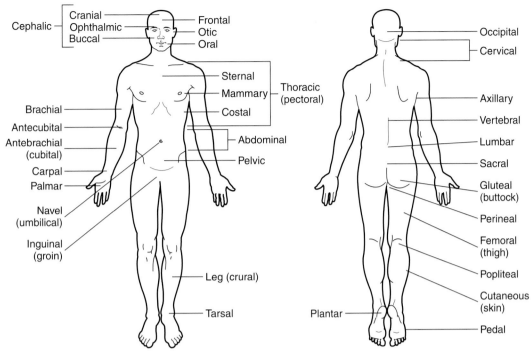

FIGURE 1.4 Regional terminology of the body.

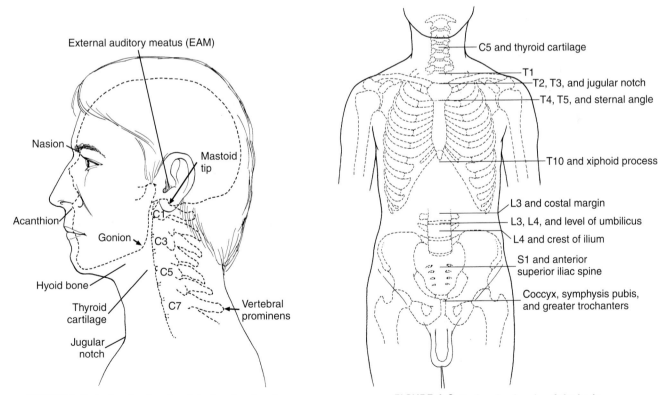

FIGURE 1.5 Surface landmarks of the head and neck.

FIGURE 1.6 Surface landmarks of the body.

TABLE 1.3	Internal Landmarks
Landmark	**Location**
Aortic arch	2.5 cm below jugular notch
Aortic bifurcation	L4-L5
Carina	T4-T5, sternal angle
Carotid bifurcation	Upper border of thyroid cartilage
Celiac trunk	4 cm above transpyloric plane
Circle of Willis	Suprasellar cistern
Common iliac vein bifurcation	Upper margin of sacroiliac joint
Conus medullaris	T12 to L1, L2
Heart—apex	5th intercostal space, left midclavicular line
Heart—base	Level of 2nd and 3rd costal cartilages behind sternum
Inferior mesenteric artery	4 cm above bifurcation of abdominal aorta
Inferior vena cava	L5
Portal vein	Posterior to pancreatic neck
Renal arteries	Anterior to L1, inferior to superior mesenteric artery
Superior mesenteric artery	2 cm above transpyloric plane
Thyroid gland	Thyroid cartilage
Vocal cords	Midway between superior and inferior border of thyroid cartilage

BODY CAVITIES

The body consists of two main cavities: the dorsal and ventral cavities. The dorsal cavity is located posteriorly and includes the cranial and spinal cavities. The ventral cavity, the largest body cavity, is subdivided into the thoracic and abdominopelvic cavities. The thoracic cavity is further subdivided into two lateral pleural cavities and a single, centrally located cavity called the mediastinum. The abdominal cavity can be subdivided into the abdominal and pelvic cavities (Figure 1.7). The structures located in each cavity are listed in Table 1.4.

ABDOMINAL AND PELVIC DIVISIONS

The abdomen is bordered superiorly by the diaphragm and inferiorly by the superior pelvic aperture (pelvic inlet). The abdomen can be divided into quadrants or regions. These divisions are useful in identifying the general location of internal organs and provide descriptive terms for the location of pain or injury in a patient's history.

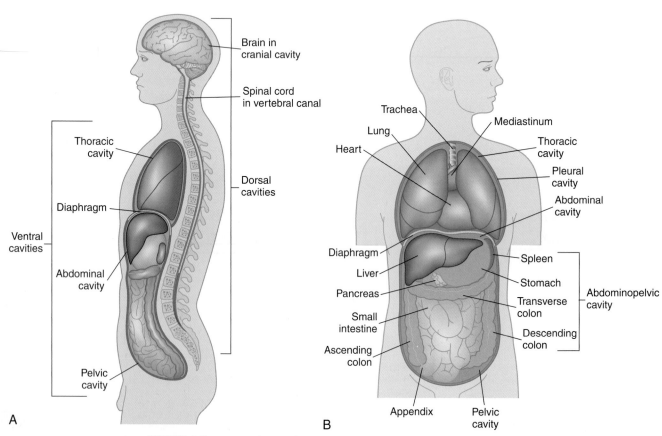

FIGURE 1.7 A, Sagittal view of body cavities. **B,** Anterior view of body cavities.

TABLE 1.4	Body Cavities
Main Body Cavities	**Contents**
Dorsal	
Cranial	• Brain
Spinal	• Spinal cord and vertebra
Ventral	
Thoracic	
• Mediastinum	• Thymus, heart, great vessels, trachea, esophagus, and pericardium
• Pleural	• Lungs, pleural membranes
Abdominal and Pelvic	
• Abdominal	• Peritoneum, liver, gallbladder, pancreas, spleen, stomach, intestines, kidneys, ureters, and blood vessels
• Pelvic	• Rectum, urinary bladder, male and female reproductive system

Quadrants

The midsagittal plane and transverse plane intersect at the umbilicus to divide the abdomen into four quadrants (Figure 1.8, *A*):

    Right upper quadrant (RUQ)
    Right lower quadrant (RLQ)
    Left upper quadrant (LUQ)
    Left lower quadrant (LLQ)

For a description of the structures located within each quadrant, see Table 1.5.

Regions

The abdomen can be further divided by four planes into nine regions. The two horizontal planes are the transpyloric and transtubercular planes. The transpyloric plane is found midway between the xiphisternal joint and the umbilicus, passing through the inferior border of the L1 vertebra. The transtubercular plane passes through the tubercles on the iliac crests, at the level of the L5 vertebral body. The two sagittal planes are the midclavicular lines. Each line runs inferiorly from the midpoint of the clavicle to the midinguinal point (Figure 1.8, *B*). The nine regions can be organized into three groups:

SUPERIOR
• Right hypochondrium
• Epigastrium
• Left hypochondrium
MIDDLE
• Right lateral
• Umbilical
• Left lateral
INFERIOR
• Right inguinal
• Hypogastrium
• Left inguinal

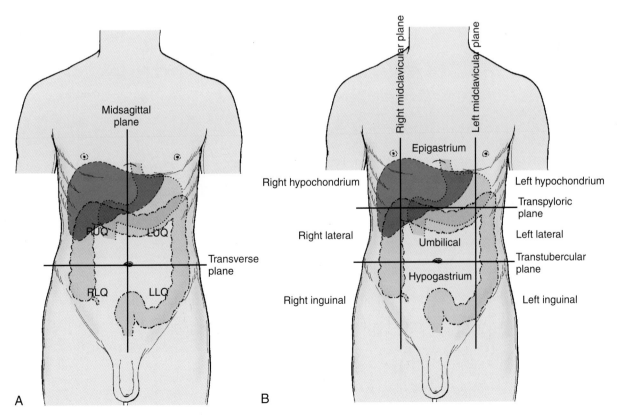

FIGURE 1.8 A, Four abdominal quadrants. B, Nine abdominal regions.

TABLE 1.5	Organs Found within Abdominopelvic Quadrants
Quadrant	**Organs**
Right upper quadrant (RUQ)	Right lobe of liver, gallbladder, right kidney, portions of stomach, small and large intestines
Left upper quadrant (LUQ)	Left lobe of liver, stomach, tail of the pancreas, left kidney, spleen, portions of large intestines
Right lower quadrant (RLQ)	Cecum, appendix, portions of small intestine, right ureter, right ovary, right spermatic cord
Left lower quadrant (LLQ)	Most of small intestine, portions of large intestine, left ureter, left ovary, left spermatic cord

IMAGE DISPLAY

Each digital image can be divided into individual regions called pixels or voxels that are then assigned a numerical value corresponding to a specific tissue property of the structure being imaged (Figure 1.9). The numerical value of each voxel is assigned a shade of gray for image display. In CT, the numerical value (CT number) is referenced to a Hounsfield unit (HU), which represents the attenuating properties or density of each tissue. Water is used as the reference tissue and is given a value of zero. A CT number greater than zero will represent tissue that is denser than water and will appear in progressively lighter shades of gray to white. Tissues with a negative CT number will appear in progressively darker shades of gray to black (Figure 1.10). In magnetic resonance (MR), the gray scale represents the specific tissue relaxation properties of T1, T2, and proton density. The gray scale in MR images can vary greatly because of inherent tissue properties and can appear different with each patient and across a series of images (Figure 1.11).

The appearance of digital images can be altered to include more or fewer shades of gray by adjusting the gray scale, a process called windowing. Windowing is used to optimize visualization of specific tissues or lesions. Window width (WW) is a parameter that allows for the adjustment of gray scale (number of shades of gray), and window level (WL) basically sets the density of the image (Figure 1.10).

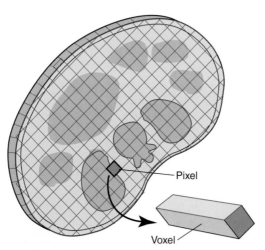

Pixel

Voxel

FIGURE 1.9 Representation of a pixel and voxel.

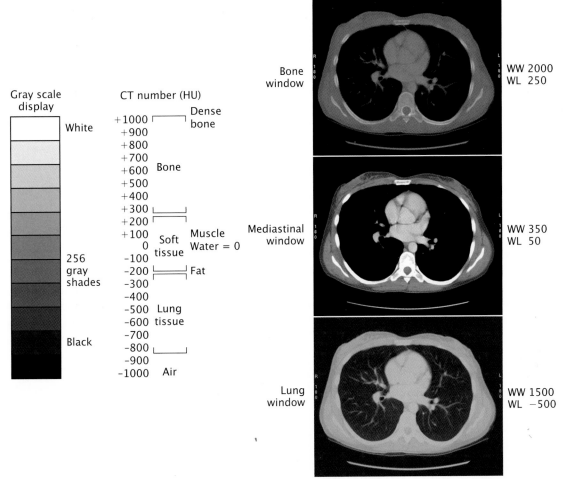

FIGURE 1.10 CT numbers and windowing on axial CT of chest.

MULTIPLANAR REFORMATION AND 3D IMAGING

Several postprocessing techniques can be applied to the original 2D digital data to provide additional 3D information for the physician. All current postprocessing techniques depend on creating a digital data stack from the original 2D images, thereby generating a cube of digital information (Figure 1.12).

Multiplanar Reformation (Reformat) (MPR)

Images reconstructed from data obtained along any projection through the cube result in a sagittal, coronal, axial, or oblique image (see Figures 1.13 and 1.14).

Curved Planar Reformation (Reformat) (CPR)

Images are reconstructed from data obtained along an arbitrary curved projection through the cube (Figure 1.15).

3D Imaging

All 3D algorithms use the principle of ray tracing in which imaginary rays are sent out from a camera viewpoint. The data are then rotated on an arbitrary axis, and the imaginary ray is passed through the data in specific increments. Depending on the method of reconstruction, unique information is projected onto the viewing plane (Figure 1.16).

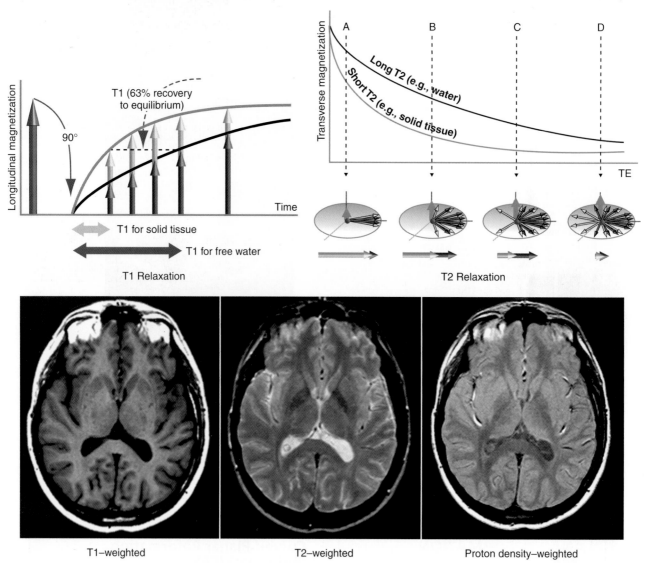

T1-weighted   T2-weighted   Proton density-weighted

FIGURE 1.11 MR tissue relaxation and image contrast.

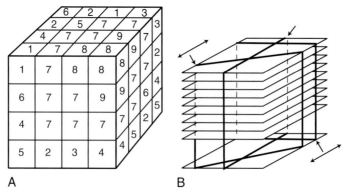

A   B

FIGURE 1.12 A, Digital cube. B, Stack of axial images.

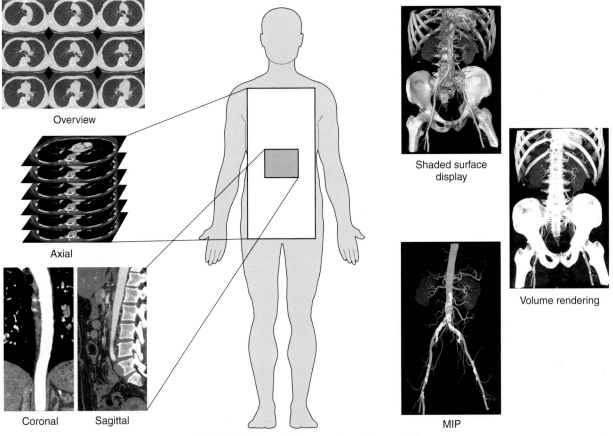

FIGURE 1.13 Multiplanar reformation and 3D.

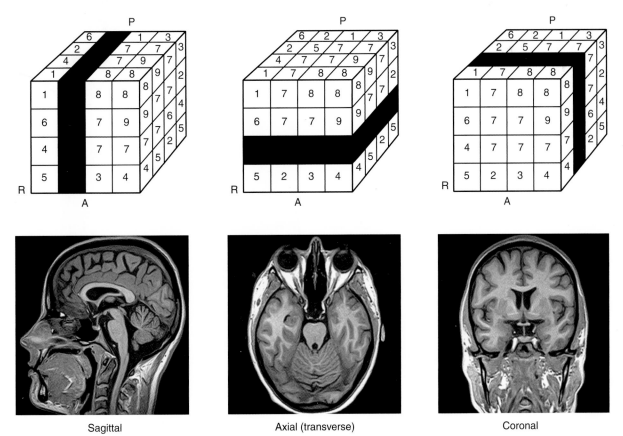

FIGURE 1.14 Multiplanar reformations of brain.

Voxels

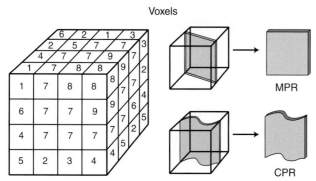

FIGURE 1.15 **Curved planar reformation. MPR,** Multiplanar reformation. **CPR,** curved planar reformation.

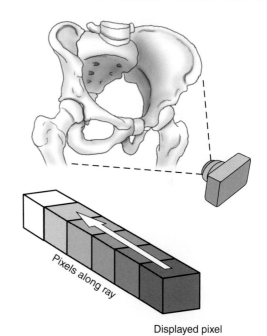

FIGURE 1.16 **Ray tracing.**

Shaded Surface Display (SSD). A ray from the camera's viewpoint is directed to stop at a particular user-defined threshold value. With this method, every voxel with a value greater than the selected threshold is rendered opaque, creating a surface. That value is then projected onto the viewing screen (Figure 1.17).

Maximum Intensity Projection (MIP). A ray from the camera's viewpoint is directed to stop at the voxel with the maximum signal intensity. With this method, only the brightest voxels will be mapped into the final image (Figure 1.18).

Volume Rendering (VR). Contributions of each voxel are summed along the course of the ray from the camera's viewpoint. The process is repeated numerous times to determine each pixel value that will be displayed in the final image (Figure 1.19).

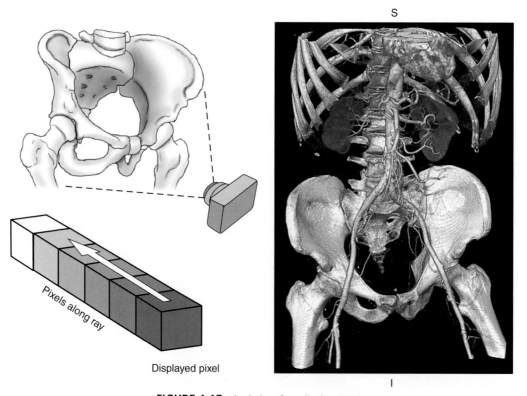

FIGURE 1.17 **Shaded surface display (SSD).**

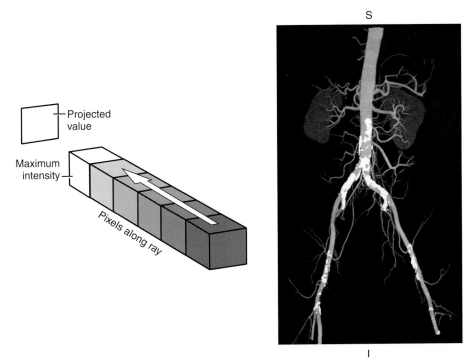

FIGURE 1.18 Maximum intensity projection (MIP).

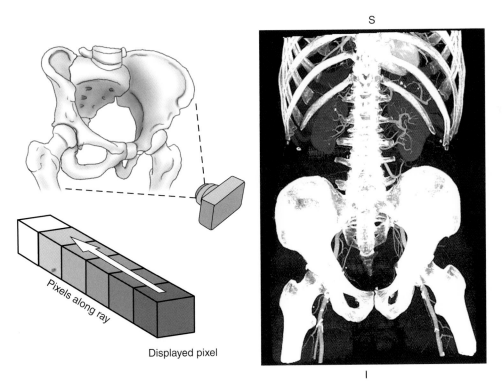

FIGURE 1.19 Volume rendering (VR).

REFERENCES

Frank E, Long B: *Radiographic positions and radiologic procedures*, ed 12, St. Louis, 2011, Mosby.

Curry RA, Tempkin BB: *Sonography: Introduction to normal structure and functional anatomy*, ed 3, St. Louis, 2010, Saunders.

Seeram E: *Computed tomography; physical principle, clinical applications, and quality control*, ed 3, Philadelphia, 2008, Saunders.

Cranium and Facial Bones

Gentlemen, damn the sphenoid bone!

Oliver Wendell Holmes (1809-1894),
Opening of anatomy lectures at Harvard Medical School

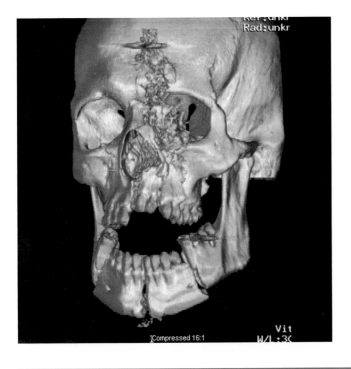

FIGURE 2.1 **3D CT of skull.** Trauma resulting from a gunshot wound.

The complex anatomy of the cranium and facial bones can be intimidating. However, with three-dimensional (3D) imaging and multiple imaging planes, the task of learning these structures can be simplified. It is important to understand normal sectional anatomy of the cranium and facial bones to identify pathologic disorders and injuries that may occur within this area (Figure 2.1). This chapter demonstrates the sectional anatomy of the following structures:

OBJECTIVES

- Define the three cranial fossae.
- Identify the location and unique structures of each cranial and facial bone.
- Identify the structures of the ear and describe their functions.
- Identify the cranial sutures.
- Describe the six fontanels in the infant cranium.
- Describe the structures that constitute the temporomandibular joint.

- Identify the location of each paranasal sinus and the meatus into which it drains.
- Identify the structures of the osteomeatal unit.
- Identify the bones that form the orbit and their associated openings.
- Describe the structures that constitute the globe of the eye.
- List the muscles of the eye and describe their functions and locations.

OUTLINE

CRANIUM

The **cranium** is composed of eight bones that surround and protect the brain. These bones include the parietal (2), frontal (1), ethmoid (1), sphenoid (1), occipital (1), and temporal (2) (Figures 2.2 through 2.5). The cranial bones are composed of two layers of compact tissue known as the internal (inner) and external (outer) tables. Located between the two tables is cancellous tissue or spongy bone called diploe (Figures 2.6 through 2.9). The base of the cranium houses three fossae called the anterior, middle, and posterior cranial fossae. The **anterior cranial fossa** (frontal fossa) is composed primarily of the frontal bone, ethmoid bone, and lesser wing of the sphenoid bone and contains the frontal lobes of the brain. The **middle cranial fossa** (temporal fossa) is formed primarily by the body of the sphenoid and temporal bones and houses the pituitary gland, hypothalamus, and temporal lobes of the brain. The **posterior cranial fossa** (infratentorial fossa) is formed by the occipital and temporal bones and contains the cerebellum and brainstem (Figures 2.6 and 2.7). For additional details of the contents found within the cranial fossa, see Table 2.1. Each cranial bone is structurally unique, and thus identification of the physical components can be challenging.

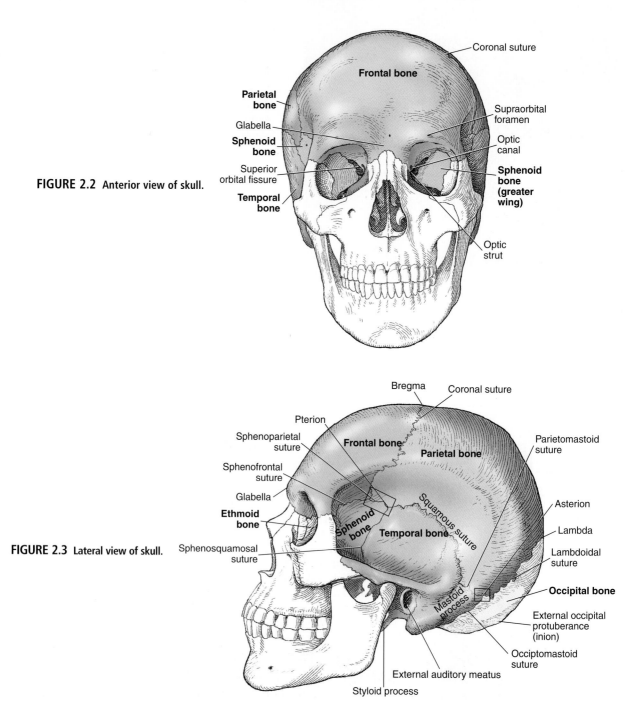

FIGURE 2.2 Anterior view of skull.

FIGURE 2.3 Lateral view of skull.

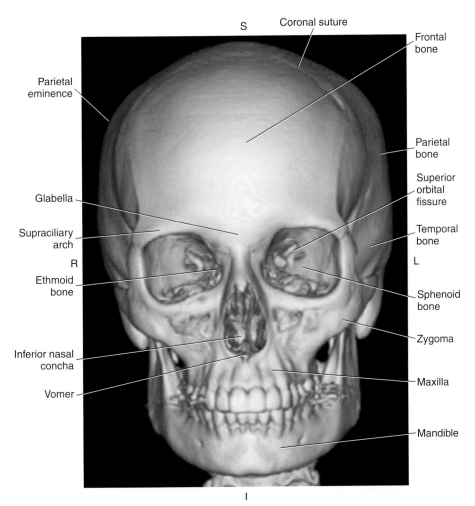

S
Coronal suture

Frontal bone

Parietal eminence

Parietal bone

Superior orbital fissure

Glabella

Temporal bone

Supraciliary arch

R

L

Ethmoid bone

Sphenoid bone

Zygoma

Inferior nasal concha

Maxilla

Vomer

Mandible

I

FIGURE 2.4 3D CT of anterior skull.

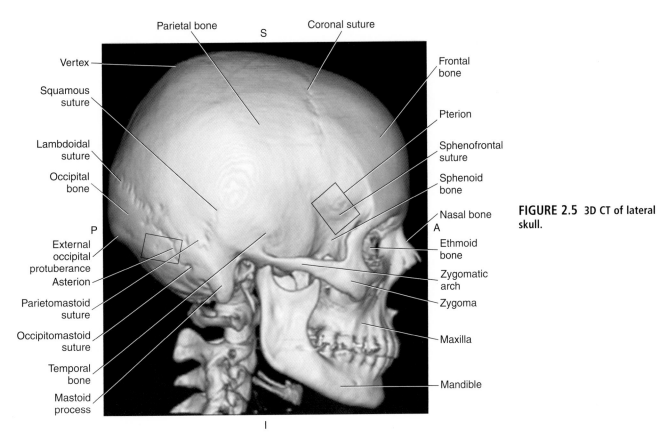

Parietal bone
S
Coronal suture

Vertex

Frontal bone

Squamous suture

Pterion

Lambdoidal suture

Sphenofrontal suture

Occipital bone

Sphenoid bone

P

Nasal bone

A

External occipital protuberance

Ethmoid bone

Asterion

Zygomatic arch

Parietomastoid suture

Zygoma

Occipitomastoid suture

Maxilla

Temporal bone

Mandible

Mastoid process

I

FIGURE 2.5 3D CT of lateral skull.

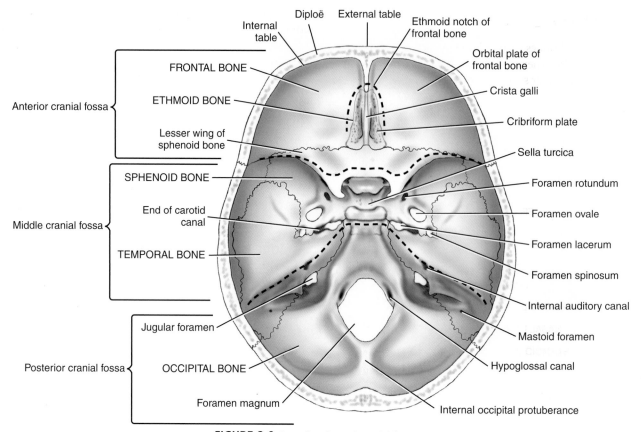

FIGURE 2.6 Superior view of cranial fossae.

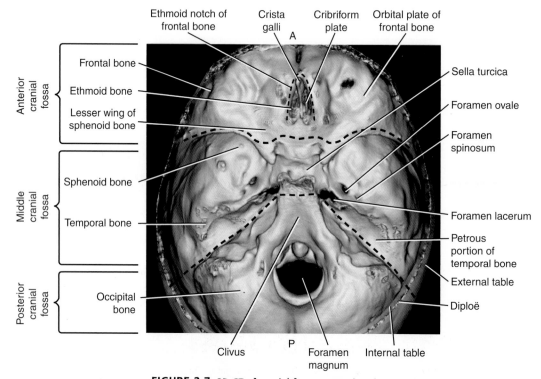

FIGURE 2.7 3D CT of cranial fossae, superior view.

Parietal Bone

The two **parietal bones** form a large portion of the sides of the cranium. Prominent markings and grooves that are found within the inner surface of the cranium are formed by corresponding meningeal vessels and cerebral gyri and sulci (Figures 2.8 and 2.9). The parietal bones articulate with the frontal, occipital, temporal, and sphenoid bones. The superior point between the parietal bones is the **vertex**, which is the highest point of the cranium (Figures 2.9 and 2.10).

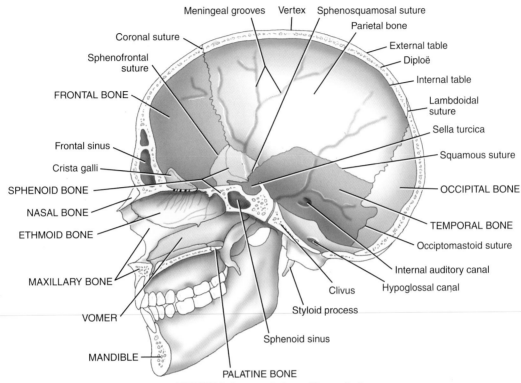

FIGURE 2.8　Lateral view of inner skull.

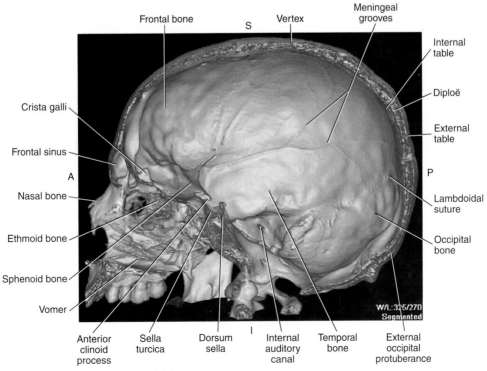

FIGURE 2.9　3D CT of inner skull, lateral view.

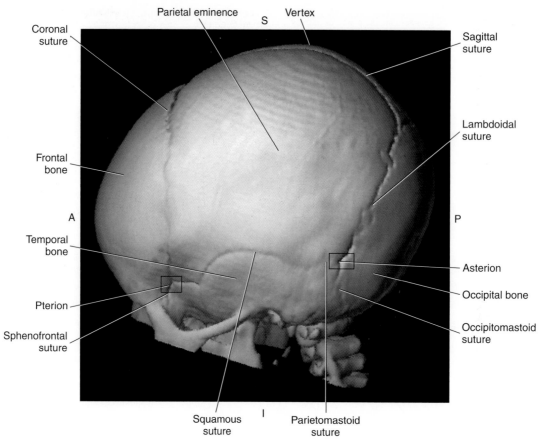

FIGURE 2.10 3D CT of lateral surface of cranium.

TABLE 2.1	Contents of the Cranial Fossae
Fossa	**Contents**
Anterior cranial fossa	Frontal lobes of cerebrum; olfactory bulbs
Middle cranial fossa	Temporal lobes of cerebrum, pituitary gland, optic nerves and chiasm, cavernous sinus, trigeminal ganglion, internal carotid artery, hypothalamus and the following cranial nerves: trigeminal, oculomotor, trochlear, abducent, and ophthalmic
Posterior cranial fossa	Cerebellum, pons, medulla oblongata, midbrain, and the following cranial nerves: facial, vestibulocochlear, glossopharyngeal, vagus, accessory, hypoglossal

Each parietal bone has a central prominent bulge on its outer surface termed the **parietal eminence** (Figure 2.4). The width of the cranium can be determined by measuring the distance between the two parietal eminences.

Frontal Bone

The **frontal bone** consists of a vertical and a horizontal portion. The **vertical** or **squamous portion** forms the forehead and anterior vault of the cranium (Figures 2.2 through 2.5). The vertical portion contains the **frontal sinuses**, which lie on either side of the midsagittal plane (Figures 2.8, 2.9, 2.11, and 2.12). Two elevated arches, the supraciliary arches, are joined to one another by a smooth area termed the glabella (Figures 2.2 and 2.4). The **horizontal portion** forms the roof over each orbit, termed the **orbital plate,** and the majority of the anterior cranial fossa (Figures 2.6, 2.7 and 2.13). Located in the superior portion of each orbit is the **supraorbital foramen,** or **notch,** which exists for the passage of the supraorbital nerve (Figures 2.2 and 2.11). Between the orbital plates is an area termed the **ethmoid notch**, which receives the cribriform plate of the ethmoid bone (Figures 2.6 and 2.7).

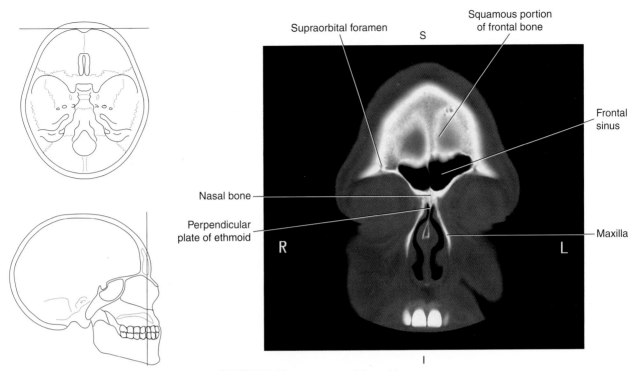

Supraorbital foramen
Squamous portion of frontal bone
S
Frontal sinus
Nasal bone
Perpendicular plate of ethmoid
Maxilla
R
L
I

FIGURE 2.11 Coronal CT of frontal bone.

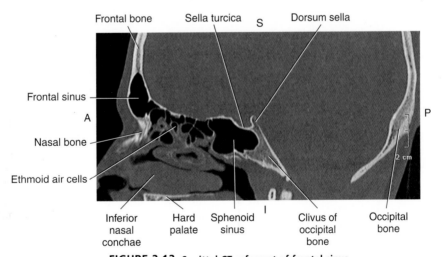

Frontal bone
Sella turcica
S
Dorsum sella
Frontal sinus
A
P
Nasal bone
Ethmoid air cells
2 cm
I
Inferior nasal conchae
Hard palate
Sphenoid sinus
Clivus of occipital bone
Occipital bone

FIGURE 2.12 Sagittal CT reformat of frontal sinus,

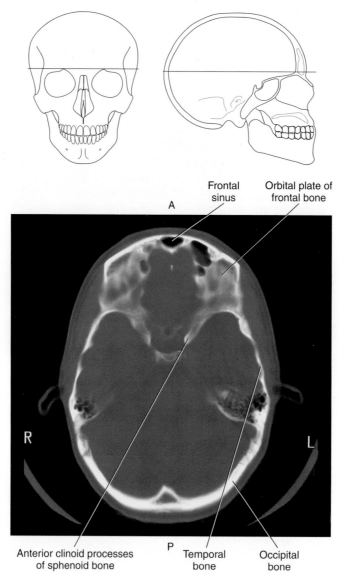

FIGURE 2.13 Axial CT of orbital plates.

Ethmoid Bone

The **ethmoid bone** is the smallest of the cranial bones and is situated in the anterior cranial fossa. This cube-shaped bone can be divided into four parts: horizontal portion, vertical portion, and two lateral masses (labyrinths) (Figures 2.14 through 2.17). The **horizontal portion**, called the **cribriform plate**, fits into the ethmoid notch of the frontal bone (Figures 2.6 and 2.7). This plate contains many foramina for the passage of olfactory nerve fibers (Figures 2.14 and 2.15). The **crista galli**, a bony projection stemming from the midline of the cribriform plate, projects superiorly to act

as an attachment for the falx cerebri, which is the connective tissue that anchors the brain to the anterior cranial fossa (Figures 2.16 and 2.17). The **vertical portion** of the ethmoid bone, called the **perpendicular plate**, projects inferiorly from the cribriform plate to form a portion of the bony nasal septum (Figure 2.16). The **lateral masses (labyrinth)** incorporate thin-walled **orbital plates** (lamina papyracea), which create a portion of the medial orbit (Figures 2.15 and 2.17). Contained within the lateral masses are many ethmoid air cells (**ethmoid sinuses**), one of the largest being the **ethmoid bulla** (Figures 2.14 through 2.17). Projecting

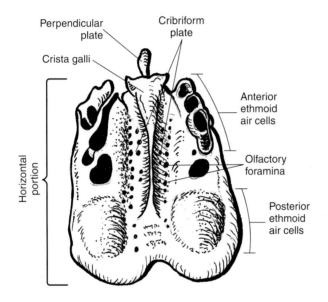

FIGURE 2.14 Superior view of ethmoid bone.

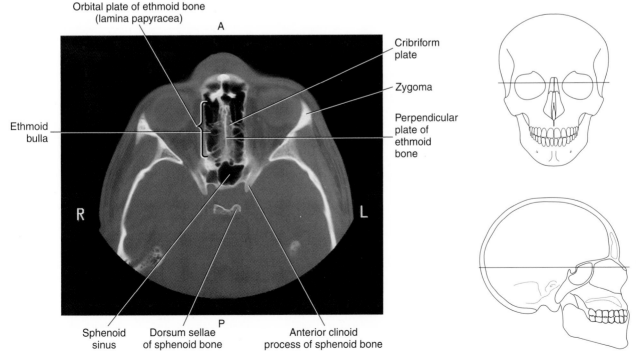

FIGURE 2.15 Axial CT of ethmoid bone.

from the lateral masses are two scroll-shaped processes called the **superior** and **middle nasal conchae** (turbinates) and the **uncinate process**. Between the uncinate process and ethmoid bulla is a narrow groove called the **infundibulum,** which is an important landmark of the paranasal sinuses (Figures 2.16 and 2.17).

The naso-orbitoethmoid (NOE) complex is the union of the ethmoid sinuses, frontal bone and sinuses, anterior cranial fossa, orbits, and nasal bones. Fractures of the NOE may cause symptoms that include nasal and forehead swelling, diplopia (double vision), and CSF rhinorrhea (leakage of cerebrospinal fluid into the nose).

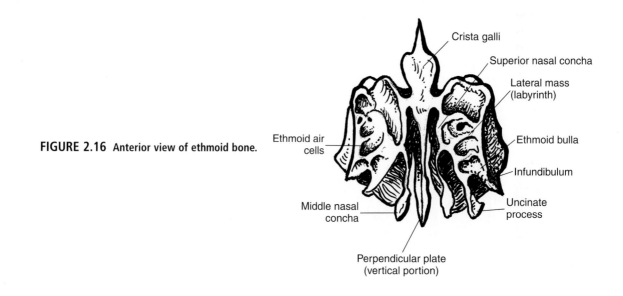

FIGURE 2.16 **Anterior view of ethmoid bone.**

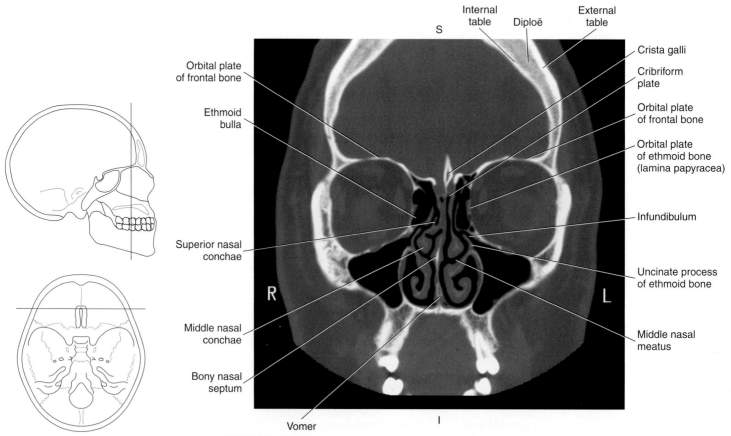

FIGURE 2.17 **Coronal CT of ethmoid bone with crista galli.**

Sphenoid Bone

The butterfly-shaped **sphenoid bone** extends completely across the floor of the middle cranial fossa (Figures 2.6 and 2.7). This bone forms the majority of the base of the skull and articulates with the occipital, temporal, parietal, frontal, and ethmoid bones. The main parts of the sphenoid bone are the body, lesser wings (2), and greater wings (2) (Figure 2.18). Located within the **body** of the sphenoid bone is a deep depression called the **sella turcica**, which houses the hypophysis (pituitary gland). Directly below the sella turcica are two air-filled cavities termed **sphenoid sinuses** (Figures 2.15 and 2.19). The anterior portion of the sella turcica is formed by the **tuberculum sellae,** and the posterior portion by the **dorsum sellae**. The dorsum sellae gives rise to the **posterior clinoid processes** (Figures 2.18,

2.20, 2.21, and 2.22). The triangular-shaped **lesser wings** attach to the superior aspect of the body and form two sharp points called **anterior clinoid processes**, which, along with the posterior clinoid processes, serve as attachment sites for the tentorium cerebelli (Figures 2.18 and 2.22). The **optic canal** is completely contained within the lesser wing and provides passage of the optic nerve and ophthalmic artery (Figure 2.22). The optic canal is separated from the superior orbital fissure by a bony root termed the **optic strut** (inferior root) (Figure 2.2, see bony orbit). The **superior orbital fissure** is a triangular-shaped opening located between the lesser and greater wings that allows for the transmission of the oculomotor, trochlear, abducens, and ophthalmic division of the trigeminal nerves, as well as the superior ophthalmic vein (Figures 2.2, 2.22, 2.24, also see

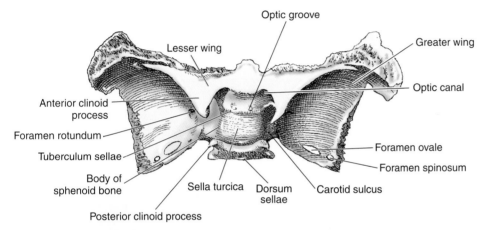

FIGURE 2.18 Superior view of sphenoid bone.

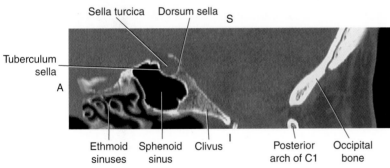

FIGURE 2.19 Sagittal CT reformat of sella turcica.

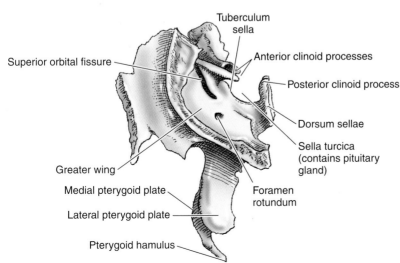

FIGURE 2.20 Lateral view of sphenoid bone.

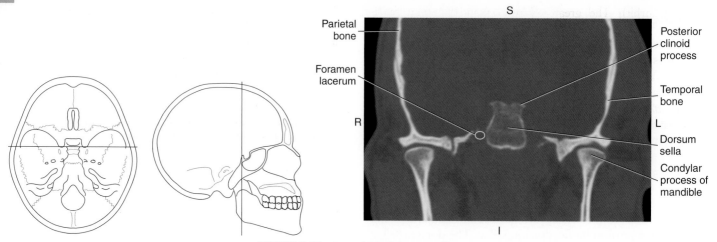

FIGURE 2.21 Coronal CT of dorsum sella.

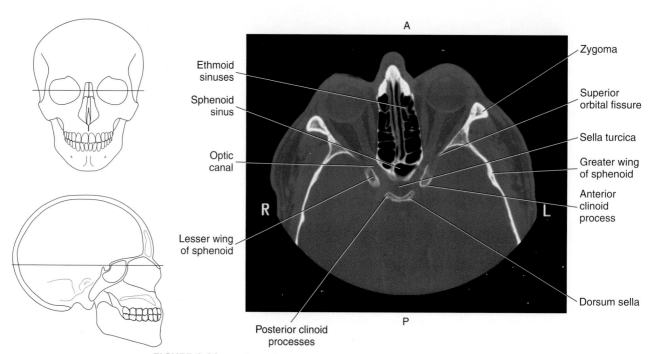

FIGURE 2.22 Axial CT of anterior clinoid processes and sphenoid bone.

bony orbit). The **greater wings** extend laterally from the sides of the body and contain three paired foramina—**rotundum, ovale,** and **spinosum**—through which nerves and blood vessels course (Figures 2.18 and 2.23 through 2.25; Table 2.2). Extending from the inferior surface of each greater wing is a **pterygoid process,** which is divided into medial and lateral pterygoid plates. The **pterygoid plates** serve as attachment sites for the pterygoid muscles used in movements of the lower jaw. The medial section is longer and has a hook-shaped projection on its inferior end termed the **pterygoid hamulus,** which provides an anchor for

gliding motion for the muscle responsible for opening the eustachian tube (Figures 2.20, 2.24, and 2.25). At the base of the pterygoid process is the **pterygoid (vidian) canal,** an opening for the passage of the petrosal nerve (Figures 2.23 through 2.25). The pterygoid processes articulate with the palatine bones and vomer to form part of the nasal cavity.

> The sphenoid bone is considered the keystone of the cranial bones because it is the only bone that articulates with all the other cranial bones.

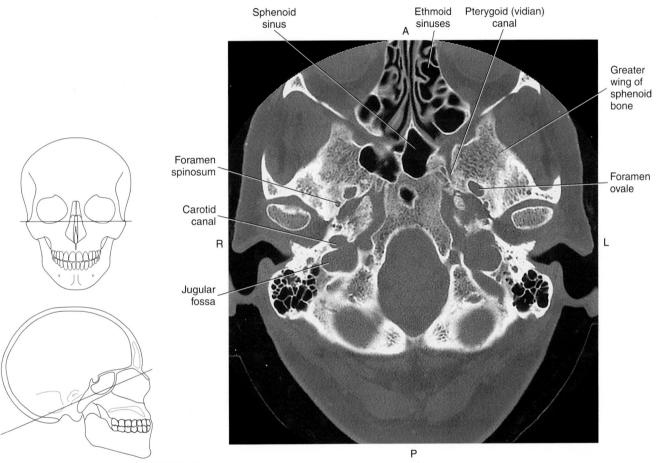

FIGURE 2.23 Axial CT of sphenoid bone with foramina ovale and spinosum.

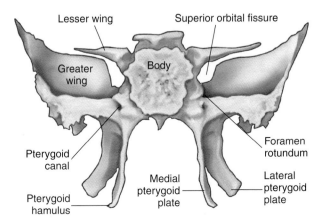

FIGURE 2.24 Anterior view of sphenoid bone.

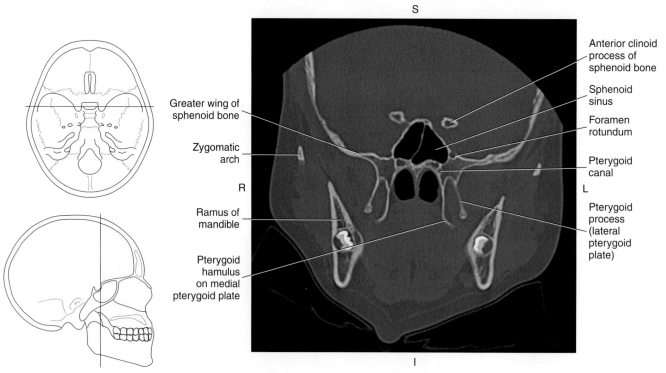

FIGURE 2.25 Coronal CT of sphenoid bone.

TABLE 2.2	Foramina and Fissures of the Skull	
Bone	**Foramen/Fissure**	**Major Structures Using Passageway**
Frontal	Supraorbital foramen (or notch)	Supraorbital nerve and artery
	Frontal foramen (or notch)	Frontal artery and nerve
Ethmoid	Cribriform plate	Olfactory nerve (I)
Sphenoid	Foramen rotundum	Maxillary branch of trigeminal nerve (V)
	Foramen ovale	Mandibular branch of trigeminal nerve (V)
	Foramen spinosum	Middle meningeal artery
	Pterygoid canal	Petrosal nerve
	Optic canal	Optic nerve and ophthalmic artery
	Superior orbital fissure	Oculomotor nerve (III), trochlear nerve (IV), ophthalmic branch of trigeminal nerve (V), abducens nerve (VI), ophthalmic vein
Sphenoid and maxillary bone	Inferior orbital fissure	Maxillary branch of trigeminal nerve (V)
Occipital	Foramen magnum	Medulla oblongata and accessory nerve (XI)
	Hypoglossal canal	Hypoglossal nerve (XII)
Temporal	Carotid canal	Internal carotid artery
	External auditory meatus	Air in canal conducts sound to tympanic membrane
	Internal auditory canal	Vestibulocochlear nerve (VIII) and facial nerve (VII)
	Stylomastoid foramen and facial nerve canal	Facial nerve (VII)
Temporal and occipital bone	Jugular foramen	Internal jugular vein, glossopharyngeal nerve (IX), vagus nerve (X), and accessory nerve (XI)
Temporal, sphenoid, and occipital bones	Foramen lacerum	Fibrocartilage, internal carotid artery as it leaves carotid canal to enter cranium, nerve of pterygoid canal and a meningeal branch from the ascending pharyngeal artery
Maxillary	Infraorbital foramen	Infraorbital nerve and maxillary branch of trigeminal nerve (V)
Lacrimal with maxilla	Lacrimal groove, nasolacrimal canal	Lacrimal sac and nasolacriminal duct
Mandible	Mental foramen	Mental artery and nerve

Occipital Bone

The **occipital bone** forms the posterior cranial fossa and the inferoposterior portion of the cranium. On the inferior portion of the occipital bone is a large oval aperture called the **foramen magnum** located at the junction of the brainstem and spinal cord (Figure 2.26). The occipital bone can be divided into four portions: lateral occipital condyles (2), basilar portion (1), and squamous portion (1) (Figure 2.27). The **occipital condyles** project inferiorly to articulate with the first cervical vertebra (atlas) at the atlantooccipital joint (Figures 2.28 and 2.29). Located obliquely at the base of the condyles and anterolateral to the foramen magnum are the **hypoglossal canals** through which the hypoglossal nerve (CN XII) courses (Figures 2.8, 2.27, 2.28, and 2.30; Table 2.2). The **basilar portion** forms the anterior margin of the foramen magnum and slopes superiorly and anteriorly to meet with the dorsum sella of the sphenoid bone to form the **clivus** (Figures 2.8, 2.27, and 2.30 through 2.32). The **squamous**

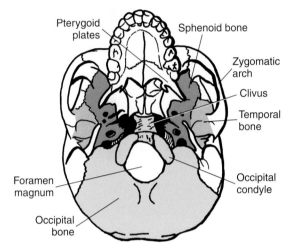

FIGURE 2.26 Inferior surface of occipital bone and cranium.

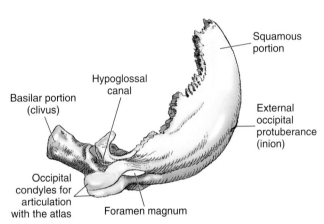

FIGURE 2.27 Lateroinferior aspect of occipital bone.

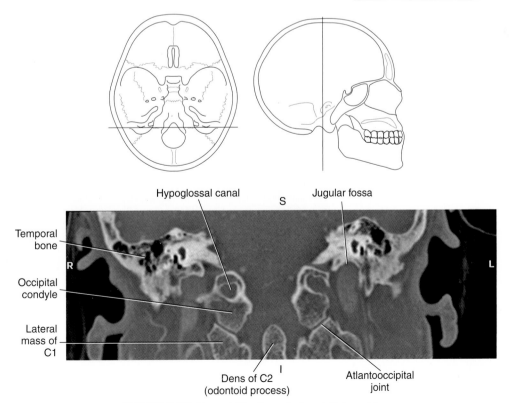

FIGURE 2.28 Coronal CT reformat of occipital condyles.

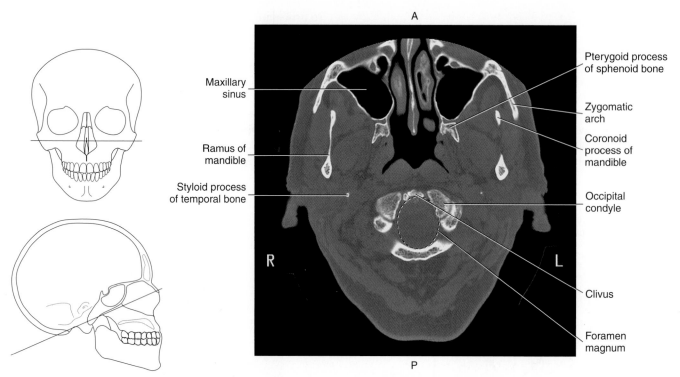

Maxillary sinus

Ramus of mandible

Styloid process of temporal bone

Pterygoid process of sphenoid bone

Zygomatic arch

Coronoid process of mandible

Occipital condyle

Clivus

Foramen magnum

R   L   A   P

FIGURE 2.29 Axial CT of occipital bone at level of foramen magnum and lateral condyles.

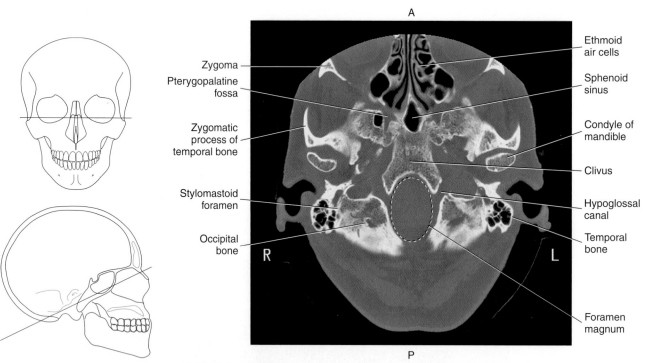

Zygoma

Pterygopalatine fossa

Zygomatic process of temporal bone

Stylomastoid foramen

Occipital bone

Ethmoid air cells

Sphenoid sinus

Condyle of mandible

Clivus

Hypoglossal canal

Temporal bone

Foramen magnum

R   L   A   P

FIGURE 2.30 Axial CT of occipital bone at level of clivus.

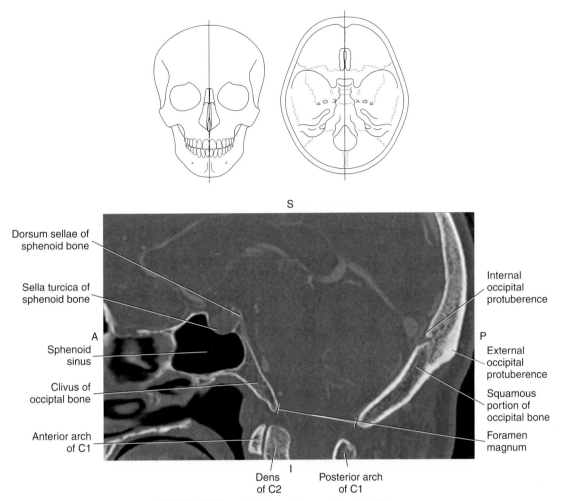

FIGURE 2.31 Sagittal CT reformat of occipital bone.

Dorsum sellae of sphenoid bone

Sella turcica of sphenoid bone

Sphenoid sinus

Clivus of occipital bone

Anterior arch of C1

Internal occipital protuberence

External occipital protuberence

Squamous portion of occipital bone

Foramen magnum

Dens of C2

Posterior arch of C1

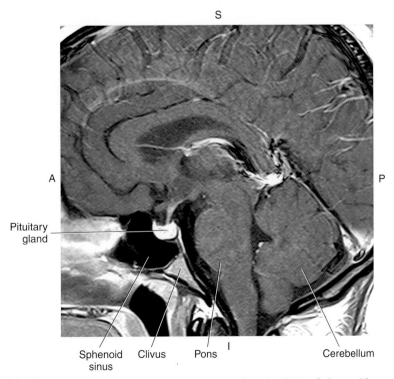

FIGURE 2.32 Sagittal, T1-weighted magnetic resonance imaging (MRI) of clivus with contrast.

Pituitary gland

Sphenoid sinus

Clivus

Pons

Cerebellum

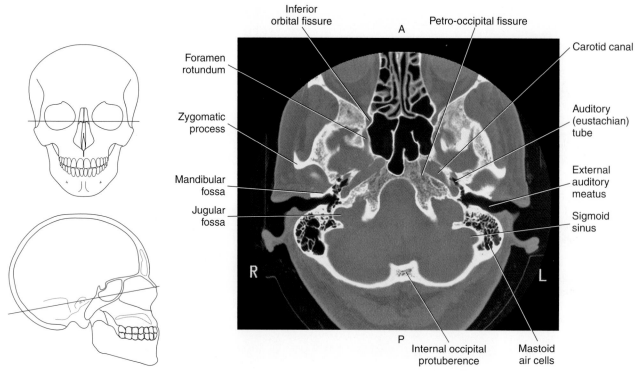

FIGURE 2.33 Axial CT of occipital bone with internal occipital protuberance.

portion curves posterosuperiorly from the foramen magnum to articulate with the parietal and temporal bones (Figure 2.3). Located on the inner surface of the squama is a bony projection termed the **internal occipital protuberance**, which marks the site where the dural venous sinuses converge (Figures 2.6 and 2.33). The **external occipital protuberance** is a projection on the external surface of the squamous part of the occipital bone in the midline. The highest point of the external occipital protuberance is termed the **inion** (Figures 2.27 and 2.31).

Temporal Bone

The two **temporal bones** contain many complex and important structures. They form part of the sides and base of the cranium, and together with the sphenoid bone create the middle cranial fossa (Figures 2.3 and 2.6). The temporal bone can be divided into four portions: squamous, tympanic, mastoid, and petrous (Figures 2.34 and 2.35). The thin **squamous portion** projects upward to form part of the sidewalls of the cranium (Figure 2.3). Extending from the squamous portion is the **zygomatic process**, which projects anteriorly to the zygoma of the face to form the **zygomatic arch** (Figures 2.25, 2.30, 2.34, and 2.36). At the base of the zygomatic process is the **articular eminence** that forms the anterior boundary of the **mandibular fossa**. The mandibular fossa is the depression that articulates with the condyloid process of the mandible, creating the

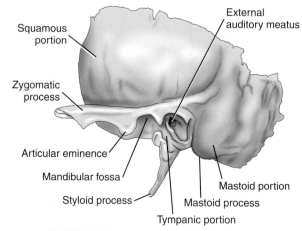

FIGURE 2.34 Sagittal view of temporal bone.

temporomandibular joint (Figures 2.34 and 2.37). The **tympanic portion** lies below the squama and forms the majority of the **external auditory meatus** (Figures 2.33 through 2.35, and 2.37). Just posterior to the tympanic portion is the **mastoid portion**, which has a prominent conical region termed the **mastoid process** (Figures 2.34, 2.37, 2.38, and 2.39). The mastoid process encloses the mastoid air cells and mastoid antrum. The **mastoid antrum** is located on the anterosuperior portion of the mastoid process. It is an air-filled cavity

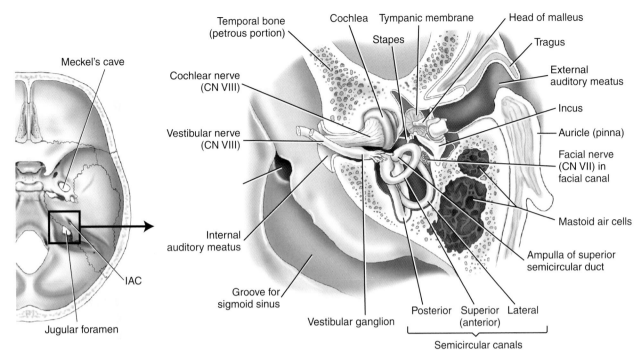

FIGURE 2.35 Superior view of petrous portion of temporal bone with middle and inner ear.

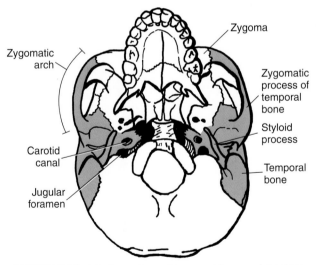

FIGURE 2.36 Inferior surface of temporal bone and cranium.

that communicates with the middle ear (tympanic cavity) (Figures 2.37 and 2.38). The **petrous portion** of the temporal bone is pyramidal in shape and situated at an angle between the sphenoid and occipital bones (Figure 2.35). The posterior surface of the petrous pyramid forms the anterior bony limit of the posterior fossa. Near the center of this surface is the opening to the **internal auditory canal**, which transmits the seventh and eighth

cranial nerves (Figures 2.35 and 2.39). Other openings associated with the posterior surface of the petrous pyramid are the **jugular foramen** and the **carotid canal**, which provide passage for the internal jugular vein and the internal carotid artery (Table 2.2). An enlargement of the jugular foramen is the **jugular fossa** (Figures 2.36, 2.40, and 2.42). Continuous in front of the jugular foramen is the **petro-occipital fissure** that separates the petrous portion of the temporal bone from the foramen magnum of the occipital bone (Figure 2.40). The carotid canal courses superiorly at its lower segment then changes direction and is seen coursing posterior to anterior (Figures 2.33 and 2.38 through 2.41). Superior to the carotid canal is an indentation on the petrous portion called **Meckel's cave** (Figures 2.35 and 2.41). Also known as the trigeminal cave, Meckel's cave is located between two layers of dura and encloses the trigeminal ganglion. It is filled with cerebrospinal fluid (CSF) and is continuous with the pontine cistern and subarachnoid space (also see trigeminal nerve in chapter 3). Between the apex of the petrous pyramid, the body of the sphenoid bone, and the basilar portion of the occipital bone is a jagged slit termed the **foramen lacerum**, which contains cartilage and allows the internal carotid artery to enter the cranium, providing small arteries that supply the inner surface of the cranium (Figure 2.40 and Table 2.2). The inferior surface of the petrous pyramid gives rise to the long slender **styloid process** that is attached to several muscles of the tongue and ligaments of the hyoid bone (Figures 2.8, 2.29, and 2.34). The **stylomastoid foramen** is situated between the mastoid process and the styloid process. This foramen constitutes the end of the **facial nerve canal** (facial canal) (Figures 2.38 and 2.42 and Table 2.2). The interior of the petrous pyramid houses the delicate middle and inner ear structures.

A basilar skull fracture is a fracture of the bones that form the base (floor) of the skull and typically involves the occipital bone, sphenoid bone, temporal bone, and/or ethmoid bone. Basilar skull fractures can cause tears in the meninges, membranes surrounding the brain. Subsequent leakage of cerebrospinal fluid (CSF) into the nasopharynx and/or nose causes the patient to experience a salty taste. Other clinical signs of a basilar skull fracture may include bruising behind the ears or around the eyes; loss of hearing, smell, or vision; and possible nerve damage resulting in weakness of the face.

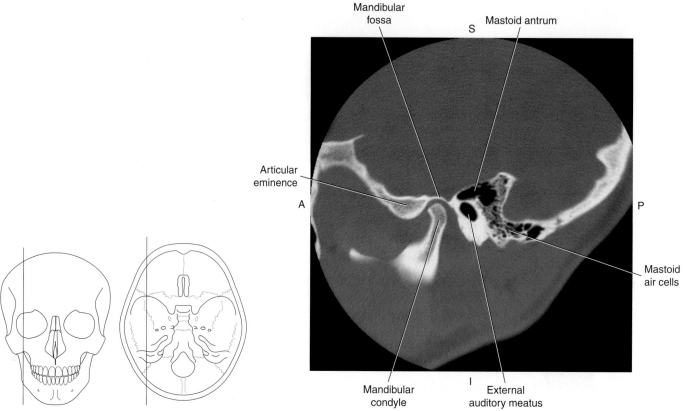

FIGURE 2.37 Sagittal CT reformat of temporal bone.

FIGURE 2.38 Coronal view of temporal bone.

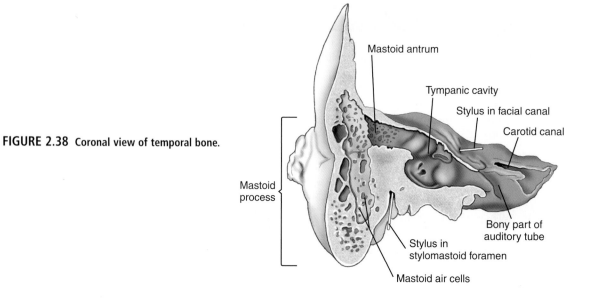

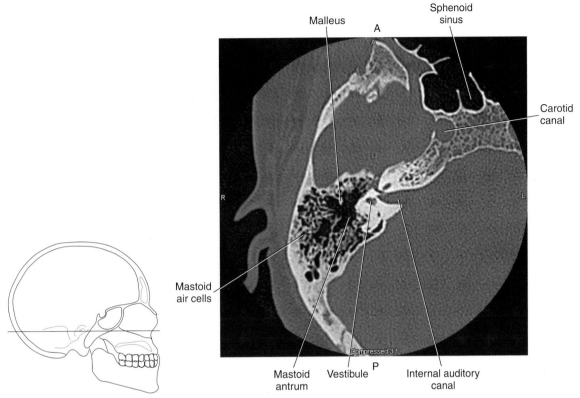

FIGURE 2.39 Axial CT of temporal bone with internal auditory canal (IAC).

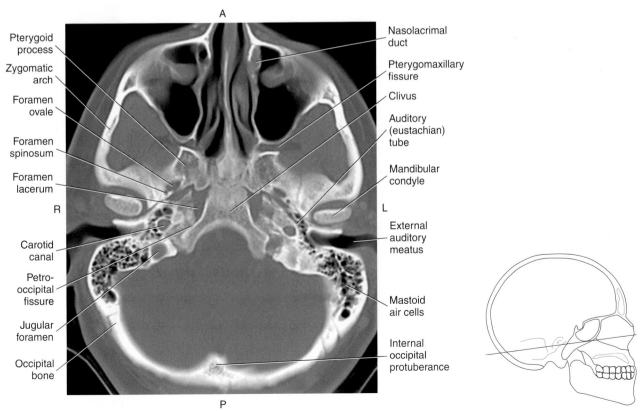

FIGURE 2.40 Axial CT of temporal bone with foramen lacerum, jugular fossa, and carotid canal.

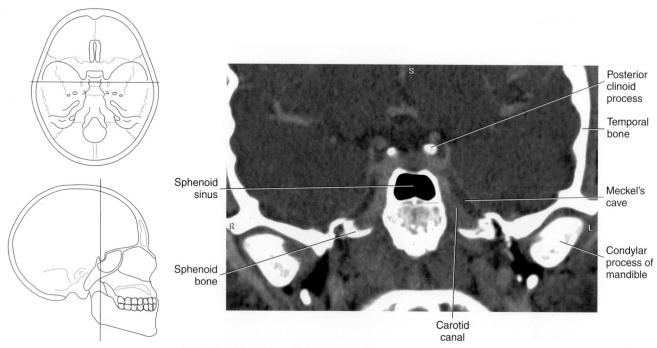

FIGURE 2.41 Coronal CT of temporal bone with Meckel's cave.

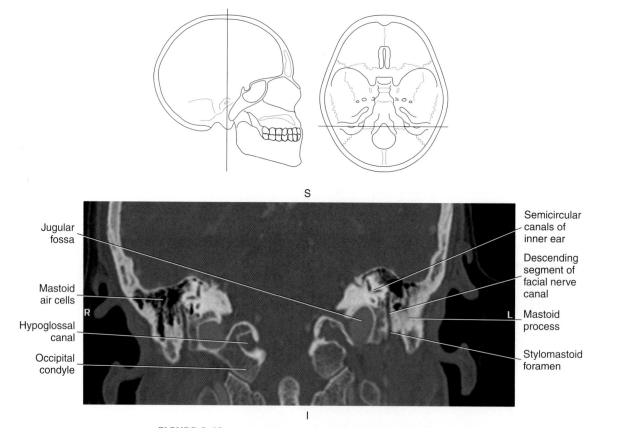

FIGURE 2.42 Coronal CT reformat of stylomastoid foramen.

Structures of the External, Middle, and Inner Ear

The structures of the ear can be divided into three main portions: external, middle, and inner (Figures 2.43 through 2.59).

The **external ear** consists of the **auricle** and the **external auditory meatus**. The external auditory meatus is a sound-conducting canal that terminates at the tympanic membrane of the middle ear (Figures 2.40 and 2.43).

The narrow, air-filled **middle ear**, or **tympanic cavity**, communicates with both the mastoid antrum and the nasopharynx. Air is conveyed from the nasopharynx to the tympanic cavity through the **eustachian tube (auditory tube)** (Figures 2.40 and 2.43). The middle ear consists of

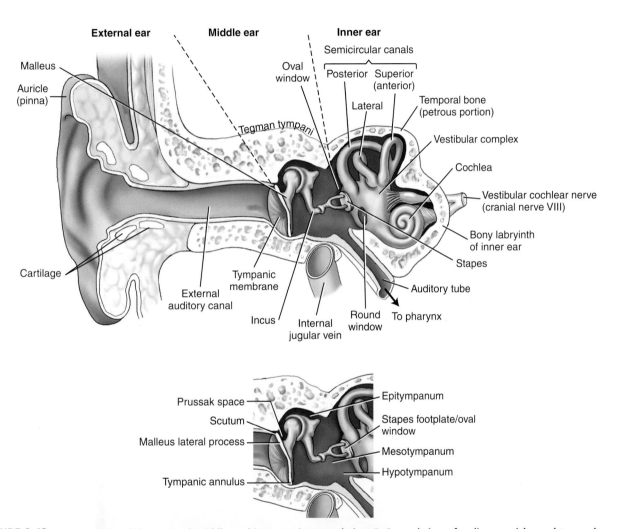

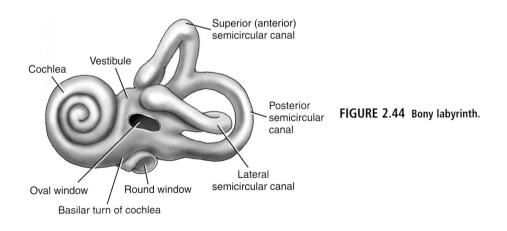

FIGURE 2.43 A, Orientation of the external, middle, and inner ear in coronal view. **B,** Coronal view of auditory ossicles and tympanic cavity.

FIGURE 2.44 Bony labyrinth.

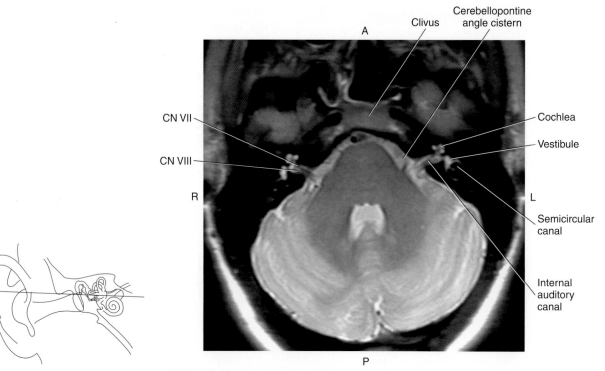

FIGURE 2.45 Axial, T2-weighted MRI of inner ear.

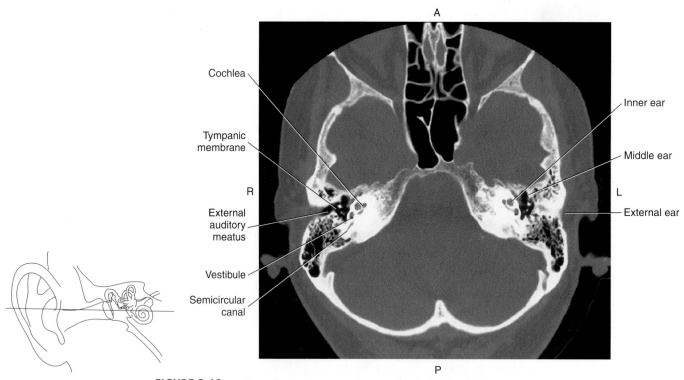

FIGURE 2.46 Axial CT of petrous portion at level of external auditory meatus.

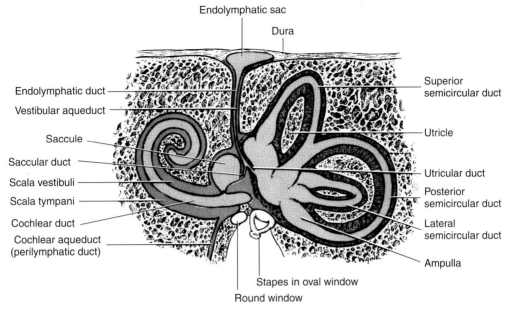

FIGURE 2.47 Membranous labyrinth.

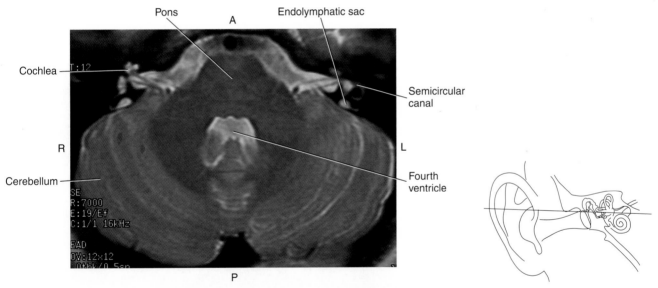

FIGURE 2.48 Axial, T2-weighted MRI with enlarged endolymphatic sac.

the **tympanic membrane** and three **auditory ossicles (malleus, incus, and stapes)** (Figure 2.43b). The tympanic membrane transmits sound vibrations to the auditory ossicles. The auditory ossicles, which are suspended in the middle ear, conduct sound vibrations from the tympanic membrane to the oval window of the inner ear (Figures 2.49 through 2.59).

The middle ear can be subdivided into the epitympanum, mesotympanum, and hypotympanum. The **epitympanum**, also called the **attic**, is located superior to the tympanic membrane and contains the head of the malleus and body of the incus. It communicates with the mastoid

air cells through a narrow opening called the **aditus ad antrum**, a potential route for the spread of infection from the middle ear to the mastoid air cells. The roof of the epitympanum is separated from the middle cranial fossa by a thin layer of bone termed the *tegmen tympani*. Two other important landmarks of the epitympanum include the scutum and Prussak's space. The scutum is a sharp, bony spur on the lateral wall of the tympanic cavity and the superior wall of the external auditory canal. The scutum provides the superior attachment site for the tympanic membrane. **Prussak's space (lateral epitympanic recess)** is bordered laterally by the tympanic membrane, superiorly by the scutum, medially by the neck of the malleus, and inferiorly by the lateral process of the malleus.

The **mesotympanum** is the portion of the middle ear that is medial to the tympanic membrane and contains the stapes, long process of the incus, handle of the malleus, and the oval and round windows.

The **hypotympanum** is the portion of the middle ear that is located inferior to the lower border of the tympanic membrane and is the site of the tympanic opening for the eustachian tube (Figures 2.49 through 2.59).

The **inner ear**, or **bony labyrinth**, contains the **vestibule** and **semicircular canals**, which control equilibrium and balance, and the **cochlea**, which is responsible for hearing (Figures 2.43 through 2.46). The vestibule is a small compartment located between the semicircular canals and the cochlea. Two openings of the vestibule are the **oval window** (Figure 2.44) for the footplate of the stapes and the **vestibular aqueduct**, which contains the endolymphatic duct (Figure 2.47). The semicircular canals are continuous with the vestibule and are easily identified because of their three separate passages (superior [anterior], posterior, and lateral) that are at right angles to each other (Figures 2.42 through 2.44). The cochlea is a conical structure with a base that lies on the **internal auditory canal** (Figure 2.45). Located within the basilar turn of the cochlea is the **round window**, which allows the fluid of the inner ear to move slightly for propagation of sound waves (Figures 2.44 and 2.47). Within the bony labyrinth is a complicated system of ducts called the **membranous labyrinth**, which is filled with **endolymph**, a fluid that helps with the propagation of sound waves. Extending from the vestibule is a slender **endolymphatic duct** that terminates as the **endolymphatic sac**, which is located between two dural layers on the posterior wall of the petrous pyramid (Figures 2.47 and 2.48). The endolymphatic duct and sac are thought to be responsible for the reabsorption of endolymph and may contribute to vestibular dysfunction. Figures 2.49 through 2.59 provide sequential computed tomography (CT) images through the external, middle, and inner ear in the axial and coronal planes, respectively.

(Text continues on page 46)

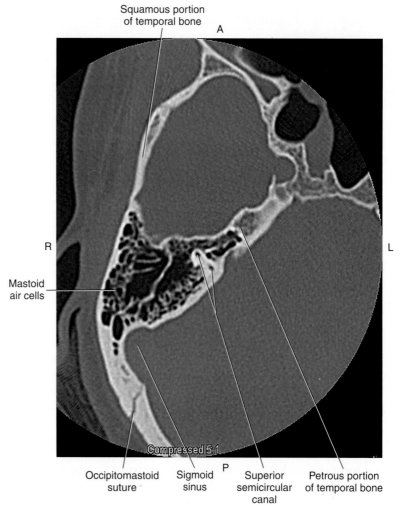

FIGURE 2.49 Axial CT of superior semicircular canal.

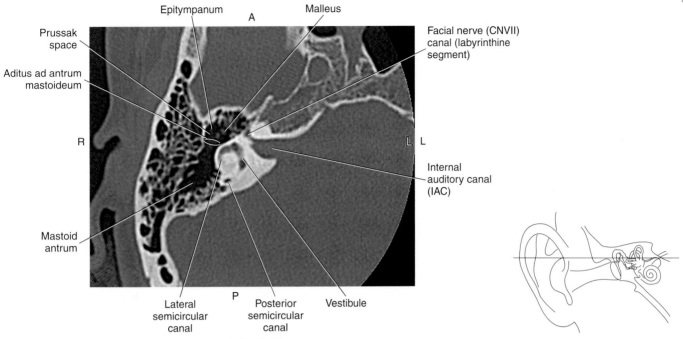

FIGURE 2.50 Axial CT of lateral semicircular canal.

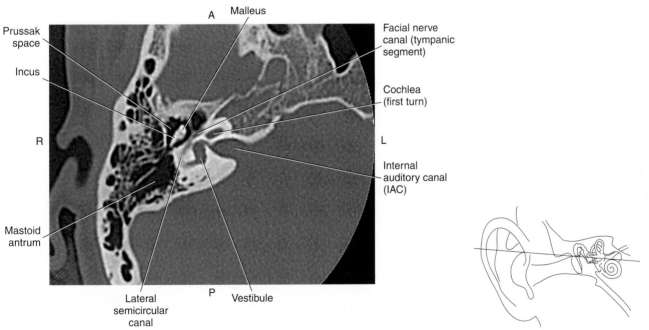

FIGURE 2.51 Axial CT of malleus and incus.

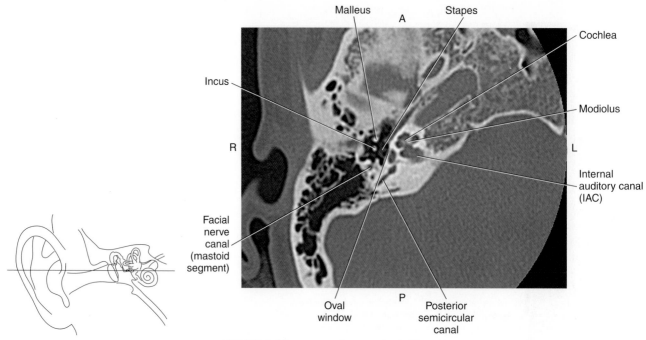

FIGURE 2.52 Axial CT of auditory ossicles.

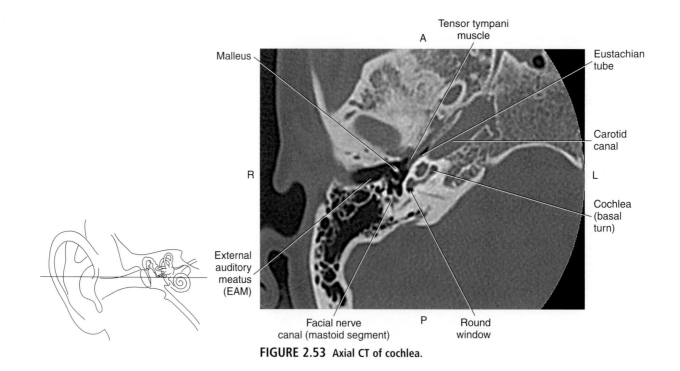

FIGURE 2.53 Axial CT of cochlea.

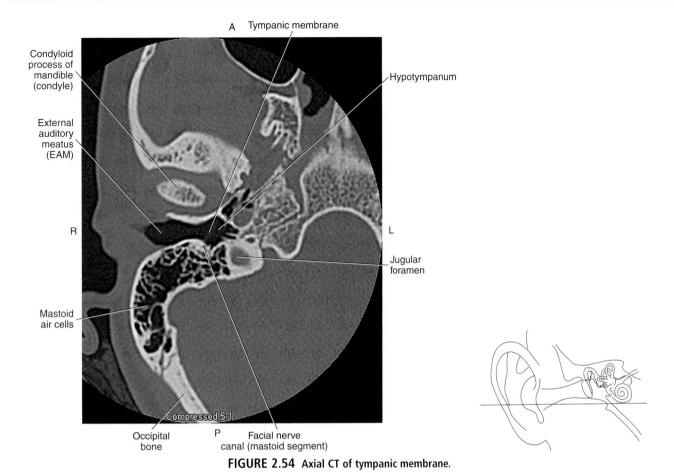

A Tympanic membrane

Condyloid process of mandible (condyle)

Hypotympanum

External auditory meatus (EAM)

R

L

Mastoid air cells

Jugular foramen

Compressed 5:1

Occipital bone

P

Facial nerve canal (mastoid segment)

FIGURE 2.54 Axial CT of tympanic membrane.

Mastoid antrum

Lateral semicircular canal

S

R

Posterior

Facial nerve canal (mastoid segment)

Stylomastoid foramen

L

Occipital condyle

Hypoglossal canal

C1

Mastoid tip

I

Jugular foramen

FIGURE 2.55 Coronal CT reformat of semicircular canals.

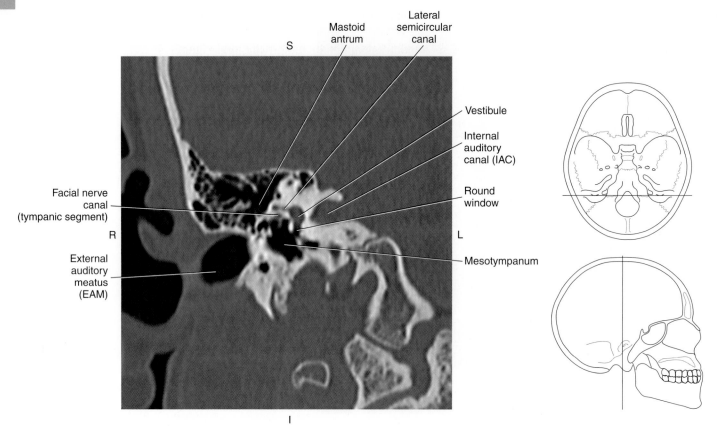

FIGURE 2.56 Coronal CT reformat of vestibule.

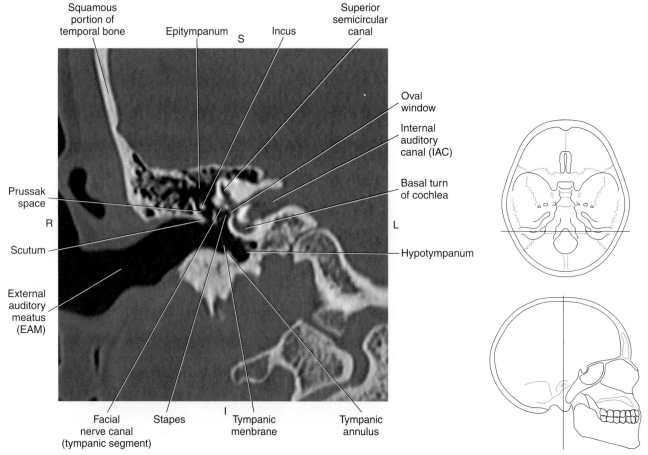

FIGURE 2.57 Coronal CT reformat of IAC.

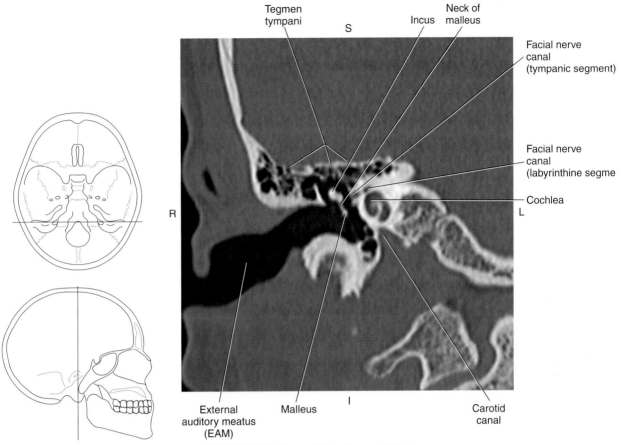

FIGURE 2.58 Coronal CT reformat of EAM.

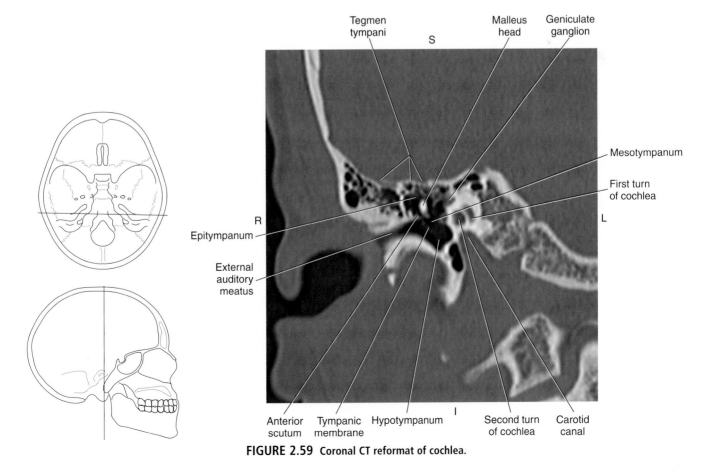

FIGURE 2.59 Coronal CT reformat of cochlea.

Meniere's disease is a disorder of the membranous labyrinth that results from a failure of the mechanism controlling the production and elimination of endolymph. In advanced cases, there is an increased accumulation of endolymph volume, resulting in an abnormal distention of the membranous labyrinth (endolymphatic hydrops). Meniere's disease is most common in middle age and may become bilateral in up to 50% of affected patients. Symptoms include episodic vertigo accompanied by nausea, fluctuating hearing loss, and a feeling of fullness in the affected ears. The success of surgical intervention in relieving Meniere's disease depends a great deal on the ability to image and evaluate the vestibular aqueduct and endolymphatic duct and sac.

Cholesteatomas are epidermoid cysts of the middle ear that can be acquired or congenital. The lumen of the cyst is filled with debris. As a cholesteatoma enlarges, it destroys the ossicles and adjacent bony structures. Cholesteatomas are usually associated with chronic infection, aural discharge, and conductive or mixed deafness. Prussak's space is the most common site of acquired cholesteatomas within the tympanic cavity.

Sutures

The cranial bones are joined by four main articulations termed **sutures**. The **squamous suture,** which is located on the side of the cranium, joins the squamous portion of the temporal bone to the parietal bone. The **coronal suture** runs transversely across the top of the cranium and is the articulation between the frontal and parietal bones. The **sagittal suture** provides the articulation between the parietal bones along the midsagittal plane. The **lambdoidal suture** is located posterior in the cranium and joins the occipital and parietal bones (Figures 2.3, 2.60 through 2.63). Sutures corresponding to the mastoid portion of the temporal bone include the **occipitomastoid** suture between the occipital bone and mastoid portion of the temporal bone and the **parietomastoid** suture between the parietal bone and mastoid portion of the temporal bone. The **asterion** is a point on the skull corresponding to the posterior end of the parietomastoid suture (Figures 2.3 and 2.60). Sutures corresponding to the sphenoid bone include the **sphenosquamousal** suture between the sphenoid bone and squamous portion of the temporal bone, the **sphenofrontal** suture between the greater wing of the sphenoid bone and the frontal bone, and the **sphenoparietal** suture located between the greater wing of the sphenoid bone and the parietal bone. The region surrounding the sphenoparietal suture where the parietal, sphenoid, temporal, and frontal bones meet is termed the **pterion,** an important landmark because it is considered the weakest part of the skull and is also the site of the anterolateral (sphenoid) fontanel in neonates (Figures 2.3 and 2.60). The **frontal (metopic) suture** divides the frontal bone into halves as it extends from the anterior fontanel or sagittal suture to the nasion in infants and children and typically disappears by the age of six (Figure 2.64).

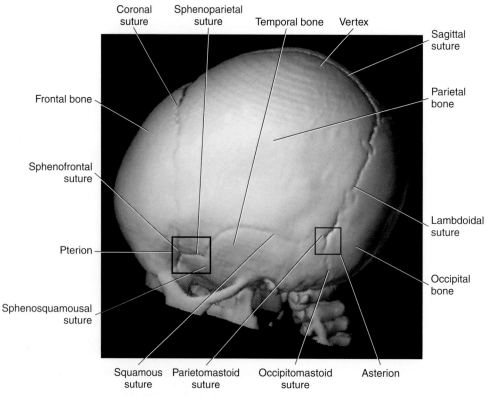

FIGURE 2.60 3D CT of lateral surface of cranium.

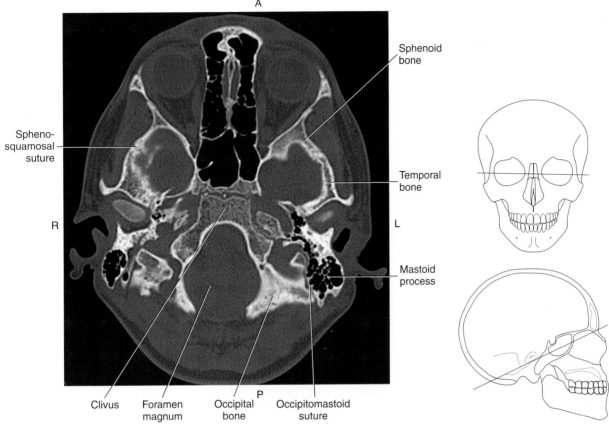

FIGURE 2.61 Axial CT of occipitomastoid suture.

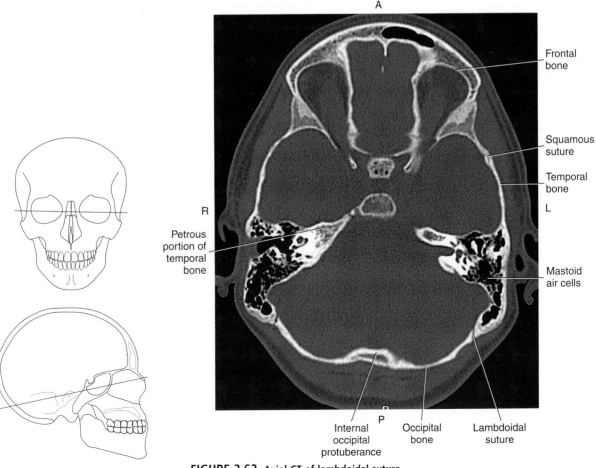

FIGURE 2.62 Axial CT of lambdoidal suture.

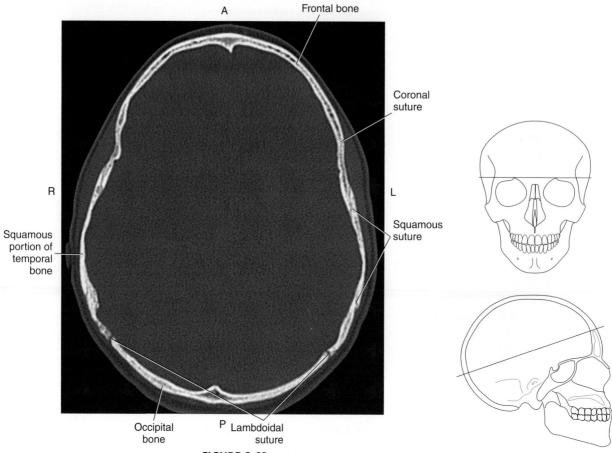

A

Frontal bone

Coronal
suture

R

L

Squamous
portion of
temporal
bone

Squamous
suture

Occipital
bone

P Lambdoidal
suture

FIGURE 2.63   Axial CT of coronal suture.

The sutures in neonates are not fully closed, allowing for growth of the head after birth. Craniosynostosis, which is the result of premature ossification of one or more of the cranial sutures, causes abnormal growth of the cranium and can limit the growth of the brain.

The pterion is known as the weakest part of the skull and is located over the anterior division of the middle meningeal artery. A severe blow to the side of the head causing a fracture and rupture of the middle meningeal artery may result in an epidural hematoma. A favored site of access for performing a burr-hole to drain the hematoma is at the pterion.

Fontanels

Within the neonatal cranium are six areas of incomplete ossification called **fontanels**. The largest is the **anterior fontanel** located at the junction of the upper parietal and frontal bones termed the **bregma** (Figure 2.64). This fontanel remains open until the age of 2. Located at the **lambda,** the junction of the parietal and occipital bones is the **posterior fontanel** (Figure 2.65). The posterior fontanel typically closes between the first and third months after birth. On the sides of the cranium are four additional fontanels, two **anterolateral (sphenoid)** and two **posterolateral (mastoid)** (Figure 2.65). The anterolateral

fontanels are located between the parietal and greater wing of the sphenoid bones. The posterolateral fontanels are located at the junction of the occipital, temporal, and parietal bones. The anterior and posterolateral fontanels ossify at approximately 2 years of age, whereas the posterior and anterolateral fontanels close between 1 and 3 months after birth (Figure 2.66).

Bulging of the anterior fontanel may indicate increased intracranial pressure, whereas a sunken fontanel may indicate dehydration.

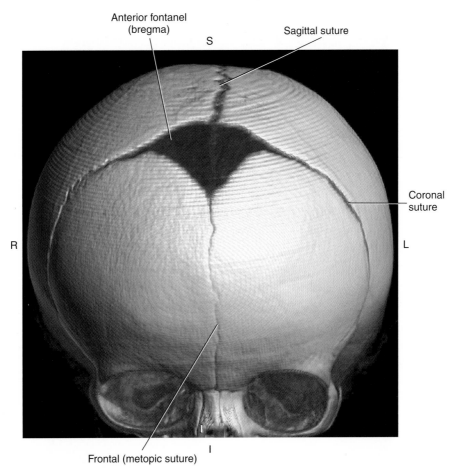

FIGURE 2.64 3D CT of infant cranium, anterior view.

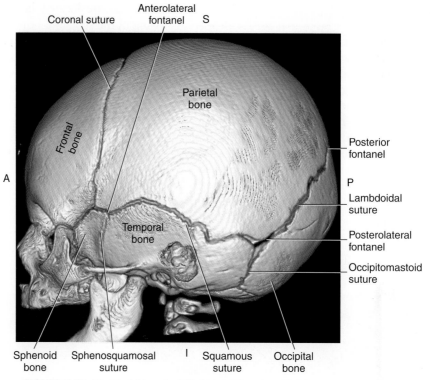

FIGURE 2.65 3D CT of 17-week old infant cranium, lateral view.

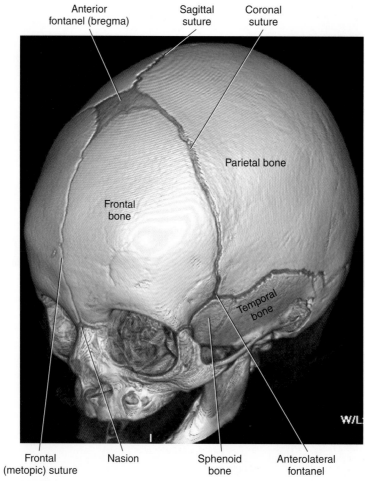

FIGURE 2.66 3D CT of 17-week old infant cranium, oblique view.

FACIAL BONES

The face is made up of 14 facial bones. The facial bones can be difficult to differentiate because of their relatively small size and irregular shape. They consist of the nasal (2), lacrimal (2), palatine (2), maxilla (2), zygoma (2), inferior nasal conchae (2), vomer (1), and mandible (1) (Figures 2.67 through 2.85).

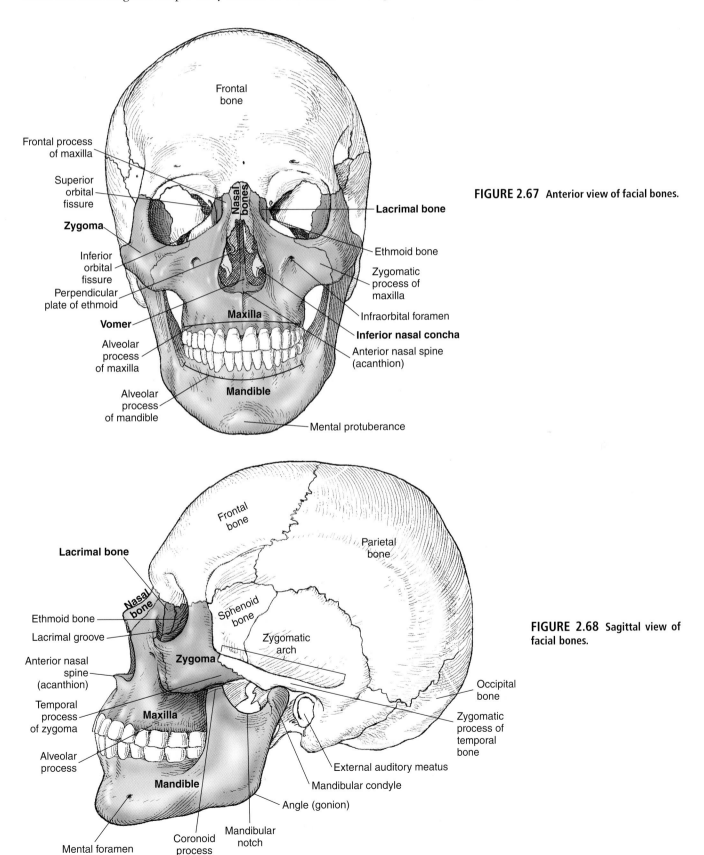

FIGURE 2.67 Anterior view of facial bones.

FIGURE 2.68 Sagittal view of facial bones.

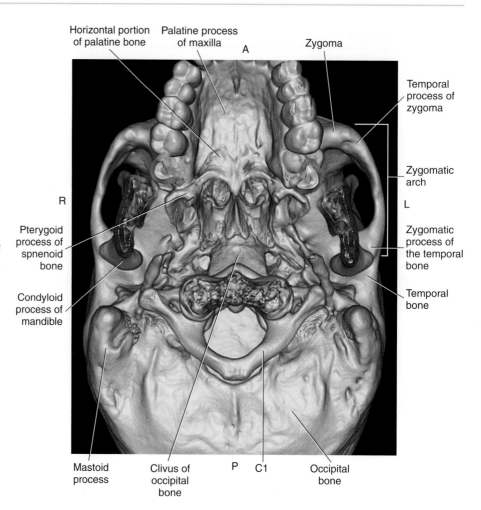

FIGURE 2.69 3D CT of inferior surface of cranial bones with mandible disarticulated.

Nasal Bones

The two **nasal bones** form the bony bridge of the nose and articulate with four bones: frontal and ethmoid bones of the cranium and the opposite nasal bone and maxilla (Figures 2.67, 2.68, 2.70, 2.71, and 2.73).

Lacrimal Bones

Posterior to the nasal bones and maxilla are the **lacrimal bones,** which are situated on the medial wall of each orbit (Figure 2.70). The junction between the lacrimal bones and the maxillae forms the **lacrimal groove,** which accommodates the **lacrimal sacs** that are part of the drainage route for excess lacrimal fluid (tears) (Figures 2.67, 2.68, 2.70, and 2.71).

Palatine Bones

The **palatine bones** are slightly L-shaped and are located in the posterior aspect of the nasal cavity between the maxilla and the pterygoid process of the sphenoid. The palatine bones consist of a horizontal portion and a perpendicular portion. The **horizontal portion** of the palatine bones joins anteriorly with the palatine process of the maxilla to form the hard palate (Figures. 2.8, 2.69, 2.74, and 2.75). The **vertical portion** extends to

form a segment of the lateral wall of the nasal cavity and the medial wall of the orbit (Figure 2.70). The **pterygopalatine fossa** is a gap between the pterygoid process of the sphenoid bone, maxilla and palatine bones. The pterygopalatine fossa contains the maxillary nerve V2 (second division of the trigeminal nerve), the pterygopalatine ganglion, and the third part of the maxillary artery (Figures 2.70 and 2.77).

Maxillary Bones

The largest immovable facial bones are the **maxillary bones,** which fuse at the midline to form a pointed process termed the **anterior nasal spine** (Figures 2.68 through 2.71). An opening on the anterior aspect of the maxilla is the **infraorbital foramen,** which transmits the infraorbital nerve and blood vessels (Figures 2.67 and 2.72). The maxillary bones contain the large **maxillary sinuses** and four processes: frontal process, zygomatic process, alveolar process, and the palatine process (Figures 2.67 and 2.72 through 2.75). The **frontal and zygomatic processes** project to articulate with the frontal bones of the cranium and the zygomatic bones of the face (Figures 2.72 and 2.73). The inferior border of the maxilla has several depressions that form the **alveolar process,** which accepts the roots of the teeth (Figures 2.67, 2.71, 2.75, and 2.76).

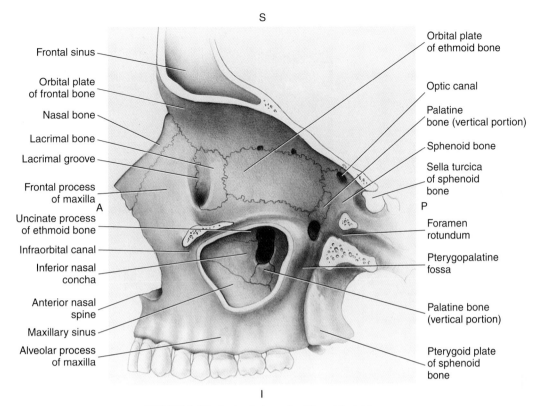

Frontal sinus

Orbital plate
of frontal bone

Nasal bone

Lacrimal bone

Lacrimal groove

Frontal process
of maxilla

Uncinate process
of ethmoid bone

Infraorbital canal

Inferior nasal
concha

Anterior nasal
spine

Maxillary sinus

Alveolar process
of maxilla

Orbital plate
of ethmoid bone

Optic canal

Palatine
bone (vertical portion)

Sphenoid bone

Sella turcica
of sphenoid
bone

Foramen
rotundum

Pterygopalatine
fossa

Palatine bone
(vertical portion)

Pterygoid plate
of sphenoid
bone

FIGURE 2.70 Sagittal view of orbit and facial bones.

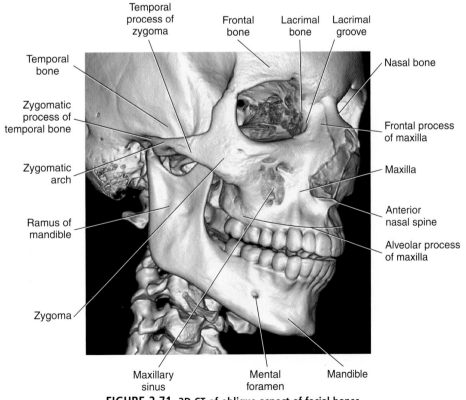

Temporal
process of
zygoma

Frontal
bone

Lacrimal
bone

Lacrimal
groove

Temporal
bone

Zygomatic
process of
temporal bone

Zygomatic
arch

Ramus of
mandible

Zygoma

Nasal bone

Frontal process
of maxilla

Maxilla

Anterior
nasal spine

Alveolar process
of maxilla

Maxillary
sinus

Mental
foramen

Mandible

FIGURE 2.71 3D CT of oblique aspect of facial bones.

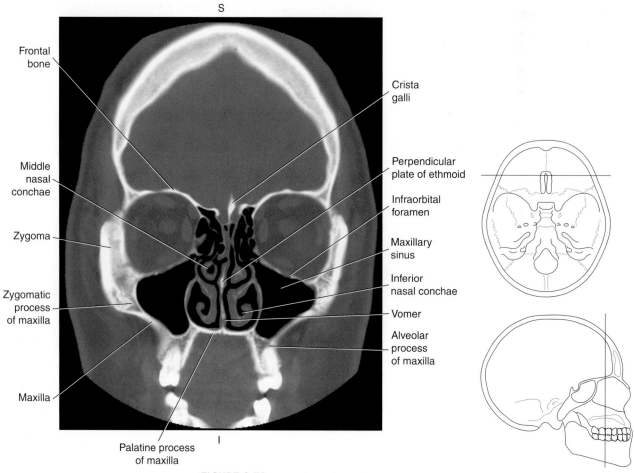

FIGURE 2.72 Coronal CT of maxilla and zygoma.

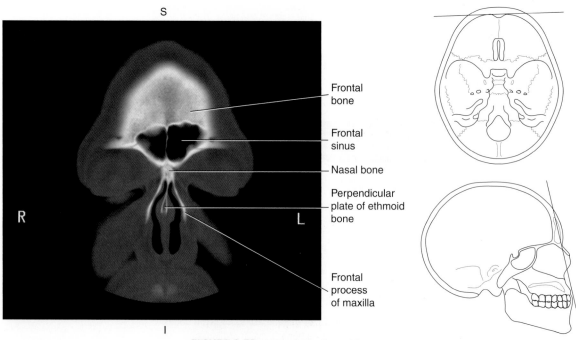

FIGURE 2.73 Coronal CT of nasal bones.

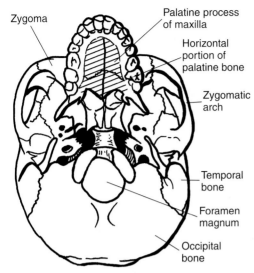

FIGURE 2.74 Inferior view of facial bones and hard palate.

The **palatine process** of the maxilla extends posteriorly to form three fourths of the **hard palate**. The posterior one fourth of the hard palate is created by the horizontal portion of the palatine bones (Figures 2.69, 2.74, and 2.75).

Zygomatic Bones

The **zygomatic bones** (zygoma or malar) create the prominence of the cheek and contribute to the lateral portion of the bony orbit (Figures 2.67, 2.71, 2.72, 2.77, and 2.78). They articulate with the maxilla, temporal, frontal, and sphenoid bones. The temporal process of the zygomatic bone extends posteriorly to join the zygomatic process of the temporal bone to form the **zygomatic arch** (Figures 2.68, 2.69, 2.71, 2.74, and 2.77).

Le Fort fractures are a result of direct anterior facial injuries. They are classified into three groups according to the facial bones that are traumatized. Type I: the alveolar process of the maxilla and the hard palate are separated from the superior part of the skull. Type II: The alveolar, zygomatic, and frontal processes of the maxilla along with the nasal bones are separated from the frontal and zygomatic bones. Type III: Virtually the entire facial skeleton, including the maxillae, nasal bones, and zygomatic bones, are separated from the frontal bone above it.

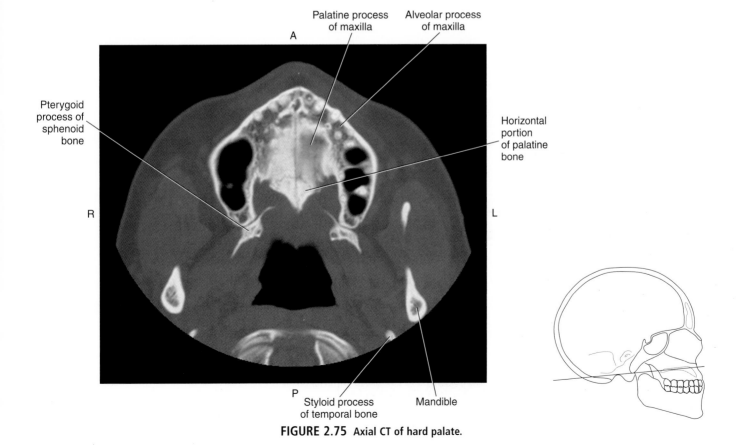

FIGURE 2.75 Axial CT of hard palate.

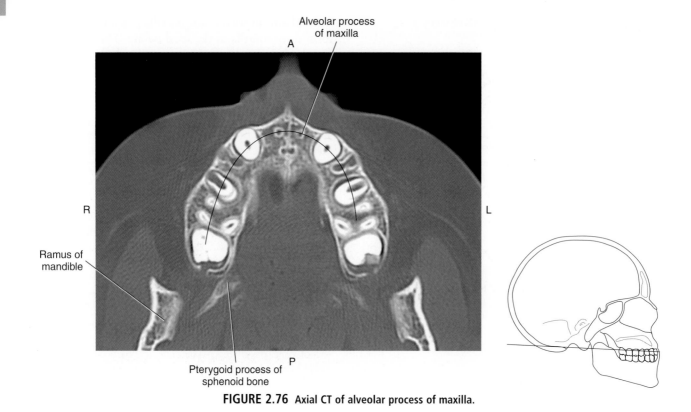

FIGURE 2.76 Axial CT of alveolar process of maxilla.

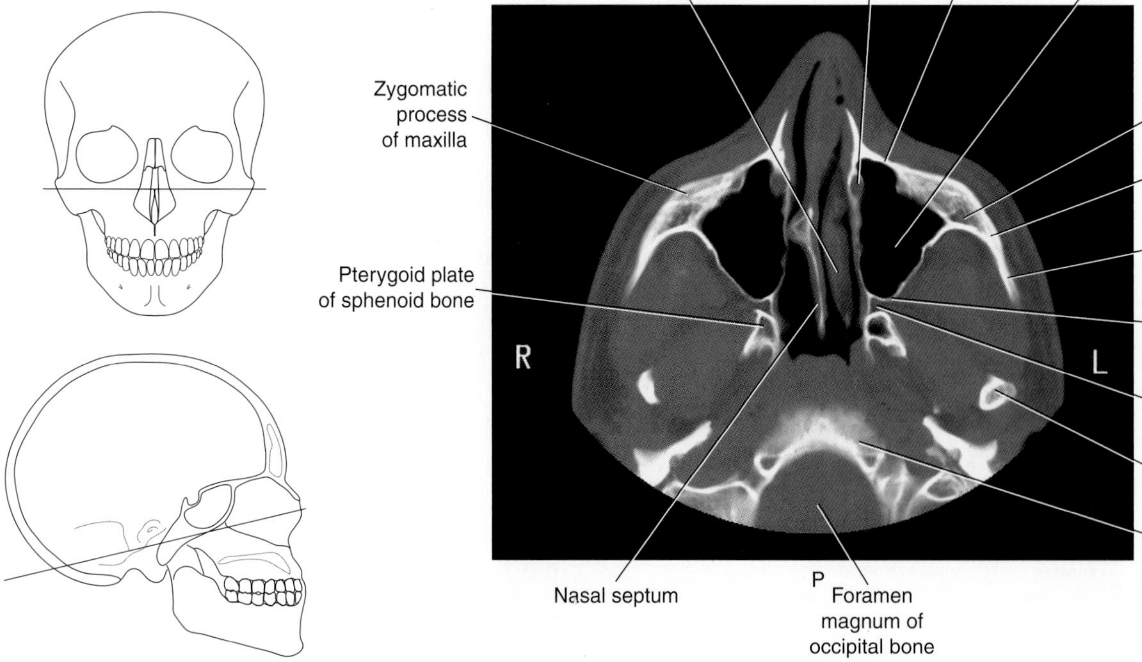

FIGURE 2.77 Axial CT of facial bones.

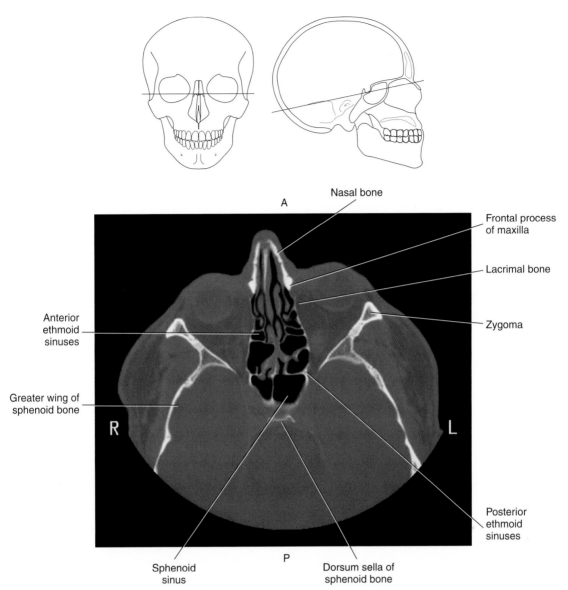

A

Nasal bone

Frontal process
of maxilla

Lacrimal bone

Zygoma

Anterior
ethmoid
sinuses

Greater wing of
sphenoid bone

R

L

Posterior
ethmoid
sinuses

Sphenoid
sinus

P

Dorsum sella of
sphenoid bone

FIGURE 2.78 Axial CT of facial bones and ethmoid sinuses.

Inferior Nasal Conchae

The **inferior nasal conchae** (inferior nasal turbinates) arise from the maxillary bones and project horizontally into the nasal cavity (Figures 2.67, 2.72, and 2.77). They can be identified by their scroll-like appearance. These conchae in conjunction with the superior and middle nasal conchae of the ethmoid bone divide the nasal cavity into three openings or **meati,** termed **superior, middle,** and **inferior** (Figures 2.79 and 2.80).

Vomer

The **vomer** is an unpaired facial bone located on the midsagittal line. The vomer forms the inferior portion of the bony **nasal septum** as it projects superiorly to articulate with the perpendicular plate of the ethmoid bone (Figures 2.8, 2.9, 2.67, and 2.72).

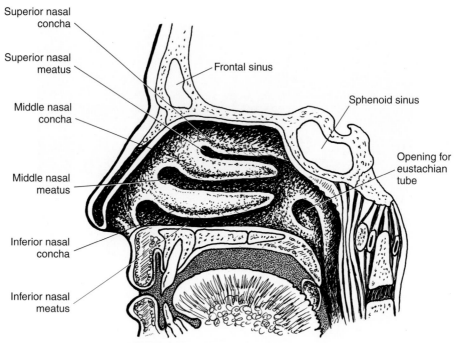

FIGURE 2.79 Sagittal view of nasal meati.

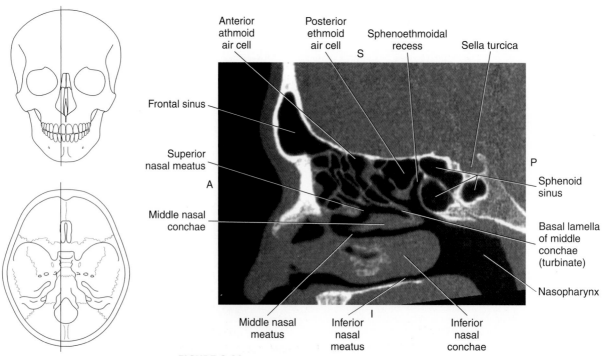

FIGURE 2.80 Sagittal CT reformat of nasal meati.

Mandible

The largest facial bone is the **mandible**. This bone is composed primarily of horizontal and vertical portions (Figures 2.81 and 2.82). The angle created by the junction of these two portions is termed the **gonion**. The curved horizontal portion, called the **body**, contains an **alveolar process** (similar to the maxilla) that receives the roots of the teeth of the lower jaw. The **mental foramina** extend through the body of the mandible and allow passage of the mental artery and nerve (Figures 2.81 and 2.82). The vertical portion of the mandible is called the **ramus** (Figures 2.71, 2.82, and 2.83). Each ramus has two processes at its superior portion: **coronoid process** and **condyloid process (condyle)** (Figures 2.81, 2.82, 2.84, and 2.85). They are separated by a concave surface called the **mandibular notch.** The coronoid process serves as an attachment site for the temporalis and masseter muscles, whereas the condyloid process articulates with the mandibular fossa of the temporal bone to form the **temporomandibular joint (TMJ)** (Figures 2.82 and 2.86).

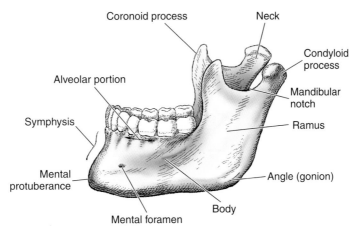

FIGURE 2.81 Lateral view of mandible.

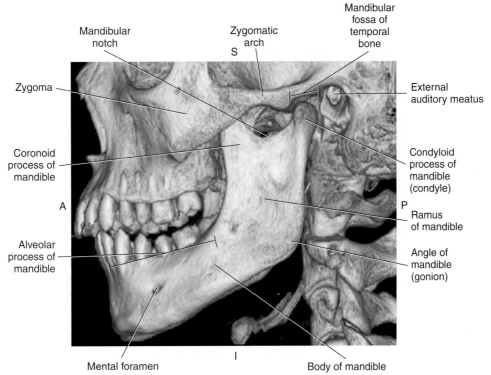

FIGURE 2.82 3D CT of lateral aspect of mandible.

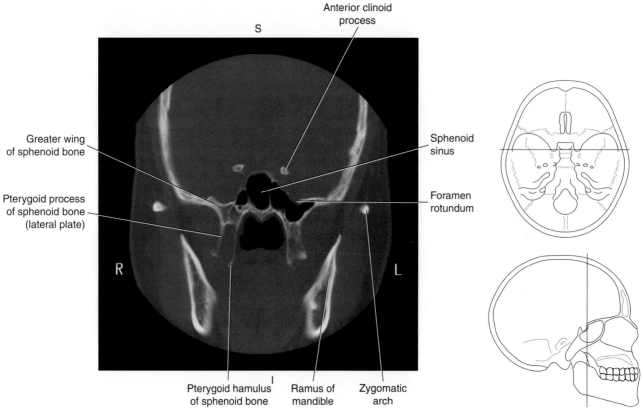

FIGURE 2.83 Coronal CT of mandibular rami.

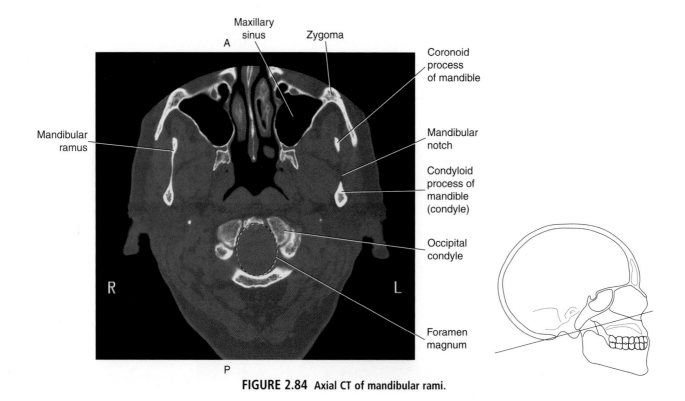

FIGURE 2.84 Axial CT of mandibular rami.

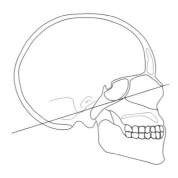

A

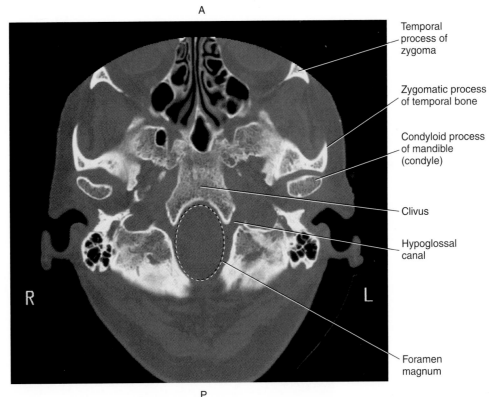

Temporal process of zygoma

Zygomatic process of temporal bone

Condyloid process of mandible (condyle)

Clivus

Hypoglossal canal

Foramen magnum

R   L

P

FIGURE 2.85 Axial CT of mandibular condyles.

TEMPOROMANDIBULAR JOINT

The temporomandibular joint (TMJ) is a modified hinge joint that allows for the necessary motions of mastication.

Bony Anatomy

The **mandibular fossa** and **articular eminence** of the temporal bone form the superior articulating surface for the mandibular condyloid process of mandible (condyle).

The articular eminence creates the anterior boundary of the joint, preventing the forward displacement of the mandibular condyle (Figures 2.86 and 2.87).

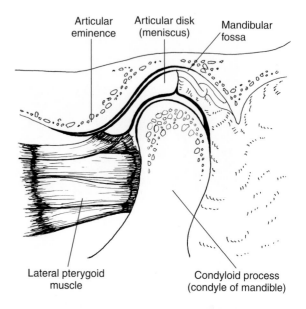

FIGURE 2.86 Lateral view of temporomandibular joint.

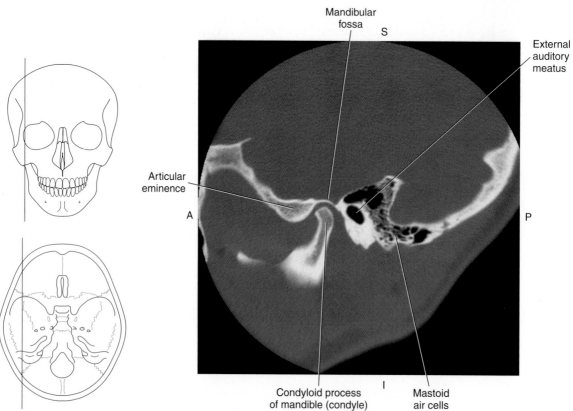

FIGURE 2.87 Sagittal CT reformat of temporomandibular joint.

Articular Disk and Ligaments

The **articular disk**, frequently called the **meniscus**, is shaped like a bowtie and is interposed between the mandibular condyle and fossa to act as a shock absorber during jaw movement (Figures 2.86, 2.88, and 2.89). The anterior and posterior portions of the meniscus are referred to as the anterior and posterior bands, respectively. The anterior band attaches to the lateral pterygoid muscle, and the posterior band has fibrous connections to both the temporal bone and the posterior aspect of the condyle. The articular disk is not tightly bound to the fossa but moves anteriorly with the condyle. Several ligaments help maintain the position of the articular disk. The articular disk is attached to the medial and lateral surfaces of the condyle by the **collateral ligaments** (Figures 2.89 and 2.90). Lateral stability is provided by the **temporomandibular ligament (lateral ligament)**, which extends from the articular eminence and zygomatic process to the posterior aspect of the articular disk and the condylar head and neck (Figure 2.91). Additionally, this ligament restricts the posterior movement of the condyle and articular disk.

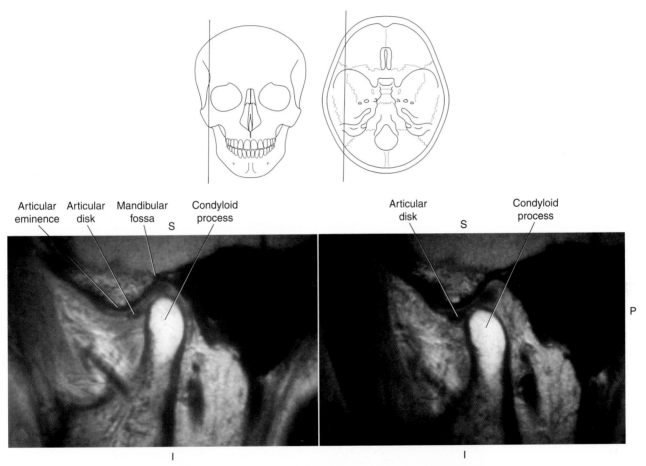

FIGURE 2.88 Sagittal, T1-weighted MRI of temporomandibular joint and articular disk. A, closed. B, open.

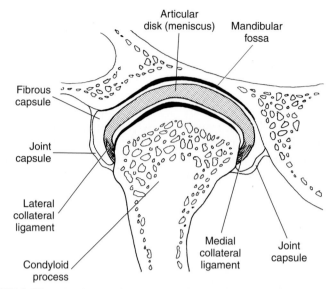

FIGURE 2.89 Coronal view of temporomandibular joint and collateral ligaments.

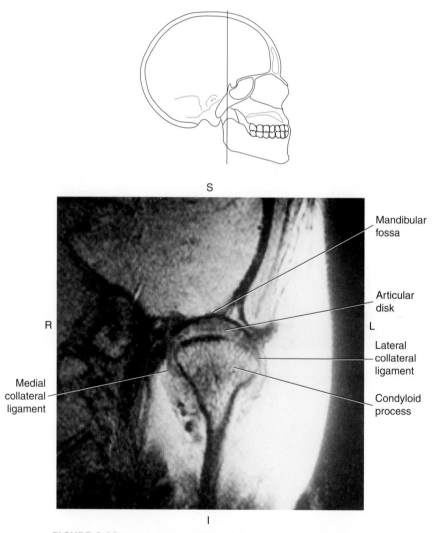

FIGURE 2.90 Coronal, T1-weighted MRI of temporomandibular joint.

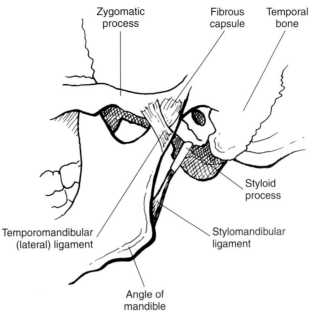

Zygomatic process

Fibrous capsule

Temporal bone

Styloid process

Temporomandibular (lateral) ligament

Stylomandibular ligament

Angle of mandible

FIGURE 2.91 Sagittal view of temporomandibular joint and lateral ligament.

Muscles

The cooperative actions of four muscles located on each side of the TMJ provide the movement of the mandible and are collectively referred to as the **muscles of mastication** (Figure 2.92). The fan-shaped **temporalis muscle** originates on the temporal fossa, inserts on the coronoid process of the mandible, and elevates the mandible. The **masseter muscle** is the strongest muscle of the jaw, arising from the zygomatic arch and inserting on the ramus and angle of the mandible. Its actions include elevation of the mandible (Figures 2.92 and 2.93). The pterygoid muscles (medial and lateral) originate from the pterygoid processes of the sphenoid bone and insert on the angle of the mandible and condylar process, respectively. The **medial pterygoid muscle** acts to close the jaw, whereas the **lateral pterygoid muscle** opens the jaw and protrudes and moves the mandible from side to side (Figures 2.92, 2.94, and 2.95).

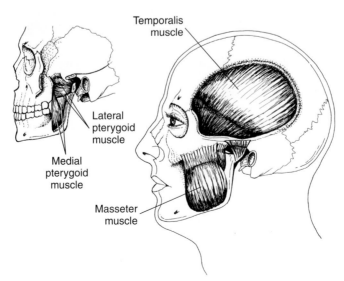

Temporalis muscle

Lateral pterygoid muscle

Medial pterygoid muscle

Masseter muscle

FIGURE 2.92 Muscles of mastication.

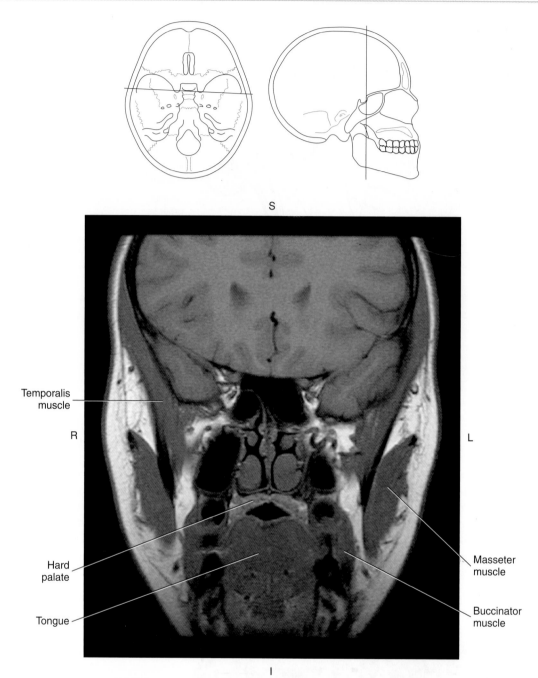

FIGURE 2.93 Coronal, T1-weighted MRI of muscles of mastication.

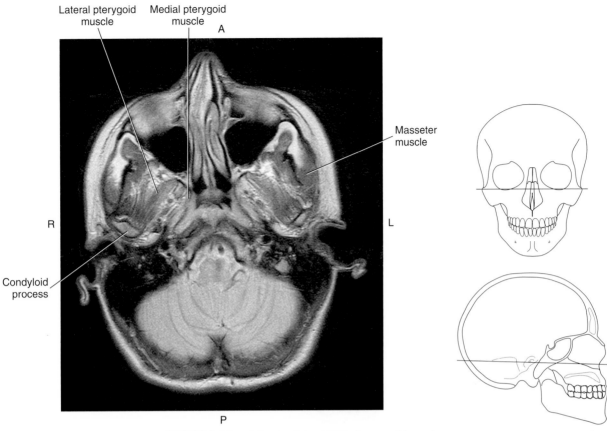

FIGURE 2.94 Axial, T1-weighted MRI of pterygoid muscles.

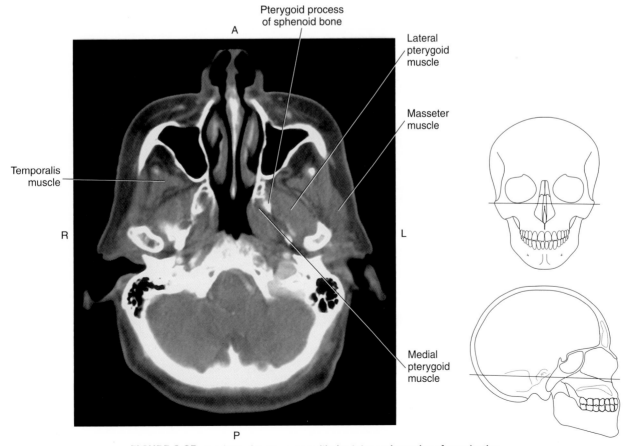

FIGURE 2.95 Axial CT of temporomandibular joint and muscles of mastication.

PARANASAL SINUSES

The **paranasal sinuses** are air-containing cavities within the facial bones and skull that communicate with the nasal cavity. The nasal cavity is lined by nasal mucosa and is responsible for filtering airborne particles as it warms and humidifies air going into the lungs. The sinuses are named after the bones in which they originate: **ethmoid, maxillary, sphenoid, and frontal.** There is great variance in the size, shape, and development of these sinuses within each individual (Figures 2.96 and 2.97).

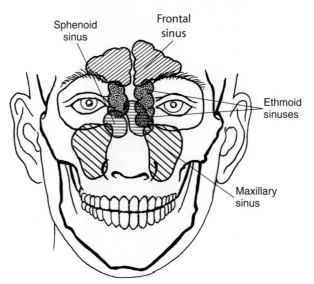

FIGURE 2.96 Anterior view of paranasal sinuses.

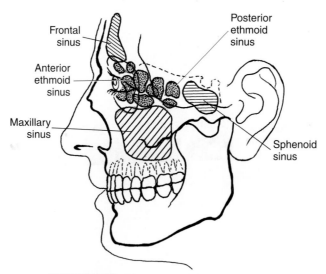

FIGURE 2.97 Lateral view of paranasal sinuses.

Ethmoid

The **ethmoid sinuses** are contained within the **lateral masses (labyrinths)** of the ethmoid bone and number in the adult between 3 to 18 cells. They are present at birth and continue to grow and honeycomb into a varying number of air cells through puberty. The ethmoid sinuses are divided into **anterior** and **posterior groups** by the basal lamella of the middle conchae (turbinate). The **basal lamella** is the lateral attachment of the middle nasal conchae to the lamina papyracea (Figure 2.80). The anterior group drains into the **middle nasal meatus,** and the posterior group drains into the **superior nasal meatus** (Figures 2.96 through 2.100 and Table 2.3).

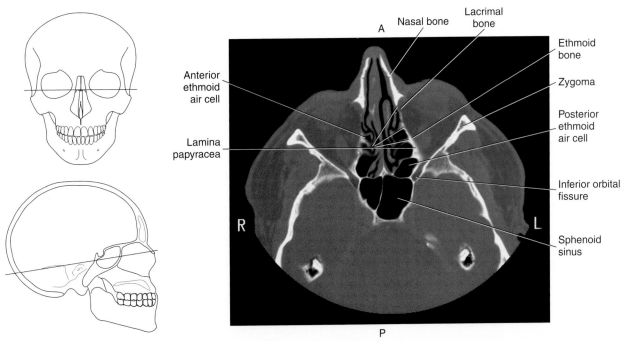

FIGURE 2.98 Axial CT of sphenoid and ethmoid sinuses.

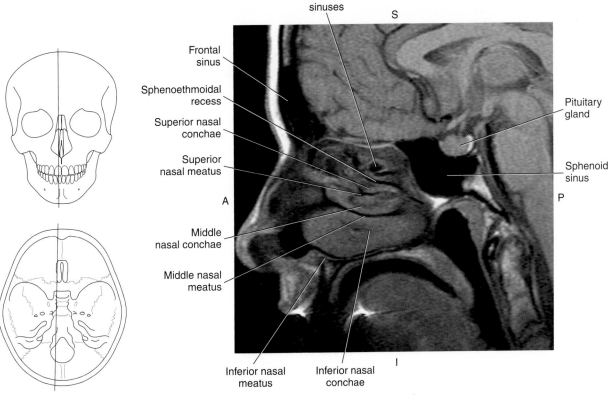

FIGURE 2.99 Sagittal, T1-weighted MRI of sphenoid sinus.

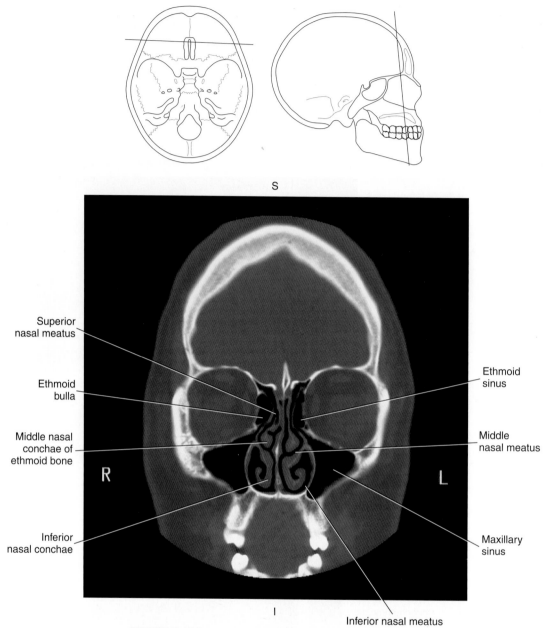

FIGURE 2.100 Coronal CT of ethmoid and maxillary sinuses.

TABLE 2.3	Paranasal Sinus Drainage Location
Sinus	**Drainage Location**
Ethmoid: anterior	Middle nasal meatus
Ethmoid: posterior	Superior nasal meatus
Maxillary	Middle nasal meatus
Sphenoid	Sphenoethmoidal recess
Frontal	Middle nasal meatus

Maxillary

The paired **maxillary sinuses (antrum of Highmore)** are located within the body of the maxilla, below the orbit and lateral to the nose. These triangular cavities are the largest of the paranasal sinuses in adults but are just small cavities at birth. Their growth stops at approximately the age of 15. The roots of the teeth and the maxillary sinuses are separated by a very thin layer of bone. Often it is difficult to differentiate between the symptoms of sinusitis and infection of the teeth. The maxillary sinuses drain into the middle nasal meatus (Figures 2.96, 2.97, 2.100, and 2.101, and Table 2.3).

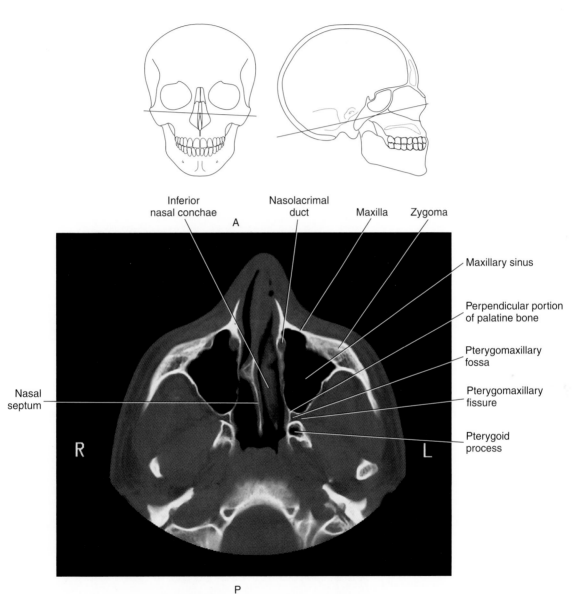

FIGURE 2.101 Axial CT of maxillary sinuses.

Sphenoid

The **sphenoid sinuses** are present at birth but contain red marrow and are therefore devoid of air. Pneumatization of the sphenoid sinuses may be seen as early as 2 years of age. Major growth of the sinuses occur in the third to fifth year, and typically assume adult configuration between 10 and 14 years of age.

Sphenoid sinuses are normally paired and occupy the body of the sphenoid bone just below the **sella turcica**. Each sphenoid sinus opens into the **sphenoethmoidal recess** directly above the **superior concha** and drains into the superior nasal meatus (Figures 2.96 through 2.99, 2.102, and 2.103, and Table 2.3).

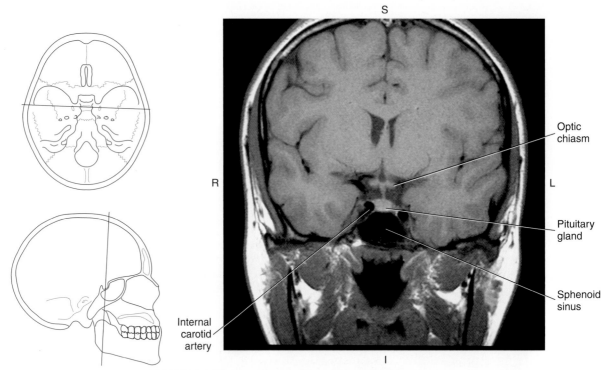

FIGURE 2.102 Coronal, T1-weighted MRI of sphenoid sinuses.

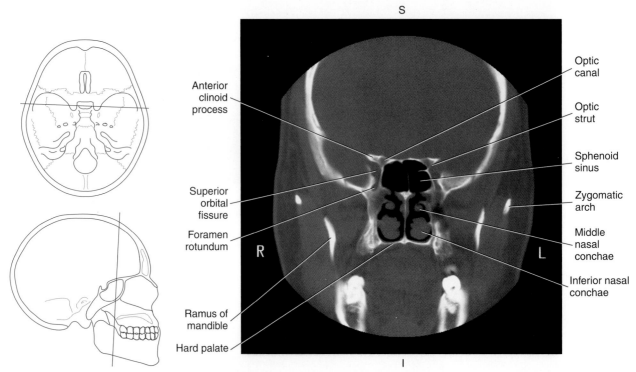

FIGURE 2.103 Coronal CT of sphenoid sinuses.

Frontal

The **frontal sinuses** are located within the vertical portion of the frontal bone (Figures 2.96, 2.97, and 2.99). These sinuses are typically paired and are separated along the sagittal plane by a **septum** (Figure 2.104). The frontal sinuses are rarely symmetric, vary greatly in size, and can contain numerous septa. These sinuses do not form or become aerated in the frontal bone until approximately age 6 making them the only paranasal sinuses that are absent at birth. The frontal sinuses drain into the middle nasal meatus (Figures 2.99 and 2.100, and Table 2.3).

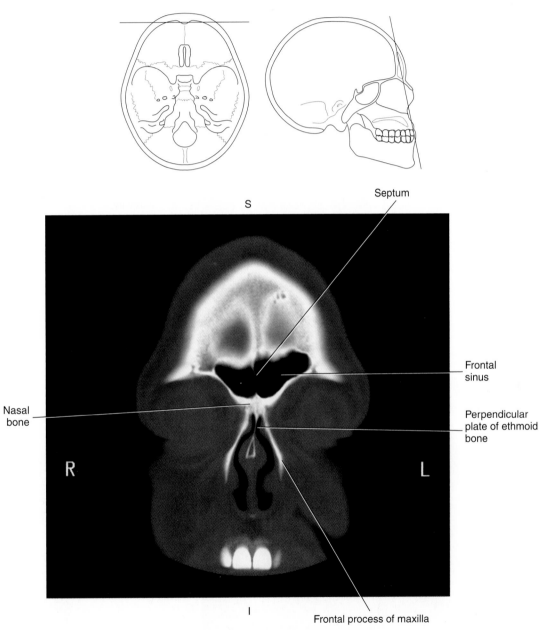

FIGURE 2.104 Coronal CT of frontal sinuses.

Osteomeatal Unit

Drainage of the paranasal sinuses occurs through various openings or ostia. The major drainage pathways and structures of these osteomeatal channels form the **osteomeatal unit** (OMU) (Figures 2.105 through 2.107). There are two osteomeatal channels: the anterior OMU and posterior OMU. The **anterior OMU** includes the ostia for the frontal and maxillary sinuses, frontal recess, infundibulum, and middle meatus. The anterior OMU provides communication between the frontal, anterior ethmoid, and maxillary sinuses. The **posterior OMU** consists of the sphenoethmoidal recess and the superior nasal meatus, which communicate with the posterior ethmoid air cells. The sphenoethmoidal recess lies just lateral to the nasal septum, above the superior nasal concha, and drains the sphenoid sinuses. Key OMU structures to identify include the infundibulum, middle meatus, uncinate process, semilunar hiatus, and ethmoid bulla. The **infundibulum** is a narrow oblong canal that serves as the primary drainage pathway from the maxillary sinuses into the middle meatus. The medial wall of the infundibulum is created by the uncinate process. The **uncinate process** is a thin, hook-shaped bony plate that

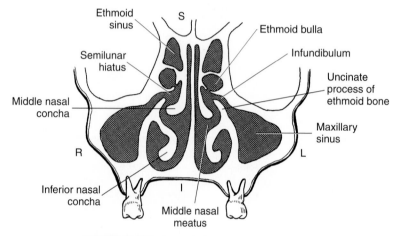

FIGURE 2.105 Coronal view of osteomeatal unit.

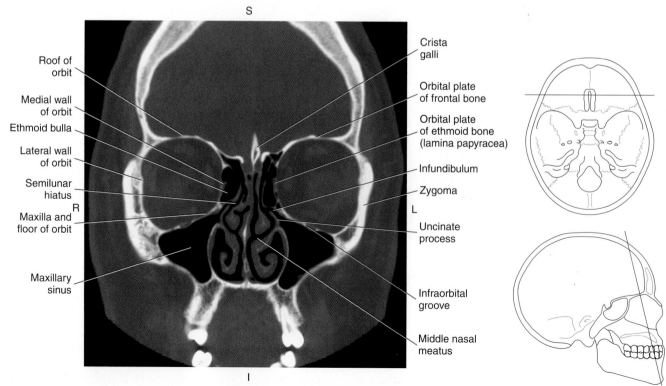

FIGURE 2.106 Coronal CT of osteomeatal unit.

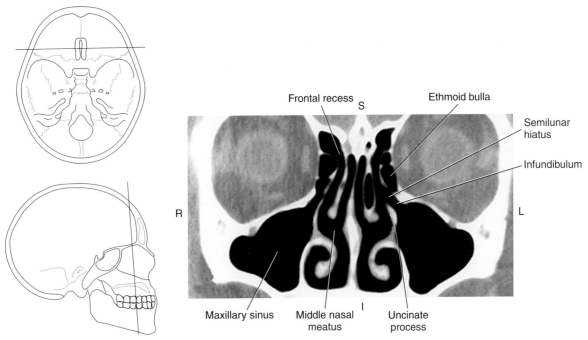

Frontal recess S   Ethmoid bulla

Semilunar hiatus

Infundibulum

R   L

Maxillary sinus   Middle nasal   I   Uncinate
                  meatus   process

FIGURE 2.107 Coronal CT of frontal recess.

arises from the floor of the anterior ethmoid sinuses and projects posteriorly and inferiorly, ending in a free edge. The free edge of the uncinate process forms the semilunar hiatus, which opens directly into the middle meatus. The **semilunar hiatus** is a gap located between the ethmoid bulla and uncinate process that forms the opening of the infundibulum. Also draining into the middle meatus is the ethmoid bulla, located superior and posterior to the infundibulum, which receives drainage from the anterior ethmoid air cells (Figures 2.105, 2.106, and 2.107).

ORBIT

Bony Orbit

The **bony orbits** are cone-shaped recesses that contain the globes, extraocular muscles, blood vessels, nerves, adipose and connective tissues, and most of the lacrimal apparatus. The junction of the frontal, sphenoid, and ethmoid bones of the cranium and the lacrimal, maxillary, palatine, and zygomatic bones of the face forms the orbit (Figures 2.108 and 2.109). Each orbit presents a roof, floor, medial wall, lateral wall, and an apex. The **roof** of the orbit is composed of the orbital plate of the frontal bone and most of the lesser wing of the sphenoid bone. On the anterolateral surface of the roof is the **lacrimal fossa** in which lies the lacrimal gland (Figures 2.108 and 2.109). The **medial wall** is exceedingly thin and is formed by a portion of the frontal process of the maxilla, the lacrimal bone, ethmoid bone, and body of the sphenoid bone (Figures 2.106, 2.108, 2.110, and 2.111). On the anterior surface of the medial wall is the **lacrimal groove** for the lacrimal

sac (Figures 2.108 through 2.110). The **floor** of the orbit, which is also the roof of the maxillary sinus, is made up of the maxilla, zygoma, and palatine bone. The **lateral wall** is the thickest wall and is formed by the greater wing of the sphenoid bone and the zygoma (Figures 2.106, 2.108, and 2.111). The posterior portion of the orbit or the apex is basically formed by the **optic canal (optic foramen)** and the superior orbital fissure. The optic canal and the superior and inferior orbital fissures allow various structures to enter and exit the orbit and establish communication between the orbit and middle cranial fossa. The optic canal forms an angle of about 37 degrees with the sagittal plane of the head; it is bound medially by the body, superiorly by the lesser wing, and inferiorly and laterally by the **optic strut (inferior root)** of the sphenoid bone (Figures 2.108 through 2.112). Coursing through the optic canal are the ophthalmic artery and optic nerve. The **superior orbital fissure**, a triangular opening located between the greater and lesser wings of the sphenoid bone, allows the passage of cranial nerves, oculomotor (III), trochlear (IV), ophthalmic branch of the trigeminal (V), and abducens (VI) as well as the ophthalmic veins (Figures 2.108, 2.109, 2.111, and 2.112). At the orbital apex, the inferior and lateral walls of the orbit are separated by the **inferior orbital fissure** through which the maxillary branch of the trigeminal nerve (V) courses (Figures 2.108 and 2.113). The medial lip of the inferior orbital fissure is notched by the infraorbital groove, which passes forward in the orbital floor to become the infraorbital canal that opens on the anterior surface of the maxilla as the **infraorbital foramen** (Figures 2.106 and 2.108 through 2.110).

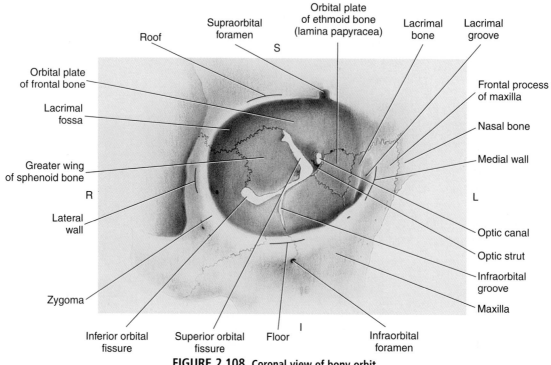

FIGURE 2.108 Coronal view of bony orbit.

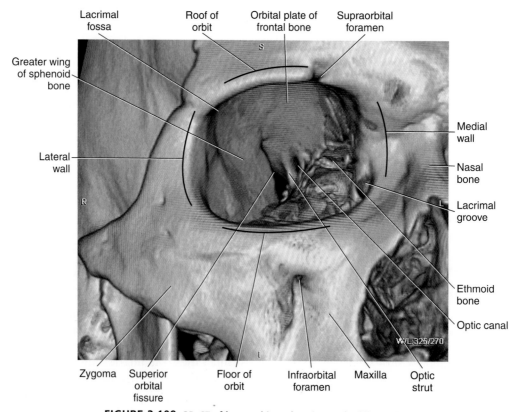

FIGURE 2.109 3D CT of bony orbit and optic canal, oblique view.

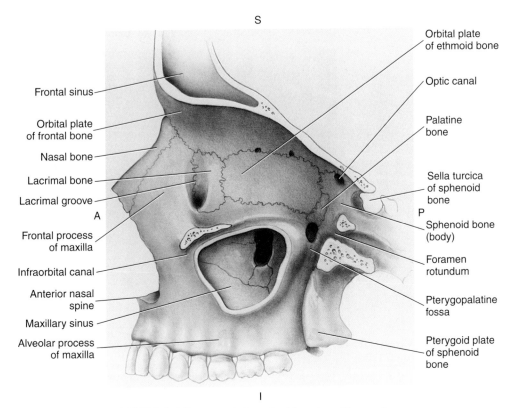

FIGURE 2.110 Sagittal view of orbit and maxillary region.

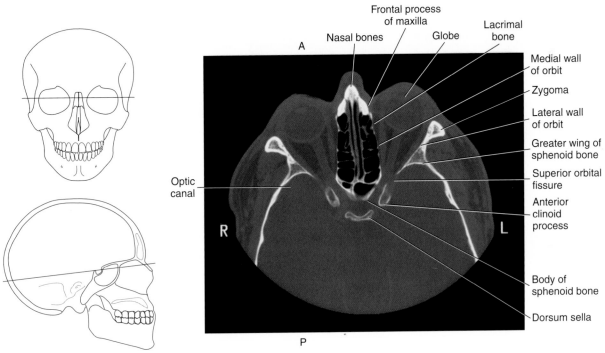

FIGURE 2.111 Axial CT of optic canal.

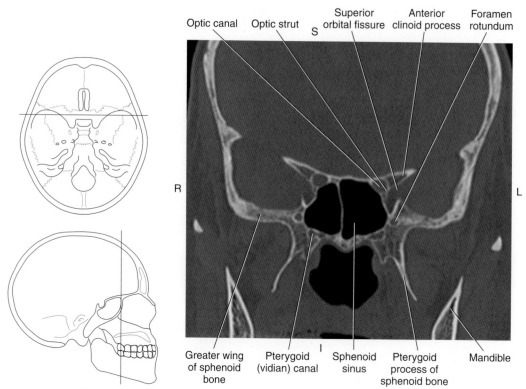

FIGURE 2.112 Coronal CT reformat of superior orbital fissure and optic canal.

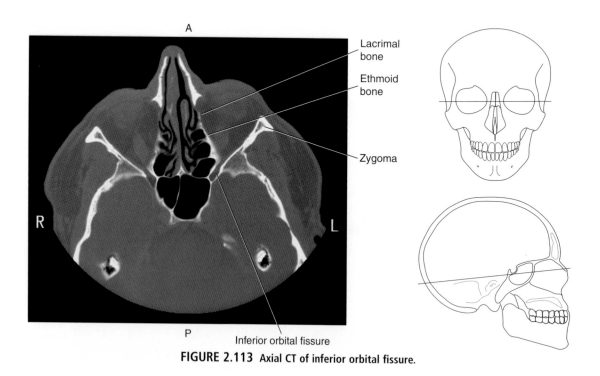

FIGURE 2.113 Axial CT of inferior orbital fissure.

Soft Tissue Structures

The globe of the eye has an irregular, spherical shape and sits in the socket of the bony orbit. The **globe** is divided into **anterior** and **posterior compartments** (Figure 2.114). The anterior compartment is a small cavity located anterior to the **lens**. It contains the **cornea** and **iris** and is filled with **aqueous humor** that helps maintain intraorbital pressure. The larger posterior compartment is located behind the lens and is surrounded by the **retina**. The retina consists of layers of tissue that include the photoreceptors responsible for vision. The posterior chamber contains a jelly-like substance called the **vitreous humor** that helps maintain the shape of the globe (Figures 2.114 through 2.116).

Direct trauma to the globe will commonly result in a blowout fracture of the orbit. These fractures most commonly involve the floor of the orbit causing orbital content herniation, which results in diplopia. A medial blowout fracture involving the orbital plate of the ethmoid bone is much less common but may cause open communication between the frontal and ethmoid sinuses and the orbit.

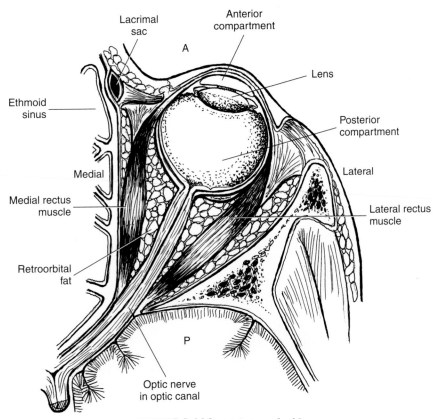

FIGURE 2.114 Axial view of orbit.

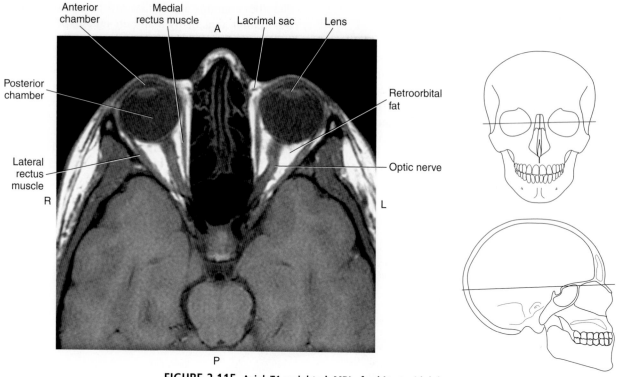

FIGURE 2.115 Axial, T1-weighted, MRI of orbit at midglobe.

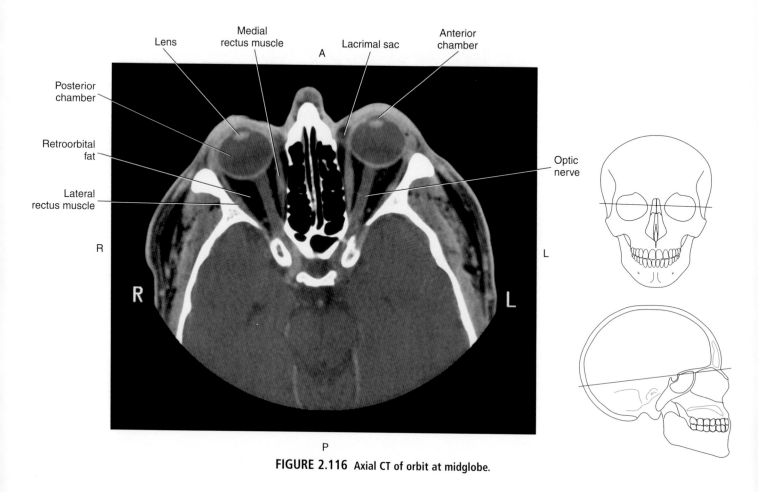

FIGURE 2.116 Axial CT of orbit at midglobe.

Optic Nerve

The **optic nerve** is the nerve of sight. It commences at the posterior surface of the globe and courses posteromedially to exit the orbit through the optic canal and is entirely surrounded by dura mater, which is continuous with the meninges of the brain (Figures 2.114 through 2.116). The **ophthalmic artery** courses adjacent to the optic nerve as it exits through the optic canal. The **superior ophthalmic vein** is located inferior to the superior rectus muscle and courses obliquely from the medial orbit to the superior orbital fissure (Figures 2.117 through 2.119). **Retroorbital fat,** which allows for better visualization of structures in cross-sectional imaging, surrounds the muscular and vascular structures within the orbit (Figures 2.114 through 2.121).

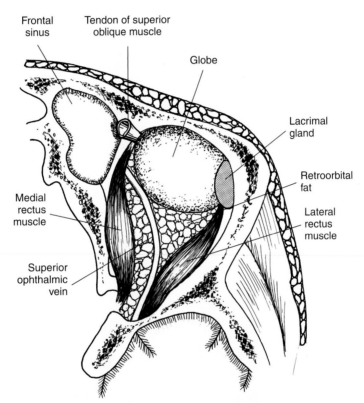

FIGURE 2.117 Axial view of orbit with lacrimal gland.

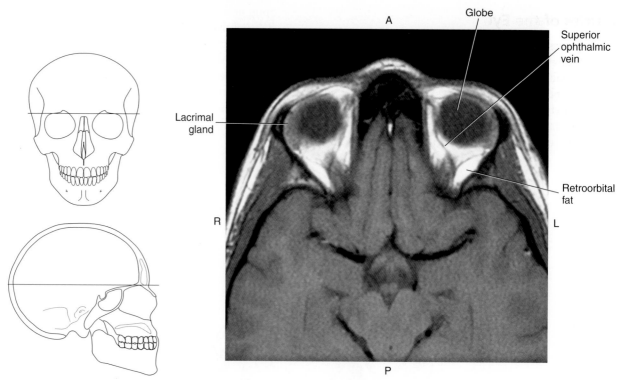

FIGURE 2.118 Axial, T1-weighted, MRI of orbit with lacrimal gland and superior ophthalmic vein.

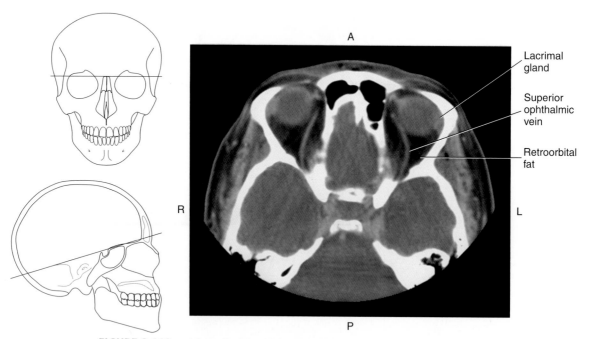

FIGURE 2.119 Axial CT of orbit with lacrimal gland and superior ophthalmic vein.

Muscles of the Eye

Six major muscles work together to control the movement of the eye. The **rectus muscle group** consists of four muscles that arise from a common tendinous ring surrounding the optic nerve and is located at the medial portion of the superior orbital fissure. The **superior, inferior, medial,** and **lateral rectus muscles** act to abduct and adduct the globe (Figures 2.114 through 2.117 and 2.120 through 2.125). Two **oblique muscles, superior** and **inferior,** abduct and rotate the globe. The superior oblique is located medial to the superior rectus muscle, and the inferior oblique lies below and anterior to the inferior rectus muscle. The upper eyelid is controlled by the **superior levator palpebrae muscle,** which originates from the orbital roof near the origin of the superior rectus muscle (Figures 2.120 through 2.125).

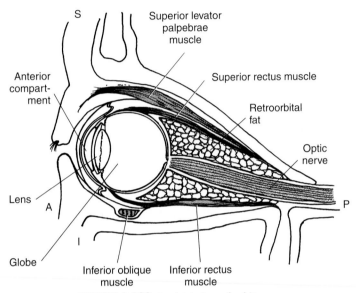

FIGURE 2.120 Sagittal view of orbit.

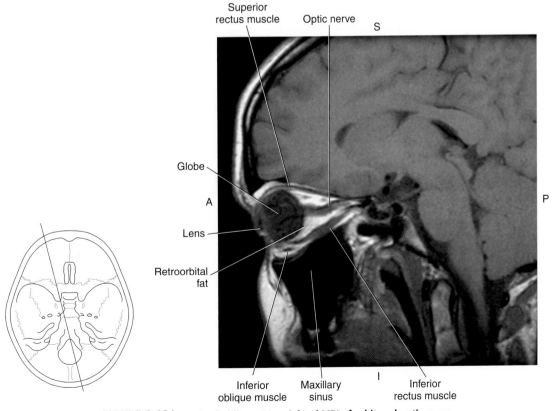

FIGURE 2.121 Sagittal oblique, T1-weighted MRI of orbit and optic nerve.

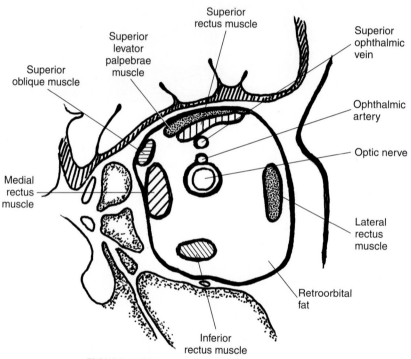

FIGURE 2.122 Coronal view of orbit and optic nerve.

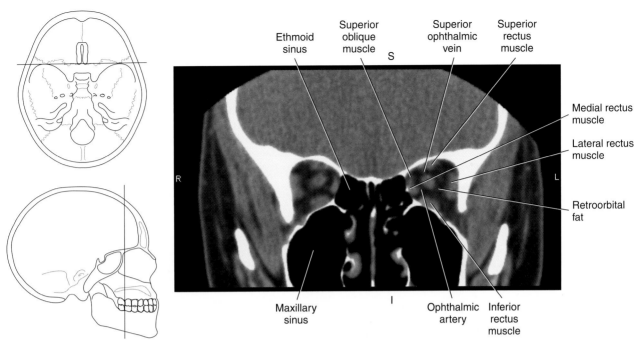

FIGURE 2.123 Coronal CT of orbit with optic nerve and vessels.

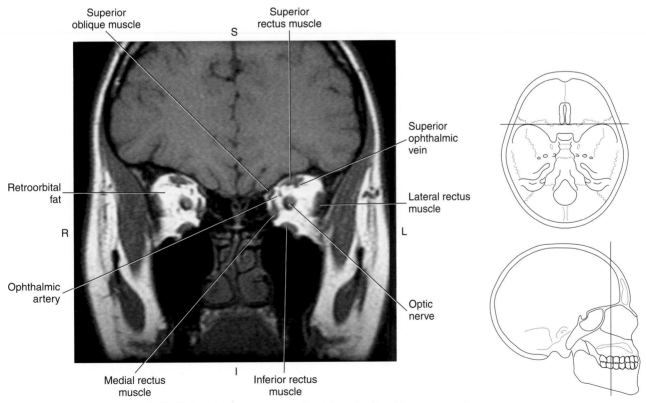

FIGURE 2.124 Coronal, T1-weighted MRI of orbit with rectus muscle group.

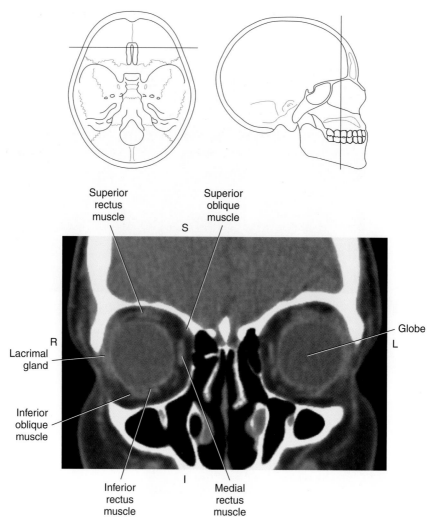

FIGURE 2.125 Coronal CT of globe and lacrimal gland.

Lacrimal Apparatus

Each **lacrimal apparatus** consists of a lacrimal gland, lacrimal canaliculi, lacrimal sac, and nasolacrimal duct and is responsible for the production and distribution of tears. Tears are important for keeping the eye moist and clean, removing waste, preventing bacterial infections, and providing nutrients and oxygen to portions of the eye. The almond-shaped **lacrimal gland** is located in the lacrimal groove, superior and lateral to the globe, where it provides most of the tear volume (Figures 2.117 through 2.119, 2.125, and 2.126). On blinking, tears collect in the area of the medial canthus and subsequently empty into small canals termed **lacrimal canaliculi** that lead to the **lacrimal sac**. The lacrimal sac, found within the lacrimal groove of the orbit, continues inferiorly to form the **nasolacrimal duct,** which passes through the nasolacrimal canal of the maxillary and lacrimal bones to empty into the **inferior nasal meatus** (Figures 2.115, 2.116, 2.126, and 2.127).

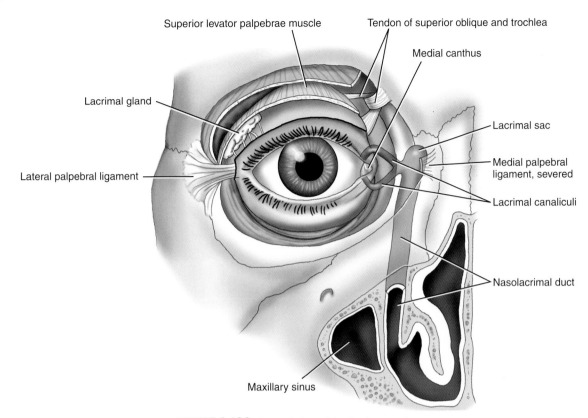

FIGURE 2.126 Coronal view of lacrimal apparatus.

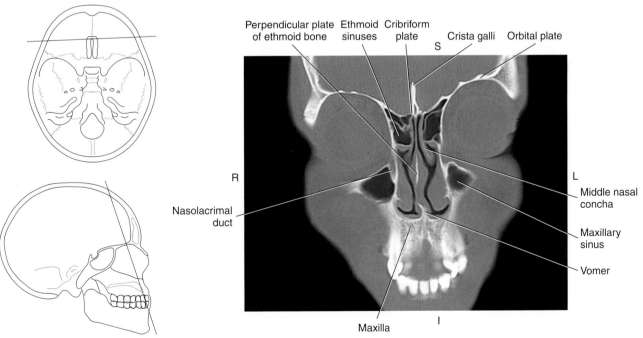

FIGURE 2.127 Coronal CT with nasolacrimal duct.

REFERENCES

Abrahams PH, Marks SC Jr, Hutchings RT: *McMinn's color atlas of human anatomy,* ed 5, St. Louis, 2003, Mosby.

Frank G: *Merrill's atlas of radiographic positioning and procedures,* ed 12, St. Louis, 2012, Mosby.

Gray H: *Gray's anatomy,* ed 15, New York, 1995, Barnes & Noble.

Harnsberger HR: *Handbook of head and neck imaging,* ed 2, St. Louis, 1995, Mosby.

Mosby's dictionary of medicine, nursing, and health professions, ed 8, St. Louis, 2008, Mosby.

Seidel HM, Ball JW, Dains JE, et al: *Mosby's guide to physical examination,* ed 7, St. Louis, 2010, Mosby.

Som PM, Curtin HD: *Head and neck imaging,* ed 5, St. Louis, 2011, Mosby.

Weir J: *Imaging atlas of human anatomy,* ed 4, St. Louis, 2010, Mosby.

3

Brain

From the brain, and from the brain only, arise our pleasures, joys, laughter and jests, as well as our sorrows, pains, griefs, and tears.

Hippocrates (460?-377? BC), The Sacred Disease

The brain regulates and coordinates many critical functions, from thought processes to bodily movements. For this reason, it is important to identify the anatomy of the brain (Figure 3.1).

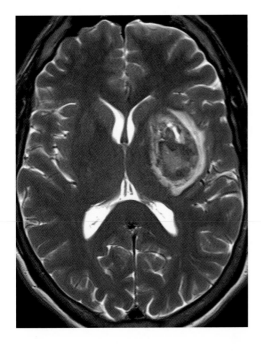

FIGURE 3.1 Axial, T2-weighted MRI of brain with intraparenchymal hematoma in left basal nuclei.

OBJECTIVES

- Describe the meninges.
- Describe the production and absorption of cerebrospinal fluid.
- Identify the components of the ventricular system.
- Identify the basal cisterns.
- List the structures of the diencephalon.
- Describe the location and function of the components of the cerebrum, brainstem, and cerebellum.
- Identify the structures of the limbic system and describe their function.
- Identify the major arteries of the cerebrum and list the structures they supply.
- List the arteries that constitute the circle of Willis.
- Identify the superficial cortical veins, deep veins, and dural sinuses of the cerebrum.
- Identify the function and course of the cranial nerves.

OUTLINE

MENINGES

The brain is a delicate organ that is surrounded and protected by three membranes called the **meninges** (Figure 3.2). The outermost membrane, the **dura mater** (tough mother), is the strongest. This double-layered membrane is continuous with the periosteum of the cranium. Located between the dura mater and the cranium are the meningeal vessels, which supply blood to the cranium and meninges. There is also a potential space between the dura and the cranium called the **epidural (extradural) space**. Located between the two layers of dura mater are the dural sinuses, which provide venous drainage from the brain. Folds of dura mater help to separate the structures of the brain and provide additional cushioning and support. The dural folds include the falx cerebri, tentorium cerebelli, and the falx cerebelli. The **falx cerebri** separates the cerebral hemispheres, whereas the **tentorium cerebelli**, which spreads out like a tent, forms a partition between the cerebrum and cerebellum. An oval opening in the tentorium cerebelli forms the **tentorial notch (incisura)**, which surrounds the midbrain and provides the only communication between the supratentorial and infratentorial spaces within the brain (Figures 3.3 through 3.6). The **falx cerebelli** separates the two cerebellar hemispheres. The middle membrane, known as the **arachnoid membrane** (spiderlike),

Transtentorial herniation is the protrusion of brain tissue through the tentorial notch. It can occur as a result of increased intracranial pressure resulting from edema, hemorrhage, or tumor.

is a delicate, transparent membrane that is separated from the dura mater by a potential space called the **subdural space**. The arachnoid membrane follows the contour of the dura mater. The inner layer, or **pia mater** (delicate, tender mother), is a highly vascular layer that adheres closely to the contours of the brain. The **subarachnoid space** separates the pia mater from the arachnoid mater. This space contains cerebrospinal fluid that circulates around the brain and spinal cord and provides further protection to the central nervous system (CNS) (Figure 3.2).

Skull fractures with rupture of the meningeal arteries can cause a life-threatening condition known as an epidural hematoma (EDH), which causes accumulation of blood in the epidural space between the dura and cranium. A subdural hematoma (SDH) is a collection of blood from ruptured vessels located in the subdural space.

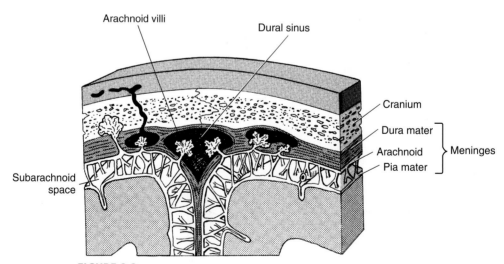

FIGURE 3.2 Coronal cross section of meninges and subarachnoid space.

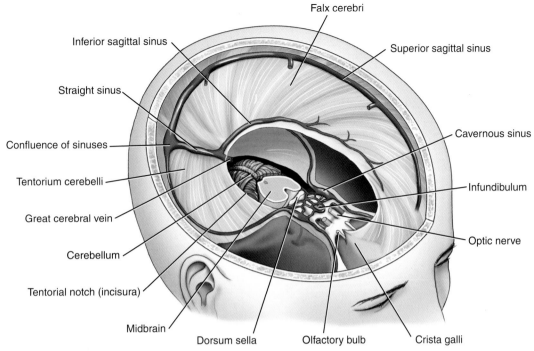

FIGURE 3.3 Dural reflections and venous sinuses.

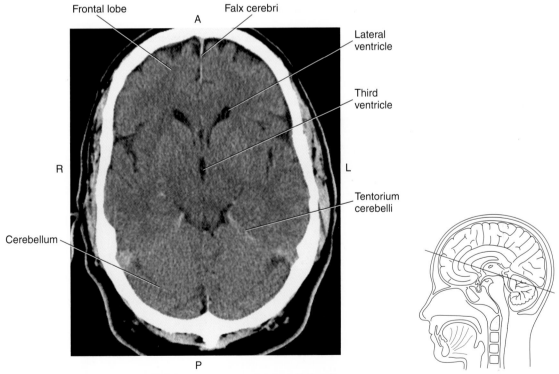

FIGURE 3.4 Axial CT of falx cerebri and tentorium cerebelli.

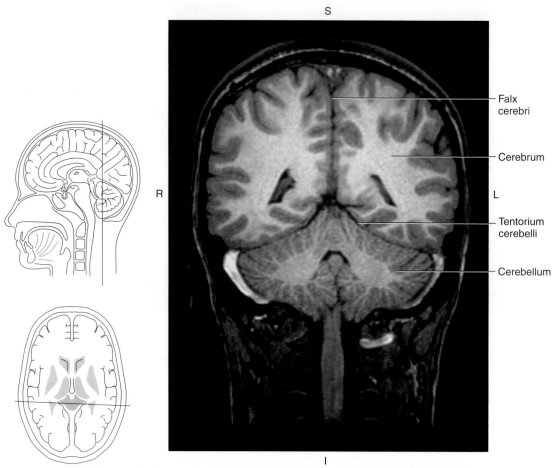

FIGURE 3.5 Coronal, T1-weighted MRI of falx cerebri and tentorium cerebelli.

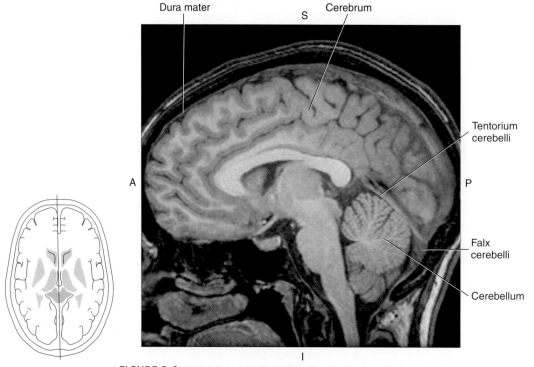

FIGURE 3.6 Sagittal, T1-weighted MRI of tentorium cerebelli.

VENTRICULAR SYSTEM

Ventricles

The **ventricular system** provides a pathway for the circulation of the cerebral spinal fluid (CSF) throughout the CNS. A major portion of the ventricular system is composed of four fluid-filled cavities (**ventricles**) located deep within the brain (Figures 3.7 through 3.9). The two most superior cavities are the **right** and **left lateral ventricles**. These ventricles lie within each cerebral hemisphere and are separated at the midline by a thin membrane known as the **septum pellucidum** (Figures 3.10 and 3.11). The lateral ventricles consist of a central portion called the body and three extensions: the **frontal (anterior)**, **occipital (posterior)**, and **temporal (inferior) horns** (Figures 3.7 through 3.16). The junction of the body and the occipital and temporal horns form a triangular area termed the **trigone (atria)**. The lateral ventricles communicate inferiorly with the third ventricle via the paired **interventricular foramen (foramen of Monro)** (Figures 3.8 and 3.10). The **third ventricle** is a thin slitlike structure, located midline just inferior to the lateral ventricles (Figures 3.7 through 3.11). The anterior wall of the third ventricle is formed by a thin membrane termed the **lamina terminalis**, and the lateral walls are formed by the thalamus. The third ventricle communicates with the fourth ventricle via a long, narrow passageway termed the **cerebral aqueduct (aqueduct of Sylvius)**. The cerebral aqueduct reaches the fourth ventricle by traversing the posterior portion of the midbrain (Figures 3.7, 3.8, and 3.13). The **fourth ventricle** is a diamond-shaped cavity located anterior to the cerebellum and posterior to the pons (Figures 3.12, 3.13, 3.14, and 3.16). Separating the fourth ventricle from the cerebellum is a thin membrane forming the **superior** and **inferior medullary velum** (Figure 3.13). CSF exits the ventricular system through foramina in the fourth ventricle to communicate with the subarachnoid space within the basal cisterns. The major exit route is the **median aperture (foramen of Magendie)**, located on the posterior wall of the fourth ventricle, which communicates with the cisterna magna (Figure 3.17). There are two **lateral apertures**, termed the **foramen of Luschka**, which communicate with the cerebellopontine angle cistern. From the fourth ventricle, CSF continues into the spinal cord via the central canal (Figures 3.8 and 3.17).

> The septum pellucidum is frequently used as a landmark to determine if the midline of the brain has shifted as a result of trauma or pressure.

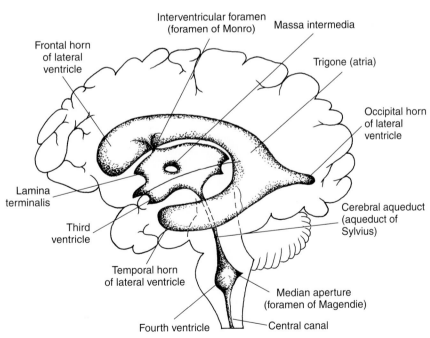

FIGURE 3.7 Lateral view of ventricular system.

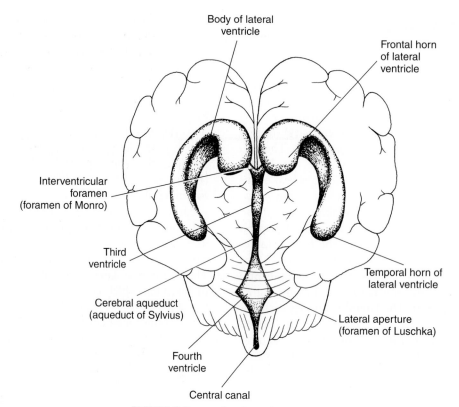

FIGURE 3.8 **Anterior view of ventricles.**

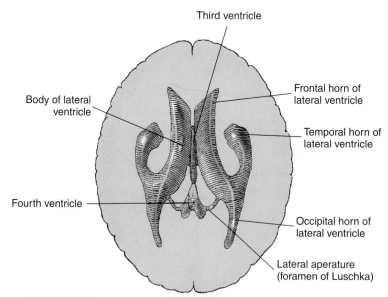

FIGURE 3.9 Superior view of ventricles in relation to surface of brain.

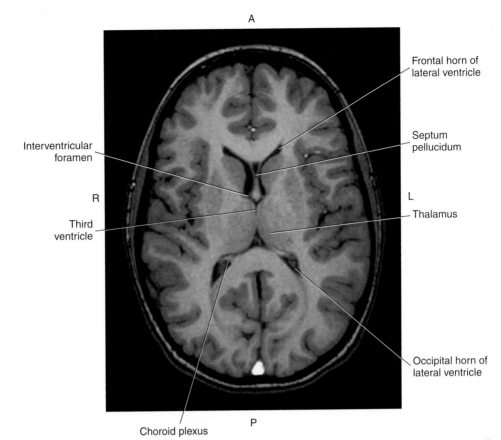

A

Frontal horn of
lateral ventricle

Septum
pellucidum

Interventricular
foramen

R   L

Thalamus

Third
ventricle

Occipital horn of
lateral ventricle

Choroid plexus   P

FIGURE 3.10 Axial, T1-weighted MRI of lateral and third ventricles.

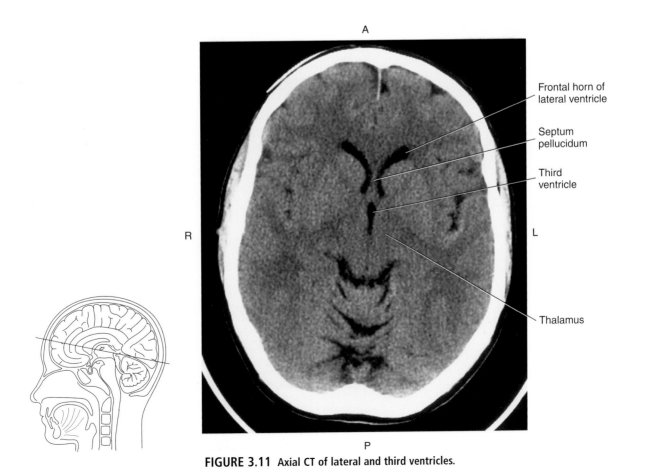

A

Frontal horn of
lateral ventricle

Septum
pellucidum

Third
ventricle

R   L

Thalamus

P

FIGURE 3.11 Axial CT of lateral and third ventricles.

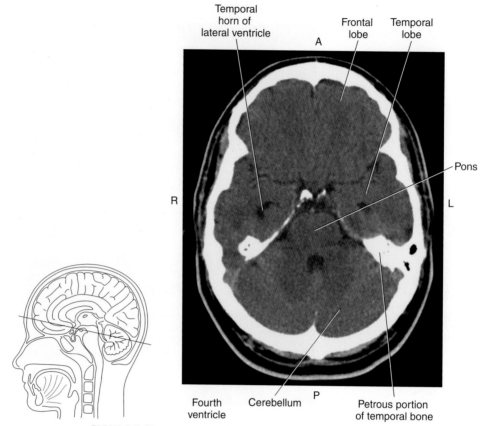

FIGURE 3.12 Axial CT of temporal horns of the lateral ventricles.

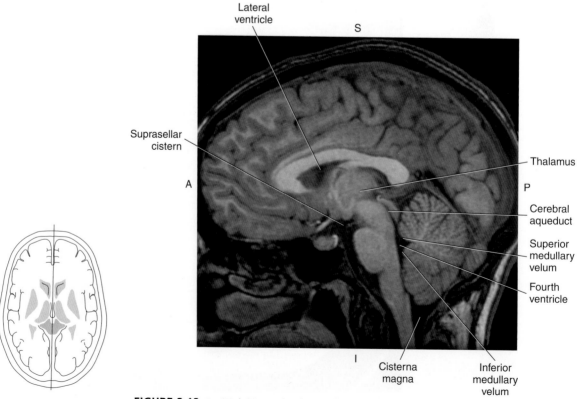

FIGURE 3.13 Sagittal, T1-weighted MRI of ventricular system.

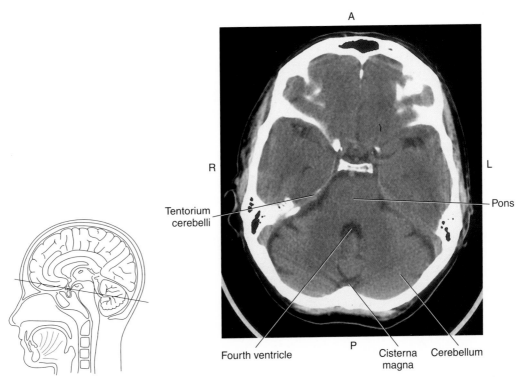

A

R   L

Tentorium
cerebelli   Pons

Fourth ventricle   P   Cisterna   Cerebellum
                                      magna

FIGURE 3.14 Axial CT of fourth ventricle.

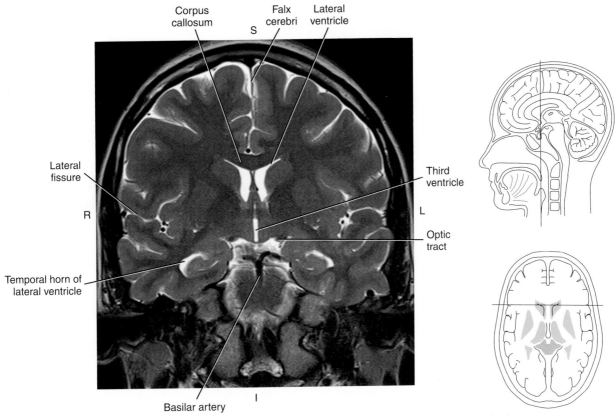

Corpus   Falx   Lateral
callosum   cerebri   ventricle
                   S

Lateral
fissure   Third
                                                ventricle
R   L
                                                Optic
                                                tract
Temporal horn of
lateral ventricle

Basilar artery   I

FIGURE 3.15 Coronal, T2-weighted MRI of temporal horns of the lateral ventricles.

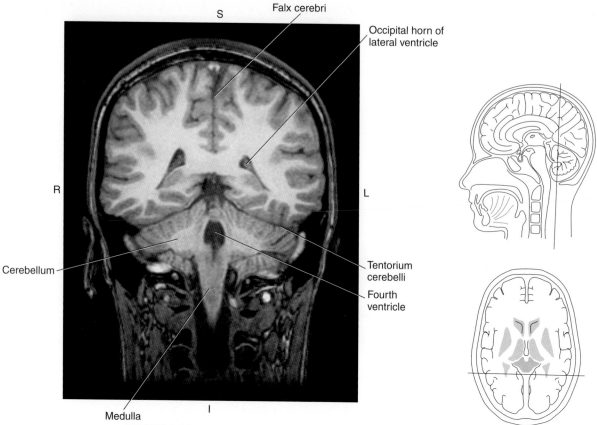

FIGURE 3.16 Coronal, T1-weighted MRI of lateral and fourth ventricles.

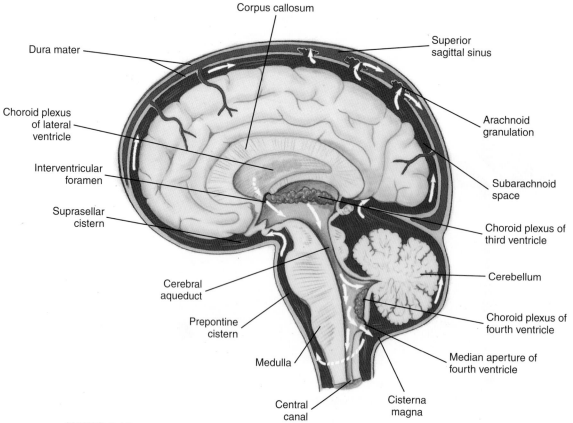

FIGURE 3.17 Sagittal view of choroid plexus and flow of CSF through the ventricular system.

Located within the ventricular system is a network of blood vessels and nerve cells termed the **choroid plexus**, which produces CSF. The choroid plexus lines the floor of the lateral ventricles, roof of the third ventricle, and inferior medullary velum of the fourth ventricle (Figure 3.17). Frequently, the choroid plexus is partially calcified, making it more noticeable on computed tomography (CT) images (Figure 3.18 and 3.19).

There exists a continuous circulation of CSF in and around the brain. Excess CSF is reabsorbed in the dural sinuses by way of **arachnoid villi**. These villi are berry-like projections of arachnoid that penetrate the dura mater (Figure 3.2 and 3.17). Enlargements of the arachnoid villi are termed granulations. Within the calvaria, these granulations can cause pitting or depressions, which are variations of normal anatomy.

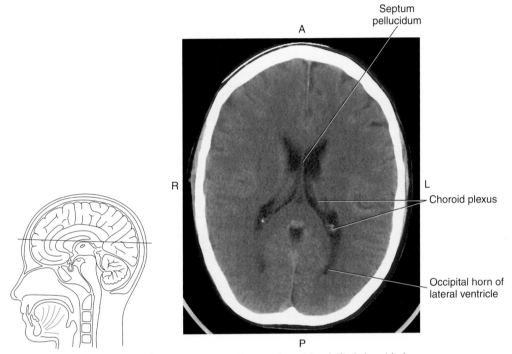

FIGURE 3.18 Axial CT of lateral ventricles with calcified choroid plexus.

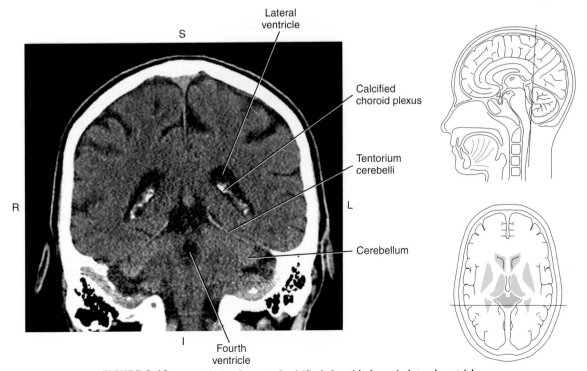

FIGURE 3.19 Coronal CT reformat of calcified choroid plexus in lateral ventricles.

Cisterns

The **subarachnoid space** is a relatively narrow, fluid-filled space surrounding the brain and spinal cord. There are locations, primarily around the base of the brain, where the subarachnoid space becomes widened (Figure 3.17). The combined term for these widened areas or pools of CSF is the **basal (subarachnoid) cisterns** (Figure 3.20). Each cistern is generally named after the brain structure it borders.

One of the largest cisterns is the **cisterna magna**. It is located in the lower posterior fossa among the medulla oblongata, cerebellar hemispheres, and occipital bone. It is continuous with the subarachnoid space of the spinal canal (Figures 3.13, 3.14, and 3.17). The **interpeduncular cistern** is located between the peduncles of the midbrain and communicates inferiorly with the **prepontine cistern** (Figures 3.21 and 3.22). The prepontine cistern is located just anterior and inferior to the pons and communicates laterally with the **cerebellopontine angle (CPA) cistern** (Figures 3.17, 3.23,

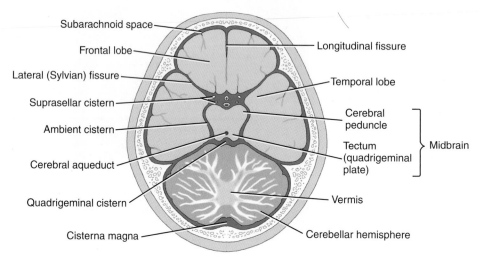

FIGURE 3.20 Axial view of basal cisterns.

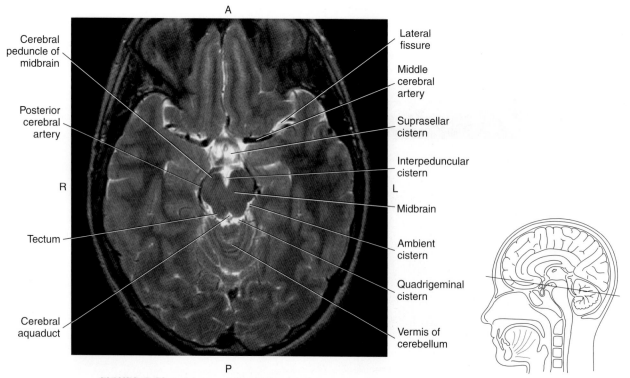

FIGURE 3.21 Axial, T2-weighted MRI of ambient, suprasellar, and interpeduncular cisterns.

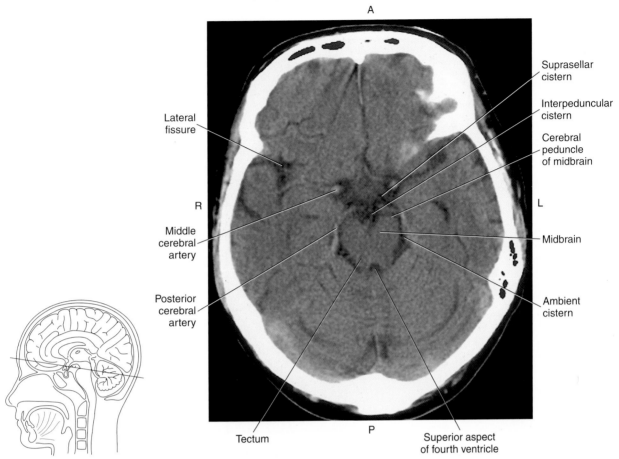

FIGURE 3.22 Axial CT of ambient, suprasellar, and interpeduncular cisterns.

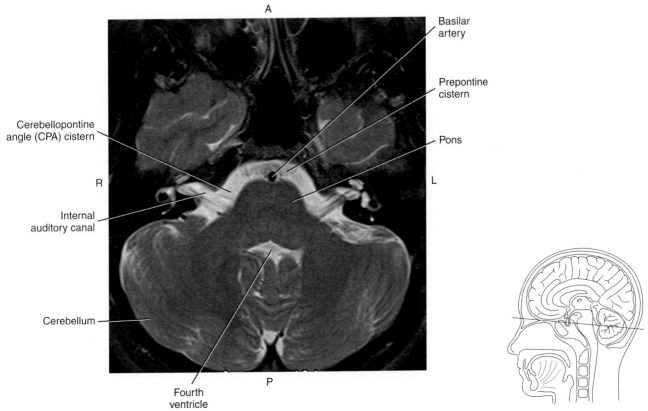

FIGURE 3.23 Axial, T2-weighted MRI of cerebellopontine angle (CPA) cistern.

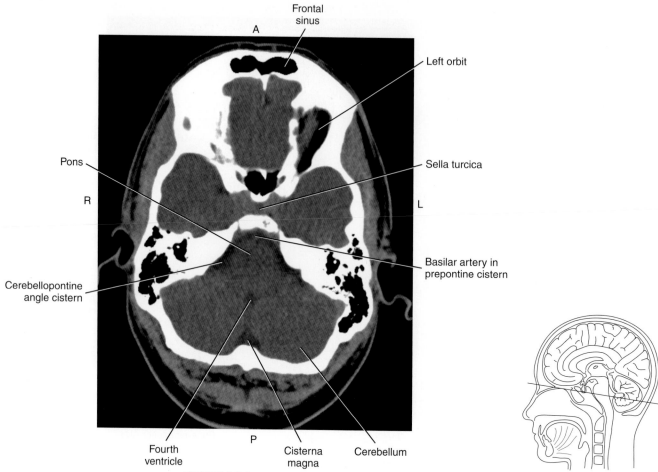

A

Frontal
sinus

Left orbit

Pons

Sella turcica

R

L

Basilar artery in
prepontine cistern

Cerebellopontine
angle cistern

Fourth
ventricle

P

Cisterna
magna

Cerebellum

FIGURE 3.24 Axial CT of cerebellopontine angle (CPA) cistern.

and 3.24). The CPA cistern is located at the junction of the pons and cerebellum. It contains important structures including cranial nerves V, VII, and VIII and the superior and anterior inferior cerebellar arteries. The **ambient cistern** courses around the lateral surface of the midbrain, connecting the interpeduncular cistern with the quadrigeminal (superior) cistern (Figures 3.20 through 3.22). The **quadrigeminal cistern** lies between the splenium of the corpus callosum and the superior surface of the cerebellum just posterior to the colliculi of the midbrain or the tectum (quadrigeminal plate) (Figures 3.20 through 3.22). Located above the sella turcica is the **suprasellar (chiasmatic) cistern,** which contains the optic chiasm and the circle of Willis (Figures 3.13, 3.17, and 3.20 through 3.22).

Bleeding within the subarachnoid space is called a subarachnoid hemorrhage (SAH). The most common cause of a SAH is a ruptured aneurysm. Patients with this condition will commonly present to the emergency department complaining of the worst headache of their lives. Blood within the subarachnoid space acts as a chemical irritant to the brain and causes an increase in intracranial pressure.

CEREBRUM

The **cerebrum** is the largest portion of the brain and is divided into **left** and **right cerebral hemispheres.** Each hemisphere contains neural tissue arranged in numerous folds called **gyri.** The gyri are separated by shallow grooves called **sulci** and by deeper grooves called **fissures.** The main sulcus that can be identified on CT and MR images of the brain is the **central sulcus,** which divides the **precentral gyrus** of the frontal lobe and **postcentral gyrus** of the parietal lobe (Figures 3.25 and 3.26). These gyri are important to identify because the precentral gyrus is considered the motor strip of the brain and the postcentral gyrus is considered the sensory strip of the brain. Other gyri important for imaging include the cingulate, parahippocampal, and superior temporal gyrus (see limbic system and temporal lobe). The two main fissures of the cerebrum are the **longitudinal fissure** and the **lateral (Sylvian fissure)** (Figures 3.27 and 3.28). The longitudinal fissure is a long, deep furrow that divides the left and right cerebral hemispheres. Located in this fissure is the falx cerebri and superior sagittal sinus. The lateral fissure is a deep furrow that separates the frontal

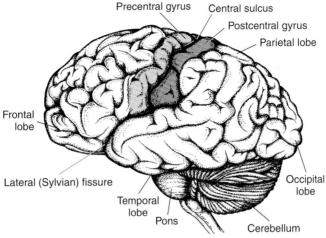

FIGURE 3.25 Lateral view of central sulcus.

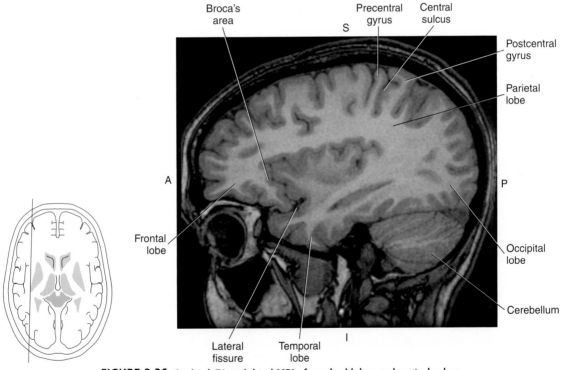

FIGURE 3.26 Sagittal, T1-weighted MRI of cerebral lobes and central sulcus.

and parietal lobes from the temporal lobe. Numerous blood vessels, primarily branches of the middle cerebral artery, follow the course of the lateral fissure (Figures 3.21, 3.22, 3.25, and 3.26 through 3.28).

Gray and White Matter Organization

The cerebrum as a whole has many critically important functions, including thought, judgment, memory, and discrimination. The cerebrum consists of **gray matter** (neuron cell bodies) and **white matter** (myelinated axons) (Figures 3.27 and 3.28). The **cerebral cortex**, the outermost portion of the cerebrum, is composed of gray matter approximately 3 to 5 mm thick. The cortex not only receives sensory input but also sends instructions to the muscles and glands for control of body movement and activity. Deep in the cortex is the white matter, which contains fibers that create pathways for the transmission of nerve impulses to and from the cortex. The largest and densest bundle of white matter fibers within

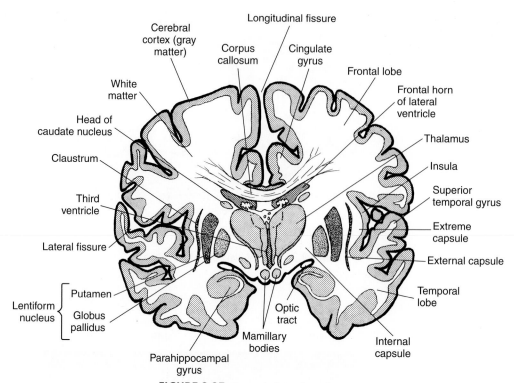

FIGURE 3.27 Coronal view of cerebrum.

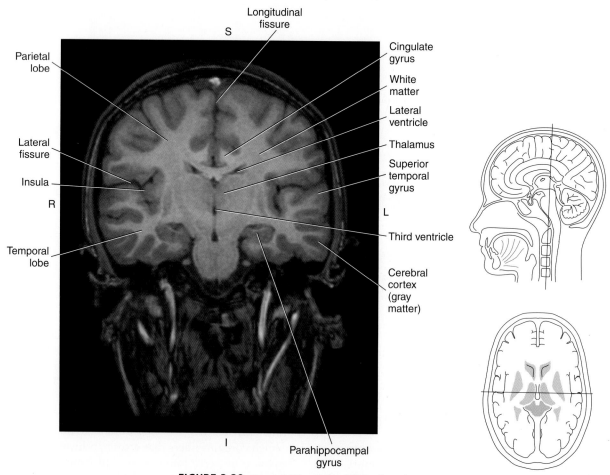

FIGURE 3.28 Coronal, T1-weighted MRI of cerebrum.

the cerebrum is the **corpus callosum**. This midline structure forms the roof of the lateral ventricles and connects the right and left cerebral hemispheres. The four parts of the corpus callosum, from anteroinferior to posterior, are the **rostrum, genu, body, and splenium** (Figures 3.29 through 3.32).

Two other important bundles of white matter fibers are the anterior and posterior commissures (Figures 3.29 and 3.30). The **anterior commissure** crosses the midline within the lamina terminalis and connects the anterior portions of each temporal lobe (Figures 3.33 and 3.34). The **posterior commissure** is a pathway made of several fibers that

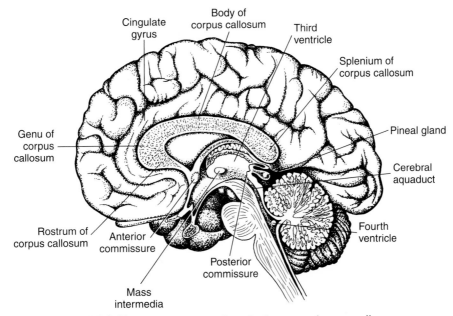

FIGURE 3.29 Midsagittal view of cerebral cortex and corpus callosum.

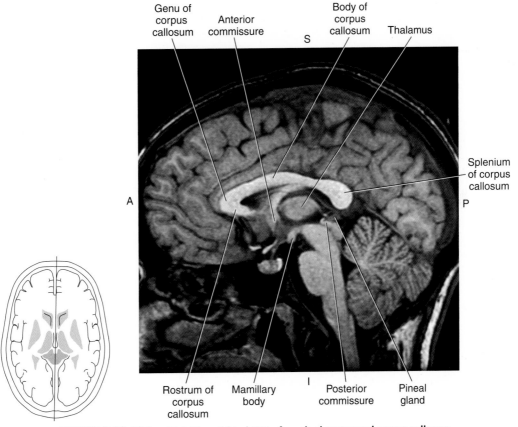

FIGURE 3.30 Midsagittal, T1-weighted MRI of cerebral cortex and corpus callosum.

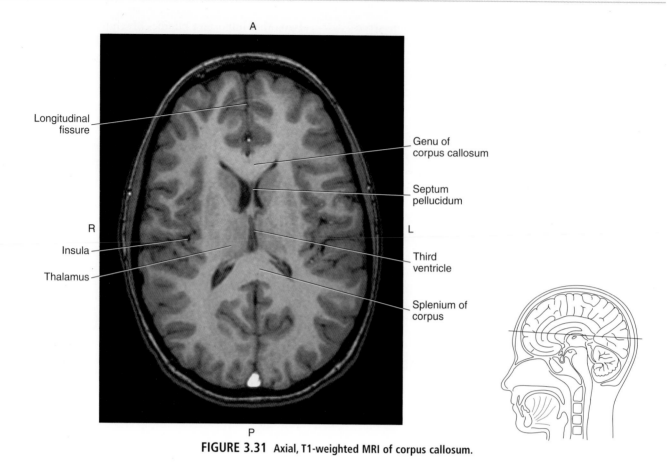

A

Longitudinal
fissure

Genu of
corpus callosum

Septum
pellucidum

R   L

Insula

Thalamus

Third
ventricle

Splenium of
corpus

P

FIGURE 3.31 Axial, T1-weighted MRI of corpus callosum.

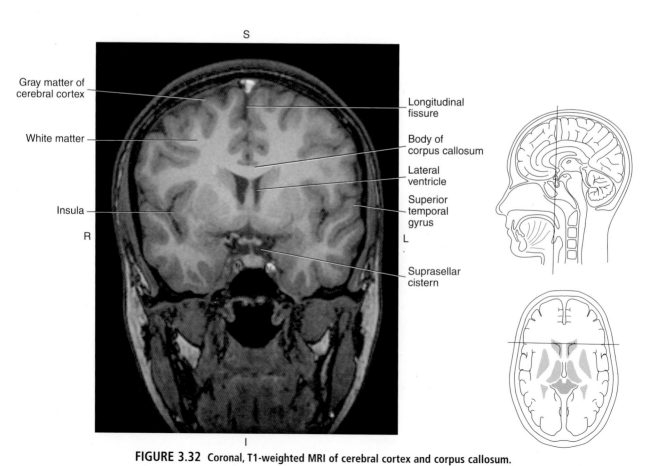

S

Gray matter of
cerebral cortex

White matter

Insula

R

Longitudinal
fissure

Body of
corpus callosum

Lateral
ventricle

Superior
temporal
gyrus

L

Suprasellar
cistern

I

FIGURE 3.32 Coronal, T1-weighted MRI of cerebral cortex and corpus callosum.

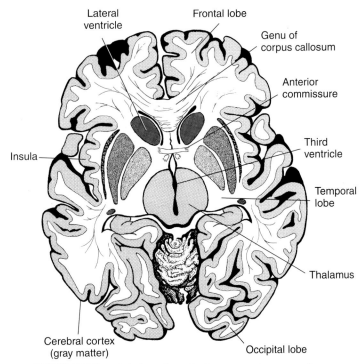

FIGURE 3.33 Axial view of cerebral cortex and corpus callosum.

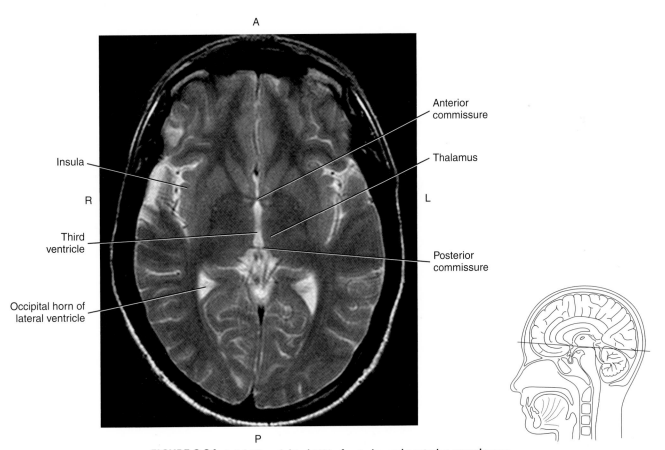

FIGURE 3.34 Axial, T2-weighted MRI of anterior and posterior commissures.

transmit nerve impulses for pupillary (consensual) light reflexes. This pathway crosses the midline posterior to the third ventricle, immediately above the cerebral aqueduct and inferior to the pineal gland (Figure 3.34).

Cerebral Lobes

The cerebral cortex of each hemisphere can be divided into four individual lobes: frontal, parietal, occipital, and temporal (Figure 3.35). These four lobes correspond in location to the cranial bones with the same name. Each lobe has critical regions that are associated with specific functions. The **frontal lobe** is the most anterior lobe of the brain. The boundaries of the frontal lobe are the central sulcus, which separates it from the parietal lobe, and the lateral fissure, which separates it from the temporal lobe (Figures 3.25, 3.26, 3.35 and 3.36). The frontal lobe mediates a wide variety of functions, such as reasoning, judgment, emotional response, planning and execution of complex actions, and control of voluntary muscle movement. The frontal lobe is also involved in speech production and contains the motor speech (language) center, **Broca's area.** Broca's area lies unilaterally on the inferior surface of the frontal lobe dominant for language, typically in the left frontal gyrus (Figure 3.35). This area is involved in the coordination or programming of motor movements for the production of speech sounds. The **parietal lobe** is located in the middle portion of each cerebral hemisphere just posterior to the central sulcus. The horizontal portion of the lateral fissure separates the parietal lobe from the temporal lobe (Figure 3.25). The parietal lobe is associated with the perception of temperature, touch, pressure, vibration, pain, and taste and is involved in writing and in some aspects of reading. The most posterior lobe, the **occipital lobe,** is separated from the parietal lobe by the parieto-occipital fissure. This lobe is involved in the conscious perception of visual stimuli. The **primary visual area** receives input from the optic tract via the optic radiations extending from the thalamus (Figure 3.36). The **temporal lobe** is anterior to the occipital lobe and is separated from the parietal lobe by the lateral fissure (Figure 3.37). Conscious perceptions of auditory and olfactory stimuli and dominance for language are functions of the temporal lobe. Memory processing occurs via the amygdala and hippocampus, clusters of gray matter located in the **parahippocampal gyrus** of the temporal lobe (Figures 3.27 and 3.28). Located on the **superior temporal gyrus** is the auditory cortex, which can be divided into primary and secondary auditory areas (Figures 3.32 and 3.35). The primary auditory area, **Heschl's gyrus,** receives the major auditory sensory information from the bilateral cochlea, whereas the secondary auditory area, **Wernicke's area,** is the center for comprehension and formulation of speech (Figure 3.35). Deep in the temporal lobe is another area of cortical gray matter termed the **insula** (island of Reil), often referred to as the fifth lobe. The insula is separated from the temporal lobe by the lateral fissure and is thought to mediate motor and sensory functions of the viscera (Figures 3.32 through 3.38).

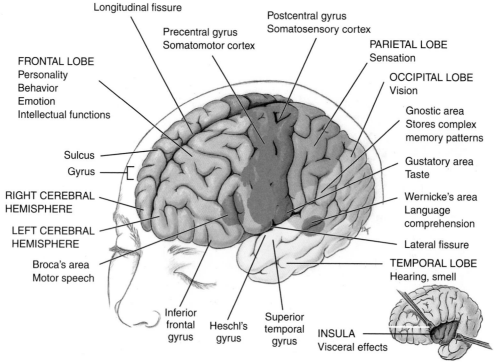

FIGURE 3.35 Lateral view of cerebral lobes.

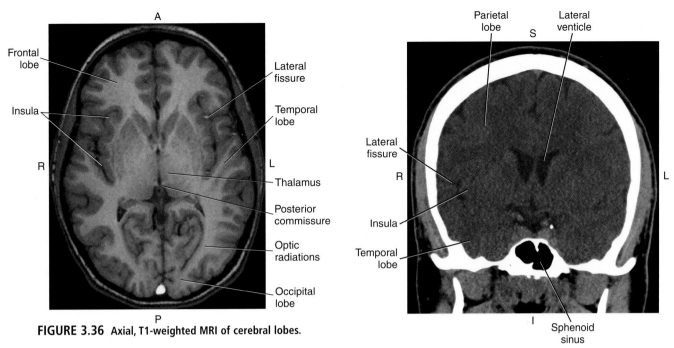

FIGURE 3.36 Axial, T1-weighted MRI of cerebral lobes.

FIGURE 3.37 Coronal CT reformat of cerebral lobes.

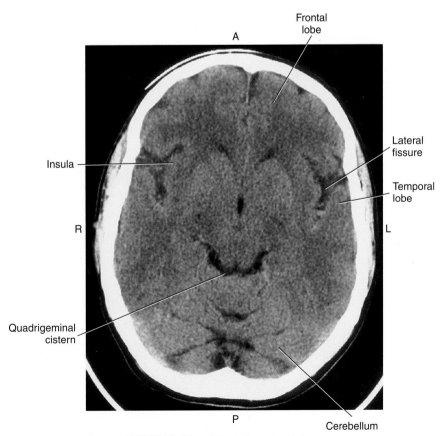

FIGURE 3.38 Axial CT of cerebral lobes.

Basal Nuclei

The **basal nuclei (ganglia)** are a collection of subcortical gray matter consisting of the caudate nucleus, lentiform nucleus, and claustrum (Figures 3.27, 3.39 and 3.40). Collectively, they contribute to the planning and programming of muscle action and movement. The largest basal nuclei are the caudate nucleus and lentiform nucleus. Both nuclei serve as relay stations between the thalamus and the cerebral cortex of the same side. The **caudate nucleus** parallels the lateral ventricle and consists of a head, body, and tail. The **head** causes an indentation to the frontal horns of the lateral ventricles, and the **tail** terminates at the amygdala in the temporal lobe (Figures 3.40 through 3.44). The **lentiform nucleus** is a biconvex lens–shaped mass of gray matter located among the insula, caudate nucleus, and thalamus. The lentiform nucleus can be further divided into the **globus pallidus** and the **putamen** (Figures 3.41 and 3.42). The **claustrum** is a thin linear layer of gray matter lying between the insula and the lentiform nucleus and is thought to be involved with the mediation of visual attention (Figures 3.41 through 3.44). Three large tracts of white matter, internal, external, and extreme capsules, separate the basal nuclei and transmit electrical impulses throughout the brain. The **internal capsule** is shaped like a boomerang and separates the thalamus and caudate nucleus from the lentiform nucleus. The **external capsule** is a thin layer of white matter that separates the claustrum from the lentiform nucleus. Another thin layer of white matter located between the claustrum and insular cortex is the **extreme capsule** (Figures 3.40 through 3.44).

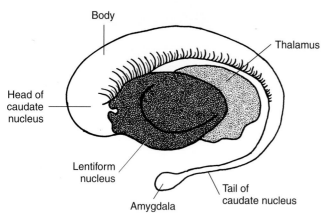

FIGURE 3.39 Lateral view of basal nuclei.

It is the control of the basal nuclei that allows for the unconscious coordination of swinging our arms in rhythm with our legs as we walk.

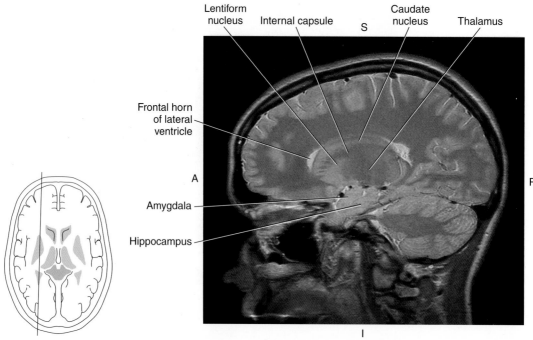

FIGURE 3.40 Sagittal, T2-weighted MRI with basal nuclei.

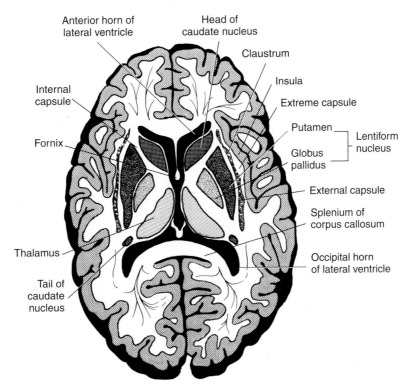

FIGURE 3.41 Axial view of basal nuclei.

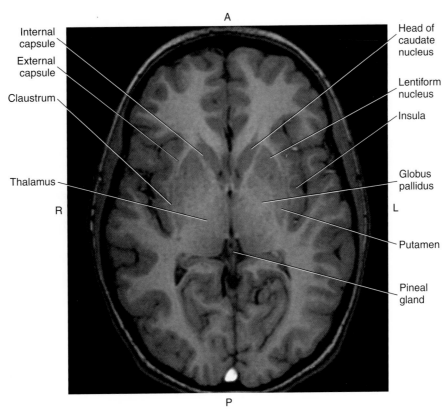

FIGURE 3.42 Axial, T1-weighted MRI of basal nuclei.

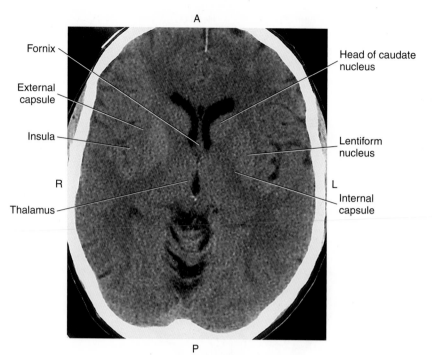

FIGURE 3.43 Axial CT of basal nuclei.

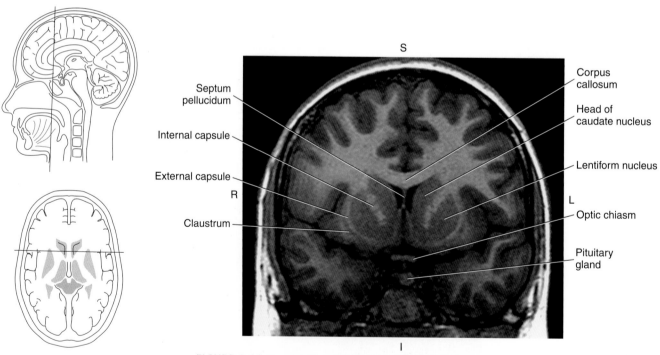

FIGURE 3.44 Coronal, T1-weighted MRI of basal nuclei.

DIENCEPHALON

The **diencephalon** is a complex of structures within the brain, whose major components are the thalamus and hypothalamus. The diencephalon functions as a relay station for sensory information, as an interactive site between the central nervous and endocrine systems, and is closely associated with the limbic system.

Thalamus

The **thalamus** consists of a pair of large oval gray masses that are interconnected with most regions of the brain and spinal cord via a vast number of fiber tracts. The thalamus makes up a portion of the walls of the third ventricle and connects through the middle of the third ventricle by adhesions known as the **massa intermedia** (Figure 3.29). The thalamus serves as a relay station to and from the cerebral cortex for all sensory stimuli, with the exception of the olfactory nerves (Figures 3.27 through 3.31, 3.28, and 3.39 through 3.43).

Hypothalamus

The **hypothalamus** consists of a cluster of small but critical nuclei located below the thalamus just posterior to the optic chiasm and forming the floor of the third ventricle. Anatomically, it includes the optic chiasm, mamillary bodies, and infundibulum and it is functionally related to the pituitary gland (Figures 3.45 and 3.46). The hypothalamus functions to integrate the activities of the autonomic, endocrine, and limbic systems by helping to maintain homeostasis as it controls regulation of temperature, appetite, sexual drive, and sleep patterns. In addition, the hypothalamus modulates the activities of the anterior and posterior lobes of the pituitary gland via the release of neurohormones, which stimulate or inhibit the release of pituitary hormones.

Pituitary Gland

The **pituitary gland (hypophysis)** is an endocrine gland connected to the hypothalamus by the infundibulum. The **infundibulum** is a slender stalk located between the optic chiasm and the mamillary bodies (Figures 3.45 and 3.46). The pituitary gland is located in the sella turcica at the base of the brain (Figures 3.46 through 3.49). The protected location of this gland suggests its importance. It is sometimes called the master gland because it controls and regulates the functions of many other glands through the action of its six major types of hormones. The pituitary gland can be broken down into an **anterior lobe (adenohypophysis)** and a **posterior lobe (neurohypophysis)**.

Epithalamus

The **epithalamus** is the most posterior portion of the diencephalon and comprises the posterior commissure and pineal gland. The **pineal gland**, an endocrine structure, secretes the hormone melatonin, which aids in the regulation of day-night cycles and reproductive functions. The pineal gland sits on the roof of the midbrain just posterior to the third ventricle and below the splenium of the corpus callosum. It is sometimes calcified, which aids in its detection on CT scans and lateral radiographs of the cranium (Figures 3.29, 3.46, 3.50, and 3.51).

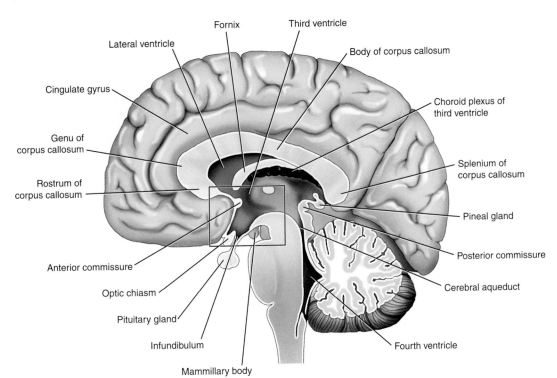

FIGURE 3.45 Sagittal view of hypothalamic nuclei. Box indicates close-up view of the hypothalamic nuclei on the next page.

(Continued)

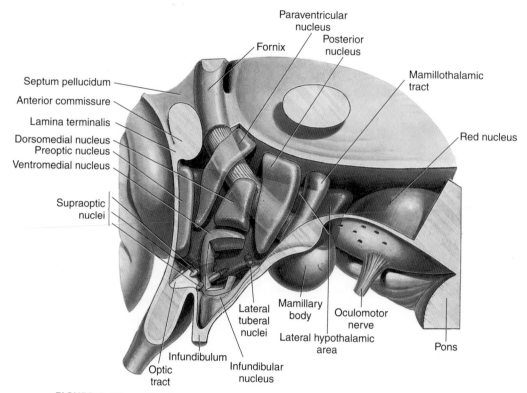

Paraventricular nucleus

Posterior nucleus

Fornix

Mamillothalamic tract

Septum pellucidum

Anterior commissure

Lamina terminalis

Dorsomedial nucleus

Preoptic nucleus

Ventromedial nucleus

Red nucleus

Supraoptic nuclei

Lateral tuberal nuclei

Mamillary body

Oculomotor nerve

Lateral hypothalamic area

Pons

Infundibulum

Optic tract

Infundibular nucleus

FIGURE 3.45 cont'd   Close-up image of hypothalamic nuclei indicated on previous page.

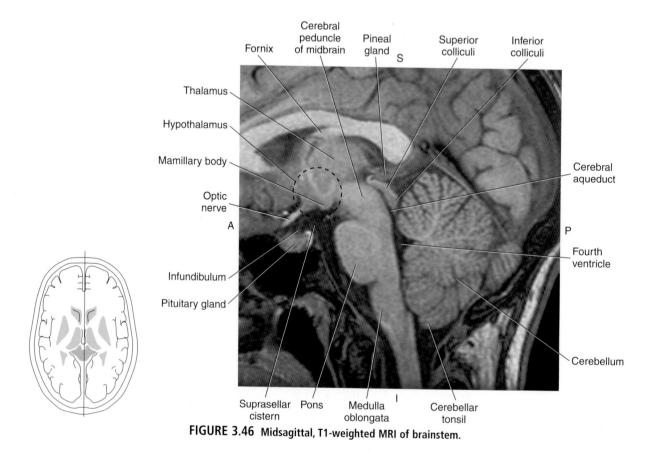

Cerebral peduncle of midbrain

Fornix

Pineal gland

Superior colliculi

Inferior colliculi

S

Thalamus

Hypothalamus

Mamillary body

Cerebral aqueduct

Optic nerve

A

P

Infundibulum

Fourth ventricle

Pituitary gland

Cerebellum

Suprasellar cistern

Pons

Medulla oblongata

I

Cerebellar tonsil

Cerebellum

FIGURE 3.46 Midsagittal, T1-weighted MRI of brainstem.

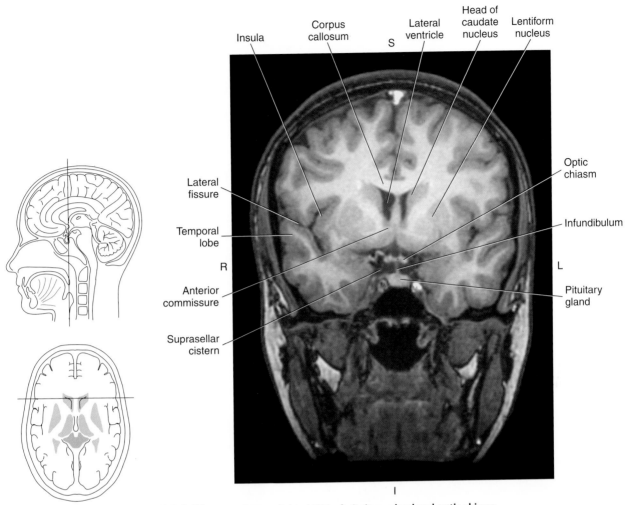

Insula
Corpus callosum
S
Lateral ventricle
Head of caudate nucleus
Lentiform nucleus
Optic chiasm
Infundibulum
Lateral fissure
Temporal lobe
Anterior commissure
Suprasellar cistern
R
L
Pituitary gland

FIGURE 3.47 Coronal, T1-weighted MRI of pituitary gland and optic chiasm.

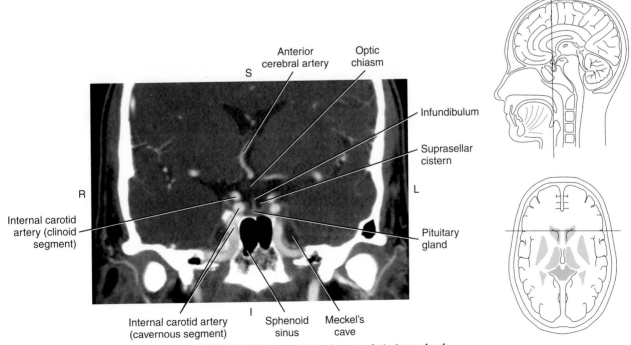

Anterior cerebral artery
Optic chiasm
S
Infundibulum
Suprasellar cistern
R
L
Internal carotid artery (clinoid segment)
Pituitary gland
Internal carotid artery (cavernous segment)
I
Sphenoid sinus
Meckel's cave

FIGURE 3.48 Coronal CT reformat of pituitary gland.

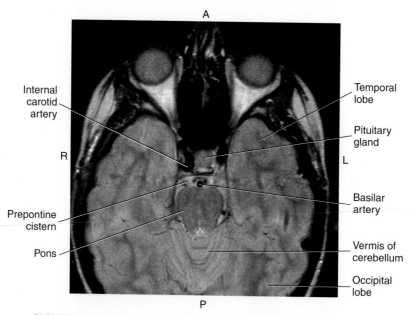

A

Internal
carotid
artery

Temporal
lobe

Pituitary
gland

R

L

Basilar
artery

Prepontine
cistern

Pons

Vermis of
cerebellum

Occipital
lobe

P

FIGURE 3.49 Axial, proton density–weighted MRI of pituitary gland.

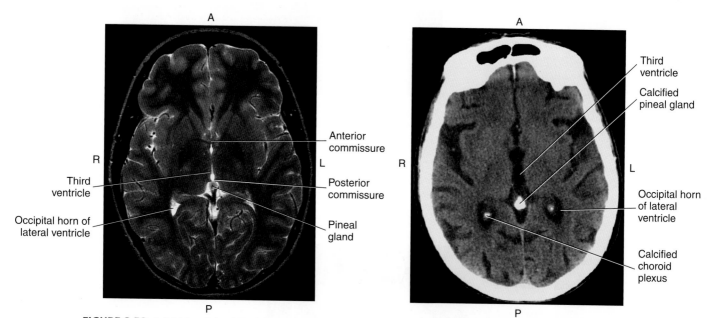

A

A

Anterior
commissure

Third
ventricle

Calcified
pineal gland

R

L

R

L

Third
ventricle

Posterior
commissure

Occipital horn
of lateral
ventricle

Occipital horn of
lateral ventricle

Pineal
gland

Calcified
choroid
plexus

P

P

FIGURE 3.50 Axial, T2-weighted MRI of pineal gland.

FIGURE 3.51 Axial CT with calcified pineal gland.

LIMBIC SYSTEM

The **limbic system** is a complex group of interconnected brain structures and fiber tracts located within and adjacent to the medial surface of the temporal lobes. They contain critical connecting pathways that extend to other areas deep within the midbrain, basal nuclei, and cerebral hemispheres (Figure 3.52). These structures have a common functional role in the emotional aspects of behavior. Particularly, the limbic system is involved in aggression, submissive and sexual behavior, memory, learning, and general emotional responses. Structures of the limbic system include the **hippocampus, amygdala, olfactory tracts, fornix, cingulate gyrus,** and **mamillary bodies.** The **parahippocampal gyrus** is the inrolled medial border of the temporal lobe and resembles the shape of a seahorse when viewed in the coronal plane. Contained within this gyrus are the hippocampus and amygdala, prominent structures involved with memory and emotion. The **hippocampus** is an important structure that has a strong role in the transition of short-term memory to long-term memory. The **amygdala** is an almond-shaped mass of gray matter located deep within the parahippocampal gyrus anterior to the hippocampus (Figures 3.40 and 3.52 through 3.54). The amygdala coordinates the actions of the autonomic and endocrine systems and is concerned with decision-making, emotional processing, and aggressive and sexual behavior. The **olfactory tracts** run underneath the frontal lobes and connect to the amygdala to bring information on the sense of smell to the limbic system (Figures 3.52 and 3.56). The limbic system is integrated with other important structures of the brain via limbic fiber tracts. The most frequently identified limbic tract is the fornix. The **fornix** is an arch-shaped structure that lies below the splenium of the corpus callosum and makes up the inferior margin of the septum pellucidum. It serves specifically to integrate the hippocampus with other functional areas of the brain (Figures 3.45, 3.46, 3.52, 3.55, and 3.57). The **cingulate gyrus** is a prominent gyrus located on the medial border of each cerebral hemisphere just superior to the corpus callosum (Figures 3.52, 3.55, and 3.57). This area is considered to be the brain's emotional control center, so it plays an important role in the limbic system. The **mamillary bodies** are two small rounded bodies in the floor of the posterior hypothalamus responsible for memory and motivation. They receive direct input from the hippocampus via the fornix and give rise to fibers that terminate in the anterior thalamus and the periaqueductal gray matter of the midbrain (Figures 3.45, 3.46, 3.52, and 3.53).

Damage to the hippocampus may result in the loss of memory. High-resolution magnetic resonance images (MRIs) of the hippocampus are useful in evaluating patients with dementia or seizures associated with hippocampal sclerosis.

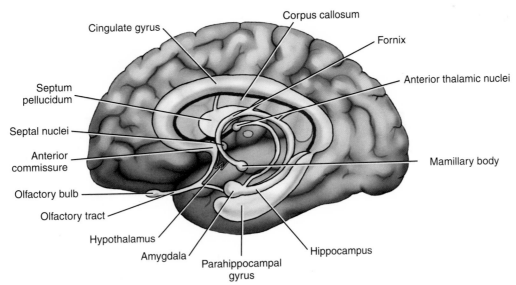

FIGURE 3.52 Lateral view of limbic system within the brain.

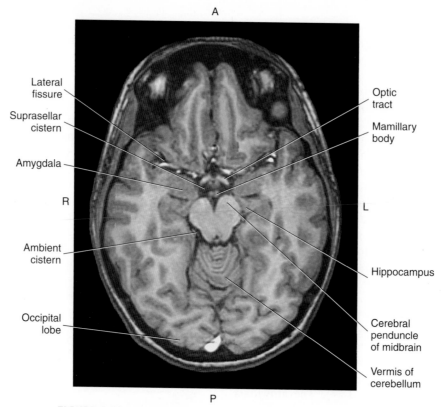

FIGURE 3.53 Axial, T1-weighted MRI of hippocampus and amygdala.

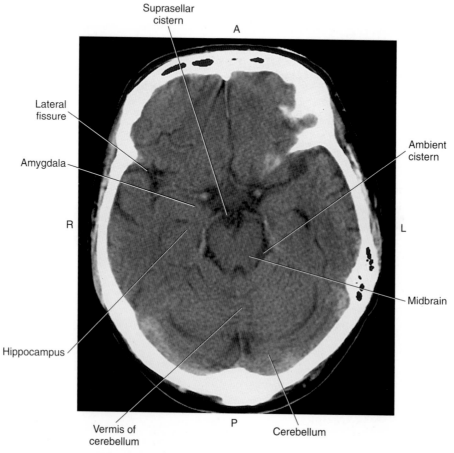

FIGURE 3.54 Axial CT of hippocampus and amygdala.

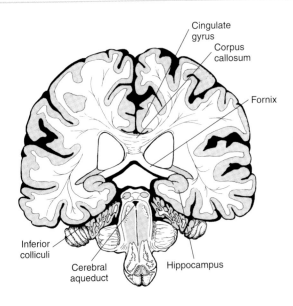

FIGURE 3.55 Coronal view of hippocampus and fornix.

Cingulate gyrus
Corpus callosum
Fornix
Inferior colliculi
Cerebral aqueduct
Hippocampus

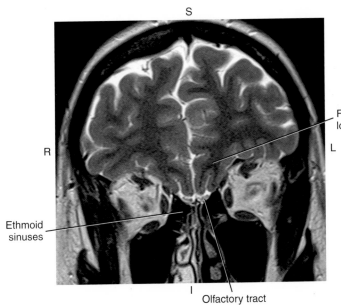

S
R
L
I
Frontal lobe
Ethmoid sinuses
Olfactory tract

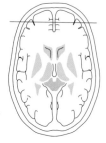

FIGURE 3.56 Coronal, T2-weighted MRI of olfactory tracts.

Lateral ventricle
Corpus callosum
Fornix
Cingulate gyrus
Thalamus
S
R
L
I
Temporal horn of lateral ventricle
Posterior commissure
Hippocampus   Third ventricle   Pons

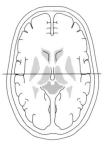

FIGURE 3.57 Coronal, T2-weighted MRI of fornix, cingulate gyrus, and hippocampus.

BRAINSTEM

The **brainstem** is a relatively small mass of tissue packed with motor and sensory nuclei, making it vital for normal brain function. Ten of the 12 cranial nerves originate from nuclei located in the brainstem. Its major segments are the midbrain, pons, and medulla oblongata (Figures 3.45, 3.46, 3.58, and 3.59). Located within the central portion of the brainstem and common to all three segments is the **tegmentum**, an area that provides integrative functions, such as complex motor patterns, aspects of respiratory and cardiovascular activity, and regulation of consciousness (Figure 3.60). The central core of the tegmentum contains the

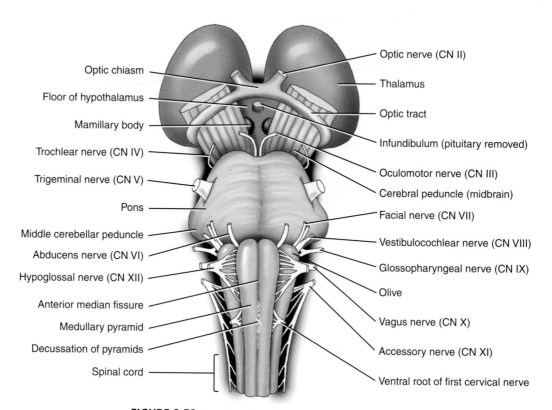

FIGURE 3.58 Anterior view of brainstem and cranial nerves.

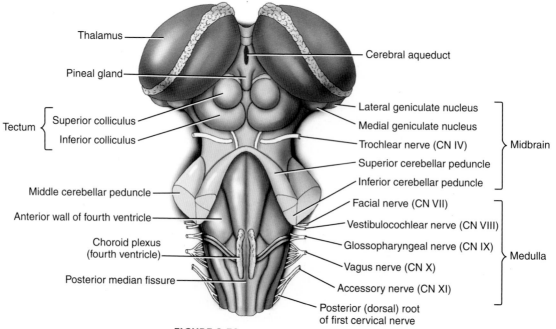

FIGURE 3.59 Posterior view of brainstem.

reticular formation, an area containing the cranial nerve nuclei and ascending and descending tracts to and from the brain. The brainstem as a whole acts as a conduit among the cerebral cortex, cerebellum, and spinal cord (Figure 3.61).

Midbrain

The **midbrain** (mesencephalon), which is located above the pons at the junction of the middle and posterior cranial fossae, is the smallest portion of the brainstem. The midbrain is primarily composed of massive bundles of nerve fiber tracts and can be divided into two major segments: **cerebral peduncles** and the **tectum** "quadrigeminal plate" (Figure 3.58). The midbrain surrounds the cerebral aqueduct, which contains CSF and connects the third and fourth ventricles. Posterior to the cerebral aqueduct is the tectum, which makes up the roof or dorsal surface of the midbrain (Figure 3.59). The tectum consists of four rounded protuberances termed **colliculi**. The upper pair, **superior colliculi**, is a center for visual reflexes that coordinate movements of the eyes with those of the head and neck. The lower pair, **inferior colliculi**, acts as a relay station for the auditory pathway, providing auditory information to the thalamus (Figures 3.46 and 3.59 through 3.65). Anterior to the cerebral aqueduct are the two large cerebral peduncles (Figures 3.46, 3.58, 3.60, 3.62, and 3.63). These ropelike bundles, composed

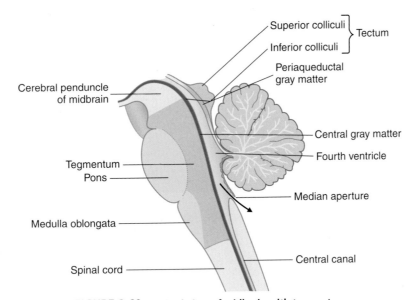

FIGURE 3.60 Sagittal view of midbrain with tegmentum.

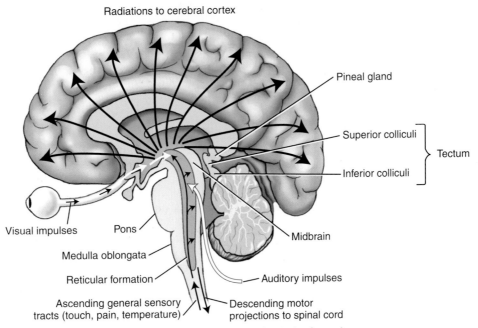

FIGURE 3.61 Sagittal view of reticular formation.

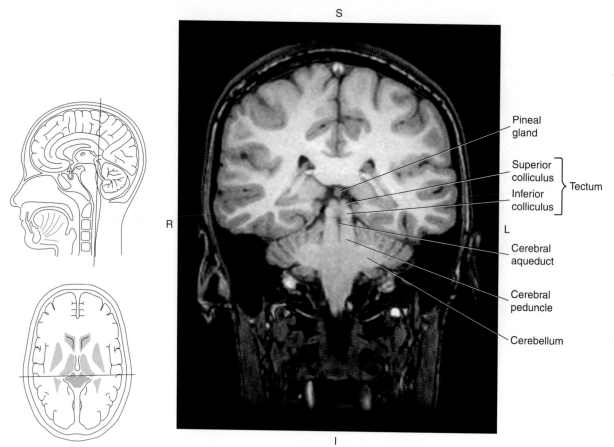

FIGURE 3.62 Coronal, T1-weighted MRI of midbrain.

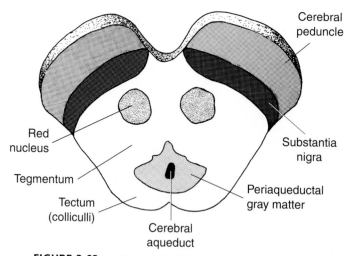

FIGURE 3.63 Axial view of midbrain and cerebral peduncles.

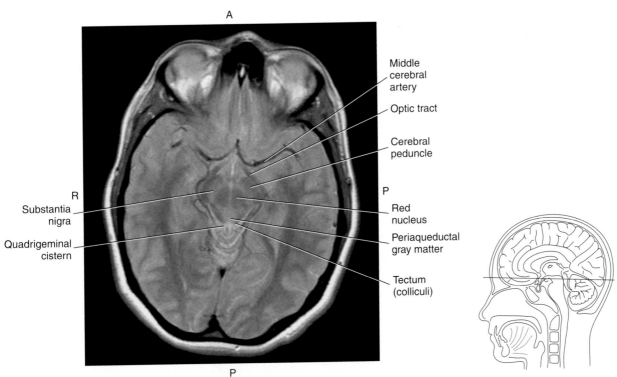

Middle cerebral artery

Optic tract

Cerebral peduncle

Red nucleus

Periaqueductal gray matter

Tectum (colliculi)

Substantia nigra

Quadrigeminal cistern

FIGURE 3.64 Axial, proton density-weighted MRI of cerebral peduncles and red nucleus.

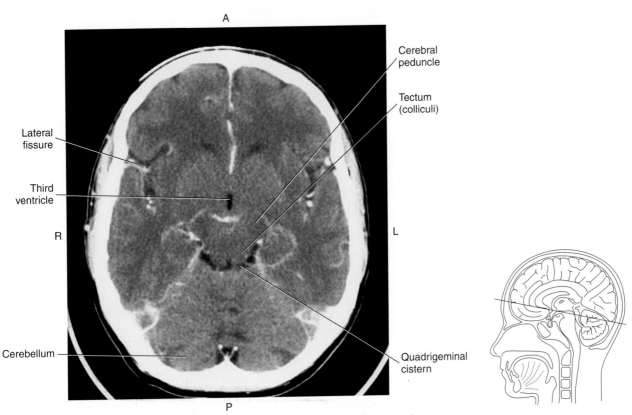

Cerebral peduncle

Tectum (colliculi)

Lateral fissure

Third ventricle

Cerebellum

Quadrigeminal cistern

FIGURE 3.65 Axial CT of cerebral peduncles and tectum.

predominantly of axons that are a direct extension of the fibers of the internal capsule, extend between the cerebral cortex to the spinal cord (Figures 3.46, 3.60, and 3.63 through 3.65). The **cerebral peduncles** are made more noticeable by the presence of the darkly pigmented substantia nigra, a broad layer of cells that contain melanin (Figures 3.63 and 3.64). The **substantia nigra** is involved with the production of dopamine, a neurotransmitter in the brain that functions in the control of muscular reflexes. Within the tegmentum of the midbrain, at the level of the superior colliculi, is the red nucleus. The **red nucleus** is composed of a tract of motor nerve fibers and serves as a relay station between the cerebellum and the cerebral hemispheres. The red nucleus contributes to the coordination of movements and the sense of balance. Another portion of the tegmentum is the **periaqueductal gray matter**, which surrounds the cerebral aqueduct. This area receives sensory input that conveys pain and temperature to the brain (Figures 3.63 and 3.64).

If neurons in the substantia nigra are damaged, dopamine production is decreased, leading to increased muscle spasticity commonly seen in Parkinson's disease.

Pons

The **pons** is a large oval-shaped expansion of the brainstem centrally located between the midbrain and medulla oblongata. The pons creates a prominent bulge as it lies just posterior to the clivus and anterior to the cerebellum. The term pons literally means bridge. This definition is appropriate because the pontine fibers relay signals between the spinal cord and the cerebral and cerebellar cortices (Figures 3.46 and 3.66 through 3.69).

Medulla Oblongata

The **medulla oblongata** extends from the pons to the foramen magnum, where it continues as the spinal cord (Figures 3.45, 3.46). The medulla oblongata contains all fiber tracts between the brain and spinal cord, as well as vital centers that regulate internal activities of the body. These centers are involved in the control of heart rate, respiratory rhythm, and blood pressure. The center of the anterior and posterior surfaces of the medulla oblongata is marked by the **anterior** and **posterior median fissures**. These two fissures divide the medulla oblongata into two symmetric halves. Located on either side of the anterior median fissure are two

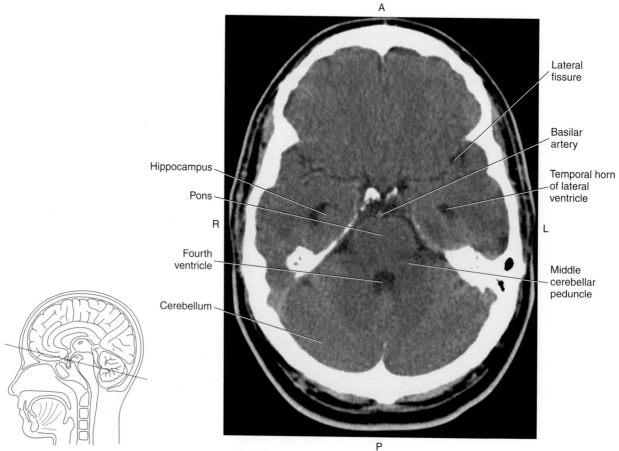

FIGURE 3.66 Axial CT of pons.

S

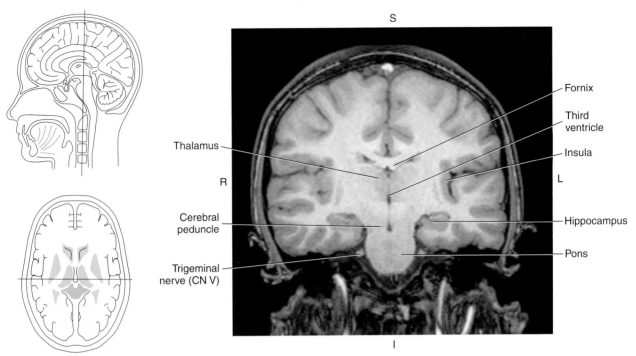

Thalamus

Fornix

Third ventricle

Insula

R

L

Cerebral peduncle

Hippocampus

Pons

Trigeminal nerve (CN V)

I

FIGURE 3.67 Coronal, T1-weighted MRI of pons.

A

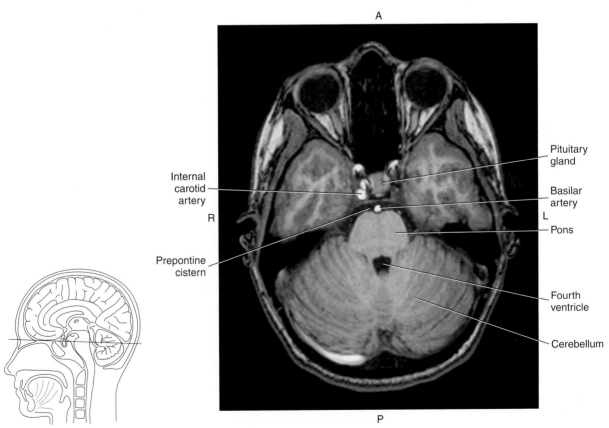

Internal carotid artery

Pituitary gland

Basilar artery

R

L

Pons

Prepontine cistern

Fourth ventricle

Cerebellum

P

FIGURE 3.68 Axial, T1-weighted MRI of pons and cerebellum.

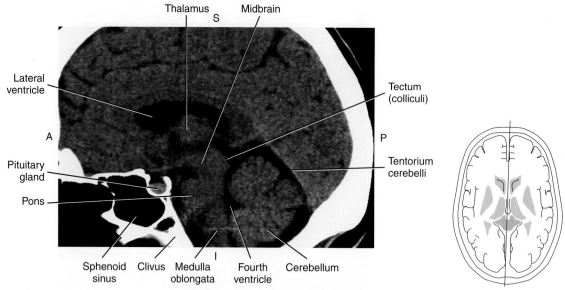

FIGURE 3.69 Sagittal CT reformat of pons.

bundles of nerve fibers called **medullary pyramids** (Figures 3.70 and 3.71). The pyramids contain nerve tracts that contribute to voluntary motor control. At the lower end of the pyramids, some of the nerve tracts cross over (decussate) to the opposite side. This decussation in part accounts for the fact that each half of the brain controls the opposite half of the body. On each lateral surface of the medulla oblongata is a rounded oval prominence called the **olive**. The olives consist of nuclei that are involved in coordination, balance, and modulation of sound impulses from the inner ear (Figures 3.70 through 3.72).

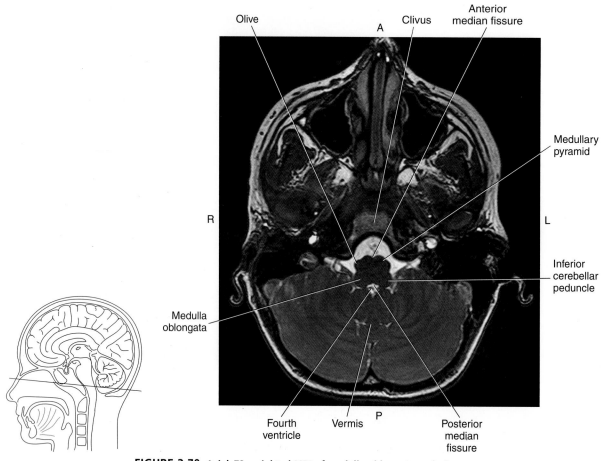

FIGURE 3.70 Axial, T2-weighted MRI of medulla oblongata and olives.

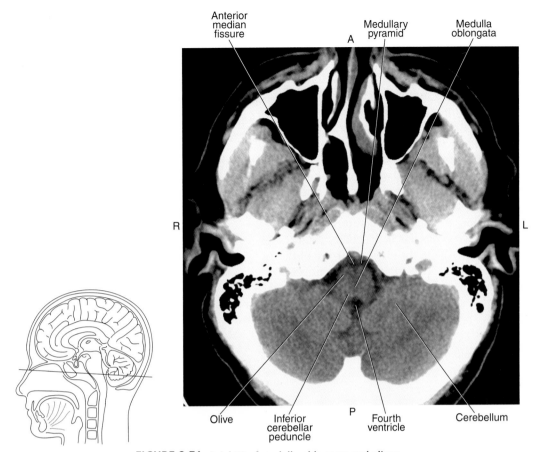

FIGURE 3.71 Axial CT of medulla oblongata and olives.

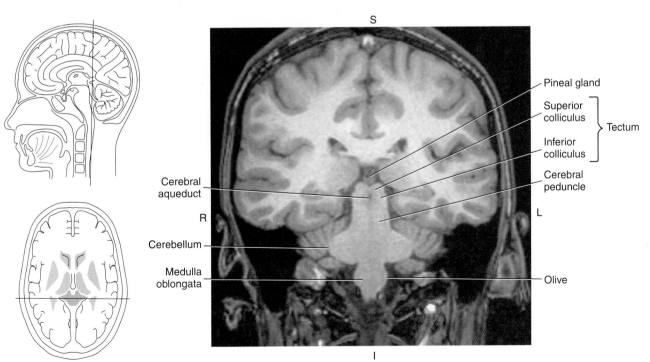

FIGURE 3.72 Coronal, T1-weighted MRI of medulla oblongata and olives.

CEREBELLUM

The **cerebellum**, which is referred to as the "little brain," attaches posteriorly to the brainstem and occupies the posterior cranial fossa (Figure 3.73). The cerebellum is the coordination center for motor functions. Although the cerebellum does not initiate actual motor functions, it uses the brainstem to connect with the cerebrum to execute a variety of movements, including maintenance of muscle tone, posture, balance, and coordination of movement. The cerebellum consists of two **cerebellar hemispheres** (lateral hemispheres). These hemispheres have an interesting appearance because the folds of gray matter resemble a cauliflower. A midline structure called the **vermis** connects the two cerebellar hemispheres (Figures 3.53, 3.54 and, 3.73, 3.74). On the inferior surface of the cerebellar hemispheres are two rounded prominences called the **cerebellar tonsils** (Figures 3.75 and 3.76).

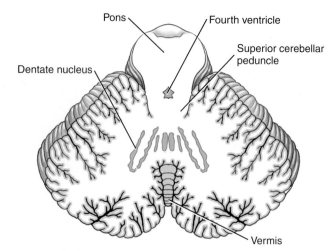

FIGURE 3.74 Axial view through cerebellum.

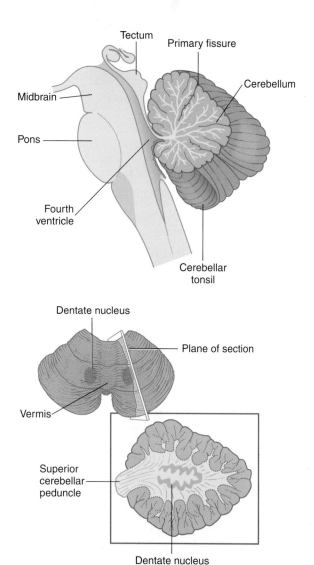

FIGURE 3.73 Midsagittal view of cerebellum and superior cerebellar peduncle.

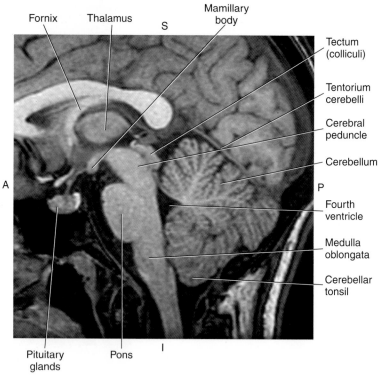

FIGURE 3.75 Sagittal, T1-weighted MRI of cerebellum.

Three pairs of nerve fiber tracts, the cerebellar peduncles, connect the cerebellum to the brainstem (Figure 3.59). The superior **cerebellar peduncles** connect the cerebellum to the midbrain. The middle cerebellar peduncles serve as attachments to the pons, and the inferior cerebellar peduncles attach to the medulla oblongata (Figures 3.77 through 3.79). All information

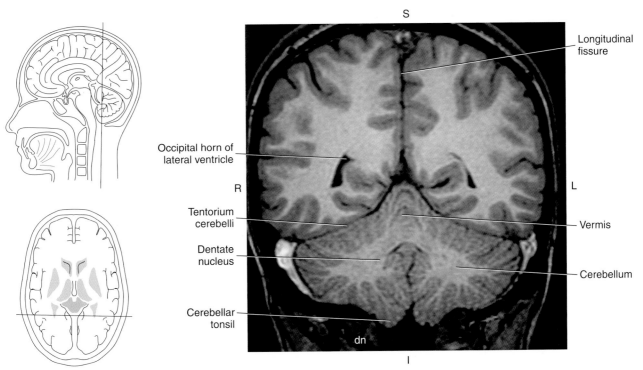

FIGURE 3.76 Coronal, T1-weighted MRI of cerebellum and dentate nucleus.

Longitudinal fissure

Occipital horn of lateral ventricle

Tentorium cerebelli

Dentate nucleus

Cerebellar tonsil

Vermis

Cerebellum

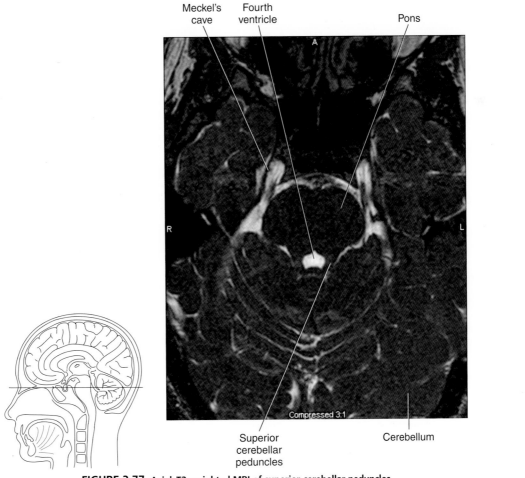

Meckel's cave

Fourth ventricle

Pons

Superior cerebellar peduncles

Cerebellum

FIGURE 3.77 Axial, T2-weighted MRI of superior cerebellar peduncles.

traveling to and from the cerebellum is routed through the cerebellar peduncles.

Deep within the center of each cerebellar hemisphere is a collection of nuclei called the **dentate nucleus**, the largest and most lateral of the deep cerebellar nuclei (Figures 3.73, 3.74 and 3.76). Fibers of the dentate nucleus project to the thalamus via the superior cerebellar peduncles. From here, the fibers travel to the motor areas of the cerebral cortex, namely the precentral gyrus, thus influencing motor control.

A defect involving downward displacement or herniation of the brainstem and cerebellum through the foramen magnum is termed Arnold-Chiari malformation (deformity) or tonsillar herniation.

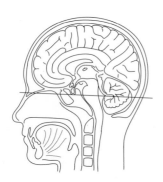

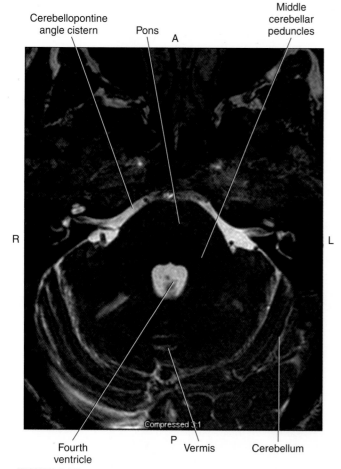

FIGURE 3.78 Axial, T2-weighted MRI of middle cerebellar peduncles.

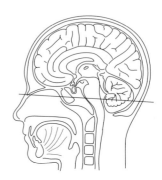

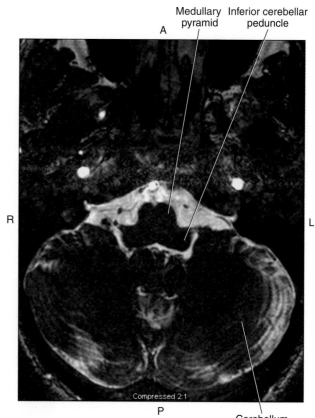

FIGURE 3.79 Axial, T2-weighted MRI of inferior cerebellar peduncles.

CEREBRAL VASCULAR SYSTEM

The vascular supply to the brain is unique. In comparison with the arteries in the body, the walls of the arteries in the brain are thin and weak, causing them to be susceptible to aneurysms and strokes. The veins of the brain do not contain valves. This lack of valves allows the blood to flow in either direction, creating a route for blood-borne pathogens to pass from the body to the head and vice versa. The capillaries of the brain are unlike those elsewhere in the body in that they do not allow movement of certain molecules from their vascular compartment into the surrounding brain tissue. This unique quality of impermeability is termed the **blood-brain barrier (BBB)**. The presence of a normal BBB prevents large amounts of contrast medium from entering the brain. Pathologic conditions can disrupt the integrity of the BBB, allowing contrast to escape from the vessel into the surrounding tissues. However, there are some structures located within the brain that do not have a BBB, so they will naturally enhance when contrast media is used. It is normal for the pituitary gland, infundibulum, pineal gland, choroid plexus, mucosal surfaces of the nasopharynx and sinuses, venous structures, and the meninges to be enhanced to varying degrees after contrast administration.

Arterial Supply

The brain receives arterial blood from two main pairs of vessels and their branches, the internal carotid arteries and the vertebral arteries, which make up the anterior and posterior circulation, respectively. Many normal variations of the arterial blood supply exist. This section focuses on the most common anatomic findings visualized in cross section (Figures 3.80 through 3.103).

Internal Carotid Arteries. The **internal carotid arteries** supply the frontal, parietal, and temporal lobes of the brain and orbital structures. These arteries arise from the bifurcation of the carotid arteries in the neck and can be divided into seven segments (Table 3.1) (Figures 3.85 and 3.86). They ascend through the base of the skull and enter the carotid canals of the temporal bones (Figures 3.80, 3.82, and 3.83). The internal carotid artery then turns forward within the cavernous sinus, then up and backward through the dura mater, forming an S shape (which is referred to as the **carotid siphon**) before it reaches the base of the brain (Figures 3.80 and 3.85 through 3.87). As the internal carotid artery exits the cavernous sinus, it branches into the **ophthalmic artery** just inferior to the anterior clinoid process (Figures 3.80 and 3.85). The internal carotid artery then runs lateral to the optic chiasm and branches into the anterior cerebral artery and the larger middle cerebral artery (Tables 3.1 and 3.2) (Figures 3.80, 3.81, and 3.84 through 3.88).

The **anterior cerebral artery** and its branches supply the anterior frontal lobe and the medial aspect of the parietal lobe (Figure 3.84). The main segments and branches of the anterior cerebral artery are the **horizontal (A1) segment, the vertical (A2) segment,** and the **distal (A3) segment** (Figures 3.84 through 3.88). The horizontal segment extends from the internal carotid artery (ICA) bifurcation to the **anterior communicating artery**. The anterior communicating artery joins the two anterior cerebral arteries just anterior to the optic chiasm (Figures 3.87 through 3.89). The vertical segment, an extension of the horizontal segment, courses superiorly toward the rostrum of the corpus callosum. The major branches of the vertical segment are the **orbitofrontal, frontopolar, pericallosal, callosomarginal, and splenial arteries** (Figures 3.84 and 3.85). The distal segment curves around the genu of the corpus callosum and continues as the **pericallosal artery** (see Tables 3.1 and 3.2) (Figures 3.80 and 3.84).

The **middle cerebral artery** is by far the largest of the cerebral arteries and is considered a direct continuation of the internal carotid artery. The middle cerebral artery gives off many branches, as it supplies much of the lateral surface of the cerebrum, insula, and anterior and lateral aspects of the temporal lobe; nearly all the basal ganglia; and the posterior and anterior internal capsule (Figures 3.80 and 3.81). The four major segments of the middle cerebral artery are the **horizontal (M1), insular (M2), opercular (M3),** and **cortical (M4)**. The horizontal segment courses from the origin at the internal carotid artery bifurcation laterally toward the insula and branches into the **lateral lenticulostriate arteries**, which supply to the lentiform nucleus, parts of the internal capsule, and caudate nucleus (Figure 3.81). The insular segment courses along the insula, continuing as the opercular segment that emerges from the lateral fissure. Upon exiting the lateral fissure, the opercular segment becomes the cortical segment, which splits into the superior and inferior groups of cortical branches that supply to nearly the entire surface of the cerebral hemispheres (Figures 3.81, 3.85 through 3.91, and Tables 3.1 and 3.2).

 Branches of the middle cerebral artery are located within the internal capsule, causing this area to be the most frequent site of strokes.

Vertebral Arteries. The **vertebral arteries** begin in the neck at the subclavian artery and ascend vertically through the transverse foramina of the cervical spine. They can be divided into four segments (see Table 3.3). The vertebral arteries curve around the atlanto-occipital joints to enter the cranium through the foramen magnum (Figure 3.92). The two vertebral arteries course along the medulla oblongata and unite ventral to the pons, to form the **basilar artery** (Figures 3.82 through 3.87 and 3.92 through 3.99). The vertebral and basilar arteries give rise to several pairs of smaller arteries that supply the cerebellum, pons, and inferior and medial surfaces of the temporal and

Artery	Segments	Location
Internal carotid artery (ICA)	Cervical (C1)	Cervical ICA
	Petrous (C2)	Carotid canal of temporal bone
	Lacerum (C3)	Base of skull to petrous apex and enters cranial vault via foramen lacerum
	Cavernous (C4)	Cavernous sinus
	Clinoid (C5)	Exits the cavernous sinus to enter the subarachnoid space near the anterior clinoid process
	Ophthalmic (supraclinoid) (C6)	Extends from C5 to the origin of the posterior communicating artery (PCoA)
	Communicating (terminal) (C7)	Origin of the PCoA to the bifurcation of the ICA into the anterior and middle cerebral arteries
Anterior cerebral artery (ACA)	Horizontal (precommunicating) (A1)	Termination of ICA to junction with anterior communicating artery (ACoA)
	Vertical (postcommunicating) (A2)	From junction with ACoA, superiorly through longitudinal fissure, to origin or callosomarginal artery
	Distal (A3)	Continues from callosomarginal artery origin as pericallosal artery
Middle cerebral artery (MCA)	Horizontal (M1)	ICA bifurcation to lateral fissure
	Insular (M2)	Courses superiorly within the lateral fissure to the insula
	Opercular (M3)	Courses inferolaterally through lateral fissure
	Cortical (M4)	Exits lateral fissure to cortex

TABLE 3.1   Segments of Internal Carotid, Anterior Cerebral, and Middle Cerebral Arteries

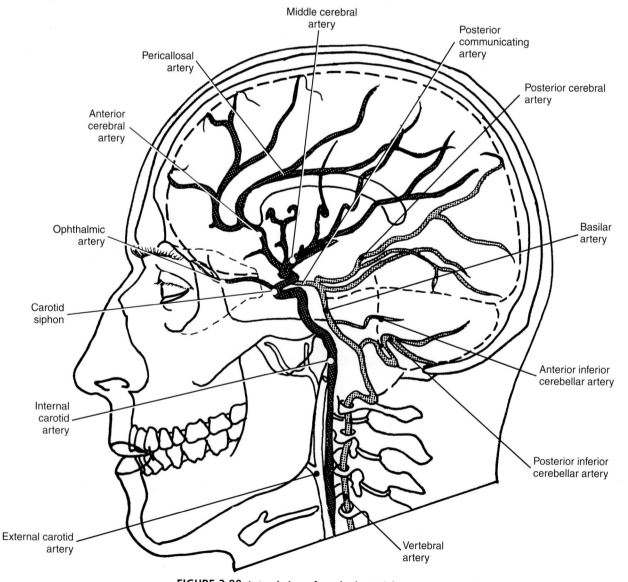

FIGURE 3.80 Lateral view of cerebral arterial system.

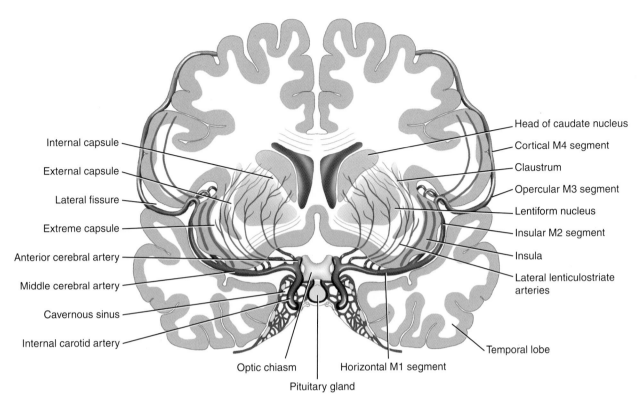

Internal capsule

External capsule

Lateral fissure

Extreme capsule

Anterior cerebral artery

Middle cerebral artery

Cavernous sinus

Internal carotid artery

Head of caudate nucleus

Cortical M4 segment

Claustrum

Opercular M3 segment

Lentiform nucleus

Insular M2 segment

Insula

Lateral lenticulostriate arteries

Temporal lobe

Optic chiasm

Horizontal M1 segment

Pituitary gland

FIGURE 3.81 Coronal view of internal carotid and middle cerebral arteries.

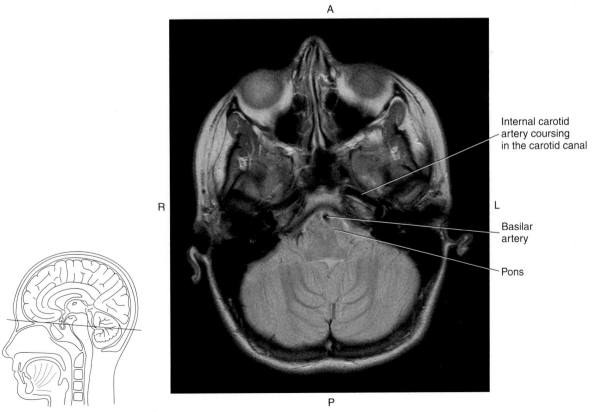

A

R

L

P

Internal carotid artery coursing in the carotid canal

Basilar artery

Pons

FIGURE 3.82 Axial, proton density-weighted MRI with carotid canal.

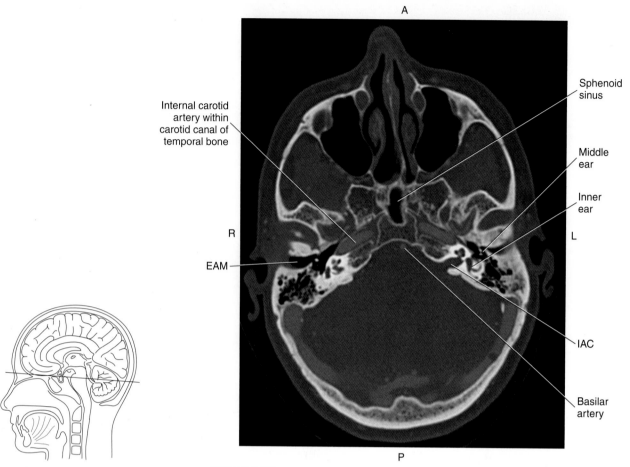

A

Internal carotid
artery within
carotid canal of
temporal bone

Sphenoid
sinus

Middle
ear

Inner
ear

R   L

EAM

IAC

Basilar
artery

P

FIGURE 3.83 Axial CT with carotid canal.

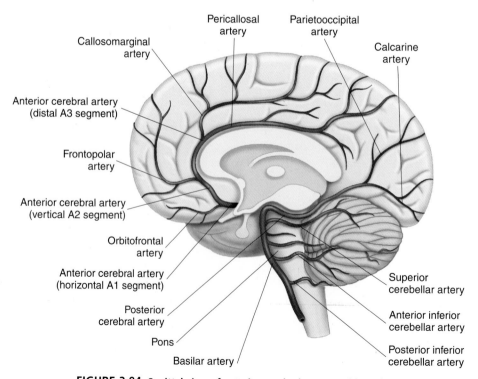

Callosomarginal
artery

Pericallosal
artery

Parietooccipital
artery

Calcarine
artery

Anterior cerebral artery
(distal A3 segment)

Frontopolar
artery

Anterior cerebral artery
(vertical A2 segment)

Orbitofrontal
artery

Anterior cerebral artery
(horizontal A1 segment)

Posterior
cerebral artery

Pons

Basilar artery

Superior
cerebellar artery

Anterior inferior
cerebellar artery

Posterior inferior
cerebellar artery

FIGURE 3.84 Sagittal view of anterior cerebral artery and branches.

TABLE 3.2	Internal Carotid Artery Branches
Artery	**Region Supplied**
Ophthalmic artery	Globe, orbit, frontal scalp, frontal, and ethmoid sinuses
Anterior cerebral artery (ACA)	Anterior frontal lobe and medial aspect of parietal lobe, head of caudate nucleus, anterior limb of the internal capsule, and anterior globus pallidus
Middle cerebral artery (MCA)	Lateral surface of the cerebrum, insula, anterior and lateral aspects of temporal lobe, nearly all the basal ganglia, and posterior and anterior internal capsules

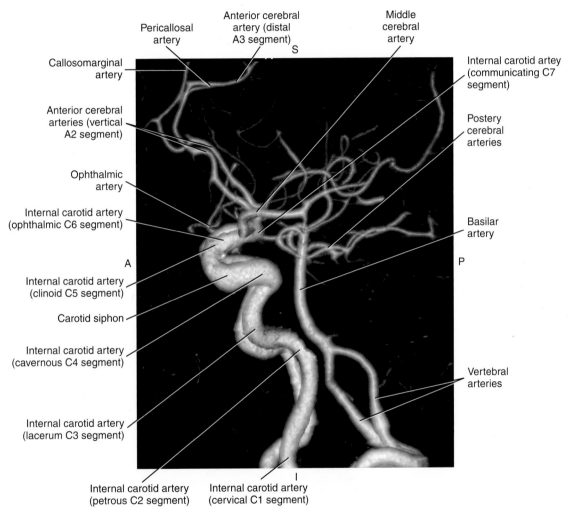

FIGURE 3.85 Lateral CTA of cerebral arteries.

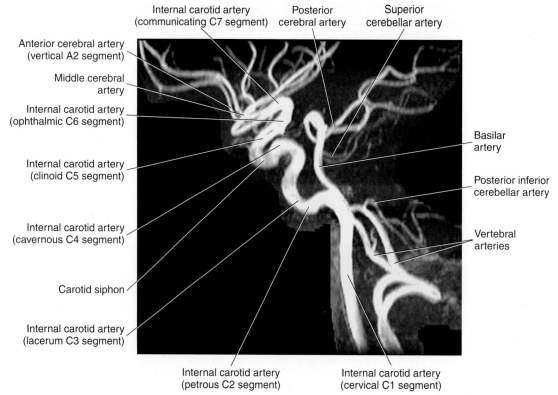

Internal carotid artery
(communicating C7 segment)

Posterior
cerebral artery

Superior
cerebellar artery

Anterior cerebral artery
(vertical A2 segment)

Middle cerebral
artery

Internal carotid artery
(ophthalmic C6 segment)

Internal carotid artery
(clinoid C5 segment)

Internal carotid artery
(cavernous C4 segment)

Carotid siphon

Internal carotid artery
(lacerum C3 segment)

Basilar
artery

Posterior inferior
cerebellar artery

Vertebral
arteries

Internal carotid artery
(petrous C2 segment)

Internal carotid artery
(cervical C1 segment)

FIGURE 3.86 Lateral MRA of cerebral arteries.

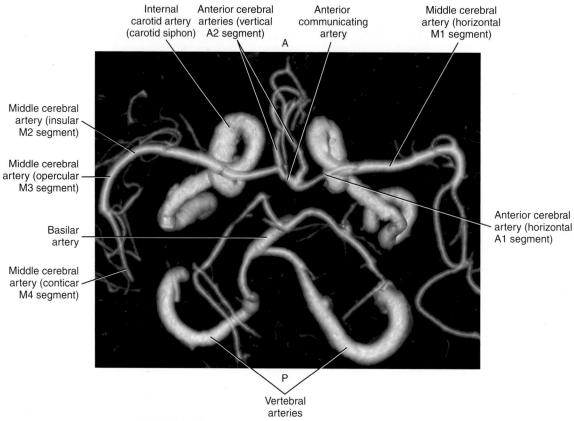

Internal
carotid artery
(carotid siphon)

Anterior cerebral
arteries (vertical
A2 segment)

Anterior
communicating
artery

Middle cerebral
artery (horizontal
M1 segment)

A

Middle cerebral
artery (insular
M2 segment)

Middle cerebral
artery (opercular
M3 segment)

Basilar
artery

Middle cerebral
artery (conticar
M4 segment)

Anterior cerebral
artery (horizontal
A1 segment)

P

Vertebral
arteries

FIGURE 3.87 Submentovertex CTA of internal carotid arteries.

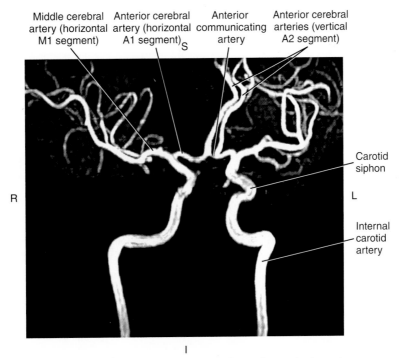

Middle cerebral artery (horizontal M1 segment)

Anterior cerebral artery (horizontal A1 segment) S

Anterior communicating artery

Anterior cerebral arteries (vertical A2 segment)

Carotid siphon

Internal carotid artery

R

L

I

FIGURE 3.88 Coronal oblique MRA of anterior cerebral arteries.

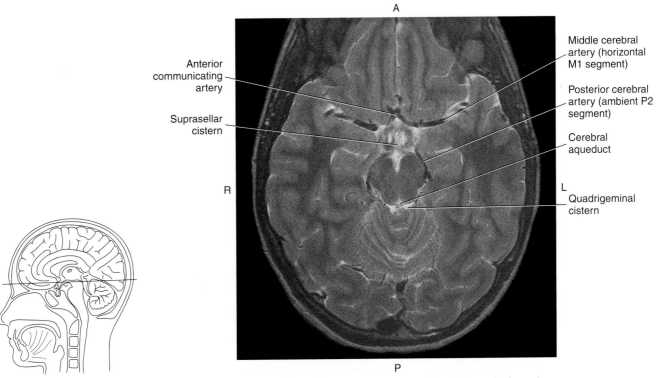

A

Anterior communicating artery

Suprasellar cistern

Middle cerebral artery (horizontal M1 segment)

Posterior cerebral artery (ambient P2 segment)

Cerebral aqueduct

R

L

Quadrigeminal cistern

P

FIGURE 3.89 Axial, T2-weighted MRI with anterior communicating and middle cerebral arteries.

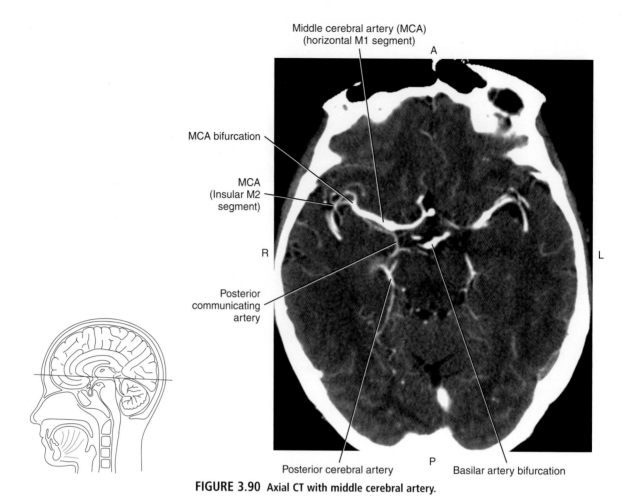

Middle cerebral artery (MCA) (horizontal M1 segment)

A

MCA bifurcation

MCA (Insular M2 segment)

R

L

Posterior communicating artery

Posterior cerebral artery

P

Basilar artery bifurcation

FIGURE 3.90 Axial CT with middle cerebral artery.

Anterior cerebral arteries

Middle cerebral artery (horizontal M1 segment)

S

Middle cerebral artery (cortical M4 segments)

Middle cerebral artery (opercular M3 segments)

Middle cerebral artery (insular M2 segments)

R

L

Internal carotid artery

I

FIGURE 3.91 Anterior MRA of middle cerebral arteries.

TABLE 3.3	Segments of Vertebral and Posterior Cerebral Arteries	
Artery	**Segment**	**Location**
Vertebral artery (VA)	Extraosseous (V1)	Subclavian artery to C6
	Foraminal (V2)	C6 to C1
	Extraspinal (V3)	C1 to Foramen magnum
	Intradural (V4)	Courses superomedially behind clivus, joins with contralateral VA to form basilar artery
Posterior cerebral artery (PCA)	Precommunicating (P1)	Extends from basilar artery bifurcation to posterior communicating artery
	Ambient (P2)	Around cerebral peduncle within ambient cistern
	Quadrigeminal (P3)	Quadrigeminal cistern
	Calcarine (P4)	In calcarine fissure on medial aspect of occipital lobe

occipital lobes. The four major pairs of arteries are listed in order from inferior to superior: **posterior inferior cerebellar (PICA), anterior inferior cerebellar (AICA), superior cerebellar (SCA),** and **posterior cerebral (PCA)** (Figures 3.92B, 3.94 through 3.97). Located between the anterior inferior cerebellar artery and superior cerebellar artery are many tiny perforating **pontine vessels.** The **posterior cerebral arteries** can be divided into four major segments: **precommunicating** or **peduncular (P1), ambient (P2), quadrigeminal (P3),** and **calcarine (P4)** (Figure 3.94). The precommunicating segment is a short segment that extends laterally from the basilar bifurcation to the posterior communicating artery (Figure 3.92C). The **posterior communicating artery** forms a connection between the posterior cerebral artery and the internal carotid artery (Figures 3.90, 3.92, 3.99, and 3.100). The ambient segment courses posteriorly in the ambient cistern around the midbrain and then continues as the quadrigeminal segment located within the quadrigeminal cistern. The calcarine P4 segment is located on the medial surface of the occipital lobe. The distal posterior cerebral artery frequently divides by bifurcation or trifurcation into many branches, including several temporal and occipital arteries (Figures 3.94, 3.101, and 3.102 and Tables 3.3 and 3.4).

Pathology involving the cerebrovascular system is the most common cause of cranial neurologic deficits. The brain needs a constant source of oxygen and glucose and is dependent on the vascular system to provide a steady supply. Any injury or disease affecting the cerebrovascular system can result in vascular insufficiency. Vascular interruptions lasting more than a few minutes will result in necrosis of adjacent brain tissue.

Circle of Willis. The cerebral arterial circle, or **circle of Willis,** is a critically important anastomosis among the four major arteries (two vertebral and two internal carotid) feeding the brain. The circle of Willis is formed by the anterior and posterior cerebral, anterior and posterior communicating, and the internal carotid arteries. The circle is located mainly in the suprasellar cistern at the base of the brain. Many normal variations of this circle may occur in individuals. The circle of Willis functions as a means of collateral blood flow between cerebral hemispheres in the event of blockage (Figures 3.98 through 3.100).

Arteriovenous malformations are the most common type of congenital vascular malformation. They consist of a tangle of dilated arteries and veins, usually accompanied by arteriovenous shunting. Approximately 40% of individuals with AVMs will bleed by the age of 40 years.

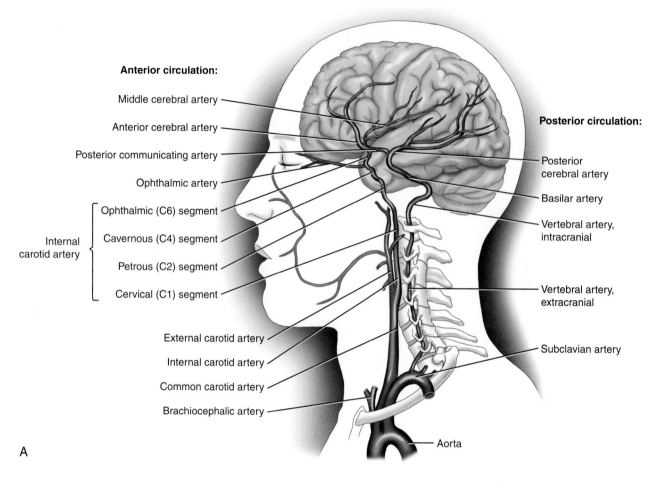

Anterior circulation:

Middle cerebral artery

Anterior cerebral artery

Posterior communicating artery

Ophthalmic artery

Internal carotid artery
- Ophthalmic (C6) segment
- Cavernous (C4) segment
- Petrous (C2) segment
- Cervical (C1) segment

External carotid artery

Internal carotid artery

Common carotid artery

Brachiocephalic artery

Posterior circulation:

Posterior cerebral artery

Basilar artery

Vertebral artery, intracranial

Vertebral artery, extracranial

Subclavian artery

Aorta

A

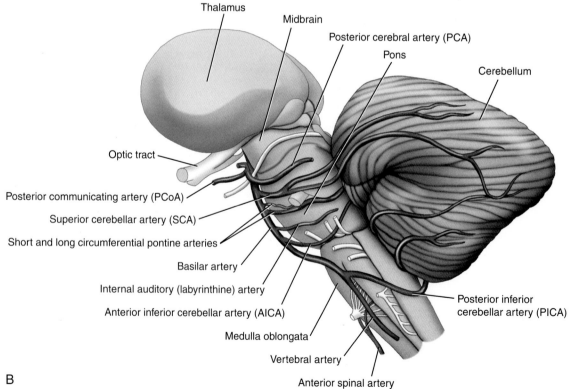

Thalamus

Midbrain

Posterior cerebral artery (PCA)

Pons

Cerebellum

Optic tract

Posterior communicating artery (PCoA)

Superior cerebellar artery (SCA)

Short and long circumferential pontine arteries

Basilar artery

Internal auditory (labyrinthine) artery

Anterior inferior cerebellar artery (AICA)

Medulla oblongata

Vertebral artery

Anterior spinal artery

Posterior inferior cerebellar artery (PICA)

B

FIGURE 3.92 Vertebrobasilar arterial system. A, Lateral view of vertebrobasilar arterial system. **B,** Lateral view of basilar artery and branches.

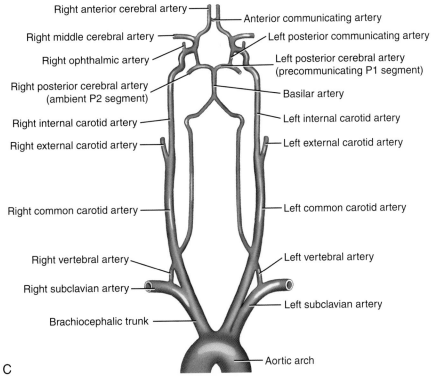

FIGURE 3.92 cont'd C, Anterior view of the internal carotid and vertebral arteries.

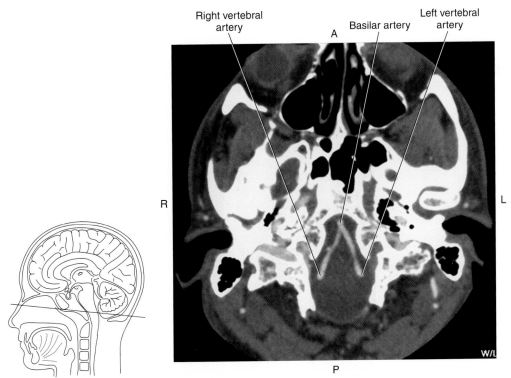

FIGURE 3.93 Axial CT of vertebral and basilar arteries.

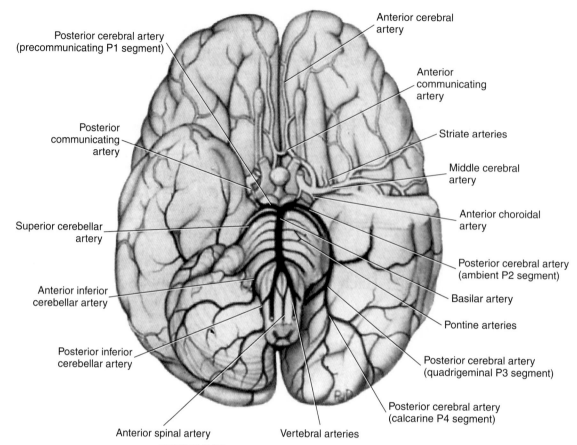

Posterior cerebral artery
(precommunicating P1 segment)

Anterior cerebral
artery

Anterior
communicating
artery

Posterior
communicating
artery

Striate arteries

Middle cerebral
artery

Superior cerebellar
artery

Anterior choroidal
artery

Posterior cerebral artery
(ambient P2 segment)

Anterior inferior
cerebellar artery

Basilar artery

Pontine arteries

Posterior inferior
cerebellar artery

Posterior cerebral artery
(quadrigeminal P3 segment)

Posterior cerebral artery
(calcarine P4 segment)

Anterior spinal artery

Vertebral arteries

FIGURE 3.94 Inferior view of brain with basilar artery.

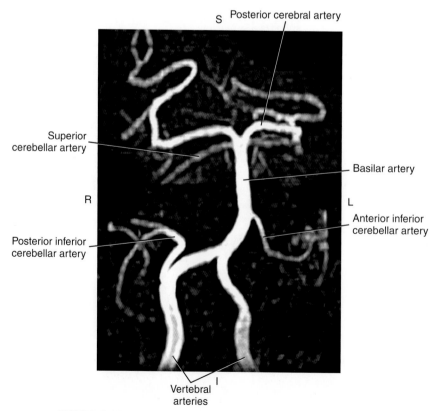

S   Posterior cerebral artery

Superior
cerebellar artery

Basilar artery

R

L

Anterior inferior
cerebellar artery

Posterior inferior
cerebellar artery

Vertebral
arteries

I

FIGURE 3.95 Coronal oblique MRA of vertebral and basilar arteries.

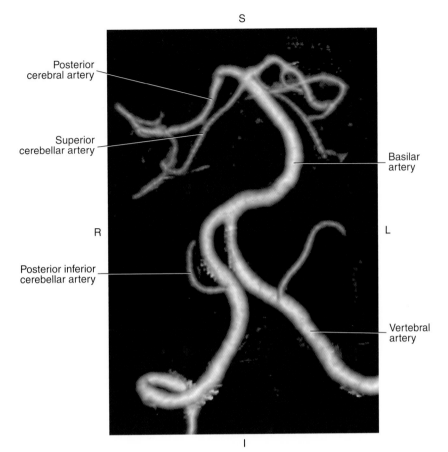

FIGURE 3.96 Anterior CTA of vertebral and basilar arteries.

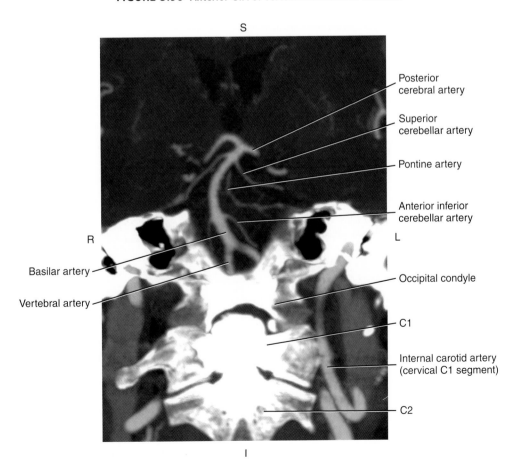

FIGURE 3.97 Coronal CT reformat of vertebral and basilar arteries.

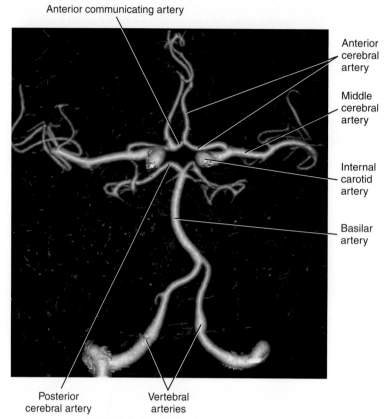

Anterior communicating artery

Anterior cerebral artery

Middle cerebral artery

Internal carotid artery

Basilar artery

Posterior cerebral artery

Vertebral arteries

FIGURE 3.98 Anterior CTA of circle of Willis.

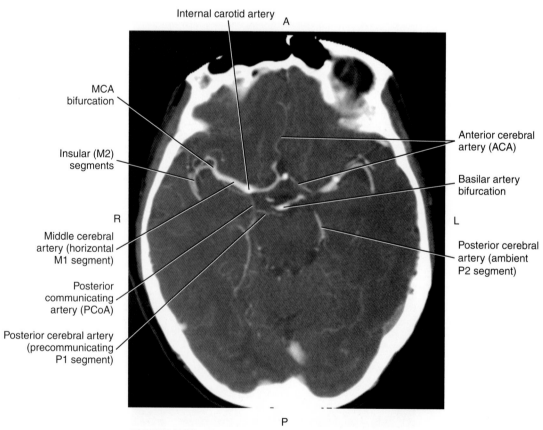

Internal carotid artery

A

MCA bifurcation

Insular (M2) segments

R

Middle cerebral artery (horizontal M1 segment)

Posterior communicating artery (PCoA)

Posterior cerebral artery (precommunicating P1 segment)

Anterior cerebral artery (ACA)

Basilar artery bifurcation

L

Posterior cerebral artery (ambient P2 segment)

P

FIGURE 3.99 Axial CT with posterior communicating artery.

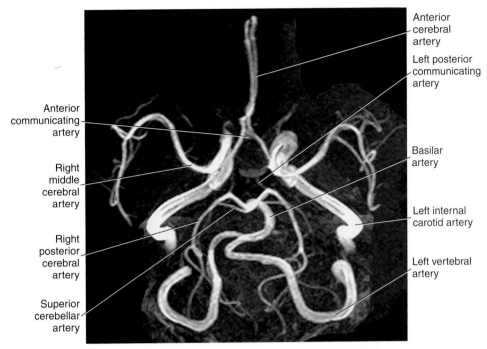

Anterior cerebral artery

Left posterior communicating artery

Anterior communicating artery

Basilar artery

Right middle cerebral artery

Left internal carotid artery

Right posterior cerebral artery

Left vertebral artery

Superior cerebellar artery

FIGURE 3.100 Submentovertex MRA of circle of Willis.

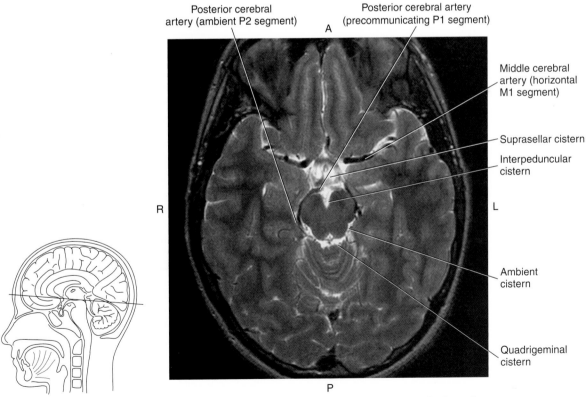

Posterior cerebral artery (ambient P2 segment)

Posterior cerebral artery (precommunicating P1 segment)

A

Middle cerebral artery (horizontal M1 segment)

Suprasellar cistern

Interpeduncular cistern

R   L

Ambient cistern

Quadrigeminal cistern

P

FIGURE 3.101 Axial, T2-weighted MRI of middle and posterior cerebral arteries.

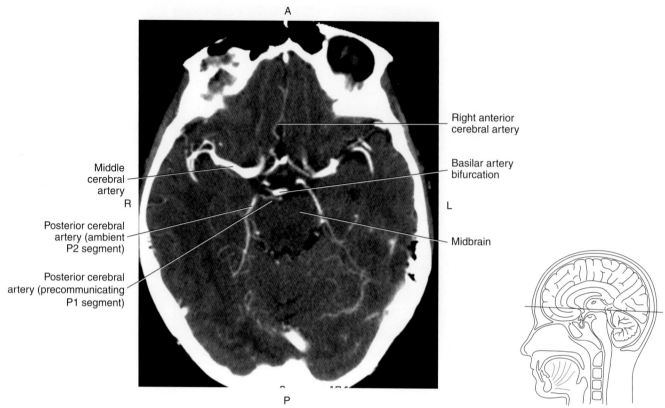

Right anterior
cerebral artery

Basilar artery
bifurcation

Midbrain

Middle
cerebral
artery

R

Posterior cerebral
artery (ambient
P2 segment)

Posterior cerebral
artery (precommunicating
P1 segment)

L

FIGURE 3.102 Axial CT of posterior cerebral arteries.

TABLE 3.4	Vertebral and Basilar Artery Branches
Artery	**Region Supplied**
Posterior inferior cerebellar (PICA)	Inferior cerebellum
Anterior inferior cerebellar (AICA)	Anterior and inferior cerebellum
Pontine vessels	Pons
Superior cerebellar (SCA)	Superior cerebellum, portions of midbrain, and pons
Posterior cerebral artery (PCA)	Occipital and temporal lobes

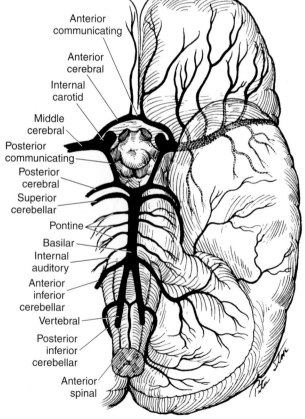

Anterior
communicating

Anterior
cerebral

Internal
carotid

Middle
cerebral

Posterior
communicating

Posterior
cerebral

Superior
cerebellar

Pontine

Basilar

Internal
auditory

Anterior
inferior
cerebellar

Vertebral

Posterior
inferior
cerebellar

Anterior
spinal

FIGURE 3.103 Inferior view of circle of Willis.

Venous Drainage

The venous system of the brain and its coverings are primarily composed of the dural sinuses, superficial cortical veins, and deep veins of the cerebrum.

Dural Sinuses. The **dural sinuses** are very large veins located within the dura mater of the brain. All the veins of the head drain into the dural sinuses and ultimately into the **internal jugular veins** of the neck. The major dural sinuses include superior and inferior sagittal, straight, transverse, sigmoid, cavernous, and petrosal (Figures 3.104 and 3.105). The **superior sagittal sinus** lies in the median plane between the falx cerebri and the calvaria. It begins at the crista galli, runs the entire length of the falx cerebri, and ends at the internal occipital protuberance of the occipital bone (Figures 3.104 through 3.108). The **inferior sagittal sinus**, which is much smaller than the superior sagittal sinus, runs posteriorly just under the free edge of the falx cerebri (Figures 3.3, 3.104, 3.105 and 3.107). The inferior sagittal sinus converges into the great cerebral vein (vein of Galen) to form the **straight sinus**. The straight sinus extends along the length of the junction of the falx cerebri and the tentorium cerebelli (Figures 3.104, 3.105, 3.107 through 3.109). The junction of the superior sagittal, transverse, and straight sinuses creates the large **confluence of the sinuses** or the **torcular herophili** (Figures 3.109 and 3.110). The **transverse sinuses** extend from the confluence between the attachment of the tentorium and the calvaria (Figures 3.111 and 3.112). As the transverse sinuses pass through the tentorium cerebelli, they become the **sigmoid sinuses**. The S-shaped sigmoid sinuses continue in the posterior cranial fossa to join the jugular bulbs of the internal jugular veins (Figures 3.110 and 3.112).

The **cavernous sinuses**, located on each side of the sella turcica and body of the sphenoid bone, are formed by numerous interconnected venous channels. They envelop the internal carotid arteries and third through sixth cranial nerves. Each cavernous sinus receives blood from the superior and inferior **ophthalmic veins** and communicates with the transverse sinuses via the **petrosal sinuses** (Figures 3.104, 3.113 through 3.117).

Superficial Cortical and Deep Veins. The **superficial cortical veins** are located along the surface of each cerebral hemisphere and are responsible for draining the cerebral cortex and portions of the white matter. The veins drain into the dural sinuses with numerous anastomoses between the superficial and deep veins (Figure 3.118).

The **deep veins** of the cerebrum drain the white matter and include the thalamostriate, septal, internal cerebral, basal (vein of Rosenthal), and great cerebral vein (vein of Galen) (Figure 3.119). The **thalamostriate vein** runs in a groove between the thalamus and caudate nucleus, where it drains both structures. The **septal vein** runs posteriorly across the septum pellucidum and joins with the thalamostriate veins to create the paired internal cerebral veins at the inferior aspect of the interventricular foramen. The **basal vein of Rosenthal** drains the medial temporal lobe and basal nuclei as it curves posteriorly around the cerebral peduncle and quadrigeminal plate to join the great cerebral vein. Each **internal cerebral vein** runs posteriorly beneath the third ventricle to meet with the paired basal veins beneath the corpus callosum to form a short trunk, the great cerebral vein. The unpaired **great cerebral vein (vein of Galen)** is a short midline vessel running between the splenium of the corpus callosum and pineal gland, where it joins with the inferior sagittal sinus to form the straight sinus. All cerebral venous output will eventually drain into one of the dural sinuses and ultimately into the internal jugular veins (Figures 3.119 through 3.123).

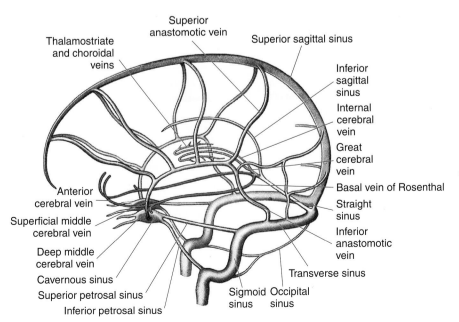

FIGURE 3.104 Sagittal view of intracranial venous system.

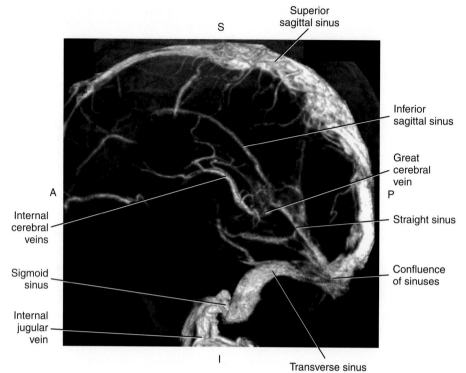

FIGURE 3.105 Lateral CT venogram of cerebral venous system.

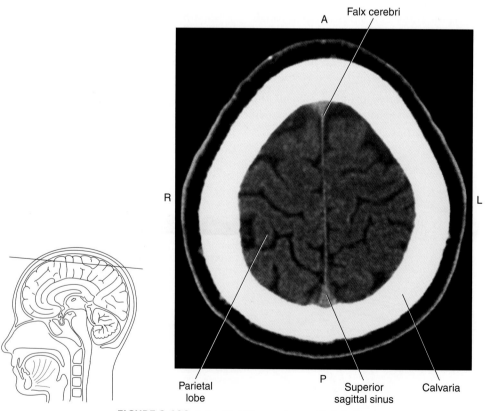

FIGURE 3.106 Axial CT with superior sagittal sinus.

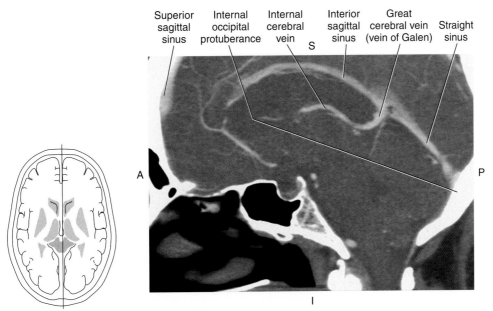

FIGURE 3.107 Sagittal CT reformat of inferior sagittal and straight sinuses.

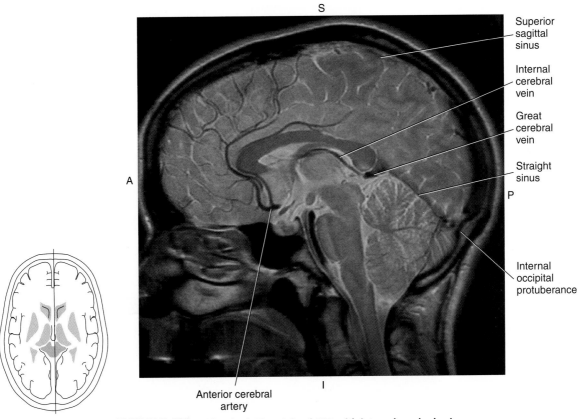

FIGURE 3.108 Midsagittal, T2-weighted MRI with internal cerebral vein.

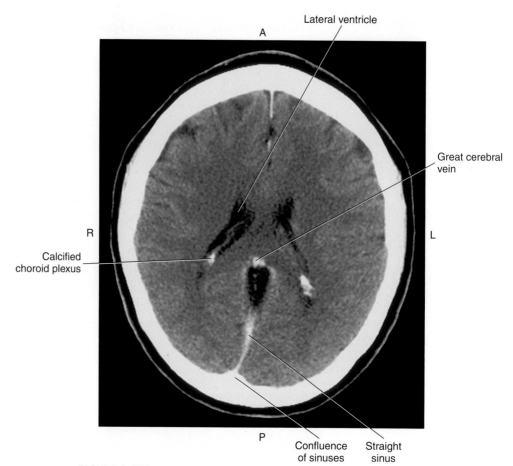

FIGURE 3.109 Axial CT of straight sinus.

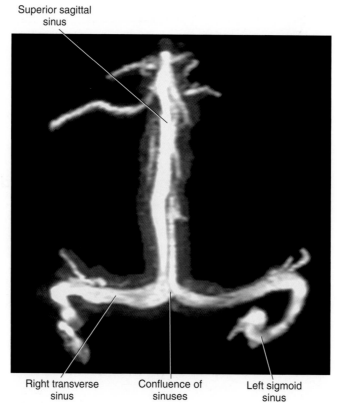

FIGURE 3.110 Coronal MRI with transverse and sigmoid sinuses.

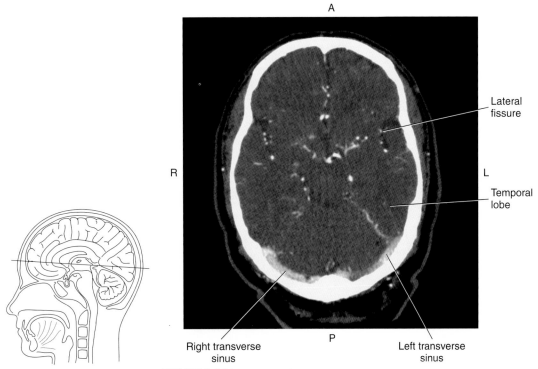

A

Lateral fissure

Temporal lobe

R

L

Right transverse sinus

P

Left transverse sinus

FIGURE 3.111 Axial CT of transverse sinuses.

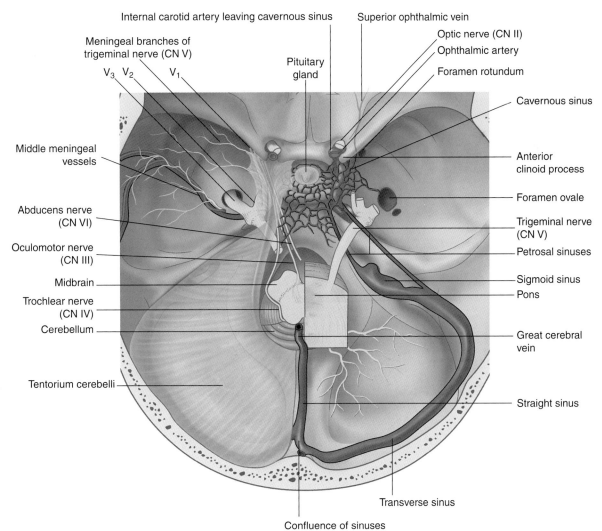

Internal carotid artery leaving cavernous sinus

Superior ophthalmic vein

Meningeal branches of trigeminal nerve (CN V)

Optic nerve (CN II)

Ophthalmic artery

Pituitary gland

Foramen rotundum

V_3 V_2 V_1

Cavernous sinus

Middle meningeal vessels

Anterior clinoid process

Foramen ovale

Abducens nerve (CN VI)

Trigeminal nerve (CN V)

Oculomotor nerve (CN III)

Petrosal sinuses

Midbrain

Sigmoid sinus

Pons

Trochlear nerve (CN IV)

Cerebellum

Great cerebral vein

Tentorium cerebelli

Straight sinus

Transverse sinus

Confluence of sinuses

FIGURE 3.112 Axial view of dural sinuses.

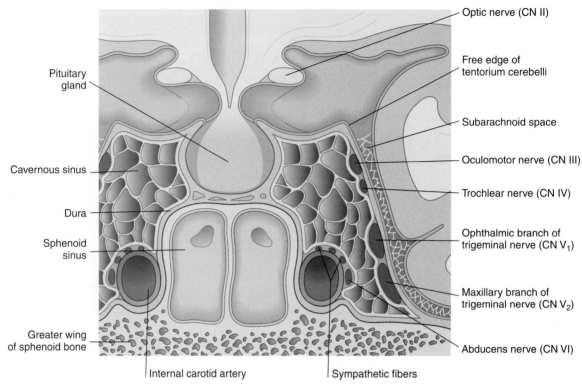

Pituitary gland

Cavernous sinus

Dura

Sphenoid sinus

Greater wing of sphenoid bone

Internal carotid artery

Sympathetic fibers

Optic nerve (CN II)

Free edge of tentorium cerebelli

Subarachnoid space

Oculomotor nerve (CN III)

Trochlear nerve (CN IV)

Ophthalmic branch of trigeminal nerve (CN V₁)

Maxillary branch of trigeminal nerve (CN V₂)

Abducens nerve (CN VI)

FIGURE 3.113 Coronal view of cavernous sinus.

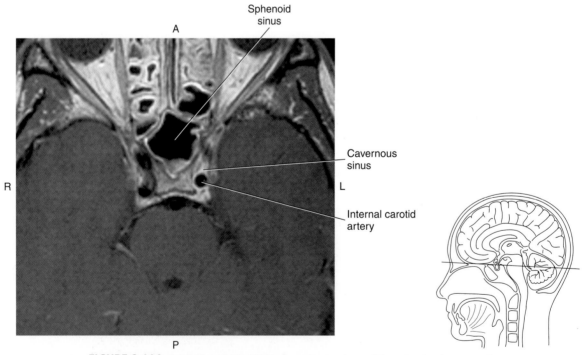

Sphenoid sinus

A

R

L

P

Cavernous sinus

Internal carotid artery

FIGURE 3.114 Axial, T1-weighted MRI of cavernous sinus with contrast enhancement.

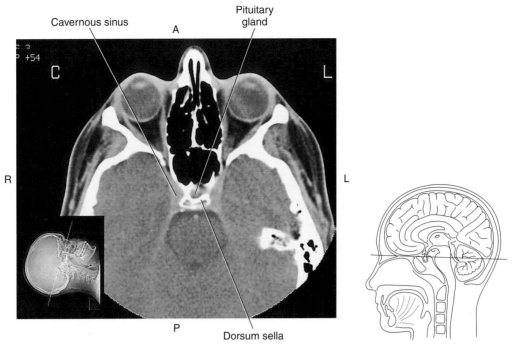

FIGURE 3.115 Axial CT of cavernous sinus with contrast enhancement.

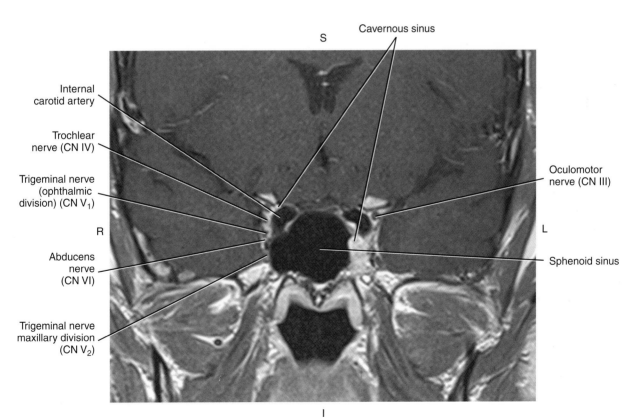

FIGURE 3.116 Coronal, T1-weighted MRI of cavernous sinus with contrast enhancement.

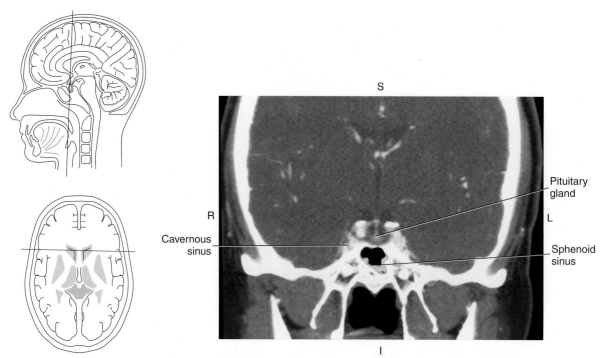

FIGURE 3.117 Coronal CT reformat of cavernous sinus with contrast enhancement.

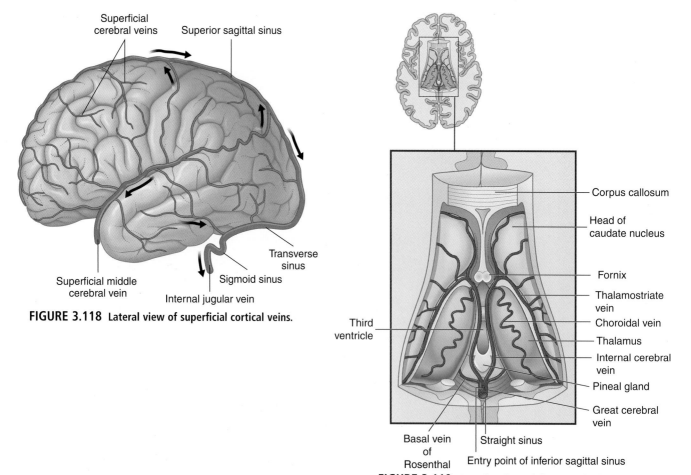

FIGURE 3.118 Lateral view of superficial cortical veins.

FIGURE 3.119 Superior view of deep cerebral veins.

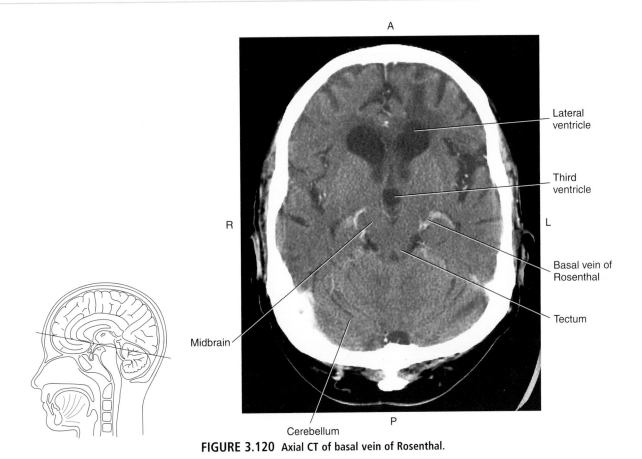

A

Lateral
ventricle

Third
ventricle

R

L

Basal vein of
Rosenthal

Tectum

Midbrain

Cerebellum

P

FIGURE 3.120 Axial CT of basal vein of Rosenthal.

A

Thalamostriate
vein

Internal
cerebral
vein

R

L

Great
cerebral
vein

Straight
sinus

P

FIGURE 3.121 Axial CT of internal cerebral and thalamostriate veins.

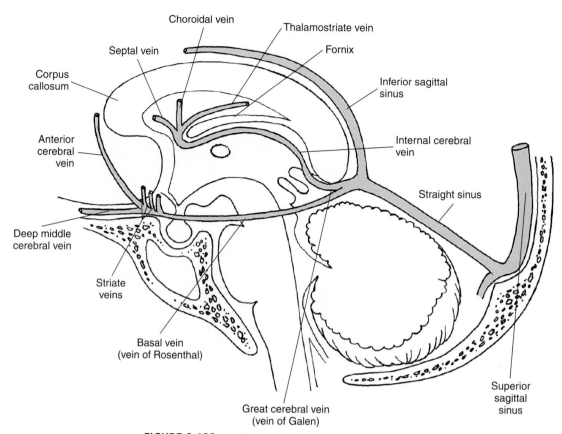

FIGURE 3.122 Sagittal view of deep cerebral veins.

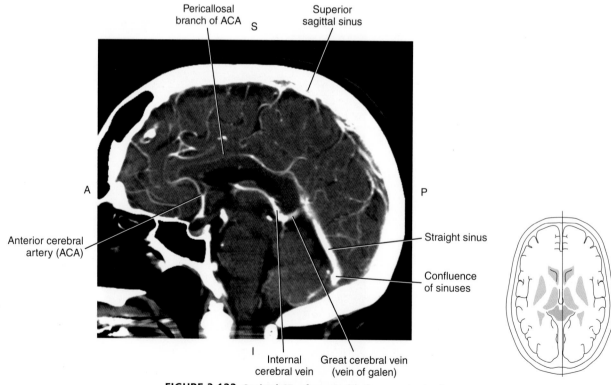

FIGURE 3.123 Sagittal CT reformat with deep cerebral veins.

CRANIAL NERVES

There are 12 cranial nerves (CNs), numbered from anterior to posterior according to their attachment to the brain. All but the first and second cranial nerves arise from the brainstem (Figures 3.58, 3.59, and 3.124). Each of these nerves corresponds to a specific function of the body (Table 3.5). It is important to recognize the adjacent brain structures that act as anatomic landmarks to localize the course of the cranial nerves in the head.

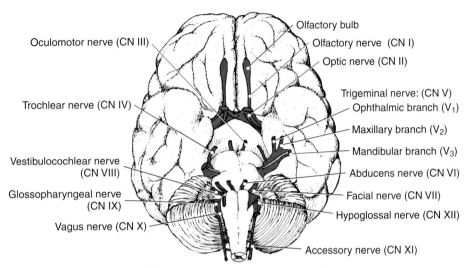

FIGURE 3.124 Inferior view of brain with cranial nerves.

TABLE 3.5	Cranial Nerves		
Cranial Nerves	**Type**	**Foramen**	**Function**
Olfactory (I)	Sensory	Olfactory foramina in cribriform plate of ethmoid bone	Smell
Optic (II)	Sensory	Optic foramen	Vision
Oculomotor (III)	Motor	Superior orbital fissure	Movement of superior, inferior, and medial rectus; inferior oblique; and levator palpebrae muscles
Trochlear (IV)	Motor	Superior orbital fissure	Movement of superior oblique muscle
Trigeminal (V)	Mixed	Meckel's cave	
Ophthalmic (V1)	Sensory	Superior orbital fissure	Sensation from cornea, scalp, eyelids, nasal cavity, forehead
Maxillary (V2)	Sensory	Foramen rotundum	Sensation from upper lip, upper jaw and teeth, maxillary sinuses, palate
Mandibular (V3)	Mixed	Foramen ovale	Movement of muscles of mastication and suprahyoid muscles Sensation from lower jaw and teeth, TMJ, anterior 2/3 of tongue
Abducens (VI)	Motor	Superior orbital fissure	Movement of lateral rectus muscle
Facial (VII)	Mixed	Internal auditory canal, facial canal, stylomastoid foramen	Movement of facial muscles and stapedius muscle of middle ear Taste from anterior 2/3 of tongue, floor of mouth and palate Sensation from EAM
Vestibulocochlear (VIII)	Sensory	Internal auditory canal	Sensation from vestibular structures for equilibrium Hearing from cochlea
Glossopharyngeal (IX)	Mixed	Jugular foramen	Movement of muscle for swallowing Sensation from parotid gland, carotid body and sinus, pharynx and middle ear Taste from posterior 1/3 of tongue
Vagus (X)	Mixed	Jugular foramen	Movement of pharyngeal and laryngeal muscles Movement of smooth muscle in trachea, bronchi, digestive tract; moderates cardiac pacemaker and vasoconstriction of coronary arteries Sensation from EAM and dura mater of posterior cranial
Accessory (XI)	Motor	Jugular foramen	Movement of SCM and trapezius muscles
Hypoglossal (XII)	Motor	Hypoglossal canal	Movement of tongue muscles

Olfactory Nerve (CN I)

The **olfactory nerve** is the nerve of smell. The olfactory neurosensory cells are located in the covering of the superior nasal concha and the superior part of the nasal septum. The axons of these cells unite to form 18 to 20 small nerve bundles that are known collectively as **olfactory nerve fibers.** The nerve fibers pass through the olfactory foramina in the cribriform plate of the ethmoid bone to synapse with the olfactory bulb in the anterior cranial fossa. The right and left olfactory tracts extend from the olfactory bulbs and run along the inferior surface of the frontal lobes to pass to the lateral hippocampal gyrus and interact with the limbic system (Figures 3.124 through 3.127). Each olfactory nerve is surrounded by the three layers of the cranial meninges.

Damage to the visual system will result in visual losses related to the location of the damage. If the optic nerve is damaged anterior to the optic chiasm, the result will be loss of vision in that eye. At the optic chiasm, damage on the medial aspect will result in loss of peripheral vision, whereas damage on the lateral aspect results in loss of the ipsilateral central (nasal) visual field. If damage occurs posterior to the optic chiasm, the result will be loss of input from the contralateral visual fields of both eyes.

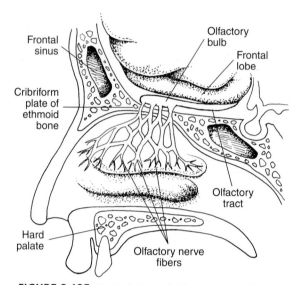

FIGURE 3.125 Sagittal view of olfactory nerve (CN I).

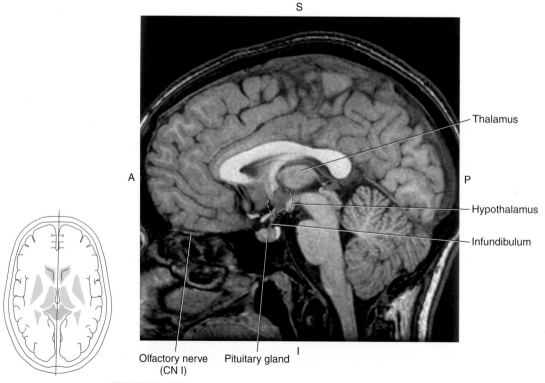

FIGURE 3.126 Sagittal, T1-weighted MRI of olfactory nerve (CN I).

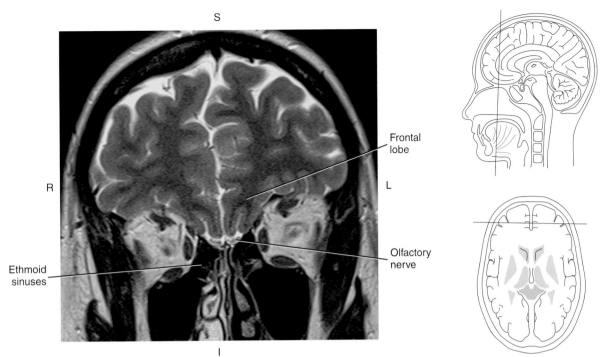

FIGURE 3.127 Coronal, T2-weighted MRI of olfactory nerves (CN I).

Optic Nerve (CN II)

The **optic nerve** is the nerve of sight. Sensory nerve cells arise from the retina and converge toward the posterior aspect of the eye. These fibers unite to form the large optic nerve that passes posteromedially through the optic canal into the middle cranial fossa to join its partner at the **optic chiasm** just anterior to the infundibulum (Figures 3.44 and 3.58). In the optic chiasm, the fibers from the medial side of the retina cross to the opposite side, and the fibers from the lateral aspect remain on the same side (Figures 3.128 through 3.130). This decussation of the medial fibers allows for binocular vision. Posterior to the optic chiasm,

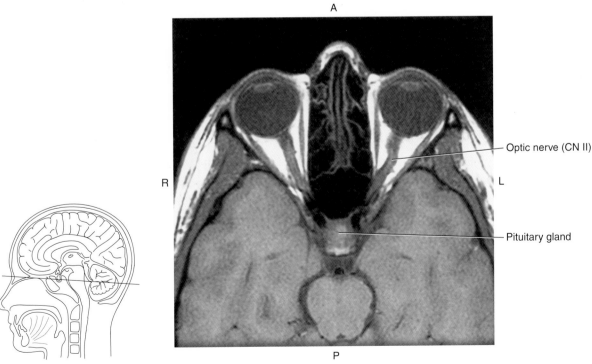

FIGURE 3.128 Axial, T1-weighted MRI of optic nerves (CN II).

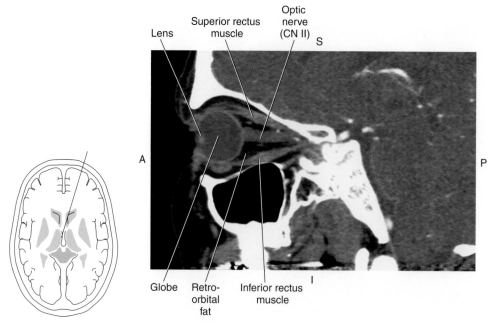

FIGURE 3.129 Sagittal oblique CT reformat of optic nerve (CN II).

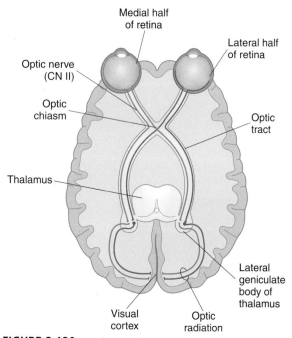

FIGURE 3.130 Axial view of optic tract and optic radiations.

the optic nerve extends as **optic tracts,** which continue around the midbrain and terminate in the posterolateral thalamus (Figures 3.15, 3.53, and 3.130). The optic pathway continues posteriorly from the thalamus as nerve axons forming **optic radiations** that are relayed to the visual cortex located in the occipital lobe (Figures 3.130 and 3.131).

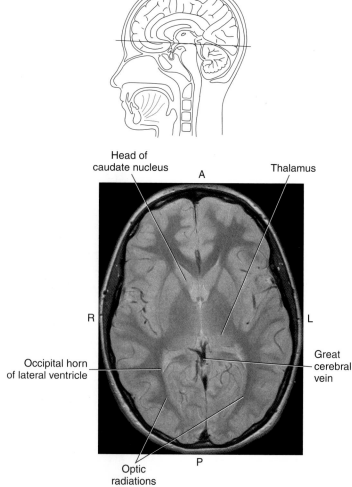

FIGURE 3.131 Axial, proton density-weighted MRI with optic radiations.

Oculomotor Nerve (CN III)

The **oculomotor nerve** moves the eye by supplying fibers to all extraocular muscles of the eye except the superior oblique and lateral rectus muscles. This nerve emerges from the midbrain and passes anteriorly into the interpeduncular cistern. It runs lateral to the posterior communicating artery through the roof of the cavernous sinus and travels in the lateral wall superolateral to the internal carotid artery. The nerve enters the orbit through the superior orbital fissure and then breaks into superior and inferior branches that innervate the superior, medial, and inferior rectus muscles, as well as the inferior oblique and levator palpebrae muscles (Figures 3.132 through 3.137).

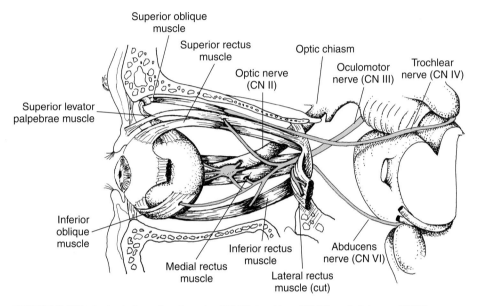

FIGURE 3.132 Sagittal view of oculomotor (CN III), trochlear (CN IV), and abducens (CN VI) nerves.

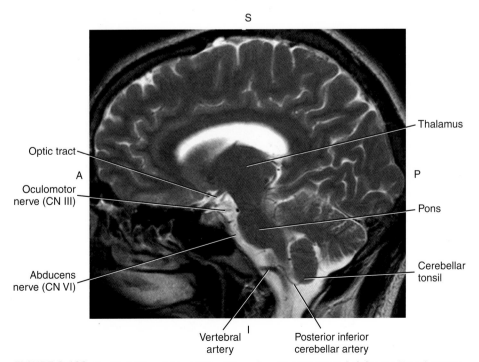

FIGURE 3.133 Sagittal, T2-weighted MRI with oculomotor (CN III) and abducens (CN VI) nerves.

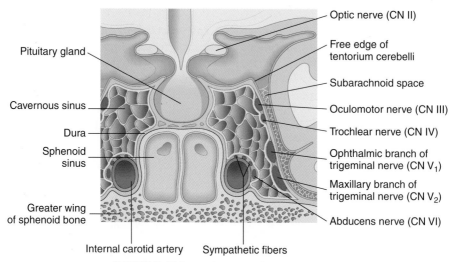

Pituitary gland

Cavernous sinus

Dura

Sphenoid sinus

Greater wing of sphenoid bone

Internal carotid artery   Sympathetic fibers

Optic nerve (CN II)

Free edge of tentorium cerebelli

Subarachnoid space

Oculomotor nerve (CN III)

Trochlear nerve (CN IV)

Ophthalmic branch of trigeminal nerve (CN V₁)

Maxillary branch of trigeminal nerve (CN V₂)

Abducens nerve (CN VI)

FIGURE 3.134 Coronal view of cavernous sinus.

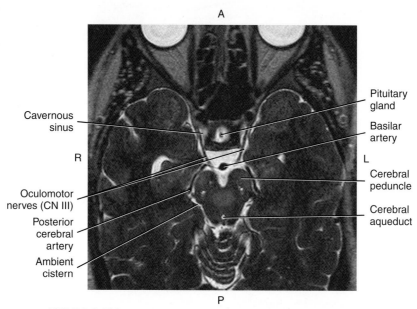

Cavernous sinus

Oculomotor nerves (CN III)

Posterior cerebral artery

Ambient cistern

Pituitary gland

Basilar artery

Cerebral peduncle

Cerebral aqueduct

FIGURE 3.135 Axial, T2-weighted MRI of oculomotor nerve (CN III).

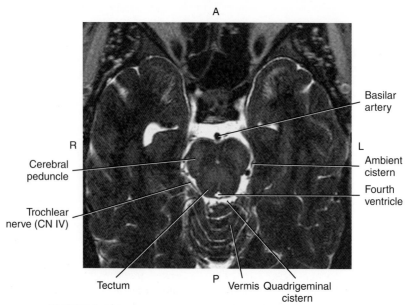

Cerebral peduncle

Trochlear nerve (CN IV)

Basilar artery

Ambient cistern

Fourth ventricle

Tectum   Vermis   Quadrigeminal cistern

FIGURE 3.136 Axial, T2-weighted MRI of trochlear nerve (CN IV).

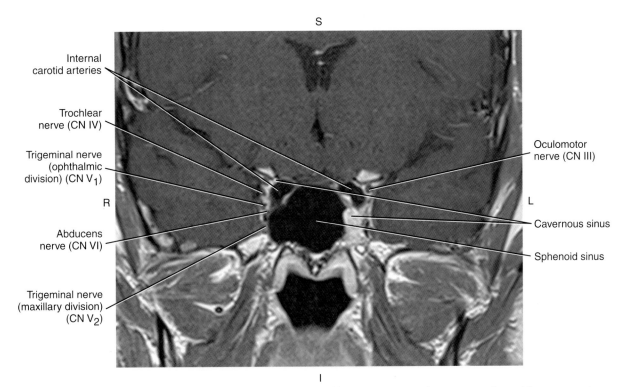

FIGURE 3.137 Coronal, T1-weighted MRI of oculomotor (CN III) and trochlear (CN IV) nerves in cavernous sinus with contrast enhancement.

Trochlear Nerve (CN IV)

The **trochlear nerve** innervates only the superior oblique muscle of the eye. It is the only cranial nerve that emerges from the posterior surface of the brainstem (Figures 3.58 and 3.136). The nerve originates in the tegmentum and exits the posterior surface of the midbrain. It travels around the brainstem to enter the cavernous sinus just below the oculomotor nerve. This nerve enters the orbit through the superior orbital fissure, where it finally reaches the superior oblique muscle (Figures 3.132, 3.134, 3.136, and 3.137).

Trigeminal Nerve (CN V)

The **trigeminal nerve**, the largest of the cranial nerves, has three major divisions: ophthalmic, maxillary, and mandibular (Figure 3.138). It is the major sensory nerve of the face and contains motor fibers for the muscles of mastication and sensory fibers from the head. The nerve exits the brain between the pons and the middle cerebellar peduncles. Before trifurcating into three branches, the nerve enters Meckel's cave and forms the trigeminal ganglion, where it is covered in dura, resulting in a CSF-filled subarachnoid space referred to as the trigeminal cistern (Figures 3.148 and 3.138 through 3.141). The **ophthalmic branch** (V_1) runs through the lateral wall of the cavernous sinus and enters the orbit through the superior orbital fissure, where it branches again to provide sensation to the lacrimal apparatus, cornea, iris, forehead, ethmoid and frontal sinuses, and nose. The **maxillary branch** (V_2) courses in the lateral wall of the cavernous

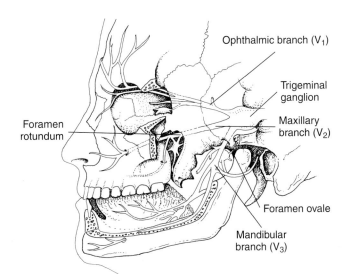

FIGURE 3.138 Sagittal view of trigeminal nerve (CN V).

sinus and exits the skull through the foramen rotundum (Figure 3.134). Branches of the maxillary nerve continue through the inferior orbital fissure and infraorbital foramen. This branch provides sensation to the cheek, sides of the nose and upper jaw, and maxillary sinuses. The **mandibular branch** (V_3) is considered a "motor" nerve and exits the skull through the foramen ovale. It innervates the muscles of mastication, ear canal, lower jaw and teeth, parotid and sublingual glands, and anterior two thirds of the tongue (Figures 3.138 through 3.141).

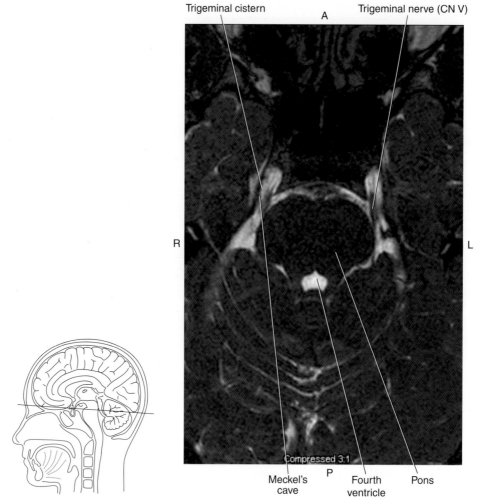

Trigeminal cistern   A   Trigeminal nerve (CN V)

R   L

Compressed 3:1

Meckel's cave   P   Fourth ventricle   Pons

FIGURE 3.139 Axial, T2-weighted MRI of trigeminal nerve (CN V).

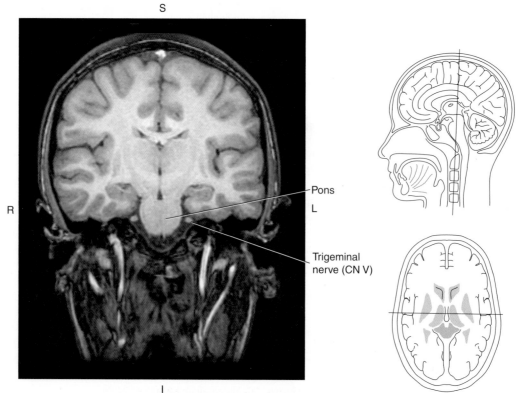

S

R   L

Pons

Trigeminal nerve (CN V)

I

FIGURE 3.140 Coronal, T1-weighted MRI of trigeminal nerve (CN V).

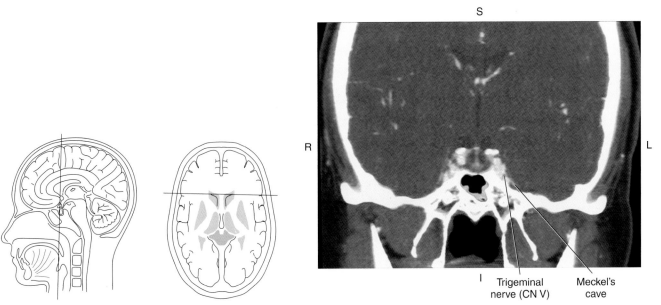

FIGURE 3.141 Coronal CT reformat of Meckel's cave.

Tic douloureux (trigeminal neuralgia) is a neurologic syndrome involving the trigeminal nerve. Usually occurring in middle age, this syndrome is characterized by short stabbing pains along the distribution of the trigeminal nerve.

Abducens Nerve (CN VI)

The **abducens nerve** supplies motor impulses to the lateral rectus muscle of the eye. It originates near the midline of the lower portion of the pons and ascends through the prepontine cistern to the cavernous sinus. Of all the cranial nerves within the cavernous sinus, the abducens nerve courses most medial. It exits the skull through the superior orbital fissure, where it meets up with the lateral rectus muscle (Figures 3.132 through 3.134, 3.137, and 3.142).

Facial Nerve (CN VII)

The **facial nerve** emerges as two distinct roots from the lower portion of the pons in a recess between the olive and inferior cerebellar peduncle and enters the internal auditory canal of

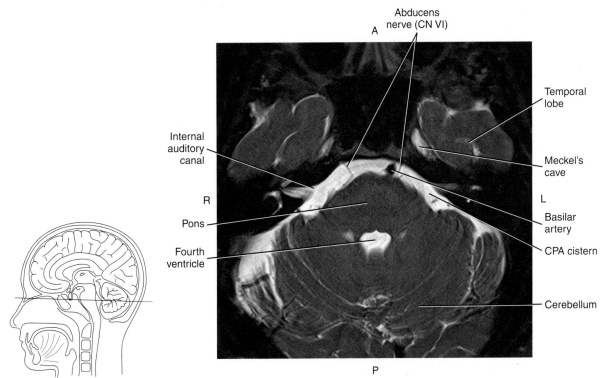

FIGURE 3.142 Axial, T2-weighted MRI of abducens nerve (CN VI).

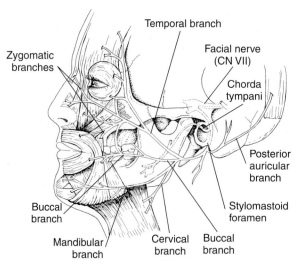

FIGURE 3.143 Sagittal view of facial nerve (CN VII) branches.

the temporal bone (Figure 3.58). After passing through the temporal bone, the nerve continues along the facial canal, where it finally emerges from the skull through the stylomastoid foramen and runs through the parotid gland (see Chapter 2, temporal bone). This nerve innervates the facial muscles, lacrimal gland, and sublingual and submandibular glands. In addition, it provides taste sensation to the anterior two thirds of the tongue (Figures 3.143 and 3.145 through 3.147).

A type of temporary facial nerve paralysis is called Bell's palsy. Many scientists believe that a viral infection may cause the facial nerve to become inflamed and to swell, causing the resultant paralysis. Symptoms include mild weakness, twitching, a drooping eyelid or corner of the mouth, excessive tearing, and drooling.

Vestibulocochlear Nerve (CN VIII)

The **vestibulocochlear nerve** exits the brainstem at the pontomedullary junction and enters the internal auditory canal behind the facial nerve (Figure 3.58). The vestibulocochlear nerve has two distinct components, vestibular and cochlear. The **vestibular branch** picks up impulses from the semicircular canals that aid in the maintenance of equilibrium. The **cochlear branch** receives impulses from the cochlea and separates these impulses into high and low frequencies for the interpretation of sound (Figures 3.144 through 3.146).

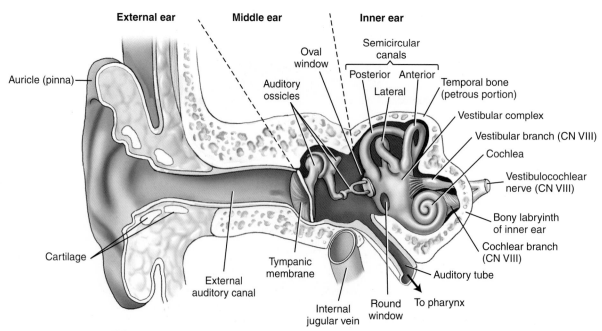

FIGURE 3.144 Coronal view of vestibulocochlear nerve (CN VIII) within inner ear.

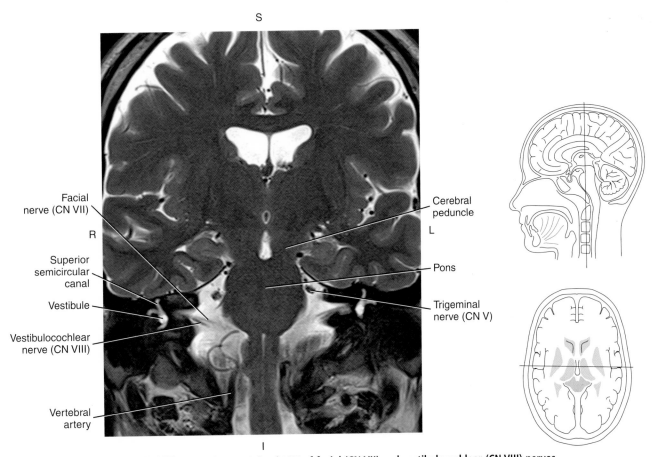

FIGURE 3.145 Coronal, T2-weighted MRI of facial (CN VII) and vestibulocochlear (CN VIII) nerves.

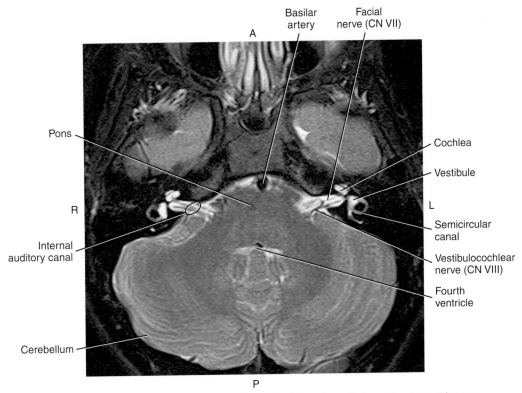

FIGURE 3.146 Axial, T2-weighted MRI of facial (CN VII) and vestibulocochlear (CN VIII) nerves.

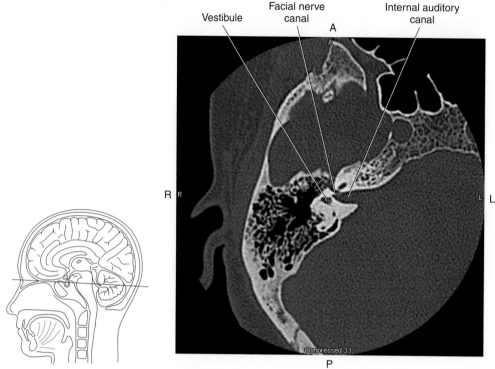

FIGURE 3.147 Axial CT of internal auditory canal.

Glossopharyngeal Nerve (CN IX)

The **glossopharyngeal nerve** supplies motor impulses to the muscles involved in swallowing. In addition, its sensory component can be divided into three groups: group 1 innervates the posterior third of the tongue, Group 2 provides sensory input of pain and temperature from the middle ear, and group 3 gathers sensory input from the carotid sinus and carotid body. The carotid sinus is a dilatation at the origin of the internal carotid artery that contains baroreceptors, which react to changes in arterial blood pressure. The carotid body, a small neurovascular structure located at the bifurcation of the common carotid artery, acts as a chemoreceptor, which senses changes in the chemical composition of blood. The glossopharyngeal nerve emerges as a series of rootlets from the medulla oblongata between the olive and inferior cerebellar peduncles (Figure 3.58). It exits the cranium through the jugular foramen and courses to the root of the tongue (Figures 3.148 through 3.150).

Vagus Nerve (CN X)

In Latin, vagus means wandering, which the **vagus nerve** does as it "wanders" inferiorly from the brainstem to the splenic flexure in the abdomen. The vagus nerve covers an extensive course to supply to areas of the neck, thorax, and abdomen. The vagus nerve arises from the medulla oblongata as 8 to 10 roots between the inferior cerebellar peduncle and the olive, eventually converging into two roots that exit the skull through the jugular

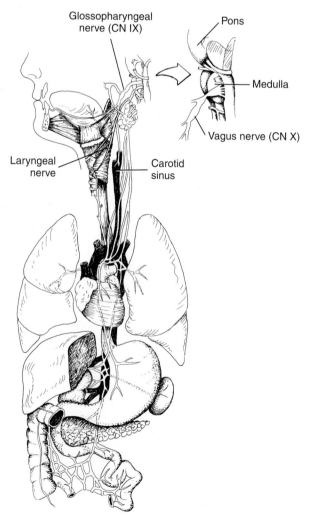

FIGURE 3.148 Glossopharyngeal (CN IX) and vagus (CN X) nerves.

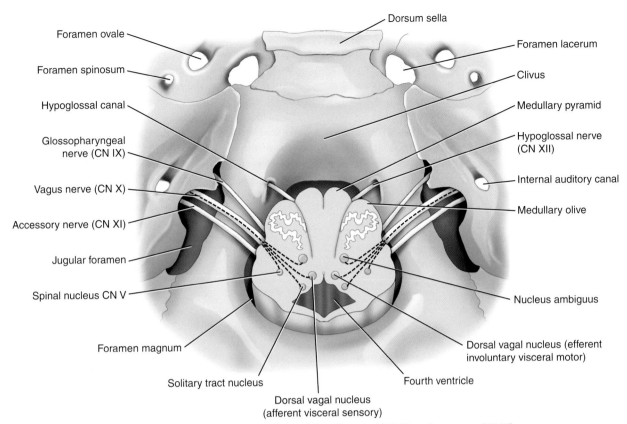

Foramen ovale

Foramen spinosum

Hypoglossal canal

Glossopharyngeal nerve (CN IX)

Vagus nerve (CN X)

Accessory nerve (CN XI)

Jugular foramen

Spinal nucleus CN V

Foramen magnum

Solitary tract nucleus

Dorsal vagal nucleus (afferent visceral sensory)

Dorsum sella

Foramen lacerum

Clivus

Medullary pyramid

Hypoglossal nerve (CN XII)

Internal auditory canal

Medullary olive

Nucleus ambiguus

Dorsal vagal nucleus (efferent involuntary visceral motor)

Fourth ventricle

FIGURE 3.149 Axial view of glossopharyngeal (CN IX), vagus (CN X), and accessory (CN XI) nerves.

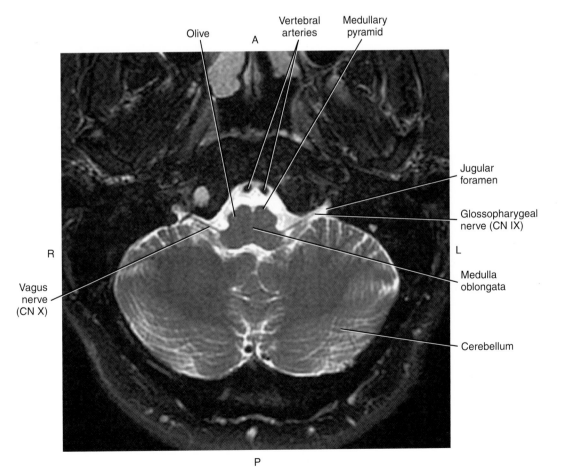

Olive

A

Vertebral arteries

Medullary pyramid

R

L

Vagus nerve (CN X)

P

Jugular foramen

Glossopharygeal nerve (CN IX)

Medulla oblongata

Cerebellum

FIGURE 3.150 Axial, T2-weighted MRI of jugular foramen and glossopharyngeal (CN IX) and vagus (CN X) nerves.

foramen (Figure 3.58). It descends through the carotid sheath while in the neck and continues inferiorly to the thorax and abdomen. At the neck, it passes through the superior thoracic aperture between the subclavian artery and brachiocephalic vein, where it continues its course toward the diaphragm behind the respective main bronchi. There are many branches of the vagus nerve that supply such structures as the dura of the posterior fossa, auricle, external auditory meatus, pharynx, soft palate, larynx, heart, stomach, liver, duodenum, and pancreas (Figures 3.148 through 3.151).

Accessory Nerve (CN XI)

The **accessory nerve** has both cranial and spinal roots. These two roots form a common stem before their exit through the jugular foramen. The cranial root, an accessory to the vagus nerve, emerges from a series of rootlets arising from the medulla oblongata (Figure 3.58). These fibers supply the skeletal muscles of the pharynx and palate. The spinal root arises from a series of rootlets from the lateral cervical cord to innervate the sternomastoid and trapezius muscles in the neck and back (Figures 3.149, 3.151, and 3.152).

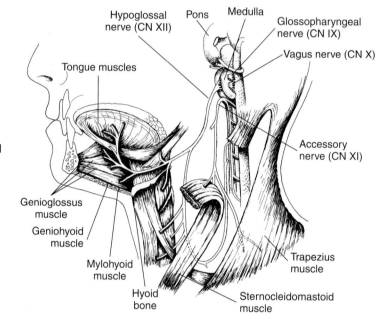

FIGURE 3.151 Sagittal view of accessory (CN XI) and hypoglossal (CN XII) nerves.

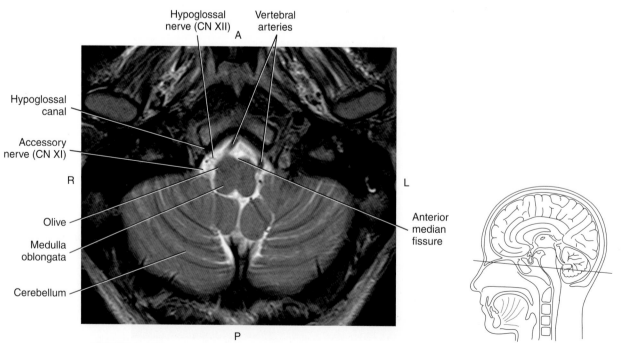

FIGURE 3.152 Axial, T2-weighted MRI of accessory (CN XI) and hypoglossal (CN XII) nerves.

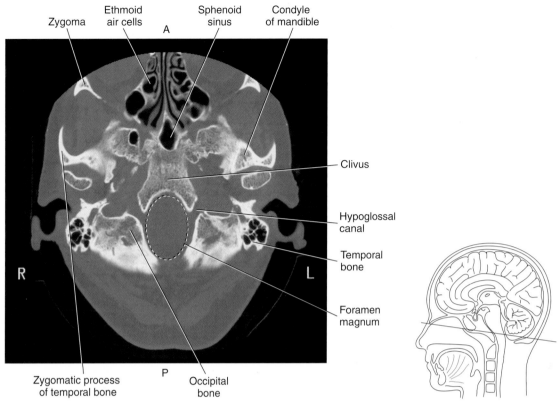

FIGURE 3.153 Axial CT of occipital condyles and hypoglossal canal.

Hypoglossal Nerve (CN XII)

All of the muscles of the tongue with the exception of one are supplied by the **hypoglossal nerve**. Several rootlets arise from the medulla oblongata between the olive and the medullary pyramids (Figure 3.58). The rootlets unite to form a trunk that passes posterior to the vertebral artery to exit the cranium through the hypoglossal canal of the occipital bone. Inferior to the skull, the hypoglossal nerve crosses lateral to the bifurcation of the common carotid artery to enter the floor of the mouth and innervate the muscles of the tongue (Figures 3.151 through 3.153).

REFERENCES

Ballinger PW: *Merrill's atlas of radiographic positions and radiologic procedures*, ed 12, St. Louis, 2012, Mosby.

Som PM, Curtin HD: *Head and neck imaging*, ed 5, St. Louis, Mosby, 2012.

Standring S: *Gray's anatomy*, ed 40, Philadelphia, 2009, Churchill Livingstone.

Spine

When you suffer an attack of
nerves you're being attacked by the nervous system.
What chance has a man got against a system?

Russell Hoban (1925-), American writer and illustrator

The spine functions to protect the delicate sensory and motor nerves that allow for peripheral sensations and body movement. Sensory or neurologic loss can be a result of injury or pathologic abnormalities of any of the many areas that constitute the normal anatomy of this region (Figure 4.1).

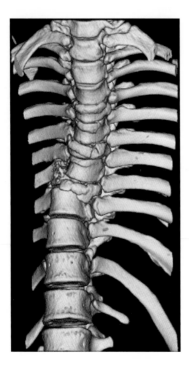

FIGURE 4.1 Posttraumatic fractures of the thoracic spine.

OBJECTIVES

- Identify the structures of a typical vertebra.
- Identify the atypical structures of the atlas and axis, thoracic vertebrae, sacrum, and coccyx.
- Identify and explain the function of the spinal ligaments.
- Define the action of and identify the muscle groups of the spine.

- Describe the components of the spinal cord and spinal nerves.
- Describe the four plexuses of the spinal cord and list the structures they innervate.
- Identify the vasculature of the spine and spinal cord.

OUTLINE

VERTEBRAL COLUMN

The **vertebral column** is a remarkable structure that supports the weight of the body, helps to maintain posture, and protects the delicate spinal cord and nerves. It is made up of 33 vertebrae, which can be separated into cervical, thoracic, lumbar, sacral, and coccygeal sections. Curvatures associated with the vertebral column provide spinal flexibility and distribute compressive forces over the spine. The cervical and lumbar sections convex forward, creating lordotic curves, and the thoracic and sacral sections convex backward, creating kyphotic curves (Figure 4.2).

Vertebrae vary in size and shape from section to section, but a typical vertebra consists of two main parts: the **body (anterior element)** and the **vertebral arch (posterior element)**. The cylindrical body is anteriorly located and functions to support body weight (Figures 4.3 and 4.4). The size of the vertebral bodies progressively increases from the superior to the inferior portion of the spine. The compact bone on the superior and inferior surfaces of the body is called the **vertebral end plate**. Located posteriorly is the ringlike arch that attaches to the sides of the body, creating a space called the **vertebral foramen**. The succession of the vertebral foramina forms the **vertebral canal**, which contains and protects the spinal cord. The vertebral arch is formed by pedicles (2), laminae (2), spinous process (1), transverse processes (2), and superior (2) and inferior (2) articular processes (Figures 4.3 through 4.6). The two **pedicles** project from the body to meet with two **laminae**, which continue posteriorly and medially to form a **spinous process**. The **transverse processes** project laterally from the approximate junction of the pedicle and lamina (Figures 4.3 and 4.4). On the upper and lower surfaces of the pedicles is a concave surface termed the **vertebral notch** (Figures 4.5 and 4.6). When the superior and inferior notches of adjacent vertebrae meet, they form **intervertebral foramina**, which allow for the transmission of spinal nerves and blood vessels (Figure 4.6). Four **articular processes**, two superior and two inferior, arise from the junctions of the pedicles and laminae to articulate with adjacent vertebrae and form the **zygapophyseal joints (facet joints)**. These joints give additional support and allow movement of the vertebral column (Figures 4.7 through 4.10). The vertebral bodies are separated by shock-absorbing cartilaginous **intervertebral disks**. These disks consist of a central mass of soft semigelatinous material called the **nucleus pulposus** and a firm outer portion termed the **annulus fibrosus** (Figures 4.9 through 4.12).

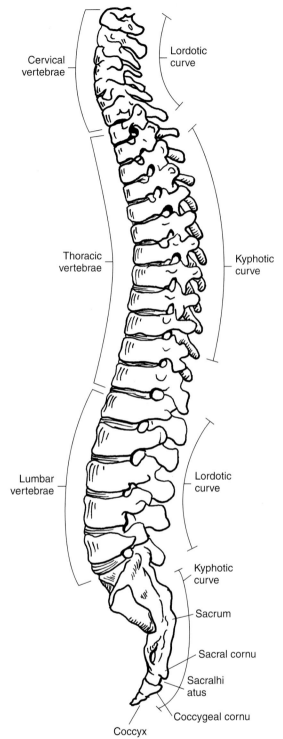

FIGURE 4.2 Lateral view of the spine.

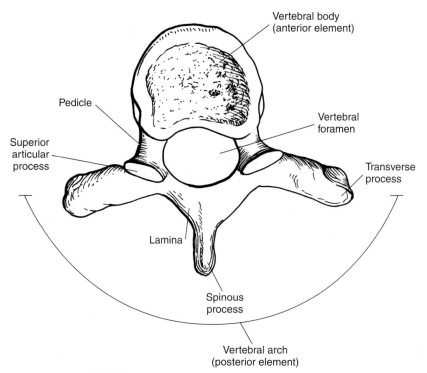

FIGURE 4.3 Superior view of the typical vertebra.

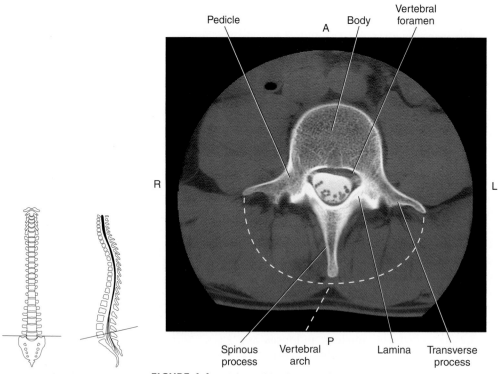

FIGURE 4.4 Axial CT of lumbar vertebra.

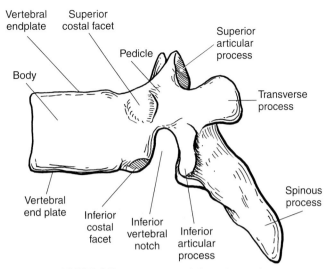

FIGURE 4.5 Lateral view of thoracic vertebra.

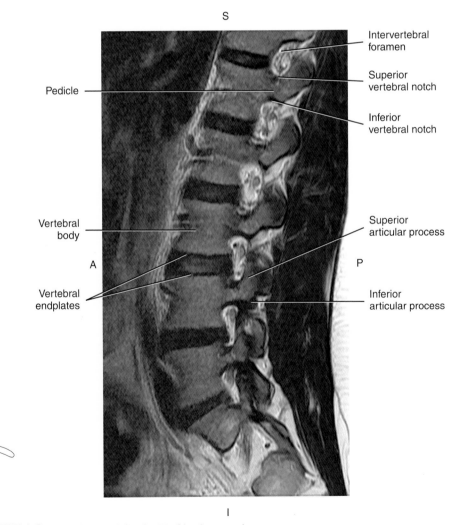

FIGURE 4.6 Sagittal, T2-weighted MRI of lumbar vertebrae.

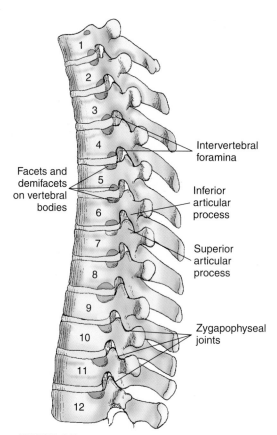

FIGURE 4.7 Lateral oblique view of thoracic spine.

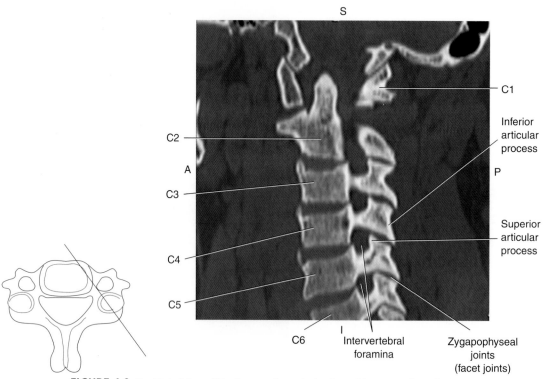

FIGURE 4.8 Sagittal oblique CT reformat of cervical spine with zygapophyseal joints.

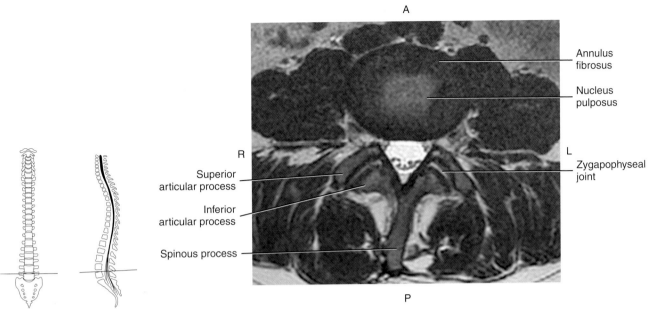

A

Annulus
fibrosus

Nucleus
pulposus

R

L

Superior
articular process

Zygapophyseal
joint

Inferior
articular process

Spinous process

P

FIGURE 4.9 Axial, T2-weighted MRI of lumbar spine with intervertebral disk and zygapophyseal joint.

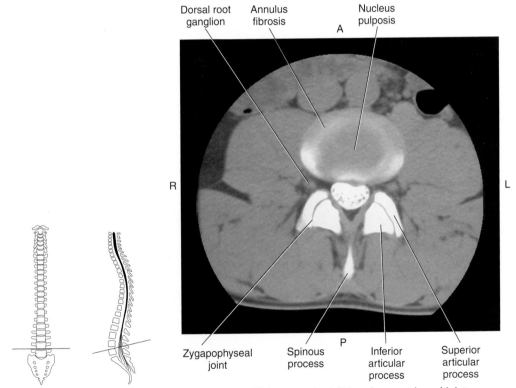

Dorsal root
ganglion

Annulus
fibrosis

Nucleus
pulposis

A

R

L

Zygapophyseal
joint

Spinous
process

P

Inferior
articular
process

Superior
articular
process

FIGURE 4.10 Axial CT of lumbar spine with intervertebral disk and zygapophyseal joint.

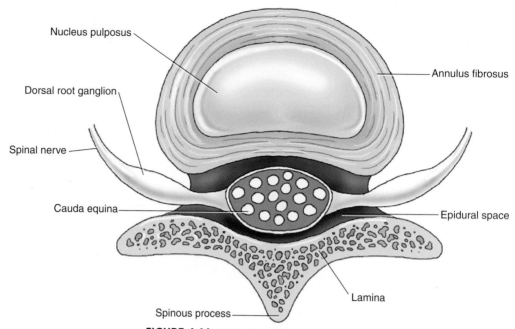

FIGURE 4.11 Axial view of intervertebral disk.

Nucleus pulposus

Annulus fibrosus

Dorsal root ganglion

Spinal nerve

Cauda equina

Epidural space

Lamina

Spinous process

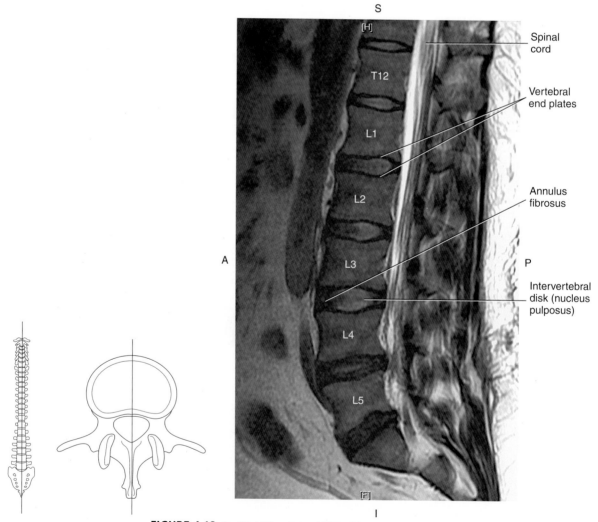

FIGURE 4.12 Sagittal, T2-weighted MRI of intervertebral disk.

S

[H]

T12

L1

L2

A   L3   P

L4

L5

[F]

I

Spinal cord

Vertebral end plates

Annulus fibrosus

Intervertebral disk (nucleus pulposus)

Cervical Vertebrae

There are seven cervical vertebrae that vary in size and shape. Within the transverse process of each cervical vertebra is a **transverse foramen** (Figures 4.13 and 4.14). These foramina allow passage of the vertebral arteries and veins as they ascend to and descend from the head. The **first cervical vertebra** is termed the **atlas** because it supports the head; its large **superior articular processes** articulate with the occipital condyles of the cranium to form the **atlantooccipital joint**. The atlas is a ringlike structure that has no body and no spinous process. It consists of an **anterior arch, posterior arch,** and two large **lateral masses** (Figures 4.13 through 4.15). The lateral masses provide the only weight-bearing articulation between the cranium and vertebral column.

The **second cervical vertebra,** the **axis,** has a large **odontoid process (dens)** that projects upward from the superior surface of the body. The odontoid process projects

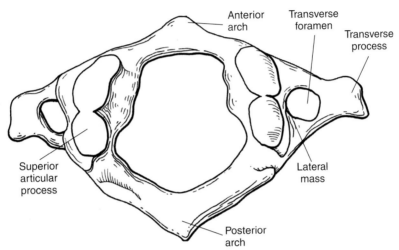

FIGURE 4.13 Superior view of C1 (atlas).

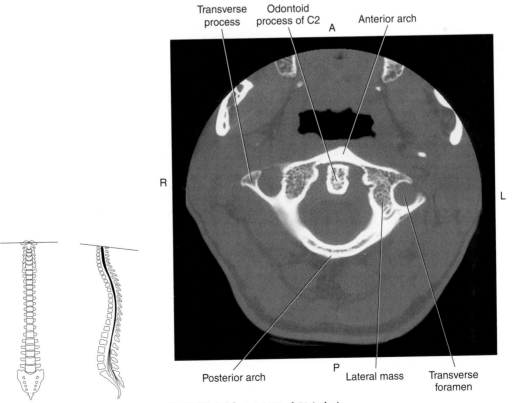

FIGURE 4.14 Axial CT of C1 (atlas).

into the anterior ring of the atlas to act as a pivot for rotational movement of the atlas (Figures 4.14 through 4.19). Lateral to the odontoid process on the upper surface of the body are the superior articular processes, on which the atlas articulates at the **atlantoaxial joint** (Figures 4.15 through 4.17 and 4.19 through 4.21). The spinous process of the axis is the first projection to be felt in the posterior groove of the neck. The cervical vertebrae C3-C6 have a unique configuration with their **bifid spinous processes** (Figures 4.22 and 4.23). The seventh cervical vertebra (**vertebra prominens**) has a long spinous process that is typically not bifid. This spinous process is easily palpable posteriorly at the base of the neck (Figures 4.24 through 4.26).

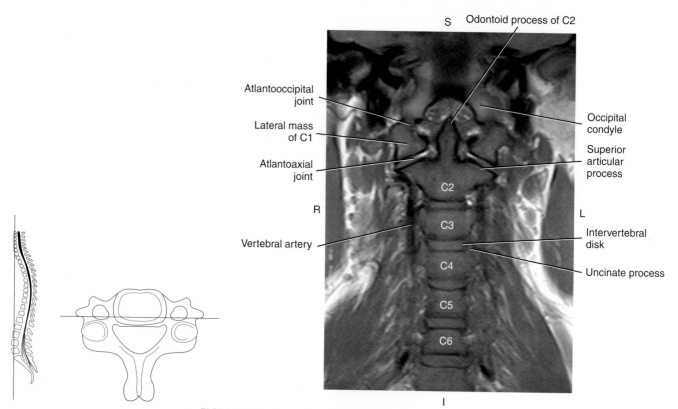

FIGURE 4.15 Coronal, T1-weighted MRI of cervical spine.

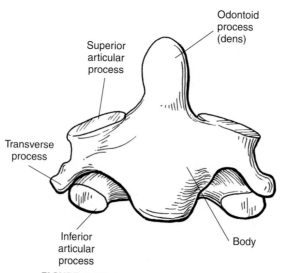

FIGURE 4.16 Anterior view of C2 (axis).

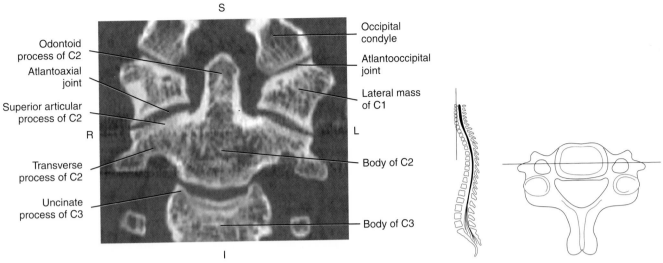

FIGURE 4.17 Coronal CT reformat of C1 (atlas) and C2 (axis).

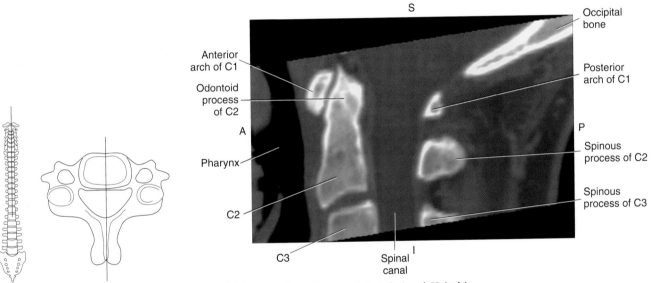

FIGURE 4.18 Sagittal CT reformat of C1 (atlas) and C2 (axis).

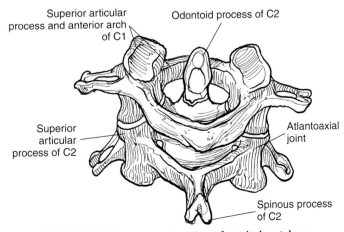

FIGURE 4.19 Posterosuperior view of cervical vertebrae.

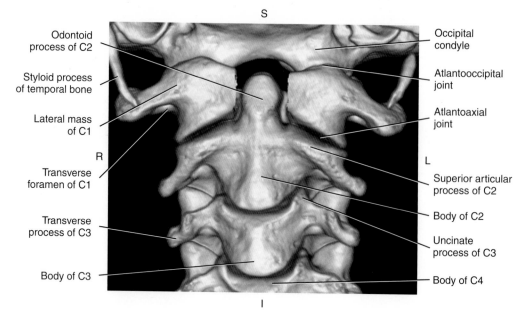

FIGURE 4.20 3D CT of cervical vertebrae, anterior view.

Odontoid process of C2

Styloid process of temporal bone

Lateral mass of C1

Transverse foramen of C1

Transverse process of C3

Body of C3

S

R

L

I

Occipital condyle

Atlantooccipital joint

Atlantoaxial joint

Superior articular process of C2

Body of C2

Uncinate process of C3

Body of C4

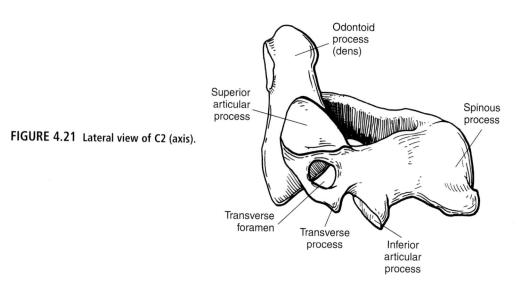

FIGURE 4.21 Lateral view of C2 (axis).

Odontoid process (dens)

Superior articular process

Spinous process

Transverse foramen

Transverse process

Inferior articular process

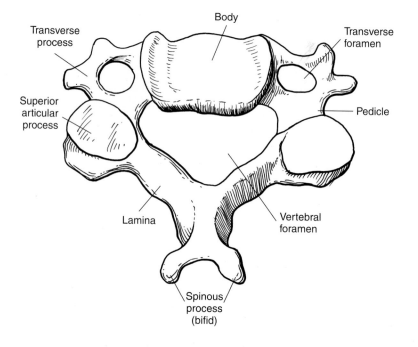

FIGURE 4.22 Superior view of cervical vertebra with bifid spinous process.

Transverse process

Body

Transverse foramen

Superior articular process

Pedicle

Lamina

Vertebral foramen

Spinous process (bifid)

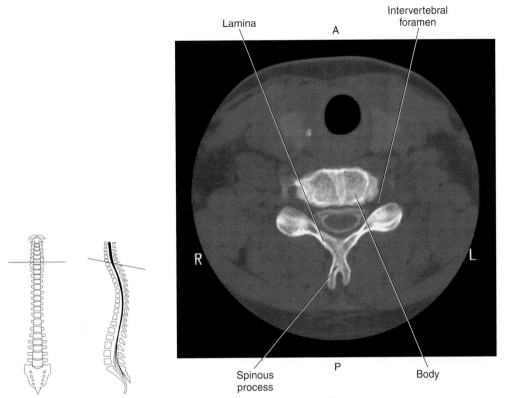

FIGURE 4.23 Axial CT of cervical vertebra with bifid spinous process.

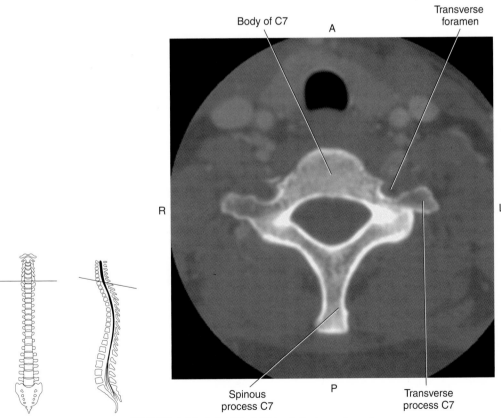

FIGURE 4.24 Axial CT of C7 (vertebral prominens).

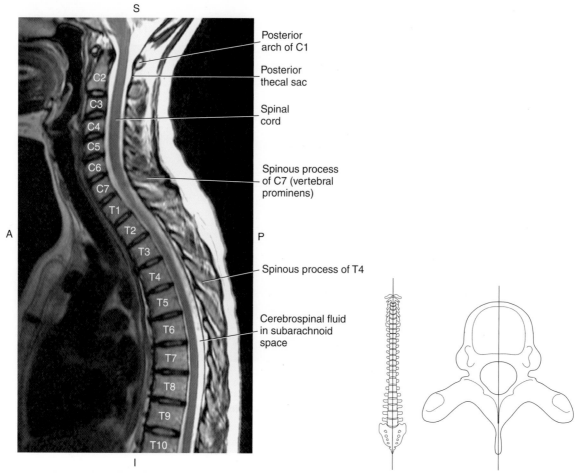

FIGURE 4.25 Midsagittal, T2-weighted MRI of cervical and thoracic spine.

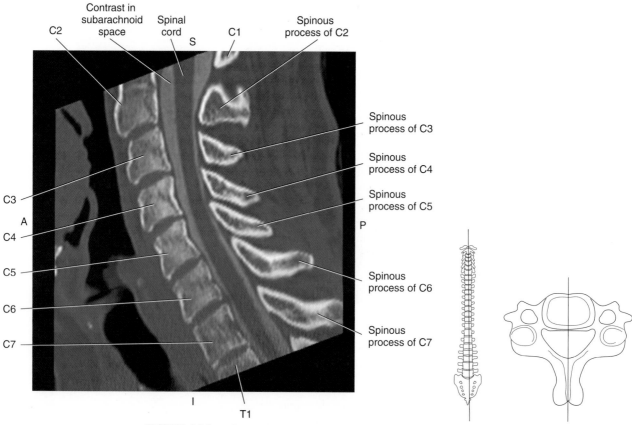

FIGURE 4.26 Midsagittal CT reformat of cervical spine, post myelogram.

Thoracic Vertebrae

Twelve vertebrae make up the thoracic section. They have typical vertebral configurations except for their characteristic **costal facets (demi facets)**, located on the body and transverse processes, that articulate with the ribs. The head of the rib articulates with the vertebral bodies at the **costovertebral joints**, whereas the tubercle of the ribs articulates with the transverse processes at the **costotransverse joints**. The spinous processes of the thoracic vertebrae are typically long and slender, projecting inferiorly over the vertebral arches of the vertebrae below (Figures 4.25, 4.27 through 4.29).

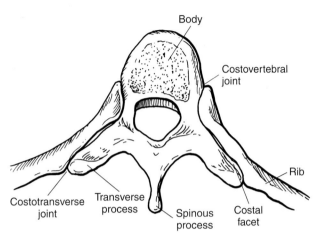

FIGURE 4.27 Superior view of thoracic vertebra.

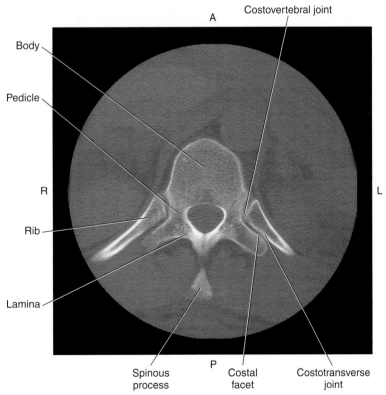

FIGURE 4.28 Axial CT of thoracic vertebra.

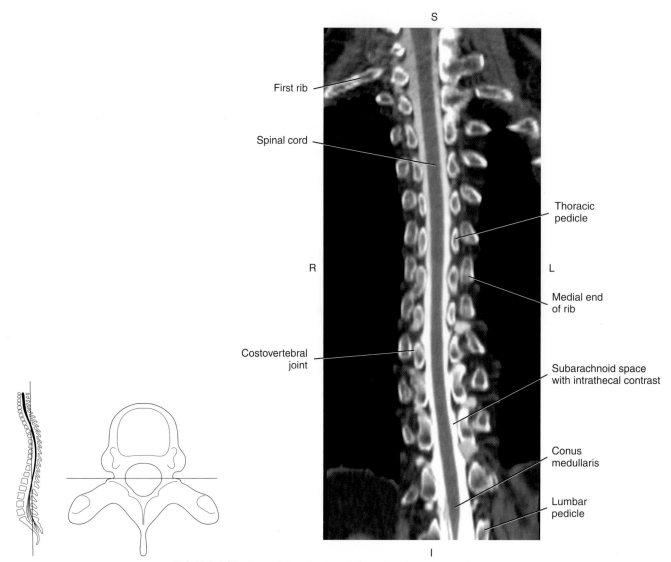

S

First rib

Spinal cord

Thoracic
pedicle

R

L

Medial end
of rib

Costovertebral
joint

Subarachnoid space
with intrathecal contrast

Conus
medullaris

Lumbar
pedicle

I

FIGURE 4.29 Coronal CT reformat of thoracic spine, post myelogram.

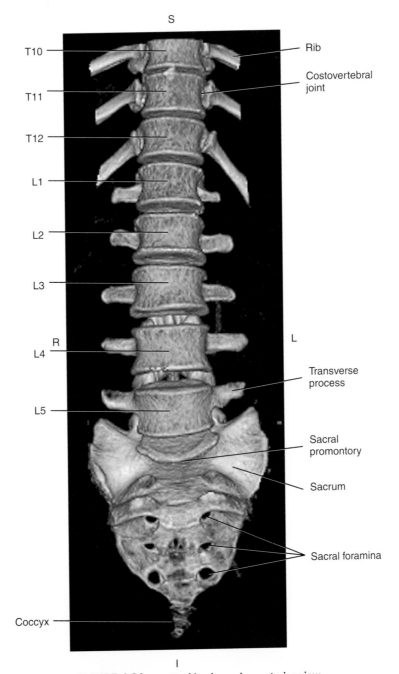

FIGURE 4.30 3D CT of lumbar spine, anterior view.

Lumbar Vertebrae

The **lumbar** section typically consists of five vertebrae. Their massive bodies increase in size from superior to inferior (Figure 4.30). The largest of the lumbar vertebrae, L5, is characterized by its massive transverse processes. The entire weight of the upper body is transferred from the fifth lumbar vertebra to the base of the sacrum across the L5-S1 intervertebral disk (Figures 4.31 through 4.35).

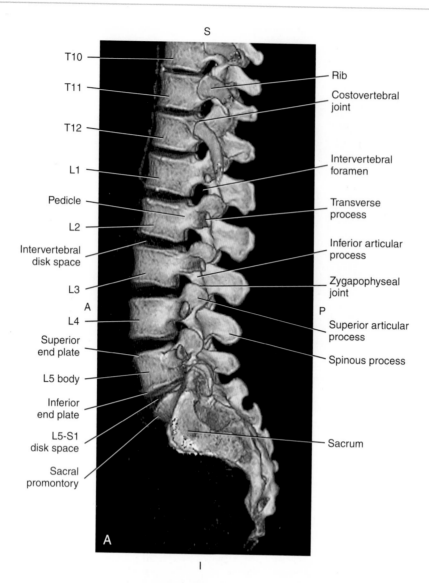

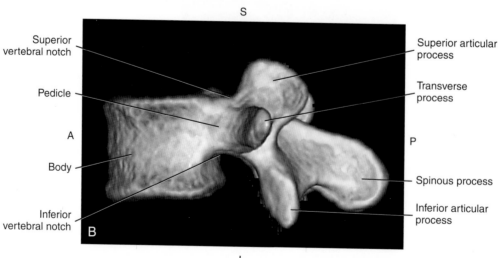

FIGURE 4.31 A, 3D CT of lumbar spine, lateral view. B, 3D CT of lumbar vertebra, lateral view.

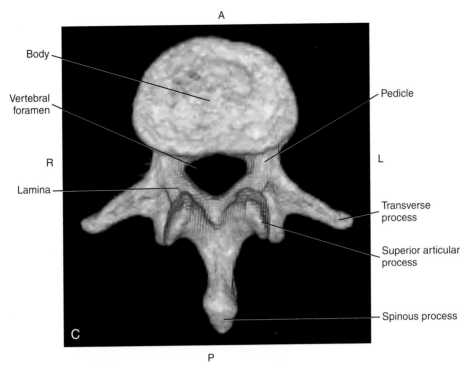

A

Body

Vertebral foramen

Pedicle

R

L

Lamina

Transverse process

Superior articular process

Spinous process

C

P

FIGURE 4.31 cont'd C, 3D CT of lumbar vertebra, superior view.

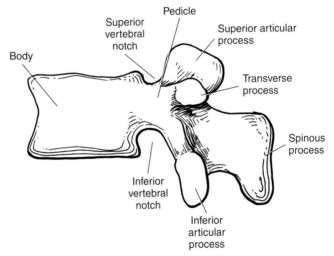

Pedicle

Superior vertebral notch

Superior articular process

Body

Transverse process

Spinous process

Inferior vertebral notch

Inferior articular process

FIGURE 4.32 Lateral view of lumbar vertebra.

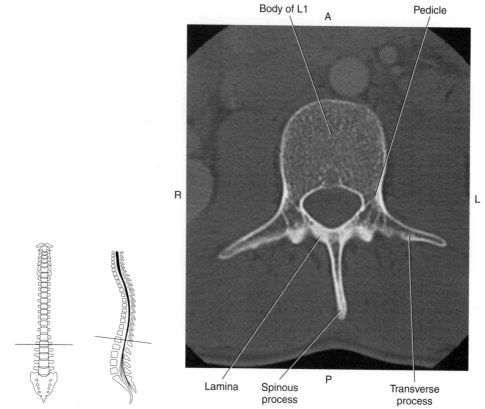

Body of L1

A

Pedicle

R

L

Lamina

Spinous
process

P

Transverse
process

FIGURE 4.33 Axial CT of lumbar vertebra.

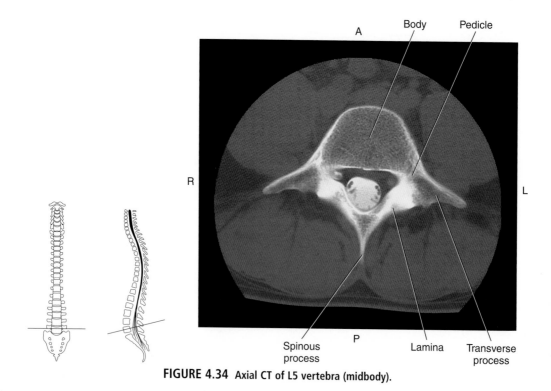

A

Body

Pedicle

R

L

Spinous
process

P

Lamina

Transverse
process

FIGURE 4.34 Axial CT of L5 vertebra (midbody).

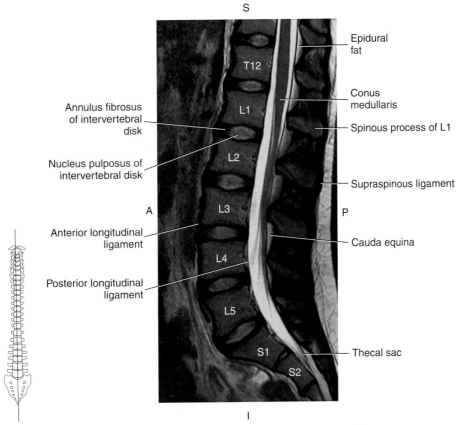

S

T12

Epidural fat

Annulus fibrosus of intervertebral disk

L1

Conus medullaris

Spinous process of L1

Nucleus pulposus of intervertebral disk

L2

A

L3

P

Supraspinous ligament

Anterior longitudinal ligament

Cauda equina

L4

Posterior longitudinal ligament

L5

S1

Thecal sac

S2

I

FIGURE 4.35 Midsagittal, T2-weighted MRI of lumbar spine.

Sacrum and Coccyx

The sacral section consists of five vertebrae that fuse to form the **sacrum**. Their transverse processes combine to form the **lateral masses (ala)**, which articulate with the pelvic bones at the **sacroiliac joints**. Located within the lateral masses are the **sacral foramina** that allow for the passage of nerves (Figures 4.30, 4.36, and 4.37). The first sacral segment has a prominent ridge located on the anterior surface of the body termed the **sacral promontory** (Figures 4.38 and 4.39). This bony landmark is used to separate the abdominal cavity from the pelvic cavity. The spinous process of the fifth sacral segment is absent, leaving an opening termed the **sacral hiatus** (Figure 4.2). Located at the sides of the sacral hiatus are

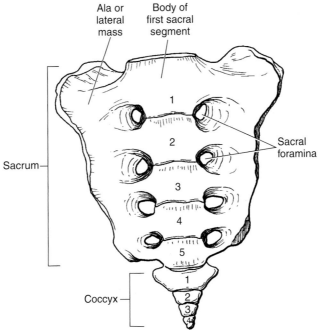

Ala or lateral mass

Body of first sacral segment

1

2

Sacral foramina

Sacrum

3

4

5

1

Coccyx

2
3
4

FIGURE 4.36 Anterior view of sacrum and coccyx.

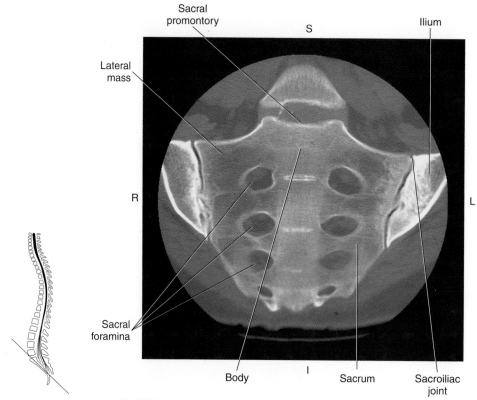

FIGURE 4.37 Coronal CT of sacrum and coccyx.

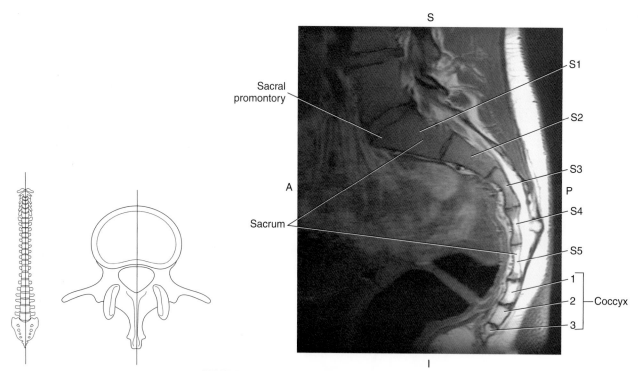

FIGURE 4.38 Sagittal, T1-weighted MRI of sacrum.

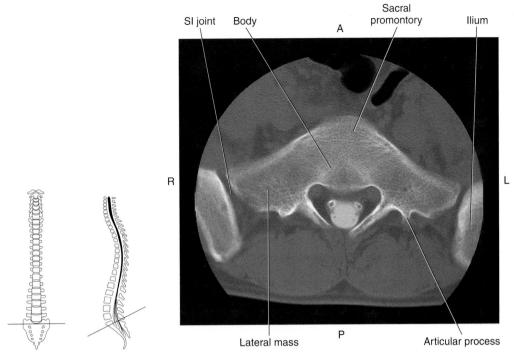

FIGURE 4.39 Axial CT of sacrum and sacroiliac joints.

the inferior articular processes of the fifth sacral segment, which project downward as the **sacral cornu**. Located inferior to the fifth sacral segment is the **coccyx**, which consists of three to five small fused bony segments (Figures 4.36 and 4.38). Superior projections off the first coccygeal segment, called **cornu**, have ligamentous attachments to the sacral cornu that provide additional stability to the articulation between the sacrum and coccyx. The coccyx represents the most inferior portion of the vertebral column.

LIGAMENTS

Specific ligaments of the spine serve to connect the cervical vertebrae and the cranium to provide mobility and protection for the head and neck. The **apical ligament** is a midline structure that connects the apex of the odontoid process to the inferior margin of the clivus (Figures 4.40 through 4.42). The **alar ligaments** are two strong bands that extend obliquely from the sides of the odontoid process, upward to the lateral margins of the occipital condyles to limit rotation and flexion of the head (Figures 4.43 and 4.44). The **transverse ligament** extends across the vertebral foramen of C1 to form a sling over the posterior surface of the odontoid process. It has a small band of longitudinal fibers that ascend to attach to the posteroinferior aspect of the clivus and inferiorly to attach to the body of the axis. The transverse ligament holds

the odontoid process of C2 against the anterior arch of C1 (Figures 4.43, 4.45, and 4.46). The transverse ligament is sometimes called the **cruciform ligament** because of its crosslike appearance when viewed in the coronal plane.

Another important ligament of the cervical region is the **ligamentum nuchae**, which serves as an attachment point for muscles. This expansive ligament extends from the external occipital protuberance of the cranium to the spinous processes of the cervical vertebrae (Figures 4.40 through 4.42). The ligamentum nuchae continues inferiorly as the supraspinous ligament. The **supraspinous ligament** is a narrow band of fibers that runs over and connects the tips of the spinous processes from the seventh cervical vertebra to the lower lumbar vertebrae. The **interspinous ligaments** extend between adjacent spinous processes throughout the spinal column (Figures 4.47 through 4.49).

In addition to the ligaments listed earlier, the stability of the suboccipital region of the spine is reinforced with the **atlantooccipital** and **tectorial membranes**. The atlantooccipital membrane consists of an anterior and posterior portion, which serve to connect the arches of the atlas with the occipital bone. The **anterior atlantooccipital membrane** passes from the anterior arch of the atlas and connects to the base of the occipital bone at its anterior margin. This ligament is the superior extension of the anterior longitudinal ligament. The **posterior atlantooccipital membrane** extends from the

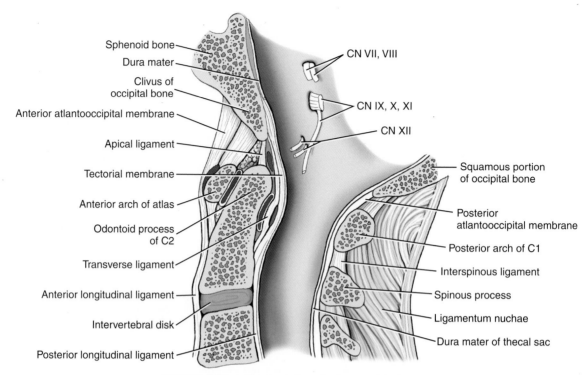

Sphenoid bone

Dura mater

Clivus of
occipital bone

Anterior atlantooccipital membrane

Apical ligament

Tectorial membrane

Anterior arch of atlas

Odontoid process
of C2

Transverse ligament

Anterior longitudinal ligament

Intervertebral disk

Posterior longitudinal ligament

CN VII, VIII

CN IX, X, XI

CN XII

Squamous portion
of occipital bone

Posterior
atlantooccipital membrane

Posterior arch of C1

Interspinous ligament

Spinous process

Ligamentum nuchae

Dura mater of thecal sac

FIGURE 4.40 Midsagittal view of atlantooccipital joint.

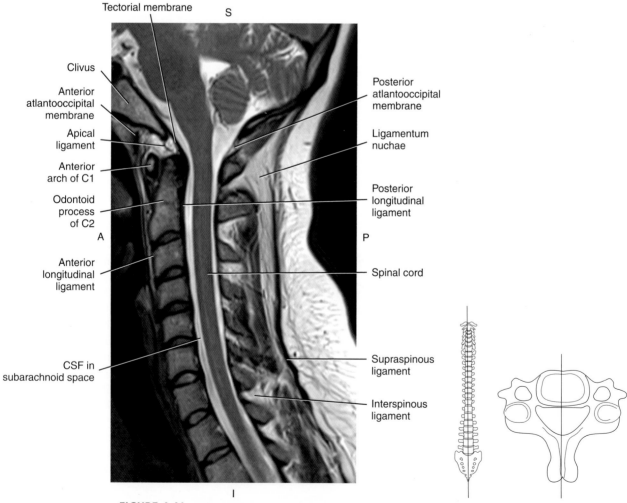

Tectorial membrane

S

Clivus

Anterior
atlantooccipital
membrane

Apical
ligament

Anterior
arch of C1

Odontoid
process
of C2

A

Anterior
longitudinal
ligament

CSF in
subarachnoid space

I

Posterior
atlantooccipital
membrane

Ligamentum
nuchae

Posterior
longitudinal
ligament

P

Spinal cord

Supraspinous
ligament

Interspinous
ligament

FIGURE 4.41 Midsagittal, T2-weighted MRI of cervical spine with spinal ligaments.

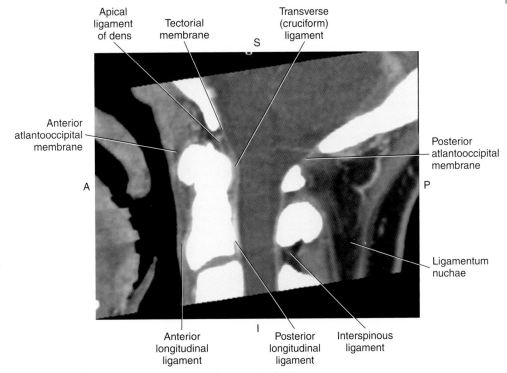

Apical ligament of dens

Tectorial membrane

Transverse (cruciform) ligament

S

Anterior atlantooccipital membrane

A

P

Posterior atlantooccipital membrane

Ligamentum nuchae

Anterior longitudinal ligament

I

Posterior longitudinal ligament

Interspinous ligament

FIGURE 4.42 Sagittal CT reformat of atlantooccipital joint.

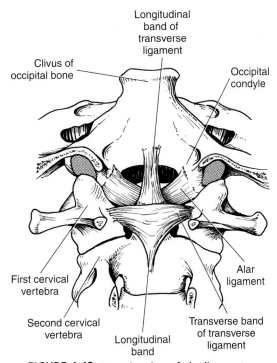

Longitudinal band of transverse ligament

Clivus of occipital bone

Occipital condyle

First cervical vertebra

Alar ligament

Second cervical vertebra

Longitudinal band

Transverse band of transverse ligament

FIGURE 4.43 Posterior view of alar ligaments.

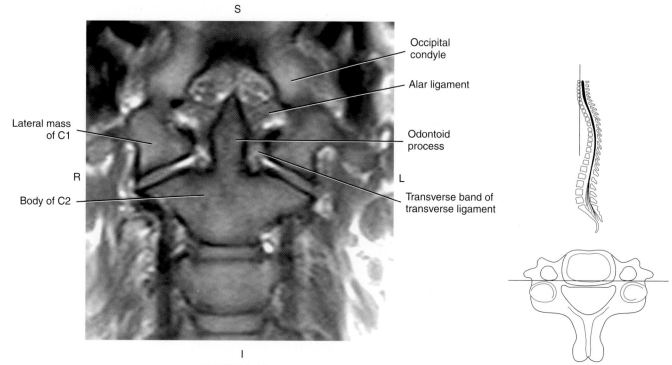

FIGURE 4.44 Coronal, T1-weighted MRI of alar ligaments.

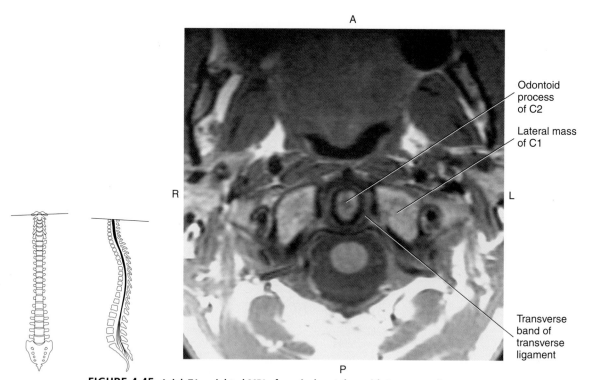

FIGURE 4.45 Axial, T1-weighted MRI of cervical vertebra with transverse ligament.

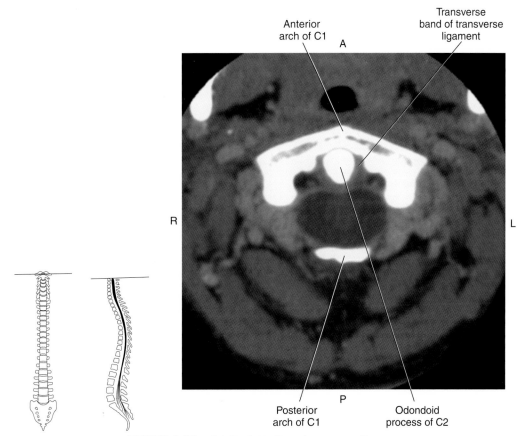

FIGURE 4.46 Axial CT of C1, C2, and transverse ligament.

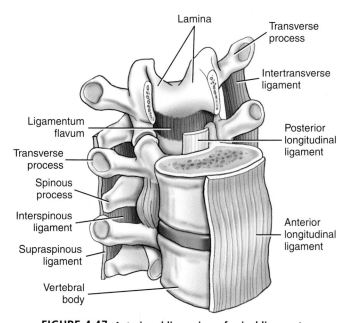

FIGURE 4.47 Anterior oblique view of spinal ligaments.

body of the axis, covering the dens, transverse, apical, and alar ligaments. The tectorial membrane forms the anterior boundary of the vertebral canal and is continuous with the posterior longitudinal ligament (Figures 4.40 through 4.42).

Several ligaments enclose the vertebral column to help protect the spinal cord and maintain stability of the vertebral column. Two of the larger ligaments are the anterior and posterior longitudinal ligaments (Figure 4.47). The **anterior longitudinal ligament** is a broad fibrous band that extends downward from C1 along the entire anterior surface of the vertebral bodies to the sacrum. This ligament connects the anterior aspects of the vertebral bodies and intervertebral disks to maintain stability of the joints and to help prevent hyperextension of the vertebral column. It is thicker in the thoracic region than in the cervical and lumbar regions, providing additional support to the thoracic spine. The **posterior longitudinal ligament** is narrower and slightly weaker than the anterior longitudinal ligament. It lies inside the vertebral canal and runs along the posterior aspect of the vertebral bodies (Figures 4.47 through 4.53). Unlike the anterior longitudinal ligament, the posterior longitudinal ligament is attached only at the intervertebral disk and adjacent margins. It is separated from the middle of each vertebra by epidural fat, which provides passage of the basivertebral veins. The posterior longitudinal

posterior arch of C1 to the occipital bone, closing the posterior portion of the vertebral canal between the cranium and C1 (Figures 4.40 through 4.42). The **tectorial membrane** is a broad ligament that extends from the clivus of the occipital bone to the posterior

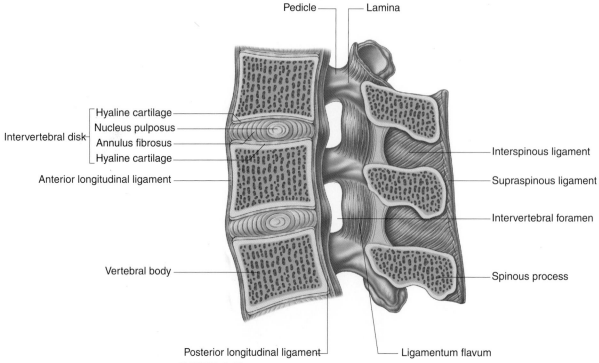

Pedicle — Lamina

Hyaline cartilage
Nucleus pulposus
Intervertebral disk
Annulus fibrosus
Hyaline cartilage

Anterior longitudinal ligament

Vertebral body

Interspinous ligament

Supraspinous ligament

Intervertebral foramen

Spinous process

Posterior longitudinal ligament — Ligamentum flavum

FIGURE 4.48 Midsagittal view of spinal ligaments.

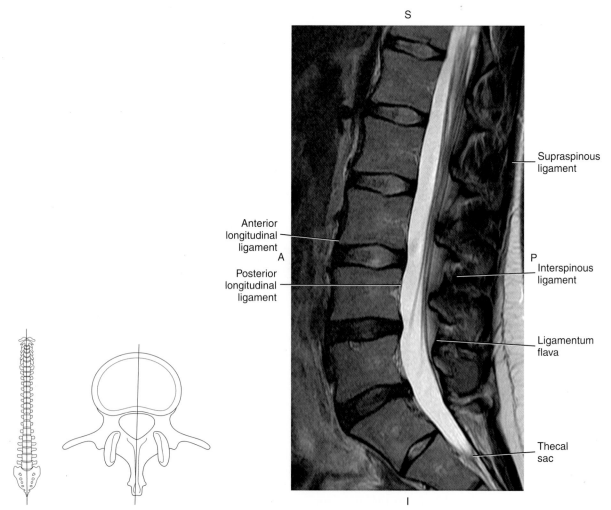

S

Anterior
longitudinal
ligament

A

Posterior
longitudinal
ligament

Supraspinous
ligament

P

Interspinous
ligament

Ligamentum
flava

Thecal
sac

I

FIGURE 4.49 Midsagittal, T2-weighted MRI of lumbar spine with spinal ligaments.

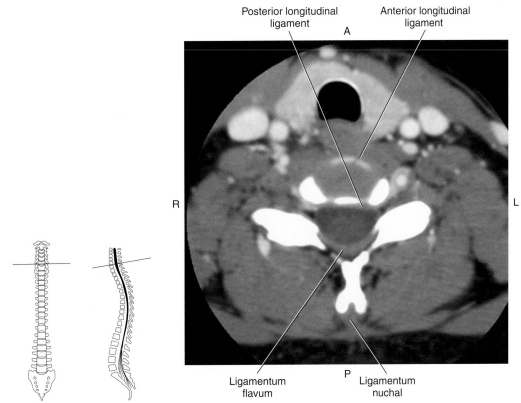

Posterior longitudinal ligament

Anterior longitudinal ligament

A

R

L

Ligamentum flavum

P Ligamentum nuchal

FIGURE 4.50 Axial CT of cervical vertebra with spinal ligaments.

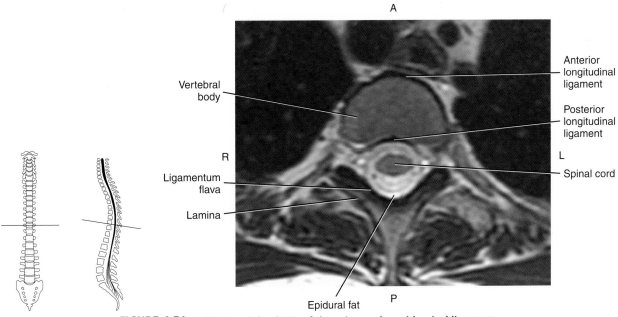

A

Vertebral body

Anterior longitudinal ligament

Posterior longitudinal ligament

R

L

Spinal cord

Ligamentum flava

Lamina

Epidural fat

P

FIGURE 4.51 Axial, T2-weighted MRI of thoracic vertebra with spinal ligaments.

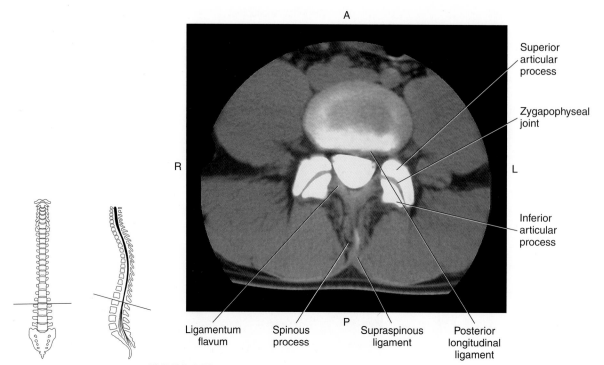

A

Superior
articular
process

Zygapophyseal
joint

R

L

Inferior
articular
process

Ligamentum   Spinous   Supraspinous   Posterior
flavum   process   ligament   longitudinal
                                             ligament

P

FIGURE 4.52 Axial CT of lumbar vertebra with spinal ligaments.

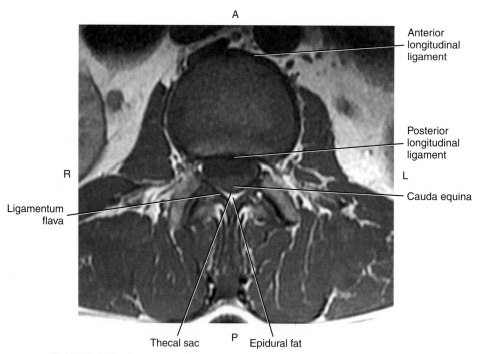

A

Anterior
longitudinal
ligament

Posterior
longitudinal
ligament

R

L

Cauda equina

Ligamentum
flava

Thecal sac   P   Epidural fat

FIGURE 4.53 Axial, T1-weighted MRI of lumbar vertebra with spinal ligaments.

ligament runs the entire length of the vertebral column beginning at C2. This ligament helps to prevent posterior protrusion of the nucleus pulposus and hyperflexion of the vertebral column.

The **ligamentum flava** are strong ligaments (consisting of yellow elastic tissue) present on either side of the spinous process. They join the laminae of adjacent vertebral arches, helping to preserve the normal curvature of the spine (Figures 4.47 through 4.53).

MUSCLES

Muscles of the back can be separated into three groupings or layers; the superficial layer (splenius muscles), the intermediate layer (erector spinae group), and the deep layer (transversospinal group). The muscle groups that run the length of the spine can be divided into regions according to their location: capitis, cervicis, thoracis, and lumborum (Table 4.1).

Superficial Layer

The **splenius muscles** are located on the lateral and posterior aspect of the cervical and upper thoracic spine. These bandage-like muscles originate on the spinous processes of C7-T6 and the inferior half of the ligamentum nuchae. They are divided into a cranial portion, **splenius capitis**, which inserts on the mastoid process of the temporal bone, and a cervical portion, **splenius cervicis**, which inserts on the transverse processes of C1-C3 (Figures 4.54 through 4.57). Together they act to extend the head and neck.

TABLE 4.1	Spinal Muscles	
Muscle	**Origin**	**Insertion**
Splenius		
Splenius capitis	Nuchal ligament and spinous processes of C7-T3	Mastoid process of temporal bone and superior nuchal line of occipital bone
Splenius cervicis		Transverse processes of C1-C3 or C4
Erector Spinae		
Iliocostalis		
Iliocostalis cervicis	Broad tendon arising from posterior iliac crest, sacrum, spinous processes of sacrum and inferior lumbar spine, and supraspinous ligament	Fibers run superiorly to cervical transverse processes and angles of lower ribs
Iliocostalis thoracis		
Iliocostalis lumborum		
Longissimus		
Longissimus capitis	Broad tendon arising from posterior iliac crest, sacrum, spinous processes of sacrum and inferior lumbar spine, and supraspinous ligament	Fibers run superiorly to mastoid process of temporal bone and to transverse processes of thoracic and cervical vertebrae
Longissimus cervicis		
Longissimus thoracis		
Spinalis		
Spinalis capitis	Broad tendon arising from posterior iliac crest, sacrum, spinous processes of sacrum and inferior lumbar spine, and supraspinous ligament	Fibers run superiorly to skull and spinous processes of upper thoracic spine
Spinalis cervicis		
Spinalis thoracis		
Transversospinal		
Semispinalis		
Semispinalis capitis	Transverse processes of cervical and thoracic spine	Fibers span 4–6 vertebral segments, running superomedially to occipital bone and spinous processes in cervical and thoracic spine
Semispinalis cervicis		
Semispinalis thoracis		
Multifidus	Sacrum, ilium, transverse processes of T1-L5 and articular processes of C4-C7	Fibers span 4–6 vertebral segments, running superomedially to spinous processes
Rotatores	Transverse processes of vertebrae, well developed in thoracic spine	Fibers run superomedially and attach to junction of lamina and transverse processes on same vertebra or spinous processes of vertebrae above their origin

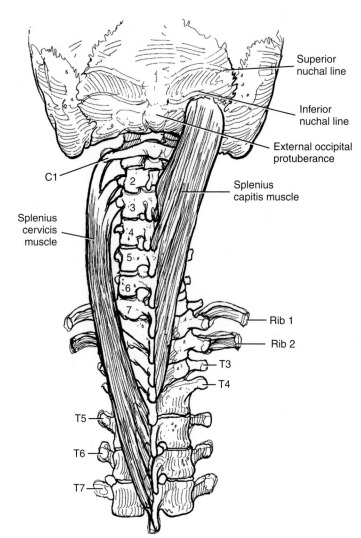

C1

2

3

4

5

6

7

Superior
nuchal line

Inferior
nuchal line

External occipital
protuberance

Splenius
capitis muscle

Splenius
cervicis
muscle

Rib 1

Rib 2

T3

T4

T5

T6

T7

FIGURE 4.54 Posterior view of splenius muscles.

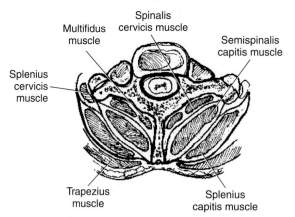

Multifidus
muscle

Spinalis
cervicis muscle

Semispinalis
capitis muscle

Splenius
cervicis
muscle

Trapezius
muscle

Splenius
capitis muscle

FIGURE 4.55 Axial view of splenius muscles.

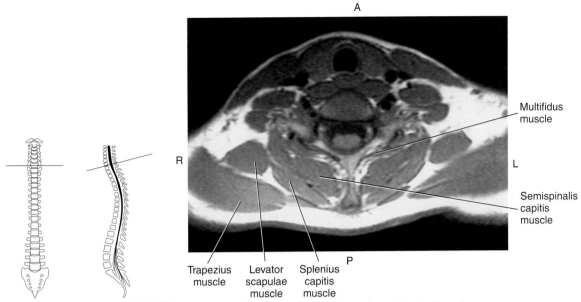

FIGURE 4.56 Axial, T1-weighted MRI of cervical vertebra with spinal muscles.

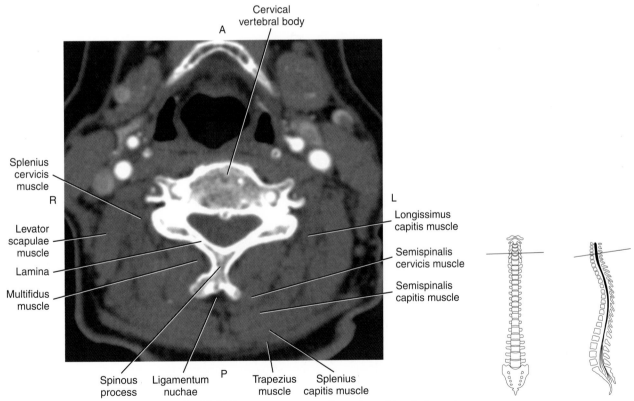

FIGURE 4.57 Axial CT of cervical vertebra with spinal muscles.

Intermediate Layer

The intermediate muscle group, the **erector spinae muscle group**, consists of massive muscles that form a prominent bulge on each side of the vertebral column. The erector spinae muscle group is the chief extensor of the vertebral column and is arranged in three vertical columns, the iliocostalis layer (lateral column), longissimus layer (intermediate column), and the spinalis layer (medial column) (Figures 4.58 and 4.59). This muscle group arises from a common broad tendon from the posterior part of the iliac crest, sacrum, and inferior lumbar spinous processes. The **iliocostalis muscles** run superiorly to attach to the angles of the ribs and transverse processes of C7 to C4. The **longissimus muscles** run superiorly to insert into the tips of the transverse processes of the thoracic and cervical regions, the angles of the ribs, and the mastoid process. The narrow **spinalis muscle group** extends from the spinous processes of the upper lumbar and lower thoracic regions to the spinous processes of the superior thoracic region and C2 (Figures 4.59 through 4.63).

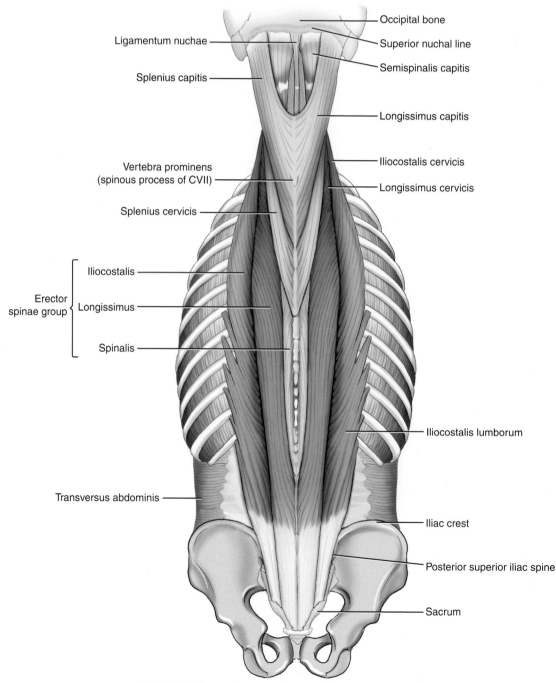

FIGURE 4.58 Posterior view of erector spinae muscle group.

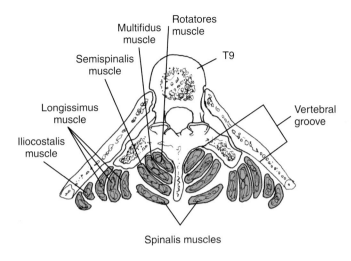

Rotatores muscle

Multifidus muscle

Semispinalis muscle

Longissimus muscle

Iliocostalis muscle

T9

Vertebral groove

Spinalis muscles

FIGURE 4.59 Axial view of erector spinae muscle group at thoracic level.

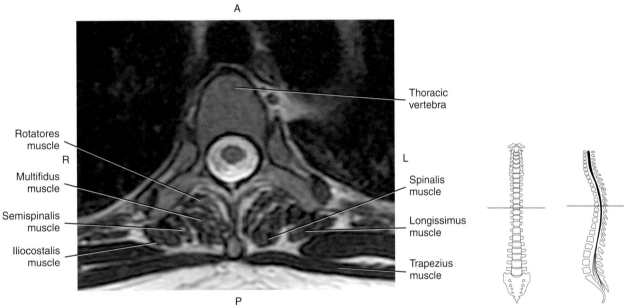

A

Thoracic vertebra

Rotatores muscle

R

Multifidus muscle

Semispinalis muscle

Iliocostalis muscle

L

Spinalis muscle

Longissimus muscle

Trapezius muscle

P

FIGURE 4.60 Axial, T2-weighted MRI of thoracic vertebra with spinal muscles.

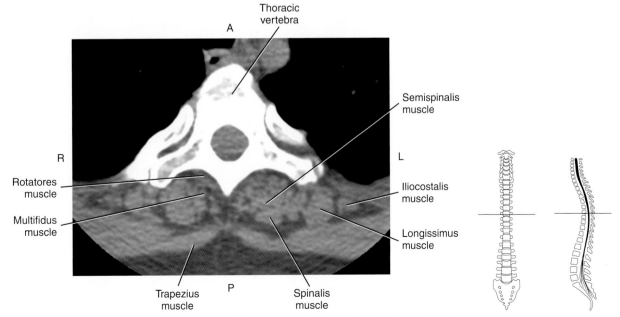

Thoracic vertebra

A

Semispinalis muscle

R

Rotatores muscle

Multifidus muscle

L

Iliocostalis muscle

Longissimus muscle

Trapezius muscle

P

Spinalis muscle

FIGURE 4.61 Axial CT of thoracic vertebra with spinal muscles.

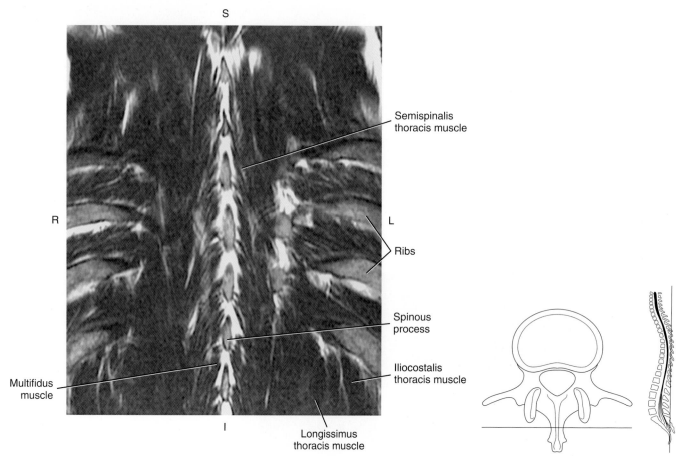

FIGURE 4.62 Coronal, T1-weighted MRI of lumbar vertebrae with spinal muscles.

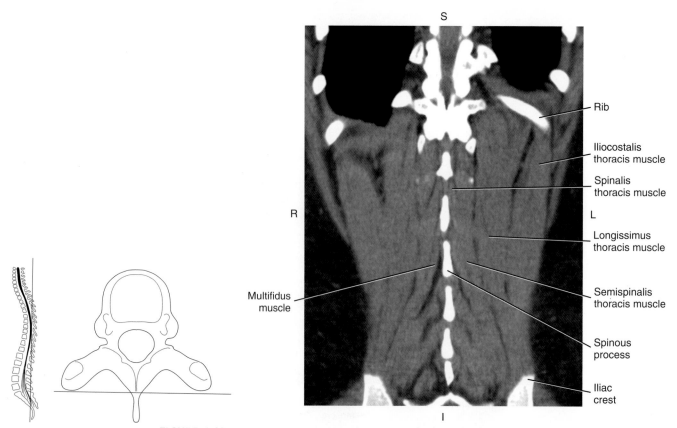

FIGURE 4.63 Coronal CT reformat of lumbar vertebrae with spinal muscles.

Deep Layer

The **transversospinal muscles** consist of several short muscles that are located in the groove between the transverse and spinous processes of the vertebrae. They can be separated into the semispinalis, multifidus, and rotatores with a primary function to flex and rotate the vertebral column (Figures 4.59 through 4.64). The **semispinalis** muscles arise from the thoracic and cervical transverse processes and insert on the occipital bone and spinous processes in the thoracic and cervical regions. The semispinalis muscles form the largest muscle mass in the posterior portion of the neck. The **multifidus** muscles consist of many fibrous bundles that extend the full length of the spine and are the most prominent in the lumbar region. The deepest of the transversospinal muscles are the rotatores, which connect the lamina of one vertebra to the transverse process of the vertebra below. They are best developed in the thoracic region.

Two additional muscles that are commonly visualized in the lumbar region of the spine are the **quadratus lumborum** and the **psoas** muscles, which are considered abdominal muscles (Figures 4.65 through 4.68). Further information on these muscles can be found in Chapter 7.

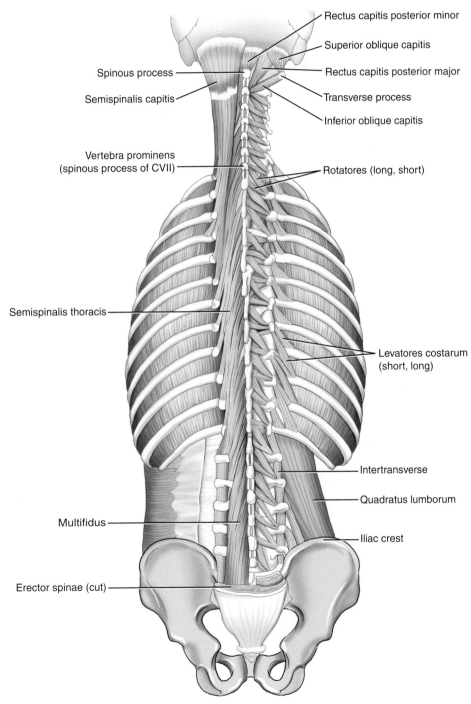

FIGURE 4.64 Posterior view of transversospinal muscle group.

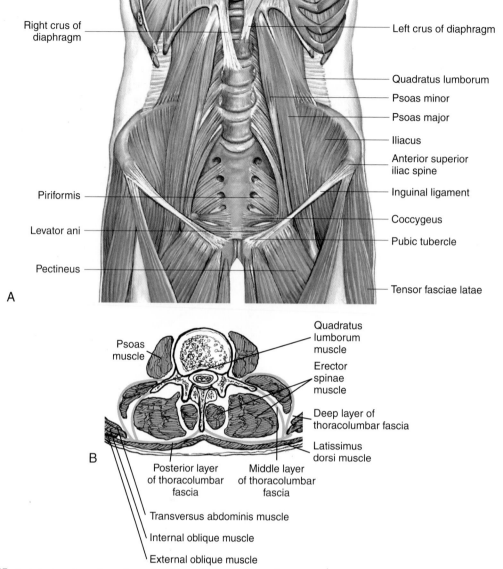

Right crus of diaphragm

Left crus of diaphragm

Quadratus lumborum

Psoas minor

Psoas major

Iliacus

Anterior superior iliac spine

Piriformis

Inguinal ligament

Levator ani

Coccygeus

Pubic tubercle

Pectineus

Tensor fasciae latae

A

Psoas muscle

Quadratus lumborum muscle

Erector spinae muscle

Deep layer of thoracolumbar fascia

Latissimus dorsi muscle

B

Posterior layer of thoracolumbar fascia

Middle layer of thoracolumbar fascia

Transversus abdominis muscle

Internal oblique muscle

External oblique muscle

FIGURE 4.65 A, Anterior view of quadratus lumborum and psoas muscles. B, Axial view of quadratus lumborum and psoas muscles.

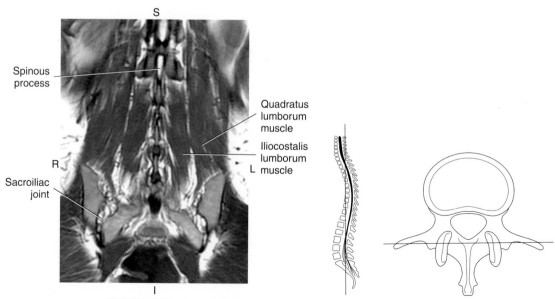

S

Spinous process

Quadratus lumborum muscle

Iliocostalis lumborum muscle

R

L

Sacroiliac joint

I

FIGURE 4.66 Coronal, T1-weighted MRI of quadratus lumborum muscle.

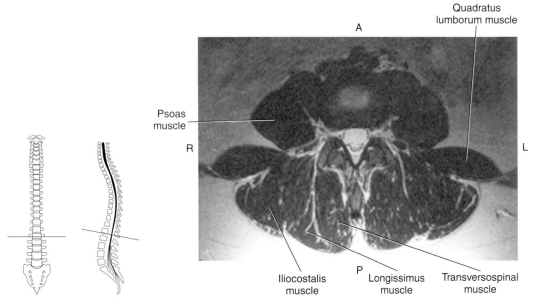

FIGURE 4.67 Axial, T2-weighted MRI of lumbar vertebra with spinal muscles.

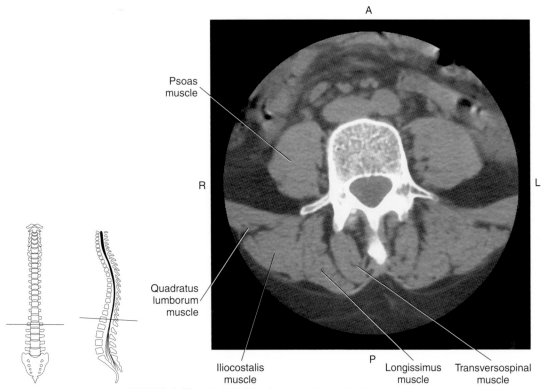

FIGURE 4.68 Axial CT of lumbar vertebra with spinal muscles.

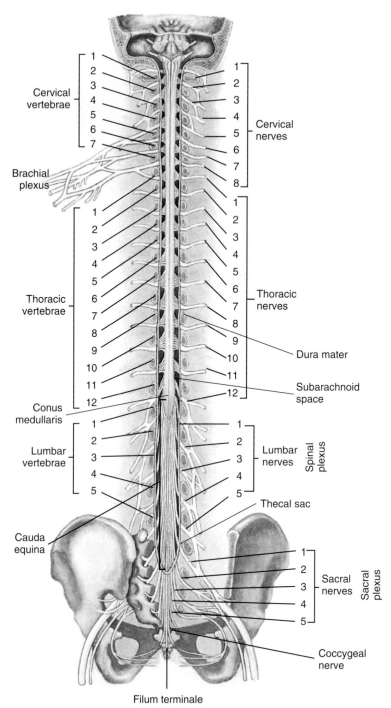

Cervical vertebrae
1
2
3
4
5
6
7

Cervical nerves
1
2
3
4
5
6
7
8

Brachial plexus

Thoracic vertebrae
1
2
3
4
5
6
7
8
9
10
11
12

Thoracic nerves
1
2
3
4
5
6
7
8
9
10
11
12

Dura mater

Subarachnoid space

Conus medullaris

Lumbar vertebrae
1
2
3
4
5

Lumbar nerves
1
2
3
4
5

Spinal plexus

Thecal sac

Cauda equina

Sacral nerves
1
2
3
4
5

Sacral plexus

Coccygeal nerve

Filum terminale

FIGURE 4.69 Posterior view of spinal meninges, thecal sac, and spinal cord.

SPINAL CORD

Spinal Meninges

Throughout its length, the delicate spinal cord is surrounded and protected by cerebrospinal fluid, which is contained in the thecal sac formed by the **spinal meninges** (Figure 4.69). The spinal meninges are continuous with the cranial meninges and can be broken into the same three layers: dura, arachnoid, and pia. The **dura** **mater** is the tough outer layer that extends to S2, creating the **thecal sac** (Figures 4.29, 4.49, 4.69 through 4.72). The anterior thecal sac adheres to the posterior longitudinal ligament and is separated from the vertebral column by an **epidural space** that contains fat and vessels. Each spinal nerve is surrounded by dura mater that extends through the intervertebral foramen called the **dural nerve root sleeve**. The **arachnoid mater** is the thin transparent membrane that is attached to the inner surface of the dura mater. A potential space called the **subdural space** runs between the arachnoid and dura mater. The arachnoid mater is connected to the pia mater by numerous delicate strands creating the spiderlike appearance associated with the arachnoid mater. The space between the arachnoid mater and pia mater is the **subarachnoid space**, which is filled with cerebrospinal fluid and the blood vessels that supply the spinal cord (Figures 4.69 through 4.74). The **pia mater** is a highly vascular layer that closely adheres to the spinal cord. At the distal end of the spinal cord, approximately L1, the pia mater continues as a long slender strand called the filum terminale. The **filum terminale** descends through the subarachnoid space to the inferior border of the thecal sac, where it is reinforced by the dura mater. After leaving the thecal sac, it eventually exits the sacral canal through the sacral

hiatus and attaches to the coccyx, providing an anchor between the spinal cord and the coccyx (Figures 4.69 and 4.70). In addition, lateral extensions of the pia mater leave the spinal cord to form pairs of **denticulate ligaments,** which attach to the dura, preventing lateral movement of the spinal cord within the thecal sac. The denticulate ligaments run between the ventral and dorsal nerve roots within the spinal column (Figures 4.73 and 4.75).

After producing chickenpox, the herpes zoster virus can lie dormant within the ventral horns of the spinal cord for years. When reactivated, the virus attacks the dorsal roots of peripheral nerves, producing a painful rash, with a distribution corresponding to the affected sensory nerve. This condition is termed shingles.

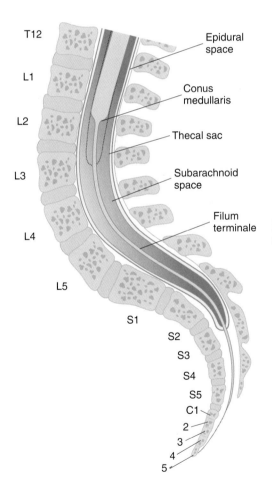

FIGURE 4.70 Midsagittal view of thecal sac, conus medullaris, and filum terminale.

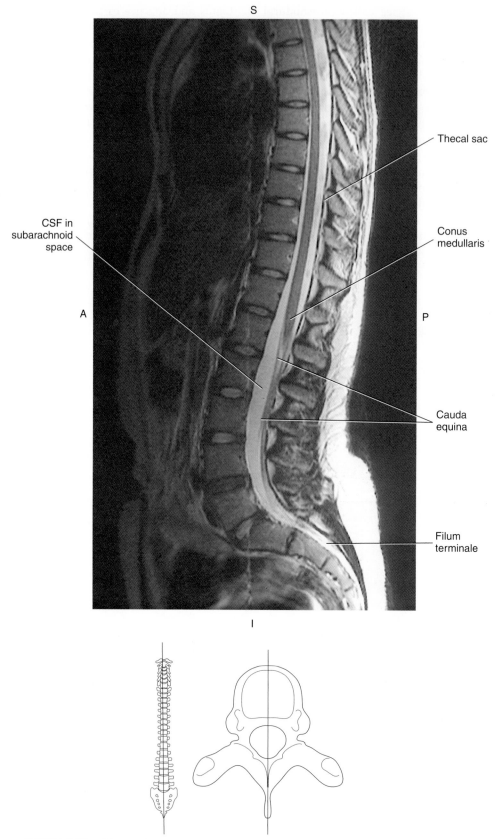

S

Thecal sac

CSF in
subarachnoid
space

Conus
medullaris

A

P

Cauda
equina

Filum
terminale

I

FIGURE 4.71 Midsagittal, T2-weighted MRI of thecal sac, conus medullaris, and filum terminale.

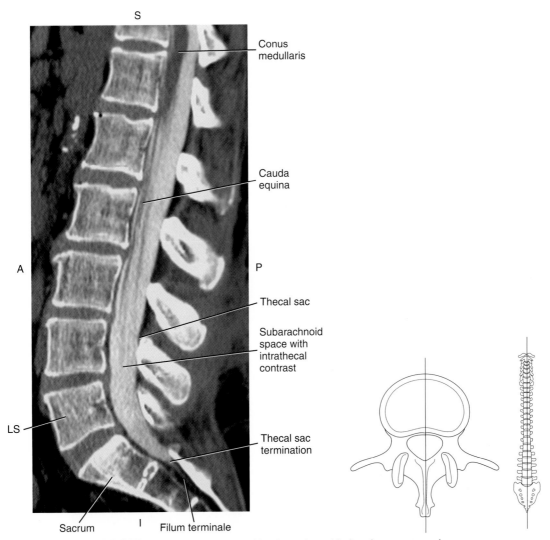

Conus medullaris

Cauda equina

Thecal sac

Subarachnoid space with intrathecal contrast

Thecal sac termination

Sacrum   I   Filum terminale

LS

A   P

S

FIGURE 4.72 Sagittal CT reformat of lumbar spine with thecal sac, post myelogram.

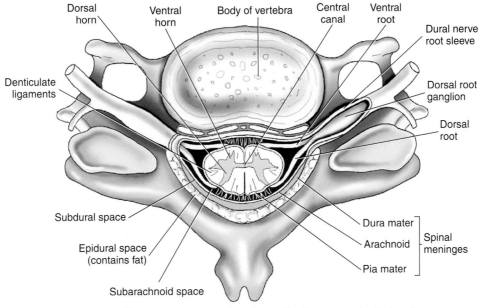

Dorsal horn

Ventral horn

Body of vertebra

Central canal

Ventral root

Dural nerve root sleeve

Dorsal root ganglion

Dorsal root

Denticulate ligaments

Subdural space

Epidural space (contains fat)

Subarachnoid space

Dura mater

Arachnoid

Pia mater

Spinal meninges

FIGURE 4.73 Axial view of spinal meninges, dural spaces, and spinal cord.

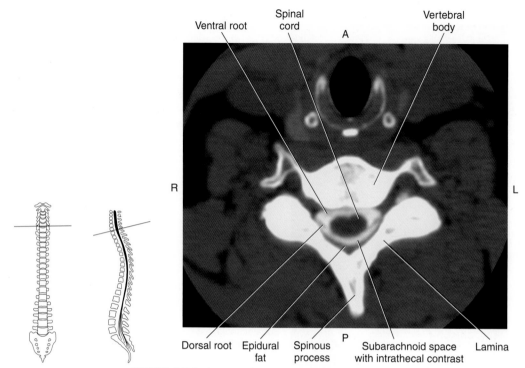

FIGURE 4.74 Axial CT of cervical spine, post myelogram.

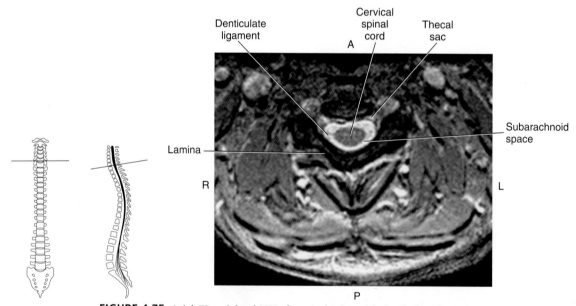

FIGURE 4.75 Axial, T2-weighted MRI of cervical spine with denticulate ligament.

Spinal Cord and Nerve Roots

The spinal cord functions as a large nerve cable that connects the brain with the body. It begins as a continuation of the medulla at the inferior margin of the brainstem and extends to approximately the first lumbar vertebra. The spinal cord tapers into a cone-shaped segment called the conus medullaris (Figures 4.69 through 4.72, and 4.76 through 4.79). The **conus medullaris** is the most inferior portion of the spinal cord and is located at approximately the level of T12–L1. At the termination of the spinal cord, nerves continue inferiorly in bundles. This grouping of nerves has the appearance of a horse's tail and is termed the cauda equina, which exits through the lumbosacral foramina (Figures 4.69, 4.76, 4.77, 4.80, and 4.81).

The spinal cord is composed of white and gray matter. The **white matter** (myelinated axons) comprises the external borders of the cord and is more abundant. The **gray matter** is composed of nerve cells and runs the entire length of the cord. It is centrally located and surrounds the **central canal**, which contains cerebrospinal fluid and is continuous with the ventricles of the brain (Figures 4.73, 4.82, and 4.91). In cross section, the gray matter has the appearance of a butterfly. The two posterior projections are the dorsal horns, and the two anterior projections are the ventral horns (Figure 4.73). The **dorsal horns** contain neurons and sensory fibers that enter the cord from the body periphery via the **dorsal roots**. These are called the afferent (sensory) nerve roots (Figures 4.74 and 4.83). The **dorsal root ganglion**, an oval enlargement of the dorsal root that contains the nerve cell bodies of the sensory neurons, is located in the intervertebral foramen (Figures 4.73 and 4.84 through 4.90). The **ventral horns** contain the nerve cell bodies of the efferent (motor) neurons. The efferent (motor) nerve roots exit the spinal cord via the ventral root to be distributed throughout the body. Just outside the intervertebral foramina, the ventral and dorsal roots unite to form the 31 pairs of **spinal nerves**. Eight of these nerve pairs correspond to the cervical region, 12 belong to the thoracic section, 5 correspond to the lumbar region, 5 correspond to the sacrum, and 1 belongs to the coccyx (Figures 4.76 and 4.91 through 4.93). Each spinal nerve provides a specific cutaneous distribution that can be demonstrated on a **dermatome map** (Figure 4.94).

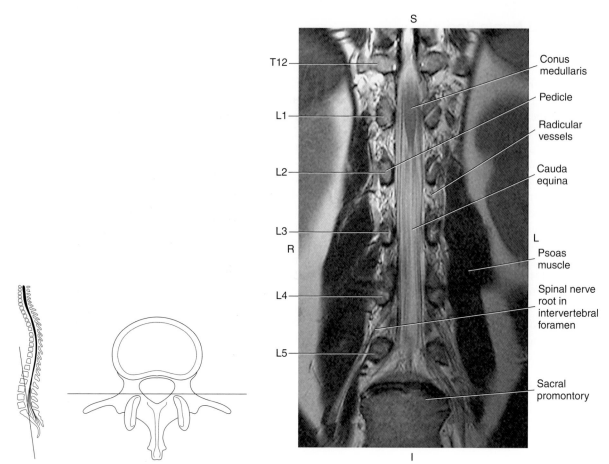

FIGURE 4.76 Coronal, T2-weighted MRI of spinal cord, conus medullaris, and cauda equina.

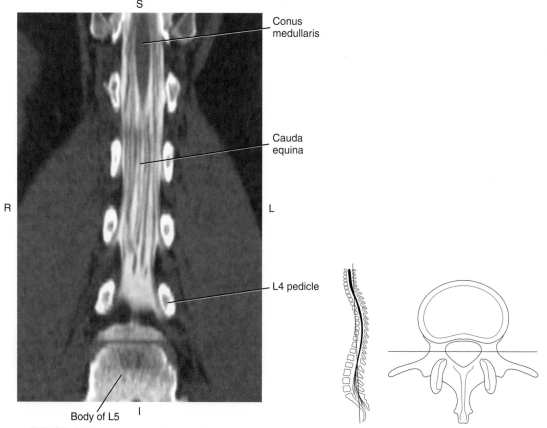

FIGURE 4.77 Coronal CT reformat of spinal cord, conus medullaris, and cauda equina, post myelogram.

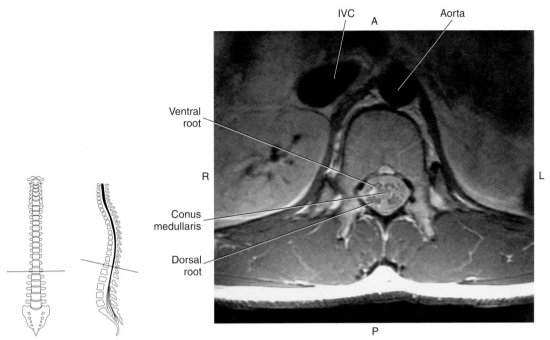

IVC   A   Aorta

Ventral root

Conus medullaris

Dorsal root

R   L

P

FIGURE 4.78 Axial, T1-weighted MRI of conus medullaris.

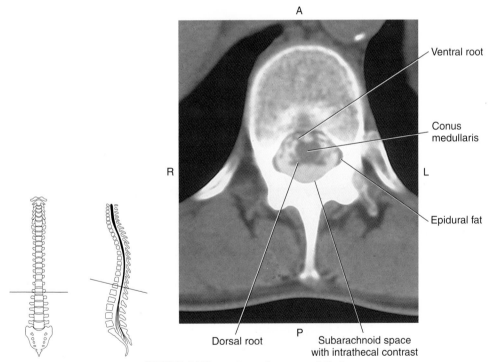

A

Ventral root

Conus medullaris

Epidural fat

R   L

Dorsal root   P   Subarachnoid space with intrathecal contrast

FIGURE 4.79 Axial CT of conus medullaris.

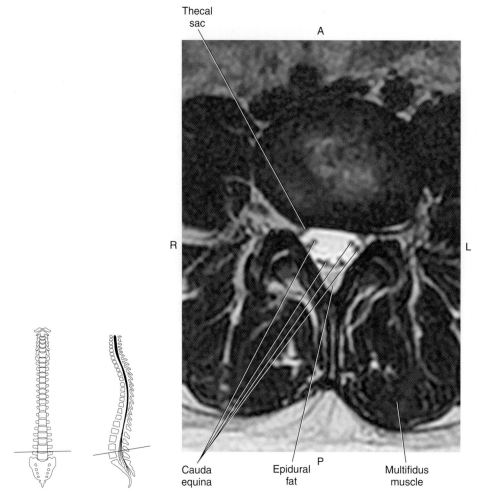

Thecal
sac

A

R

L

Cauda
equina

Epidural
fat

P

Multifidus
muscle

FIGURE 4.80 Axial, T2-weighted MRI of cauda equina.

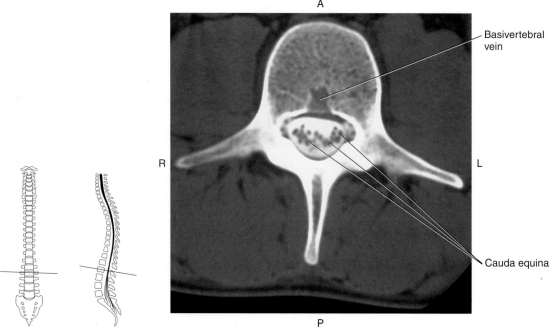

A

Basivertebral
vein

R

L

Cauda equina

P

FIGURE 4.81 Axial CT of cauda equina.

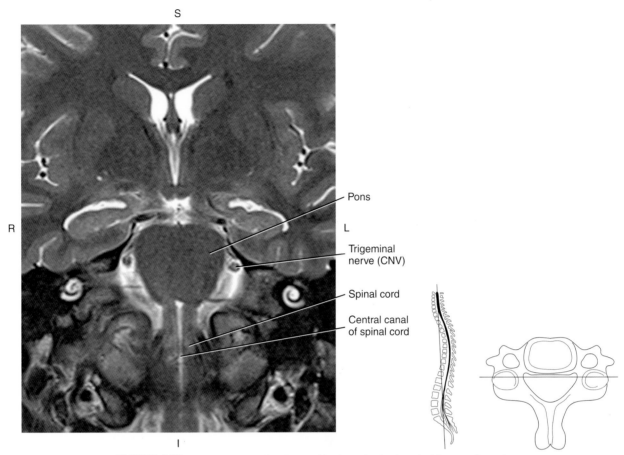

FIGURE 4.82 Coronal, T2-weighted MRI of brain and spinal cord with central canal.

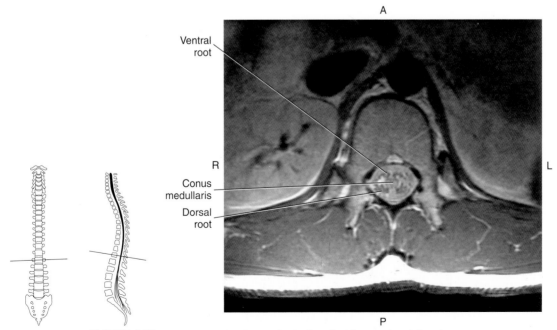

FIGURE 4.83 Axial, T1-weighted MRI of spinal cord with ventral and dorsal roots.

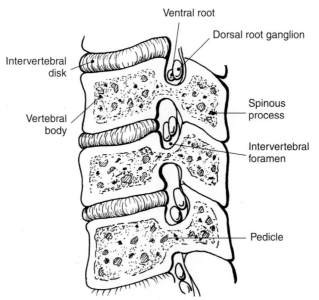

FIGURE 4.84 Sagittal view of spine with intervertebral foramina.

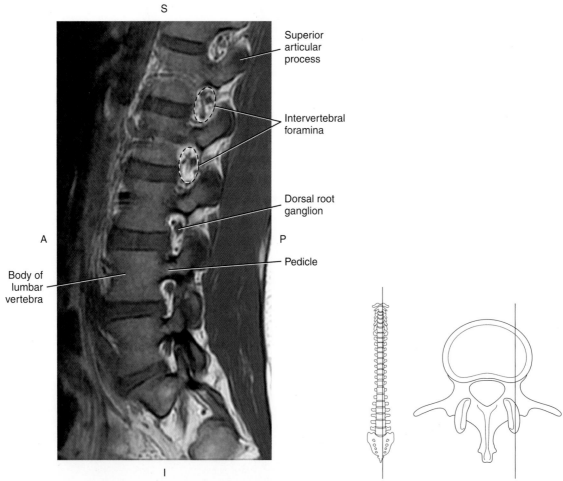

FIGURE 4.85 Sagittal, T1-weighted MRI of lumbar spine with intervertebral foramina.

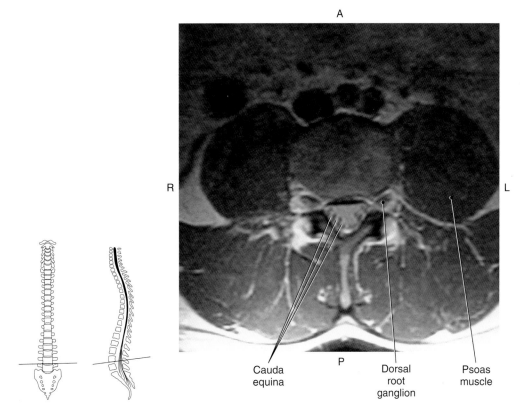

FIGURE 4.86 Axial, T1-weighted MRI of lumbar vertebra with dorsal root ganglion.

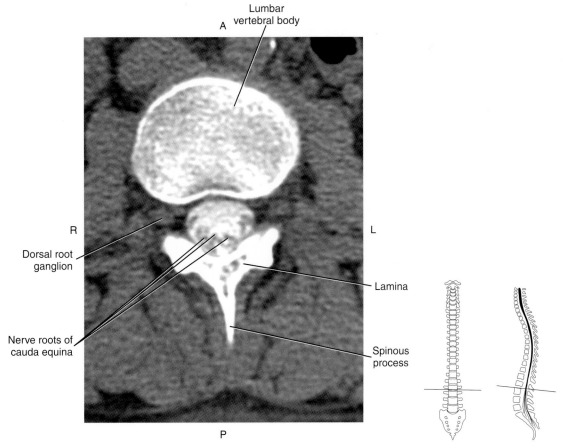

FIGURE 4.87 Axial CT of lumbar vertebra with dorsal root ganglion, post myelogram.

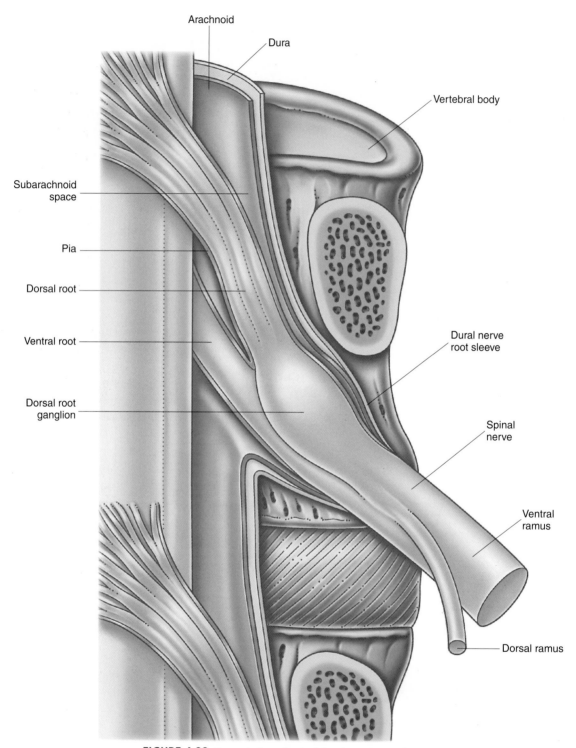

Arachnoid

Dura

Vertebral body

Subarachnoid space

Pia

Dorsal root

Ventral root

Dorsal root ganglion

Dural nerve root sleeve

Spinal nerve

Ventral ramus

Dorsal ramus

FIGURE 4.88 Coronal view of spinal dural nerve root sleeve.

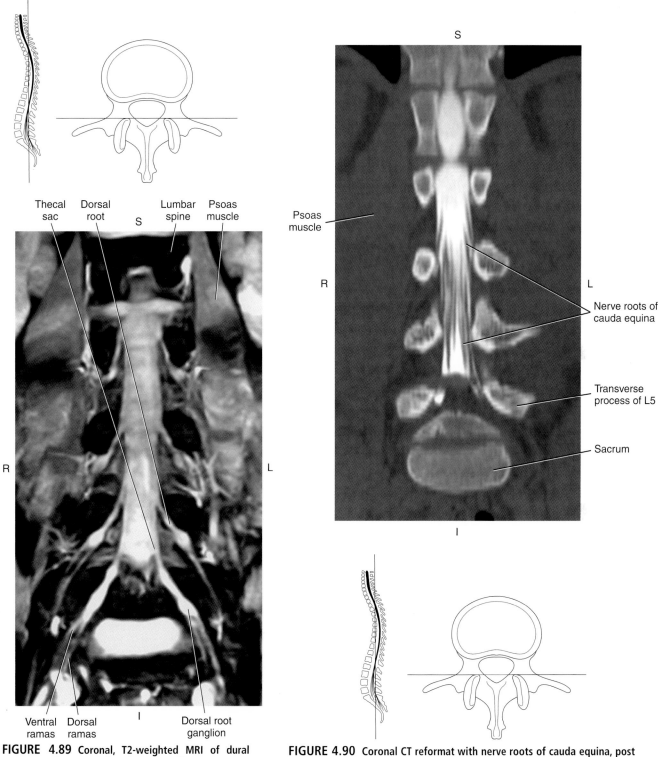

FIGURE 4.89 Coronal, T2-weighted MRI of dural nerve root sleeve and dorsal root ganglion.

FIGURE 4.90 Coronal CT reformat with nerve roots of cauda equina, post myelogram.

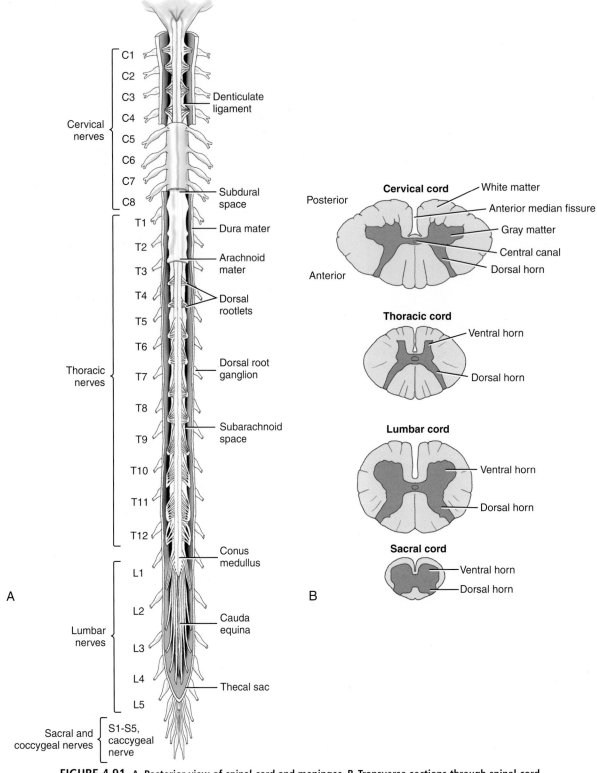

FIGURE 4.91 A, Posterior view of spinal cord and meninges. **B,** Transverse sections through spinal cord.

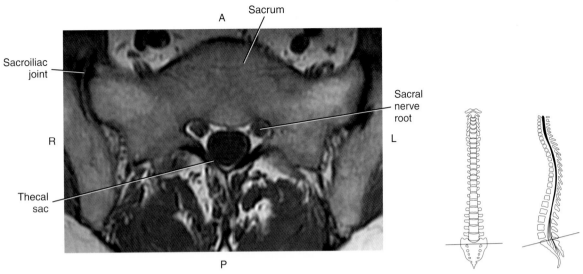

FIGURE 4.92 Axial, T1-weighted MRI of sacral nerves.

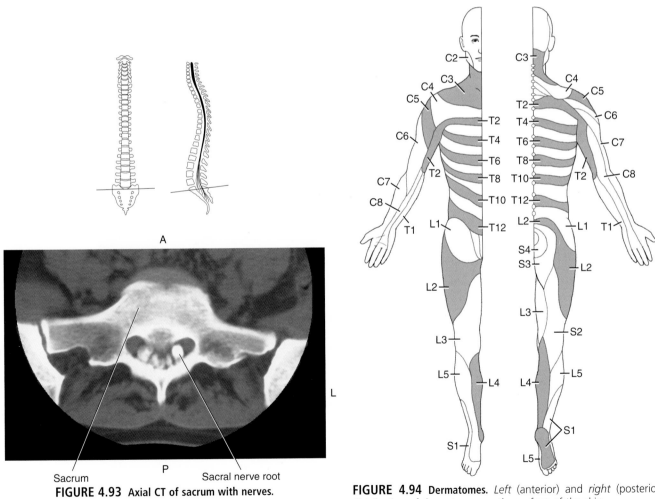

FIGURE 4.93 Axial CT of sacrum with nerves.

FIGURE 4.94 Dermatomes. *Left* (anterior) and *right* (posterior) distribution of dermatomes on the surface of the skin.

PLEXUSES

The spinal cord is enlarged in two regions by the cell bodies of nerves that extend to the extremities. The **cervical enlargement** extends from the vertebral bodies of approximately C3-C7, and the **lumbosacral enlargement** occurs within the lower thoracic region. Cross-section images of the spinal cord at various levels have considerable differences in size and shape because of the changing proportion of gray and white matter (Figures 4.91 and 4.95 through 4.100).

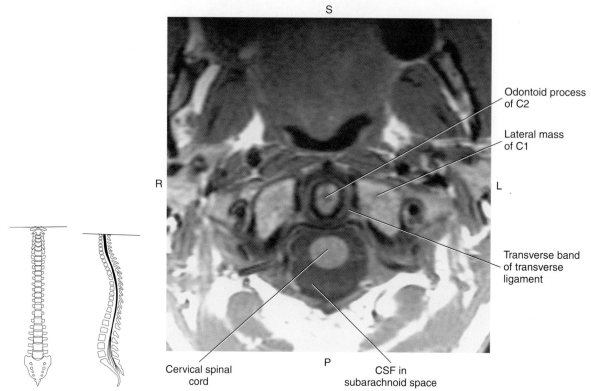

FIGURE 4.95 Axial, T1-weighted MRI of cervical spinal cord.

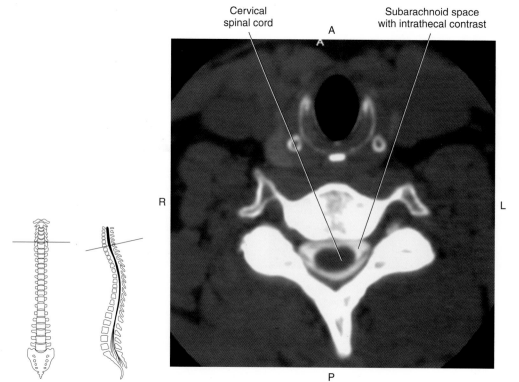

FIGURE 4.96 Axial CT of cervical spinal cord, post myelogram.

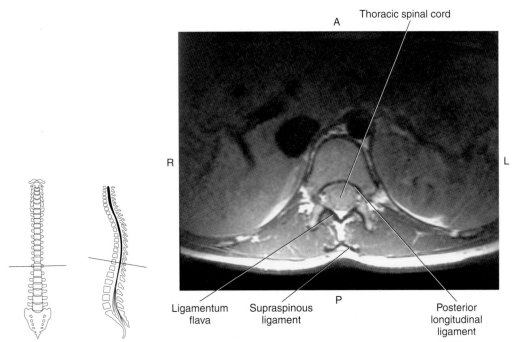

FIGURE 4.97 Axial, T1-weighted MRI of thoracic spinal cord.

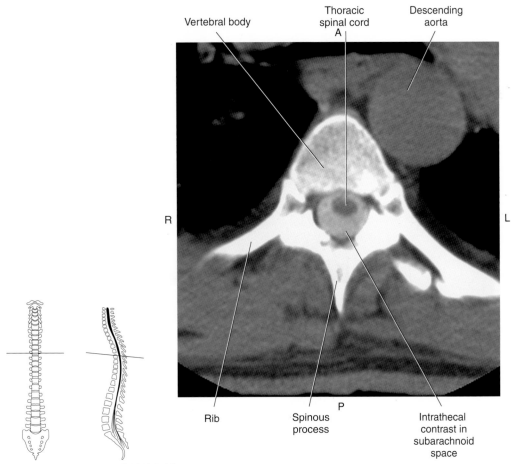

FIGURE 4.98 Axial CT of thoracic spinal cord, post myelogram.

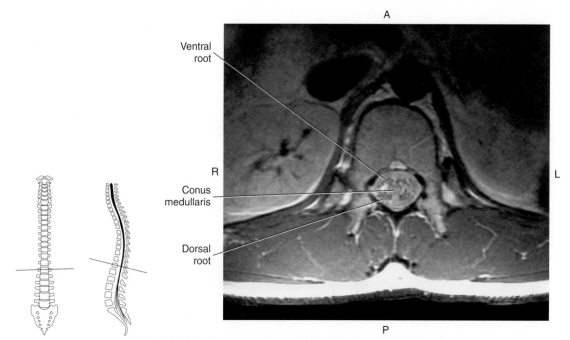

FIGURE 4.99 Axial, T1-weighted MRI of conus medullaris at T-12.

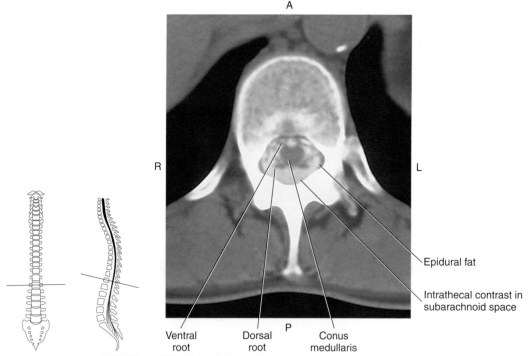

FIGURE 4.100 Axial CT of conus medullaris at T-12, post myelogram.

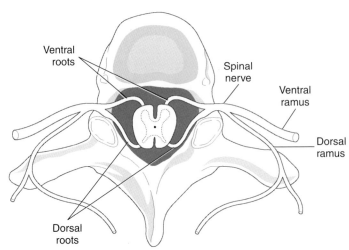

FIGURE 4.101 Distribution of ventral and dorsal rami in transverse section of spinal cord.

Shortly after emerging from the intervertebral foramen, each nerve divides into **dorsal** and **ventral rami,** which contain both motor and sensory fibers (Figure 4.101). The dorsal rami of all spinal nerves extend posteriorly to innervate the skin and muscles of the posterior trunk. The ventral rami of T2-T12 pass anteriorly as the intercostal nerves to supply the skin and muscles of the anterior and lateral trunk. The ventral rami of all other spinal nerves form complex networks of nerves called **plexuses.** These plexuses serve the motor and sensory needs of the muscles and skin of the extremities. The four major nerve plexuses are the cervical, brachial, lumbar, and sacral (Figure 4.102).

Cervical Plexus

The **cervical plexus** arises from the upper four ventral rami of C1-C4 to innervate the neck, lower part of the face and ear, the side of the scalp, and the upper thoracic area. The major motor branch of this plexus is the **phrenic nerve,** which is formed by the branches of C3, C4, and upper division of C5. This nerve descends vertically down the neck and passes into the superior thoracic aperture, where it continues inferiorly to the diaphragm (Figures 4.102 through 4.106).

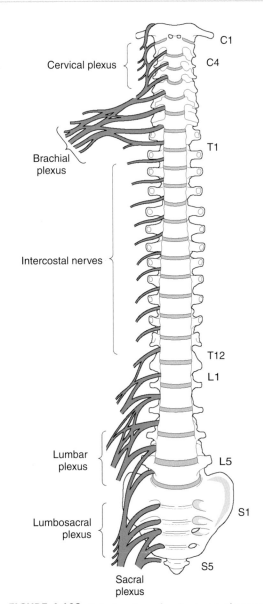

FIGURE 4.102 Anterior view of major nerve plexuses.

The phrenic nerve, which innervates the diaphragm, is formed by motor fibers from C3-C5. A primary danger of a broken neck is that an injury at or above the level of C4 may result in paralysis of respiratory muscles, resulting in breathing difficulties and impaired speech production.

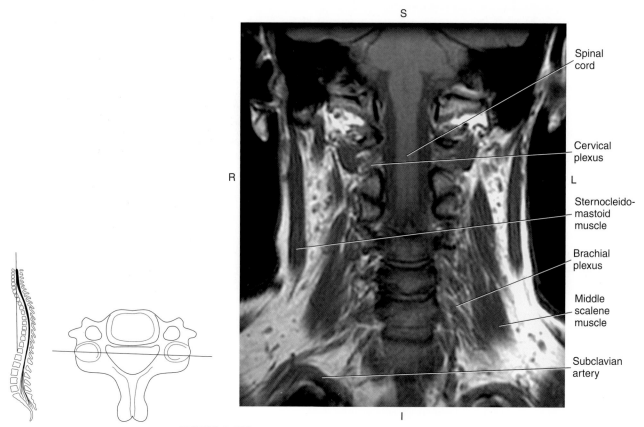

FIGURE 4.103 Coronal, T1-weighted MRI of cervical plexus.

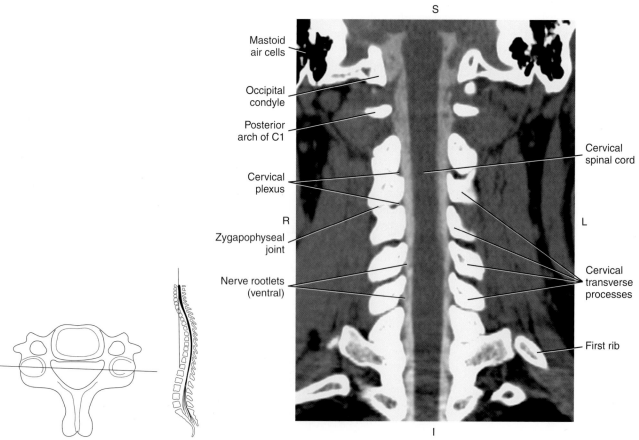

FIGURE 4.104 Coronal CT reformat of cervical plexus.

Intervertebral foramen   Nerve rootlets   Spinal cord   Spinous process

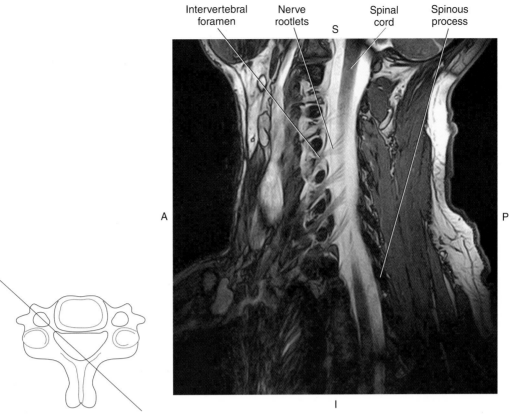

FIGURE 4.105 Sagittal, T2-weighted MRI of cervical plexus.

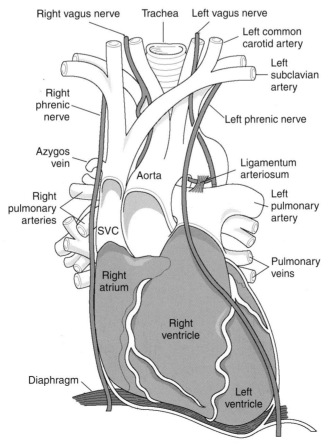

FIGURE 4.106 Coronal view of phrenic nerve in thoracic cavity.

Brachial Plexus

The **brachial plexus** is a large, complex network of nerves arising from the five ventral rami of C5-C8 and T1. The roots of the brachial plexus emerge between the anterior and middle scalene muscles, where they continue laterally and inferiorly to divide into three cords just posterior to the clavicle. The brachial plexus is located posterior to the subclavian artery as it courses toward the axillary region of the shoulder (Figures 4.107 and 4.108). The **cords** extend through the axilla to form five terminal branches: the **musculocutaneous, axillary, median, radial,** and **ulnar** nerves. These nerves provide innervation for the muscles of the upper extremity and shoulder (Figures 4.107 through 4.115).

> Herniated intervertebral disks are most common at vertebral levels C5-C6, C6-C7, L4-L5, and L5/S1.

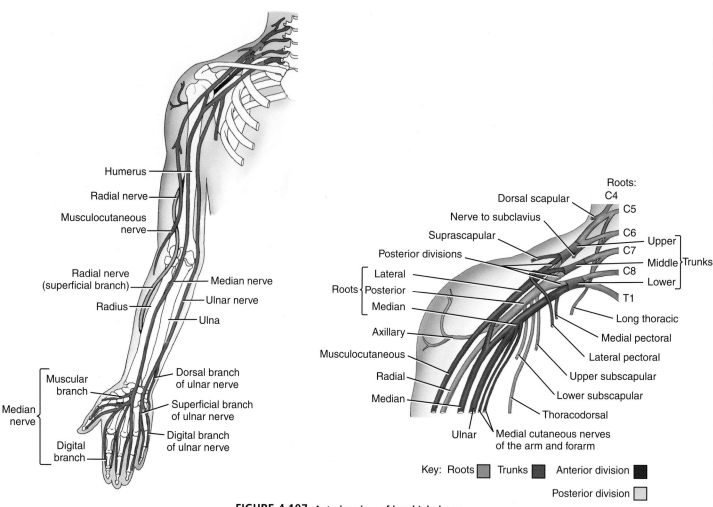

FIGURE 4.107 Anterior view of brachial plexus.

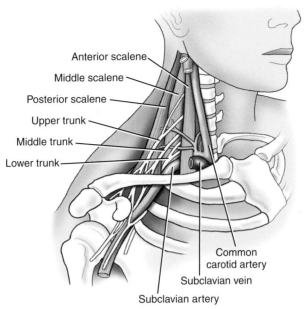

FIGURE 4.108 Anterior oblique view of brachial plexus.

Anterior scalene
Middle scalene
Posterior scalene
Upper trunk
Middle trunk
Lower trunk

Common carotid artery
Subclavian vein
Subclavian artery

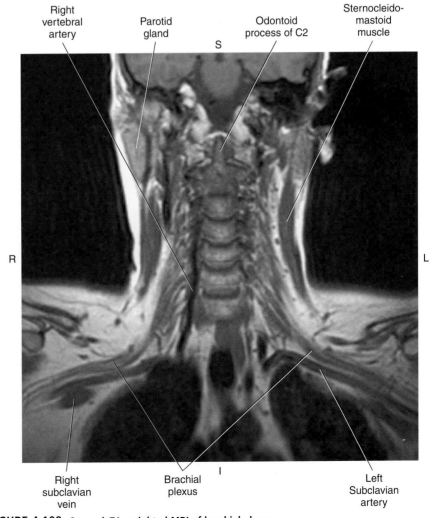

Right vertebral artery
Parotid gland
Odontoid process of C2
Sternocleido-mastoid muscle

S

R

L

Right subclavian vein
Brachial plexus
Left Subclavian artery

I

FIGURE 4.109 Coronal, T1-weighted MRI of brachial plexus.

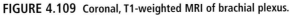

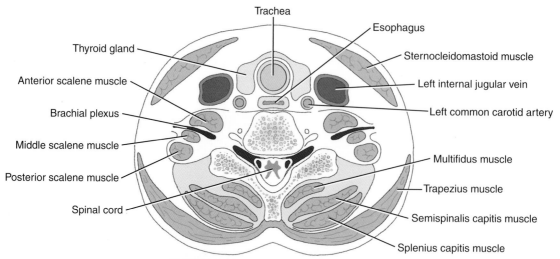

Trachea

Thyroid gland

Anterior scalene muscle

Brachial plexus

Middle scalene muscle

Posterior scalene muscle

Spinal cord

Esophagus

Sternocleidomastoid muscle

Left internal jugular vein

Left common carotid artery

Multifidus muscle

Trapezius muscle

Semispinalis capitis muscle

Splenius capitis muscle

FIGURE 4.110 Axial view of brachial plexus.

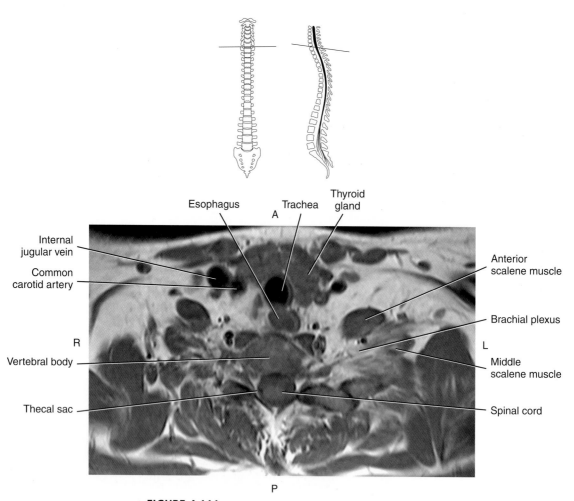

Esophagus

Trachea

Thyroid gland

A

Internal jugular vein

Common carotid artery

Anterior scalene muscle

Brachial plexus

R

L

Vertebral body

Middle scalene muscle

Thecal sac

Spinal cord

P

FIGURE 4.111 Axial, T1-weighted MRI of brachial plexus.

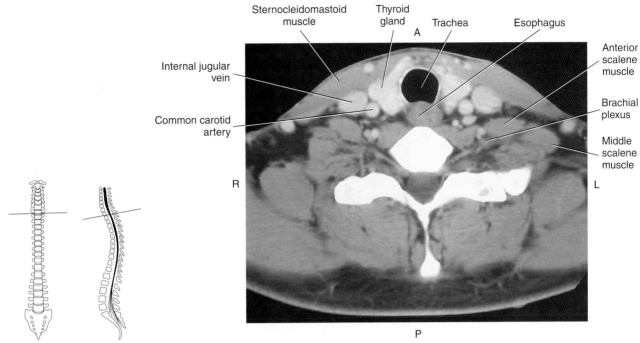

FIGURE 4.112 Axial CT of brachial plexus.

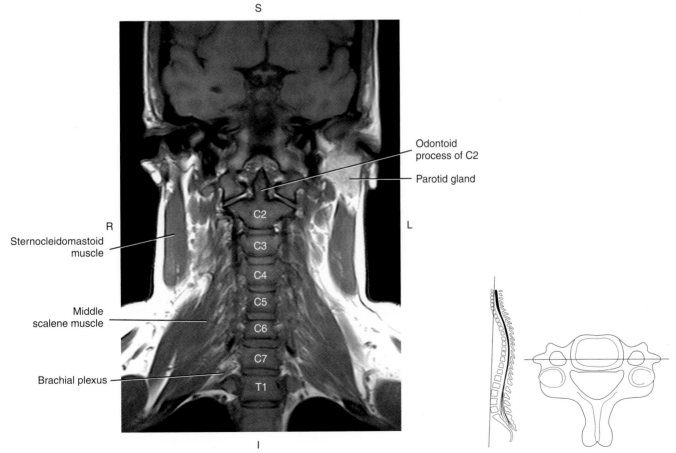

FIGURE 4.113 Coronal, T1-weighted MRI of cervical spine and brachial plexus.

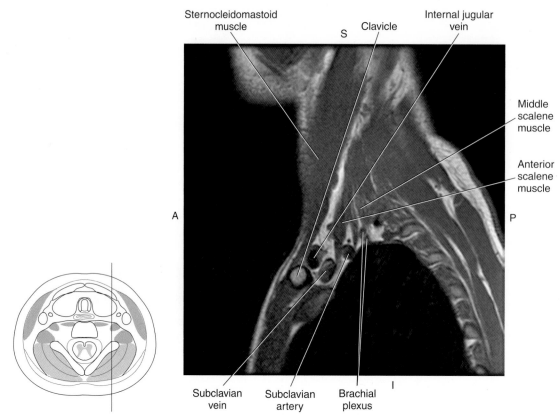

FIGURE 4.114 Sagittal, T1-weighted MRI of brachial plexus and scalene muscles.

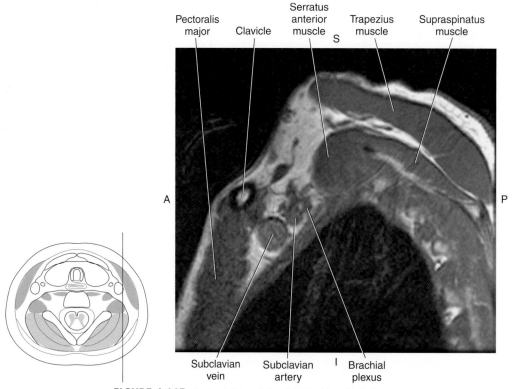

FIGURE 4.115 Sagittal, T1-weighted MRI of brachial plexus.

Lumbar Plexus

The **lumbar plexus** arises from the ventral rami of T12 and L1-L4. The lumbar plexus is situated on the posterior abdominal wall, between the psoas major muscle and the transverse processes of the lumbar vertebrae. In general, it serves the lower abdominopelvic region and anterior and medial muscles of the thigh. The **femoral nerve** is the largest branch of the lumbar plexus descending beneath the inguinal ligament.

At the level of the lesser trochanter the femoral nerve divides into several branches, the largest being the **saphenous nerve,** which descends along the medial aspect of the leg to the ankle accompanied by the great saphenous vein. The saphenous nerve innervates the anterior lower leg, some of the ankle, and part of the foot (Figures 4.116 through 4.119).

Paraplegia will result from transection of the spinal cord between the cervical and lumbosacral enlargements. Quadriplegia will result if the transection occurs above the level of C3.

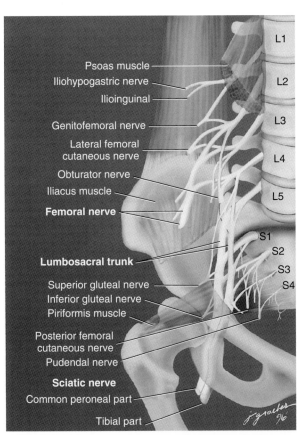

FIGURE 4.116 Anterior view of lumbar and sacral plexuses.

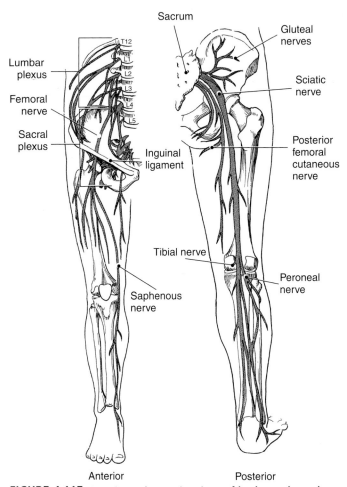

FIGURE 4.117 Anterior and posterior views of lumbar and sacral plexuses.

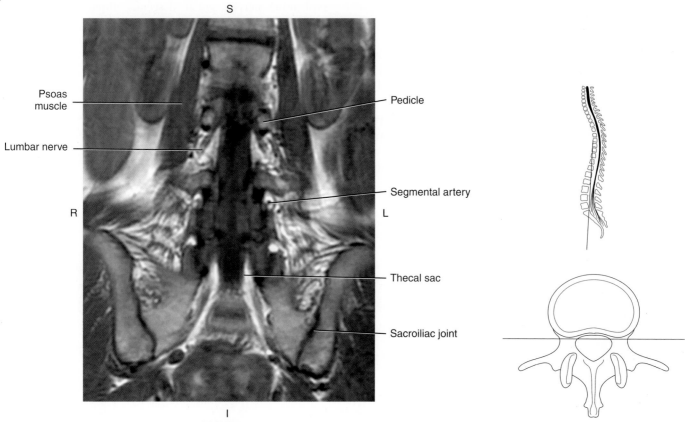

FIGURE 4.118 Coronal, T1-weighted MRI of lumbar plexus.

S

Psoas muscle

Pedicle

Lumbar nerve

Segmental artery

R

L

Thecal sac

Sacroiliac joint

I

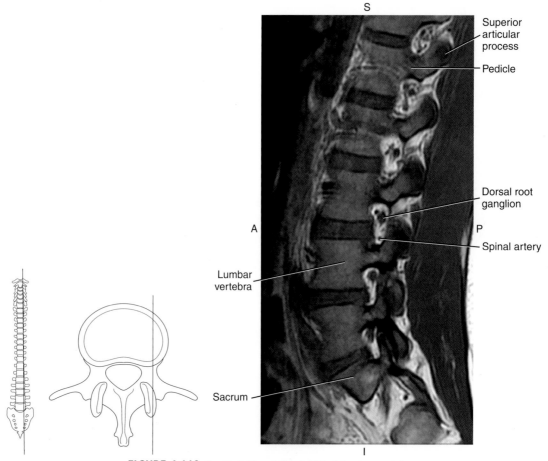

FIGURE 4.119 Sagittal, T1-weighted MRI of lumbar vertebra.

S

Superior articular process

Pedicle

A

P

Dorsal root ganglion

Spinal artery

Lumbar vertebra

Sacrum

I

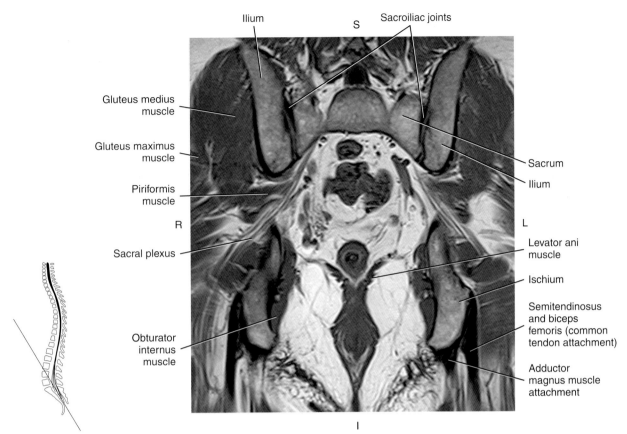

FIGURE 4.120 Coronal, T1-weighted MRI of sacroiliac joints and sacral plexus.

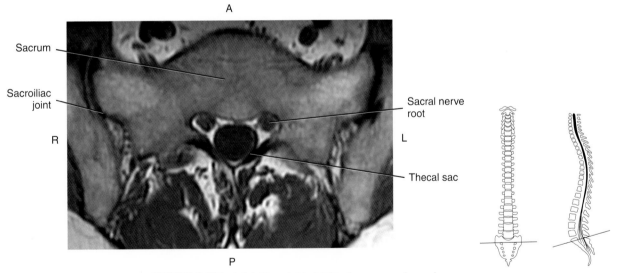

FIGURE 4.121 Axial, T1-weighted MRI of sacrum and sacral nerve.

Sacral Plexus

Arising from L4-L5 and S1-S4, the nerves of the **sacral plexus** innervate the buttocks, posterior thigh, and feet. These nerves converge toward the inferior sacral foramina to unite into a large flattened band. Most of this nerve network continues into the thigh as the **sciatic nerve,** which is the largest nerve in the body. The sciatic nerve exits the pelvis through the greater sciatic foramen and continues to descend vertically along the posterior thigh. In its course it divides into the **tibial** and **peroneal nerves,** which innervate the posterior aspect of the lower extremity. The sacral plexus lies against the posterolateral wall of the pelvis between the piriformis muscle and internal iliac vessels, just anterior to the sacroiliac joint (Figures 4.116, 4.117, and 4.120 through 4.124).

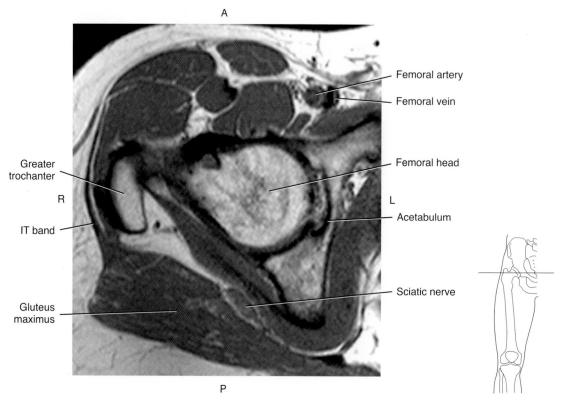

FIGURE 4.122 Axial, T1-weighted MRI of femoral head and sciatic nerve, right hip.

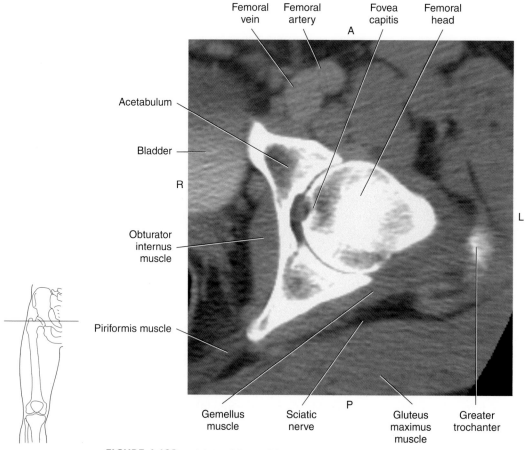

FIGURE 4.123 Axial CT of femoral head and sciatic nerve, left hip.

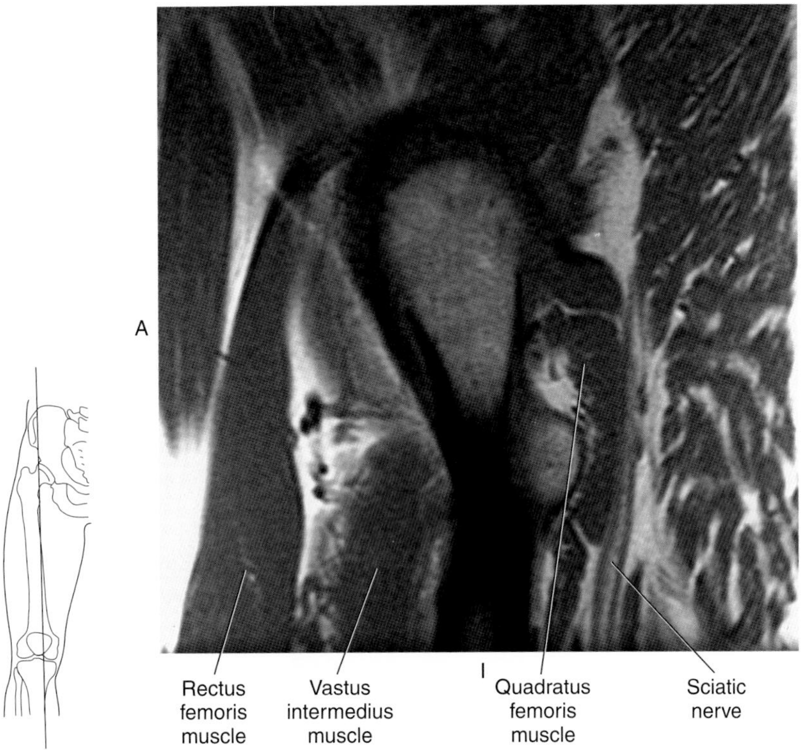

Rectus femoris muscle

Vastus intermedius muscle

Quadratus femoris muscle

Sciatic nerve

FIGURE 4.124 Sagittal, T1-weighted MRI of sciatic nerve.

VASCULATURE

Spinal Arteries

The spinal cord is supplied by a single anterior spinal artery, by paired posterior spinal arteries, and by a series of spinal branches. The **anterior spinal artery** is formed, just caudal to the basilar artery, by the union of two small branches of the vertebral arteries (Figure 4.125). It runs the entire length of the spinal cord in the anterior median fissure and supplies the anterior two thirds of the spinal cord (Figures 4.91, 4.126 and 4.127). Although the anterior spinal artery is quite small in diameter, it is widest in the cervical and lumbar enlargements and is much reduced in the thoracic region. The **posterior spinal arteries** arise as small branches of either the vertebral or the posterior inferior cerebellar arteries and descend along the dorsal surface of the spinal cord (Figure 4.128). The posterior one third of the spinal cord is supplied by the posterior spinal arteries. There exist frequent anastomoses joining the two posterior spinal arteries with each other and with the anterior spinal artery.

Arising from the posterior aspect of the descending aorta are **segmental arteries** that supply the vertebral column and spinal cord. They are termed the **intercostal** arteries in the thoracic region and **lumbar arteries** in the lumbar region. These vessels extend toward the intervertebral foramen, where they divide into spinal branches (Figures 4.128 through 4.131). After giving off an anterior and posterior branch to the walls of the vertebral column, the spinal branches divide into anterior and posterior radicular arteries that pass along the ventral and dorsal roots into the spinal cord (Figure 4.128). The **anterior radicular arteries** contribute blood to the anterior spinal artery, and the **posterior radicular arteries** contribute blood to the posterior spinal arteries. The largest of the radicular arteries is the **great anterior radicular artery (artery of Adamkiewicz)**, which arises in the lower thoracic and upper lumbar region typically between T12 and L3 (Figures 4.125 and 4.127). This vessel makes a major contribution to the anterior spinal artery and provides the main blood supply to the inferior two thirds of the spinal cord.

A rupture from an aneurysm of the great radicular artery (artery of Adamkiewicz) may result in paralysis of the lower limbs because the artery provides the main blood supply to the inferior two thirds of the spinal cord.

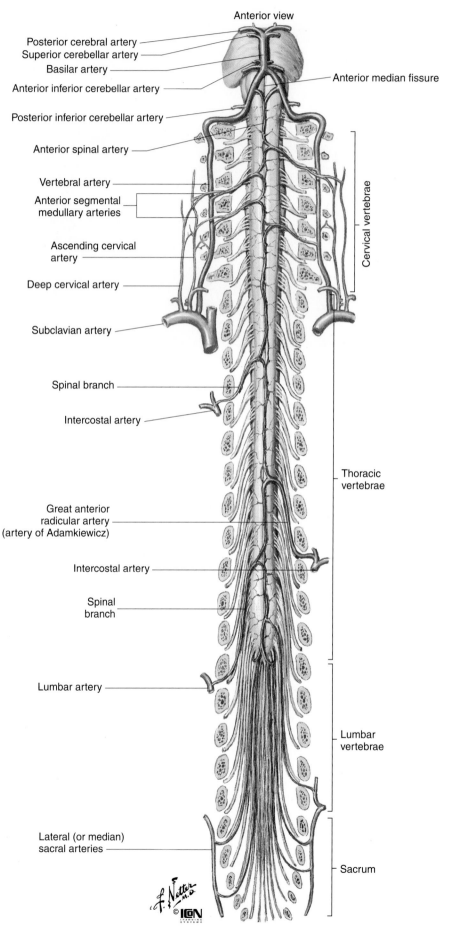

Anterior view

Posterior cerebral artery
Superior cerebellar artery
Basilar artery
Anterior inferior cerebellar artery

Posterior inferior cerebellar artery

Anterior spinal artery

Vertebral artery
Anterior segmental medullary arteries

Ascending cervical artery

Deep cervical artery

Subclavian artery

Spinal branch

Intercostal artery

Great anterior radicular artery (artery of Adamkiewicz)

Intercostal artery

Spinal branch

Lumbar artery

Lateral (or median) sacral arteries

Anterior median fissure

Cervical vertebrae

Thoracic vertebrae

Lumbar vertebrae

Sacrum

FIGURE 4.125 Anterior view of spinal arteries.

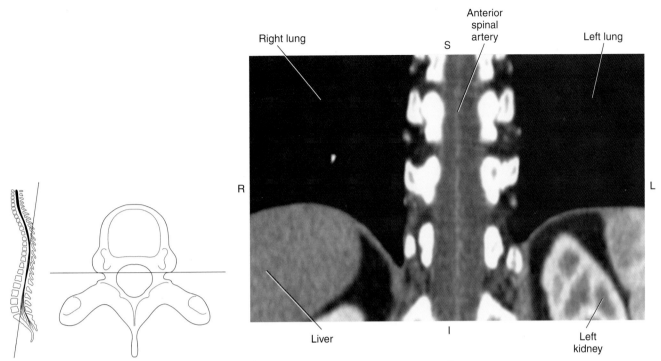

FIGURE 4.126 Coronal CT reformat with anterior spinal artery.

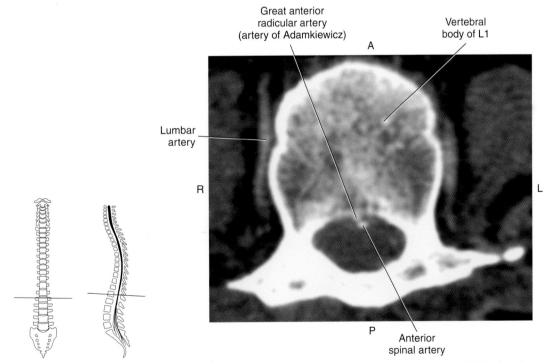

FIGURE 4.127 Axial CT with anterior spinal artery and great anterior radicular artery (artery of Adamkiewicz).

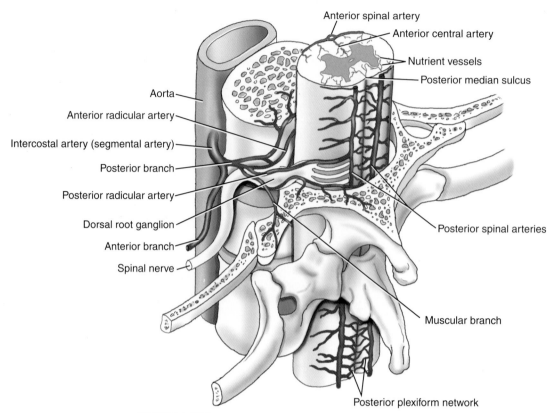

FIGURE 4.128 Posterior oblique view of radicular arteries.

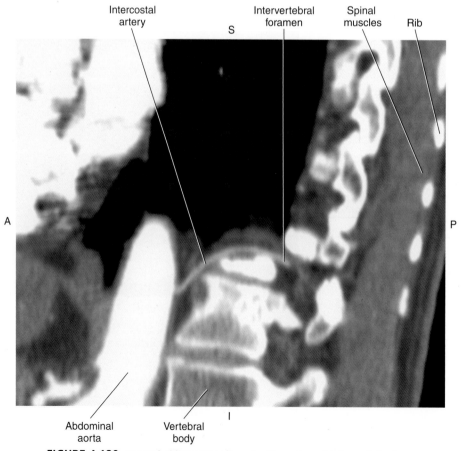

FIGURE 4.129 Coronal oblique CT reformat with aorta and intercostal artery.

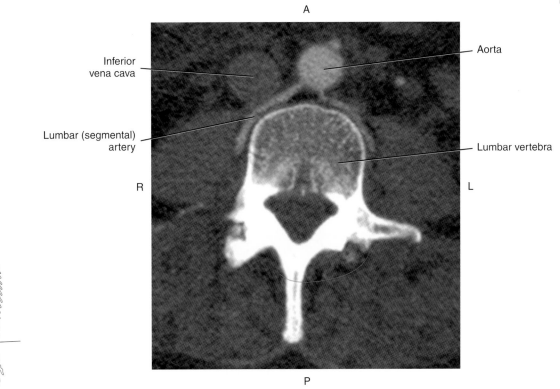

FIGURE 4.130 Axial CT of aorta and lumbar artery.

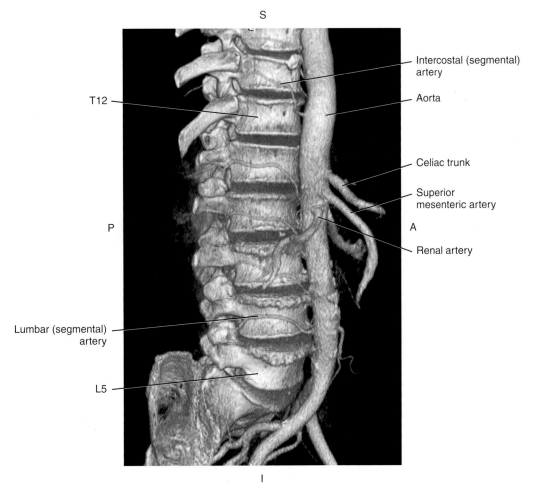

FIGURE 4.131 3D CT of lumbar spine, aorta, and segmental arteries, anterior oblique view.

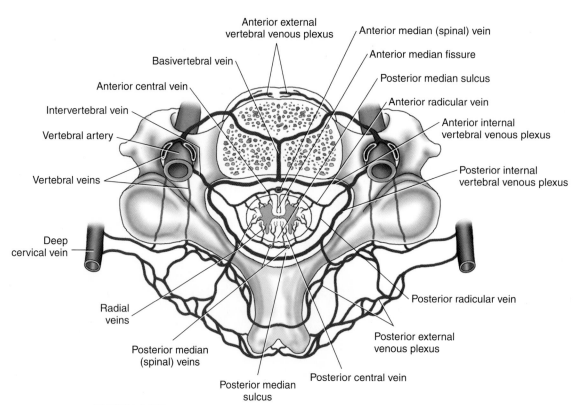

FIGURE 4.132 Axial view of venous drainage of vertebral column and spinal cord.

Spinal Veins

Veins of the Spinal Cord. The veins that drain the spinal cord follow the same segmental organization as their arterial counterparts. The central gray matter of the cord is drained by the **anterior** and **posterior central veins** located in the anterior median fissure and posterior sulcus, respectively (Figure 4.132). The outer white matter is drained by small **radial veins** that encircle the spinal cord within the pia mater. The venous blood collected by these tiny veins drains into the **anterior** and **posterior median (spinal) veins** created by the longitudinal venous channels within the pia mater on the anterior and posterior surfaces of the spinal cord (Figure 4.132). The anterior median vein parallels the anterior spinal artery, and the posterior median vein typically presents as the largest vascular structure on the posterior surface of the spinal cord. The anterior and posterior median veins drain into the **anterior** and **posterior radicular veins** that parallel the ventral and dorsal nerve roots and eventually empty into the **intervertebral veins** that accompany the spinal nerves through the intervertebral foramina.

Veins of the Vertebral Column The veins of the vertebral column form an extensive network of **internal** and **external venous plexuses**, named according to their corresponding location in the vertebral column (Figures 4.132 through 4.135). The **internal venous plexuses** lie within the vertebral canal in the epidural space and are divided into **anterior** and **posterior internal plexuses**.

The valveless **external venous plexuses** communicate freely with the vertebral veins and intracranial venous sinuses and are located at the outer surfaces of the vertebral column. They can be divided into the anterior and posterior external plexuses. The **anterior external venous plexuses** run directly in front of the vertebral bodies, and the **posterior external venous plexuses** run along the posterior aspect of the vertebral arches (Figure 4.133). The anterior sections of the internal and external plexuses communicate via a network of veins called the **basivertebral veins,** which drain the vertebral bodies. The large basivertebral veins emerge from the posterior surfaces of the vertebral bodies (Figures 4.132, 4.133, 4.136, and 4.137). The internal and external venous plexuses, along with the radicular veins, drain into the intervertebral veins, ending in the vertebral, intercostal, lumbar, and sacral veins.

Because the vertebral venous plexuses are valveless, an increase in intra-abdominal pressure (e.g., coughing, straining) may cause backflow of blood into the basivertebral veins of the spine or dural sinuses of the brain. This creates a potential pathway for metastatic disease or other pathology to spread to the central nervous system.

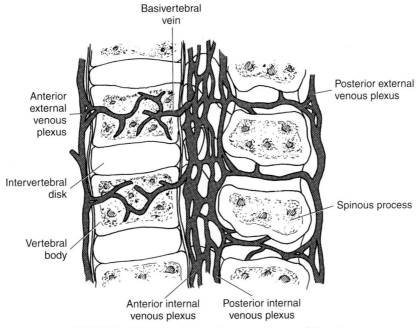

Basivertebral vein

Anterior external venous plexus

Intervertebral disk

Vertebral body

Posterior external venous plexus

Spinous process

Anterior internal venous plexus

Posterior internal venous plexus

FIGURE 4.133 Sagittal view of venous plexuses of the spine.

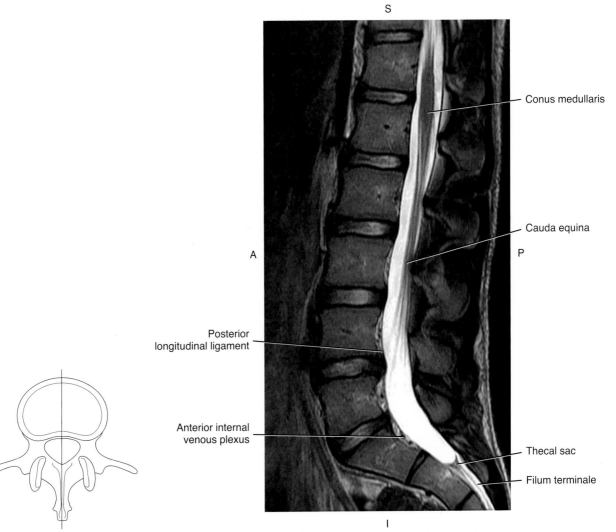

S

Conus medullaris

Cauda equina

A

P

Posterior longitudinal ligament

Anterior internal venous plexus

Thecal sac

Filum terminale

I

FIGURE 4.134 Sagittal, T2-weighted MRI of lumbar spine with anterior internal venous plexus.

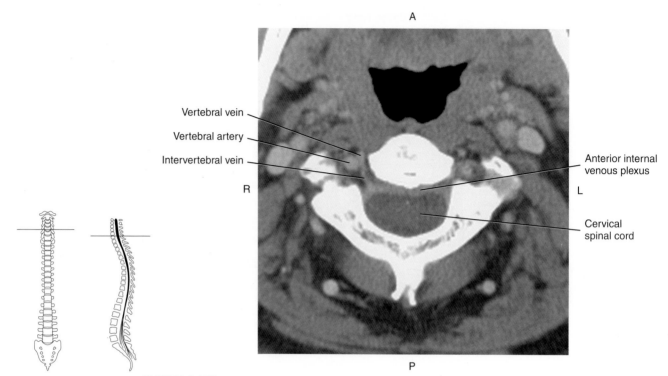

A

Vertebral vein

Vertebral artery

Intervertebral vein

R

Anterior internal
venous plexus

Cervical
spinal cord

L

P

FIGURE 4.135 Axial CT of cervical vertebra with anterior internal venous plexus.

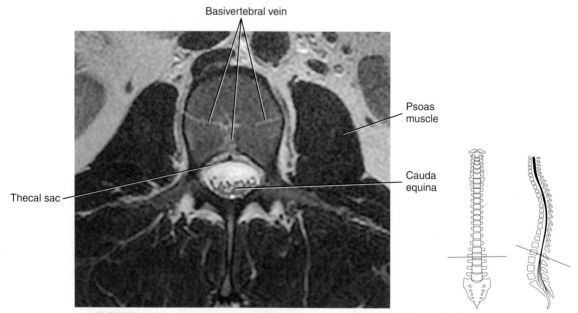

Basivertebral vein

Psoas
muscle

Cauda
equina

Thecal sac

FIGURE 4.136 Axial, T2-weighted MRI of lumbar vertebra with basivertebral vein.

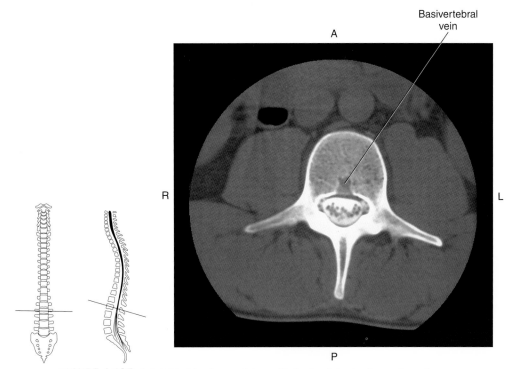

A

Basivertebral
vein

R   L

P

FIGURE 4.137 Axial CT of lumbar vertebra with basivertebral vein, post myelogram.

REFERENCES

Frank: *Merrill's atlas of radiographic positions and radiologic procedures*, ed 12, St. Louis, 2012, Mosby.

Jacob S: *Atlas of human anatomy*, Philadelphia, 2002, Churchill Livingstone.

Larsen WJ: *Anatomy: development function clinical correlations*, Philadelphia, 2002, Saunders.

Mosby's *medical, nursing, and allied health dictionary*, ed 6, St. Louis, 2002, Mosby.

Standring S: *Gray's anatomy*, ed 40, Philadelphia, 2011, Churchill Livingstone.

Som PM, Curtin HD: *Head and neck imaging*, ed 4, St. Louis, 2002, Mosby Year Book.

5

Neck

A sharp tongue and a dull mind are usually found in the same head.

Proverb

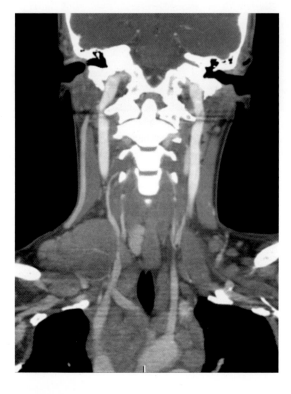

The neck has a large amount of complex anatomy situated in a relatively small area. Recent advances in medical imaging have enhanced the ability to differentiate among the structures of the neck (Figure 5.1).

FIGURE 5.1 Coronal CT reformat demonstrating massive cervical lymphadenopathy.

OBJECTIVES

- List the three anatomic sections of the pharynx.
- List and identify the laryngeal cartilages.
- Identify and describe the esophagus and trachea.
- Identify and state the function of the salivary glands.
- Describe the location and function of the thyroid gland.
- List the cervical lymph node regions.

- Identify the fascial planes and spaces.
- Identify the pharyngeal muscles.
- State the triangles of the neck and identify the muscles that divide them.
- Describe the course of the major vessels located within the neck.

OUTLINE

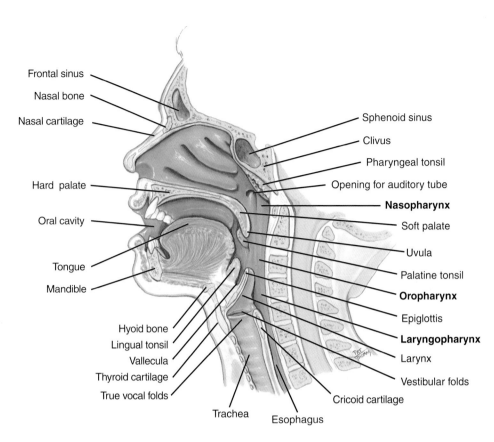

Frontal sinus

Nasal bone

Nasal cartilage

Sphenoid sinus

Clivus

Pharyngeal tonsil

Opening for auditory tube

Hard palate

Nasopharynx

Soft palate

Oral cavity

Uvula

Palatine tonsil

Tongue

Oropharynx

Mandible

Epiglottis

Laryngopharynx

Larynx

Hyoid bone

Lingual tonsil

Vallecula

Vestibular folds

Thyroid cartilage

Cricoid cartilage

True vocal folds

Trachea

Esophagus

FIGURE 5.2   Midsagittal view of the neck.

ORGANS

The structures of the neck are attached to one another by connective tissue and muscles. They are located primarily in the anterior and middle portions of the neck and include the pharynx, larynx, esophagus, trachea, salivary glands, thyroid gland, and cervical lymph nodes.

Pharynx

The **pharynx** is a funnel-shaped fibromuscular tube approximately 12 cm long that acts as an opening for both the respiratory and digestive systems. The pharynx extends from the base of the skull and ends inferiorly as the continuation of the esophagus. The pharynx is divided into three sections: nasopharynx, oropharynx, and laryngopharynx (Figures 5.2 through 5.5).

The **nasopharynx** is the most superior portion of the pharynx. It is an extension of the nasal cavities with which it shares the nasal mucosa. The nasopharynx has a respiratory function to allow for the passage of air from the nasal cavity to the larynx. Posteriorly, the boundaries of the nasopharynx are the clivus and upper cervical spine. It is bordered inferiorly by the **soft palate** and extends down to the level of the **uvula,** which is a projection on the posterior edge of the soft palate (Figures 5.2 through 5.7). In the roof and posterior wall of the nasopharynx is a collection of lymphoid tissue known as **pharyngeal tonsils,** commonly called the adenoids (Figures 5.2 through 5.5). Within the lateral wall

of the nasopharynx, posterior to the inferior nasal conchae, is the opening of the **auditory tube (eustachian tube),** which connects the middle ear to the nasopharynx (Figure 5.2).

The **oropharynx** is the posterior extension of the oral cavity and extends from the soft palate to the level of the hyoid bone (Figures 5.2, 5.4, 5.5, 5.8, and 5.9). It is separated from the larynx by the epiglottis. Two additional pairs of lymphoid tissue are found within the oropharynx: the **palatine tonsils,** which are located on the lateral walls, and the smaller **lingual tonsils,** which are situated on the base of the tongue (Figures 5.2 and 5.3). Collectively, the tonsils initiate specific defense mechanisms of the immune system by protecting against pathogens entering the nasopharynx and oropharynx. At the union of the base of the tongue and the epiglottis are two pouch-like openings called **valleculae.** The valleculae are common sites for foreign objects to become lodged within the pharynx (Figures 5.2 through 5.5, 5.10, and 5.11).

The narrow **laryngopharynx** continues from the oropharynx and lies between the hyoid bone and the entrance to the larynx and esophagus (Figures 5.2 through 5.5). It continues as the esophagus at the level of the cricoid cartilage of the larynx. Within the anterior walls of the laryngopharynx, along either side of the larynx, are two depressions or cavities termed the **piriform sinuses (recesses).** These sinuses divert food away from the entrance of the larynx and into the esophagus (Figures 5.3 and 5.12 through 5.17).

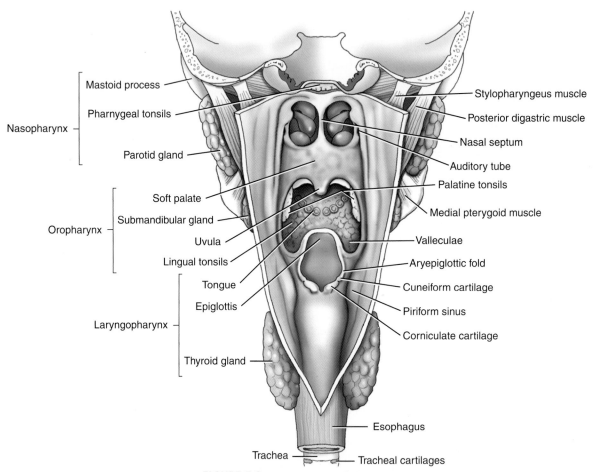

FIGURE 5.3 Posterior view of pharynx.

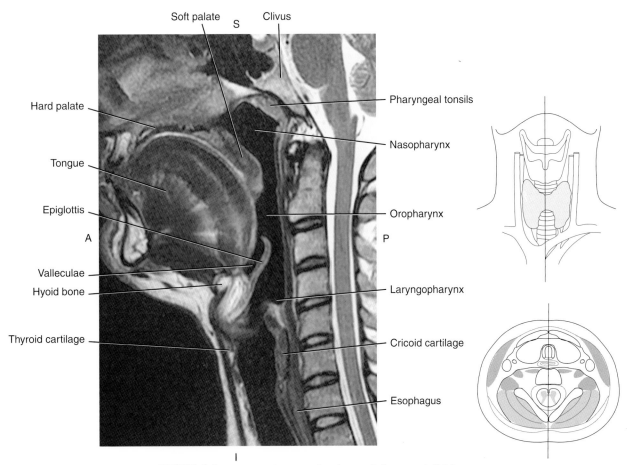

FIGURE 5.4 Midsagittal, T2-weighted MRI of pharyngeal divisions.

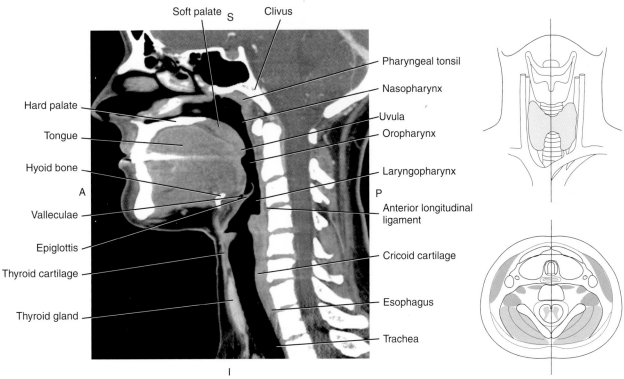

FIGURE 5.5 Sagittal CT reformat of pharynx.

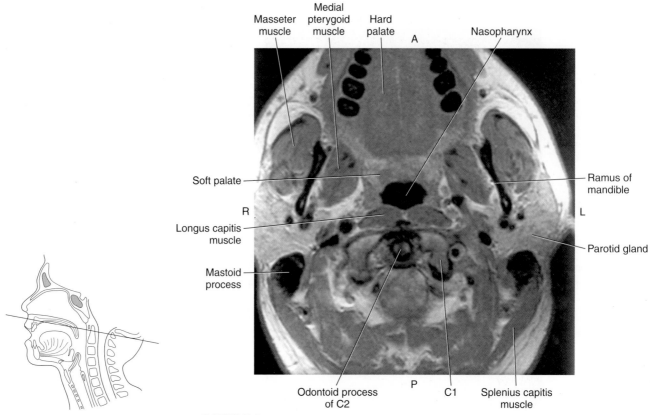

FIGURE 5.6 Axial, T1-weighted MRI of nasopharynx.

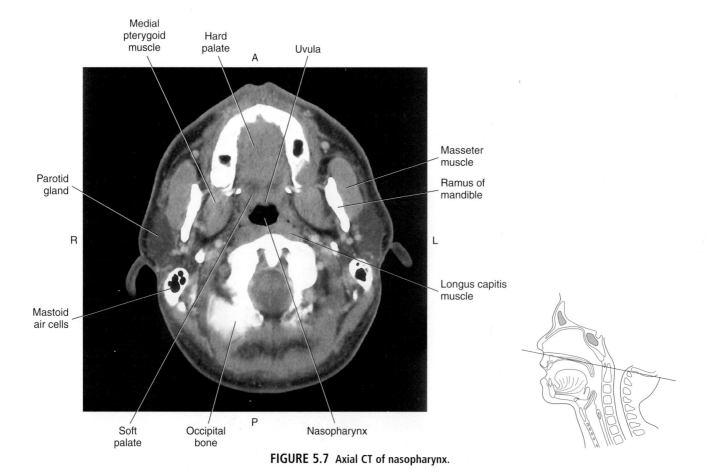

FIGURE 5.7 Axial CT of nasopharynx.

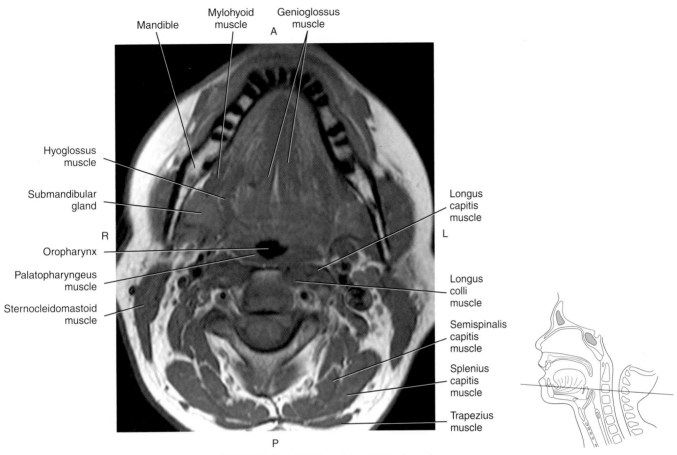

Mandible

Mylohyoid muscle

Genioglossus muscle

A

Hyoglossus muscle

Submandibular gland

R

Oropharynx

Palatopharyngeus muscle

Sternocleidomastoid muscle

Longus capitis muscle

L

Longus colli muscle

Semispinalis capitis muscle

Splenius capitis muscle

Trapezius muscle

P

FIGURE 5.8 Axial, T1-weighted MRI of oropharynx.

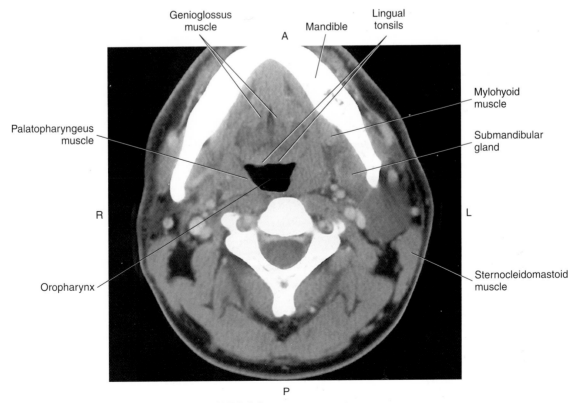

Genioglossus muscle

Mandible

Lingual tonsils

A

Palatopharyngeus muscle

Mylohyoid muscle

Submandibular gland

R

L

Oropharynx

Sternocleidomastoid muscle

P

FIGURE 5.9 Axial CT of oropharynx.

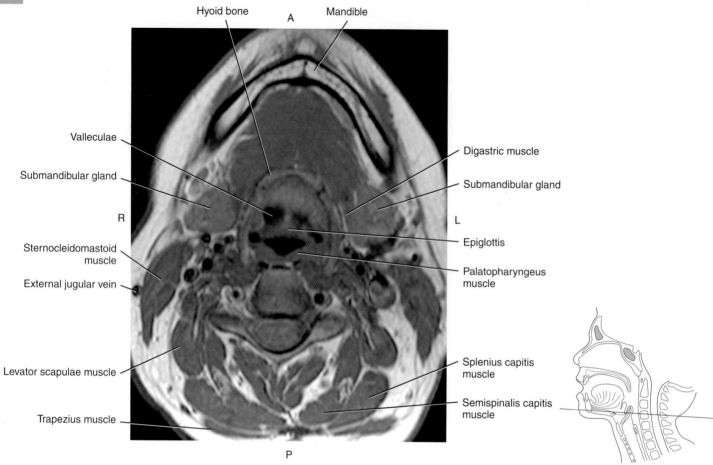

FIGURE 5.10 Axial, T1-weighted MRI of valleculae.

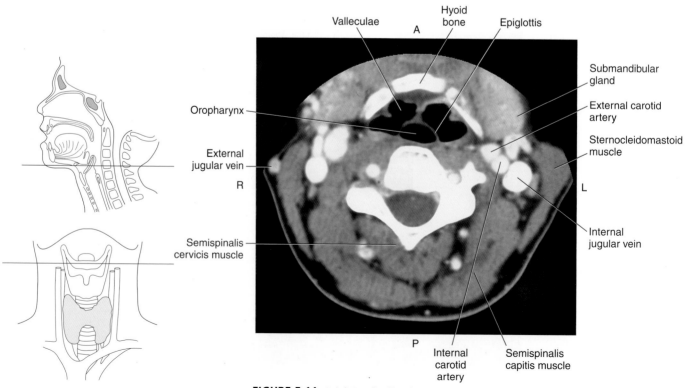

FIGURE 5.11 Axial CT of valleculae.

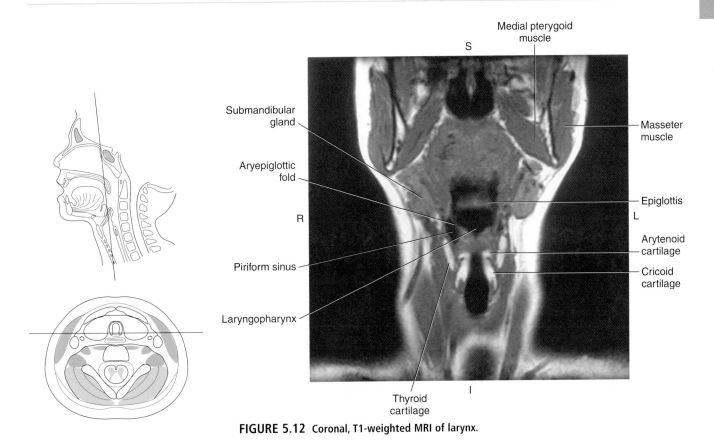

FIGURE 5.12 Coronal, T1-weighted MRI of larynx.

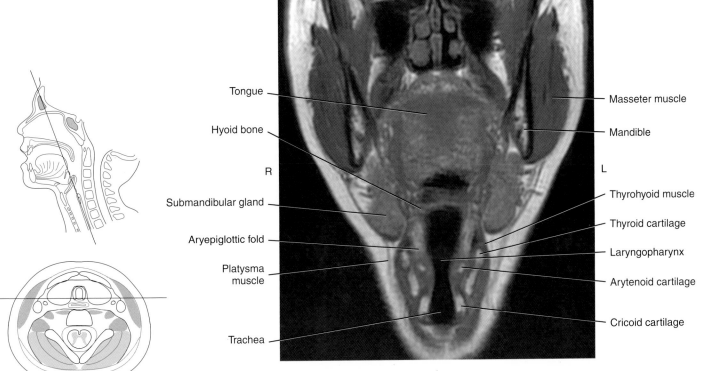

FIGURE 5.13 Coronal, T1-weighted MRI of piriform sinuses.

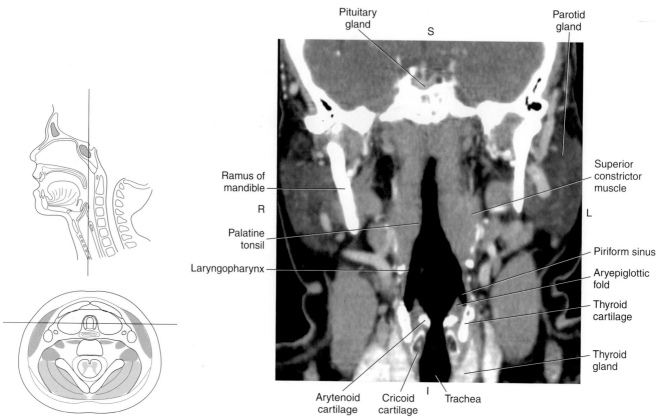

FIGURE 5.14 Coronal CT reformat of piriform sinuses.

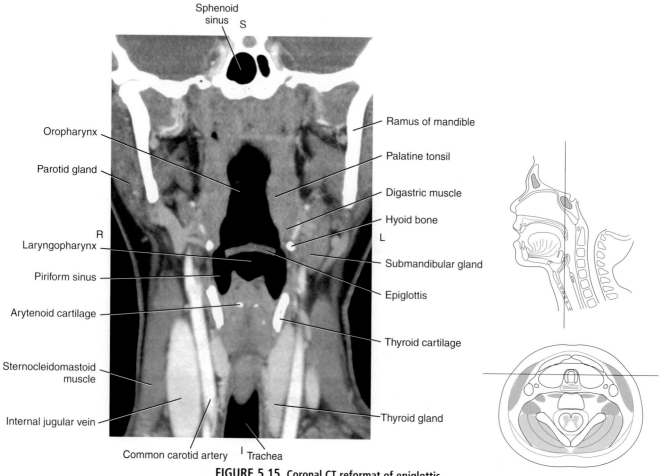

FIGURE 5.15 Coronal CT reformat of epiglottis.

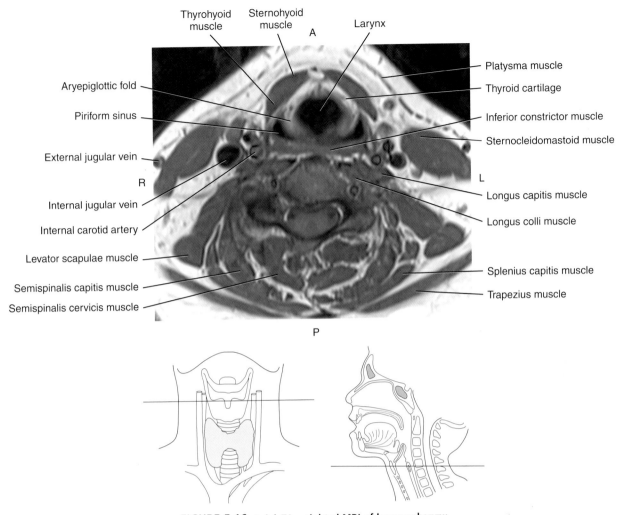

FIGURE 5.16 Axial, T1-weighted MRI of laryngopharynx.

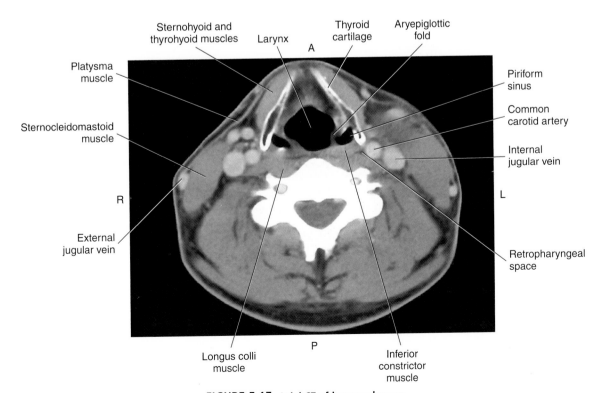

FIGURE 5.17 Axial CT of laryngopharynx.

Larynx

The **larynx** is the bony skeleton that surrounds and pro-tects the vocal cords and is commonly called the voice box. It begins at the laryngopharynx, continues to the trachea, and marks the beginning of the respiratory path-way by allowing for the passage of air into the trachea. The larynx consists of an outer skeleton made up of nine cartilages that extend from approximately the third to the sixth cervical vertebrae. These cartilages are connected to one another by ligaments and are moved by numerous muscles. Three of the cartilages are unpaired and include the thyroid, epiglottis, and cricoid. The three paired car-tilages are the arytenoid, corniculate, and cuneiform (Figures 5.18 through 5.21). The largest and most supe-rior is the **thyroid cartilage**. It consists of a right and a left lamina that unite anteriorly to form a shield to protect the vocal cords (Figures 5.19, 5.20, 5.22, and 5.23). The posterior aspect of the lamina have superior and inferior projections termed the **superior** and **inferior**

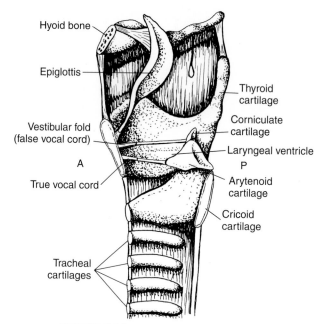

FIGURE 5.18 Midsagittal view of larynx.

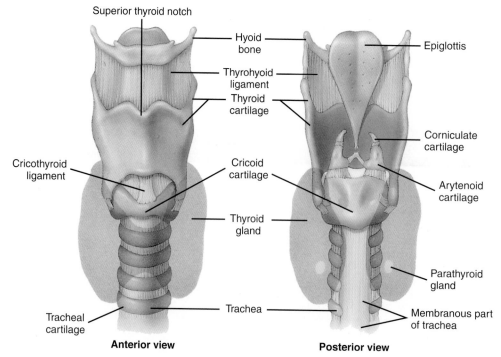

Anterior view   **Posterior view**

FIGURE 5.19 Anterior and posterior views of larynx.

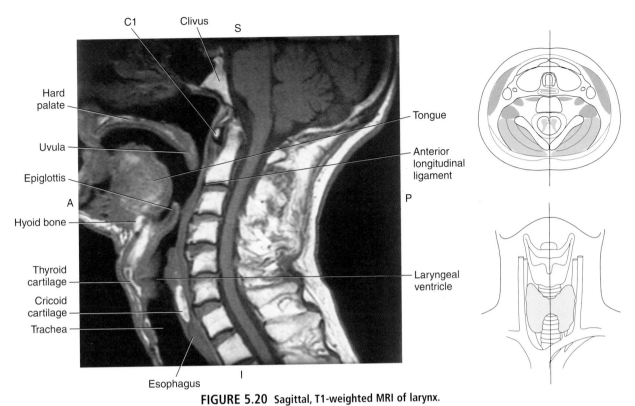

FIGURE 5.20 Sagittal, T1-weighted MRI of larynx.

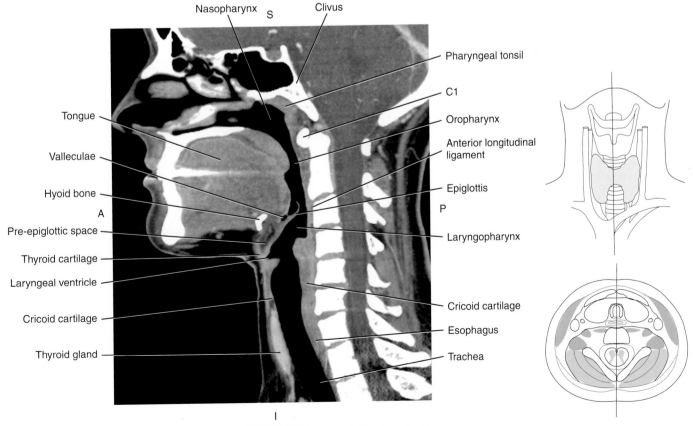

FIGURE 5.21 Sagittal CT reformat of larynx.

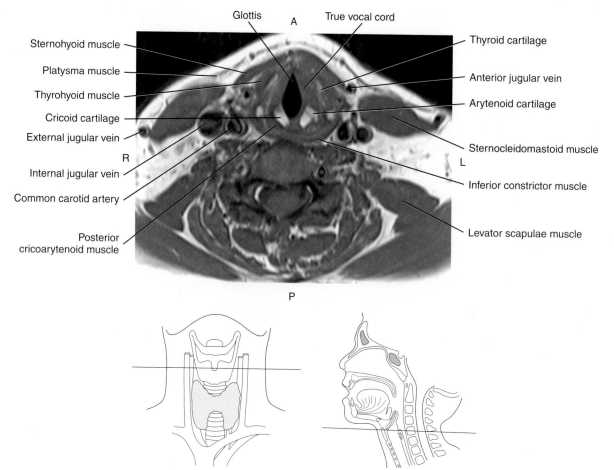

Glottis

True vocal cord

A

Sternohyoid muscle

Platysma muscle

Thyrohyoid muscle

Cricoid cartilage

External jugular vein

R

Internal jugular vein

Common carotid artery

Posterior
cricoarytenoid muscle

P

Thyroid cartilage

Anterior jugular vein

Arytenoid cartilage

Sternocleidomastoid muscle

L

Inferior constrictor muscle

Levator scapulae muscle

FIGURE 5.22 Axial, T1-weighted MRI of neck with thyroid cartilage.

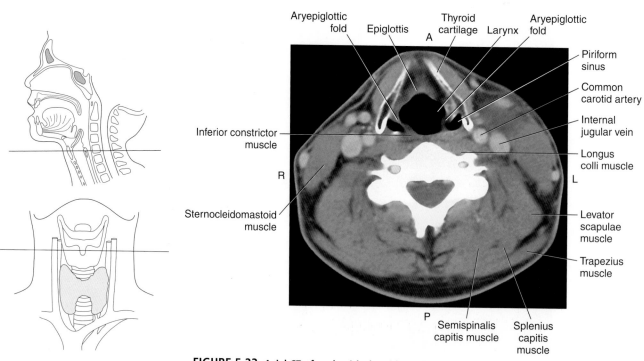

Aryepiglottic
fold

Epiglottis

Thyroid
cartilage

A

Larynx

Aryepiglottic
fold

Piriform
sinus

Common
carotid artery

Internal
jugular vein

Longus
colli muscle

Levator
scapulae
muscle

Trapezius
muscle

Inferior constrictor
muscle

R

Sternocleidomastoid
muscle

L

P

Semispinalis
capitis muscle

Splenius
capitis
muscle

FIGURE 5.23 Axial CT of neck with thyroid cartilage.

horns (cornua), respectively. The anterior union of the lamina forms a vertical projection commonly referred to as the **laryngeal prominence (Adam's apple).** Just above the laryngeal prominence is an area where the lamina do not meet, creating the superior thyroid notch. On the posterior aspect of this projection is the attachment for the epiglottis. The leaf-shaped **epiglottis** differs from the other cartilages in that it is elastic and allows for movement. It is covered with a mucus membrane and projects superiorly and posteriorly behind the tongue. It is attached to the thyroid cartilage via the thyroepiglottic ligament and to the hyoid bone via the hyoepiglottic ligament. During swallowing, the epiglottis folds back over the larynx, preventing the entry of liquids or solid food into the respiratory passageways (Figures 5.18 through 5.21, 5.24, and 5.25). The paired **arytenoid cartilages** are shaped like pyramids and are situated at the posterior aspect of the larynx just on top of the cricoid cartilage (Figures 5.18, 5.19, 5.22, 5.26, and 5.27). Articulating with the superior surface of the arytenoid cartilages are the small, horn-shaped **corniculate cartilages.** These cartilages are involved in the movement of the vocal cords for the production of sound. The small, curved **cuneiform cartilages** lie within the folds of tissue termed the *aryepiglottic folds* that extend between the lateral aspect of the arytenoid cartilage and epiglottis (Figure 5.3). The **cricoid cartilage** is a complete ring that forms the base of the larynx on which the other laryngeal cartilages rest. The posterior portion of the cricoid is broader than the anterior portion.The cricoid cartilage marks the junction between the larynx and the trachea and the beginning of the esophagus (Figures 5.2, 5.28, and 5.29).

Resultant swelling of the epiglottis because of bacterial or viral infection can be very dangerous (acute epiglottitis). This condition can result in closure of the glottis and suffocation.

The inner structures of the larynx include the false and true vocal cords and the aryepiglottic folds. The false and true vocal cords consist of two pair of ligaments that extend from the arytenoid cartilages to the posterior laminal surface of the thyroid cartilage and are separated by a space termed the **laryngeal ventricle** (Figures 5.18, 5.20 and 5.21). The superior pair of ligaments is called the **vestibular folds or false vocal cords** because they are not directly concerned in the production of sound. The inferior pair is the **true vocal cords** named accordingly for their involvement in the production of sound (Figure 5.18). The true vocal cords extend toward the midline in a closed position during phonation. With quiet respiration the true vocal cords are in a relaxed position, creating an opening between them called the **glottis** (Figures 5.18, 5.26, 5.27, 5.30, and 5.31). The glottis is the part of the larynx most directly involved with voice production. The **aryepiglottic folds** consist of tissue projecting off the arytenoid cartilages to the inferior margin of the epiglottis. These folds form the lateral margins of the entrance to the larynx. Located lateral to these folds, between the larynx and thyroid cartilage, are two mucosal pouches called the piriform sinuses whose medial borders form the lateral walls of the larynx (Figures 5.3, 5.12 through 5.17).

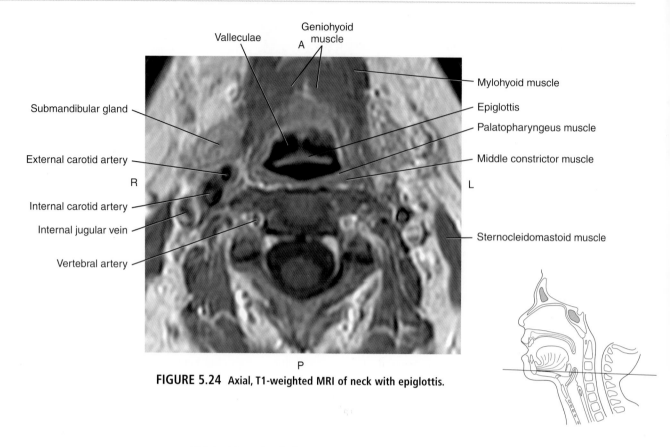

Valleculae

Geniohyoid muscle

A

Submandibular gland

External carotid artery

R

Internal carotid artery

Internal jugular vein

Vertebral artery

Mylohyoid muscle

Epiglottis

Palatopharyngeus muscle

Middle constrictor muscle

L

Sternocleidomastoid muscle

P

FIGURE 5.24 Axial, T1-weighted MRI of neck with epiglottis.

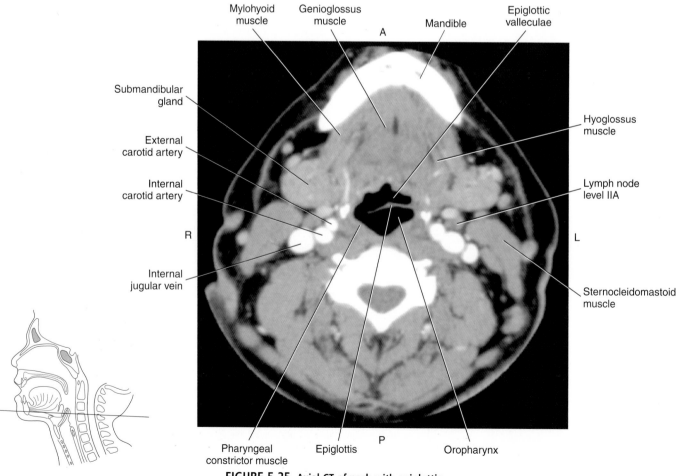

Mylohyoid muscle

Genioglossus muscle

A

Mandible

Epiglottic valleculae

Submandibular gland

External carotid artery

Internal carotid artery

R

Internal jugular vein

Hyoglossus muscle

Lymph node level IIA

L

Sternocleidomastoid muscle

Pharyngeal constrictor muscle

Epiglottis

P

Oropharynx

FIGURE 5.25 Axial CT of neck with epiglottis.

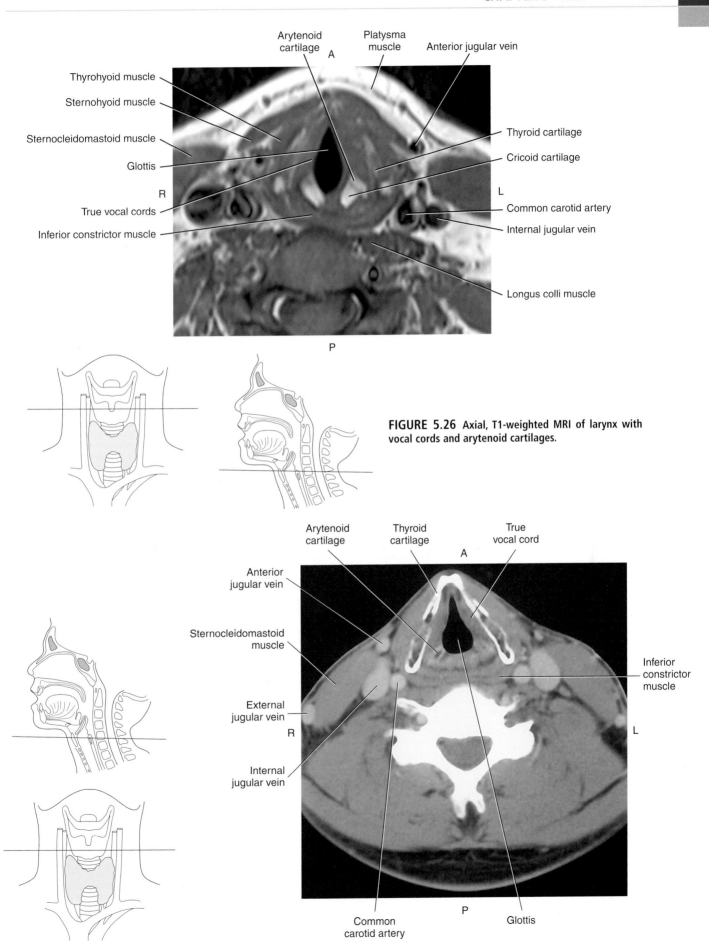

Arytenoid cartilage
Platysma muscle
Anterior jugular vein
Thyrohyoid muscle
Sternohyoid muscle
Sternocleidomastoid muscle
Glottis
True vocal cords
Inferior constrictor muscle
Thyroid cartilage
Cricoid cartilage
Common carotid artery
Internal jugular vein
Longus colli muscle
A
R
L
P

FIGURE 5.26 Axial, T1-weighted MRI of larynx with vocal cords and arytenoid cartilages.

Arytenoid cartilage
Thyroid cartilage
True vocal cord
Anterior jugular vein
Sternocleidomastoid muscle
External jugular vein
Internal jugular vein
Inferior constrictor muscle
Common carotid artery
Glottis
A
R
L
P

FIGURE 5.27 Axial CT of larynx with vocal cords and arytenoid cartilages.

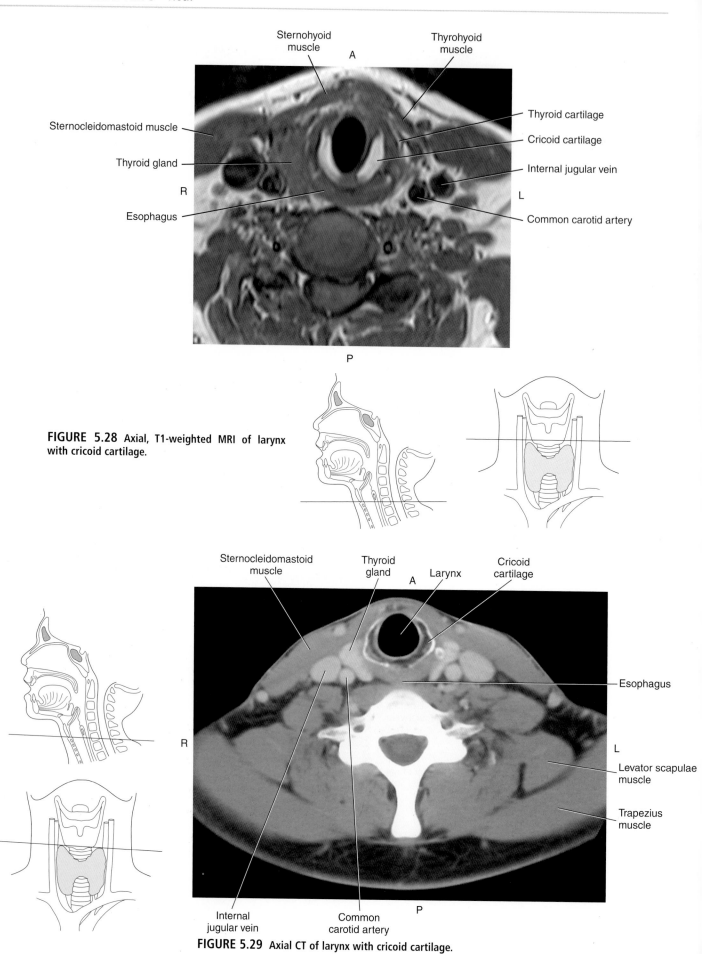

Sternohyoid muscle

Thyrohyoid muscle

A

Sternocleidomastoid muscle

Thyroid gland

Esophagus

R

Thyroid cartilage

Cricoid cartilage

Internal jugular vein

Common carotid artery

L

P

FIGURE 5.28 Axial, T1-weighted MRI of larynx with cricoid cartilage.

Sternocleidomastoid muscle

Thyroid gland

A   Larynx

Cricoid cartilage

R

Esophagus

L

Levator scapulae muscle

Trapezius muscle

Internal jugular vein

Common carotid artery

P

FIGURE 5.29 Axial CT of larynx with cricoid cartilage.

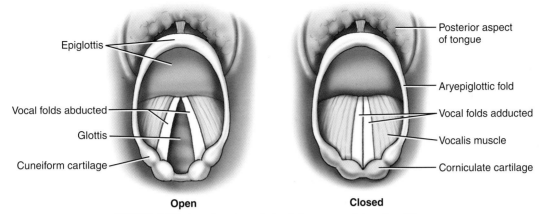

Epiglottis

Posterior aspect of tongue

Aryepiglottic fold

Vocal folds abducted

Vocal folds adducted

Glottis

Vocalis muscle

Cuneiform cartilage

Corniculate cartilage

Open   **Closed**

FIGURE 5.30 Superior view of glottis in open and closed positions.

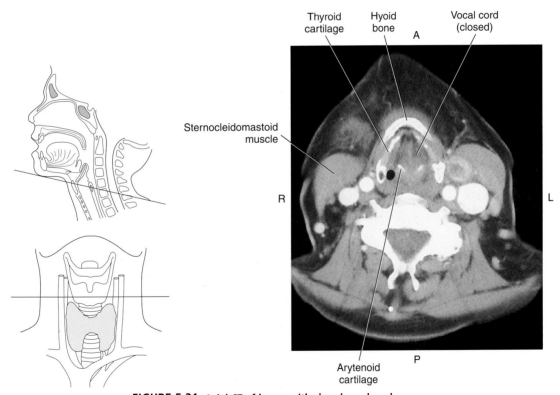

Thyroid cartilage

Hyoid bone

A

Vocal cord (closed)

Sternocleidomastoid muscle

R   L

P

Arytenoid cartilage

FIGURE 5.31 Axial CT of larynx with closed vocal cords.

Esophagus and Trachea

The **esophagus** is a muscular tube that extends down from the laryngopharynx to the cardiac orifice of the stomach (Figures 5.32 through 5.34). It begins posterior to the cricoid cartilage and descends through the thoracic cavity between the trachea and anterior longitudinal ligament of the vertebrae (Figures 5.20 and 5.21). The esophagus then enters the abdominal cavity through an opening in the diaphragm termed the **esophageal hiatus** to join the stomach (Figure 5.32). There are two narrowed areas, or sphincters, of the esophagus: esophageal and cardiac. The esophageal sphincter is situated at the entrance of the esophagus and functions to prevent air from entering the esophagus. The inferior or cardiac sphincter prevents reflux from the stomach into the esophagus. The **trachea**, considered the airway, extends from the larynx to the lungs and lies immediately anterior to the esophagus (Figures 5.20, 5.21, and 5.32 through 5.34). Considered an elastic tube, the trachea is reinforced by approximately 16-20 C-shaped pieces of cartilage that maintain an open passageway for air. The cartilages are closed posteriorly by elastic connective tissue that allows for the passage of food through the esophagus. At approximately the level of T5, the trachea bifurcates at a level termed the **carina** into the right and left mainstem bronchi.

The tracheostomy is one of the most frequently performed procedures today and is one of the oldest described surgical procedures dating back at least 3,500 years. It is an operative procedure that creates a surgical airway in the trachea via an incision in the neck and insertion of a tracheostomy tube between the second and third tracheal rings.

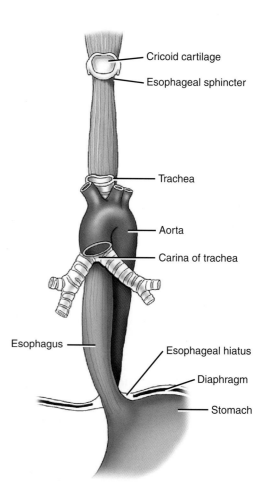

FIGURE 5.32 Anterior view of esophagus.

- Cricoid cartilage
- Esophageal sphincter
- Trachea
- Aorta
- Carina of trachea
- Esophagus
- Esophageal hiatus
- Diaphragm
- Stomach

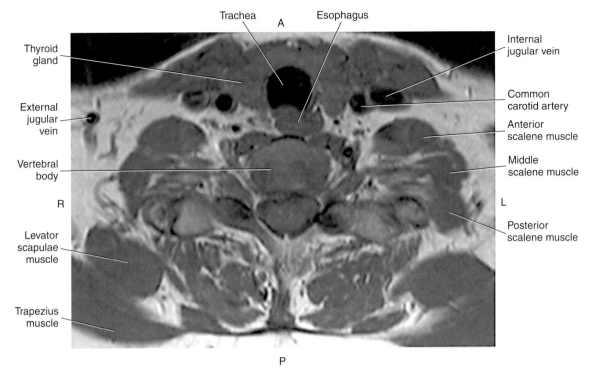

Trachea
A
Esophagus

Thyroid
gland

Internal
jugular vein

External
jugular
vein

Common
carotid artery

Anterior
scalene muscle

Vertebral
body

Middle
scalene muscle

R

L

Levator
scapulae
muscle

Posterior
scalene muscle

Trapezius
muscle

P

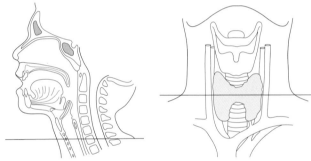

FIGURE 5.33 Axial, T1-weighted MRI of esophagus and trachea.

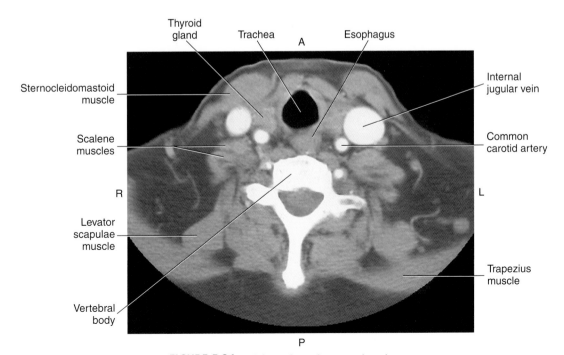

Thyroid
gland
Trachea
A
Esophagus

Sternocleidomastoid
muscle

Internal
jugular vein

Scalene
muscles

Common
carotid artery

R

L

Levator
scapulae
muscle

Trapezius
muscle

Vertebral
body

P

FIGURE 5.34 Axial CT of esophagus and trachea.

Salivary Glands

The **salivary glands** collectively produce and empty saliva into the oral cavity via ducts to begin the process of digestion. Each pair of salivary glands has a distinctive cellular organization and produces saliva with slightly different properties. There are three large paired salivary glands: parotid, submandibular, and sublingual (Figure 5.35). The largest of these are the **parotid glands**, which are situated in front of the auricle, wedged between the ramus of the mandible and the sternocleidomastoid muscle (Figures 5.36 through 5.39). The parotid glands extend inferiorly from the level of the external auditory meatus to the angle of the mandible. Their appearance differs from that of the other salivary glands because of the fatty tissue and intraglandular lymph nodes they contain. The **parotid duct (Stensen's duct)** emerges from the anterior edge of the gland. It passes under the zygomatic arch to enter the oral cavity opposite the second upper molar. The **submandibular glands** border the posterior half of the mandible, extending from the angle of the mandible to the level of the hyoid bone (Figures 5.40 through 5.42). The **submandibular duct (Wharton's duct)** opens into the oral cavity on either side of the lingual frenulum immediately posterior to the teeth. The **sublingual glands** are the smallest of the salivary glands and lie under the tongue on the floor of the mouth (Figures 5.43 and 5.44). Numerous (10-20) **sublingual ducts (Rivinus's ducts)** open in a line along the floor of the mouth. Some of these ducts may fuse to form Bartholin's duct, which opens into or adjacent to the submandibular duct (Figure 5.35).

More than 750 minor salivary glands are scattered throughout the mouth and throat. They can be found in the mucosa of the oral cavity, palate, paranasal sinuses, pharynx, trachea, and bronchi. They consist of both mucous and serous glands that help with the total production of saliva. The most common tumor site among the minor salivary glands is the palate.

The mumps virus often targets the salivary glands, most commonly the parotid gland. Infection usually occurs between 5 and 9 years of age. Because of an effective mumps vaccine, the incidence of this disease has been dramatically reduced.

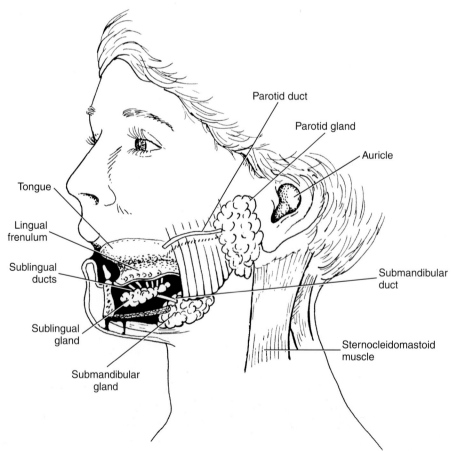

FIGURE 5.35 Lateral view of salivary glands and lymph nodes.

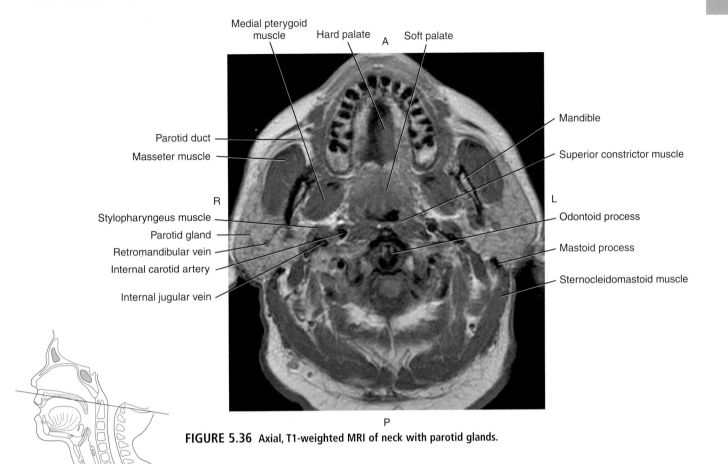

FIGURE 5.36 Axial, T1-weighted MRI of neck with parotid glands.

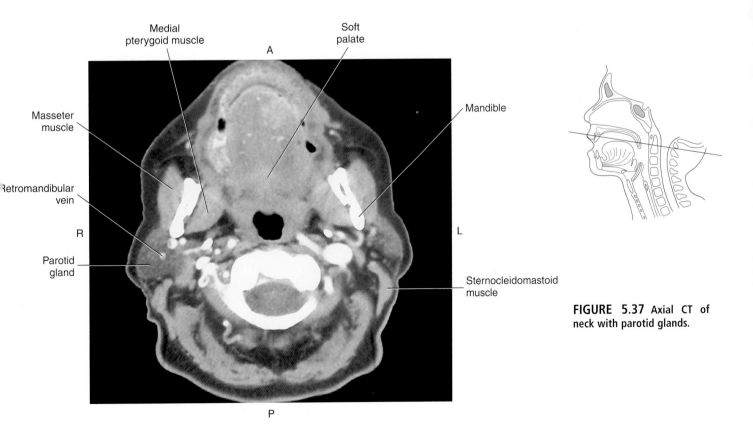

FIGURE 5.37 Axial CT of neck with parotid glands.

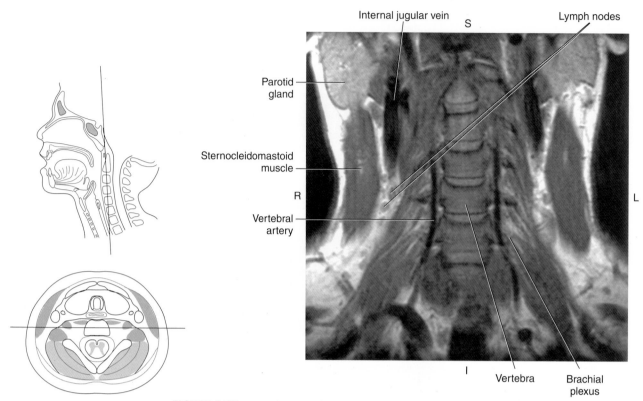

FIGURE 5.38 Coronal, T1-weighted MRI of parotid glands.

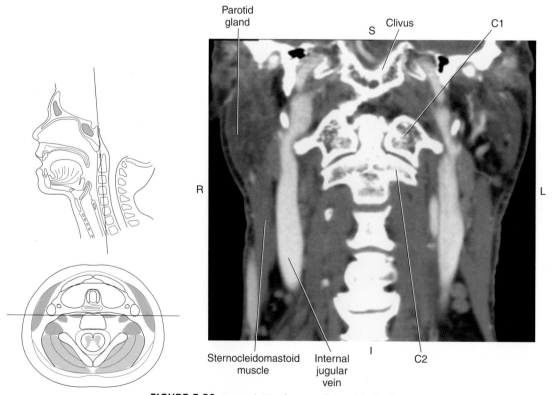

FIGURE 5.39 Coronal CT reformat of parotid glands.

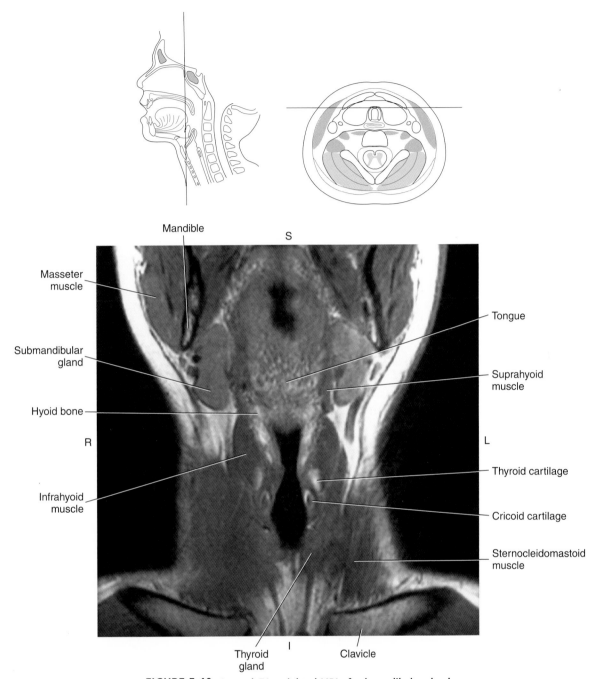

Mandible

S

Masseter
muscle

Tongue

Submandibular
gland

Suprahyoid
muscle

Hyoid bone

R   L

Thyroid cartilage

Cricoid cartilage

Infrahyoid
muscle

Sternocleidomastoid
muscle

Thyroid
gland

I

Clavicle

FIGURE 5.40 Coronal, T1-weighted MRI of submandibular glands.

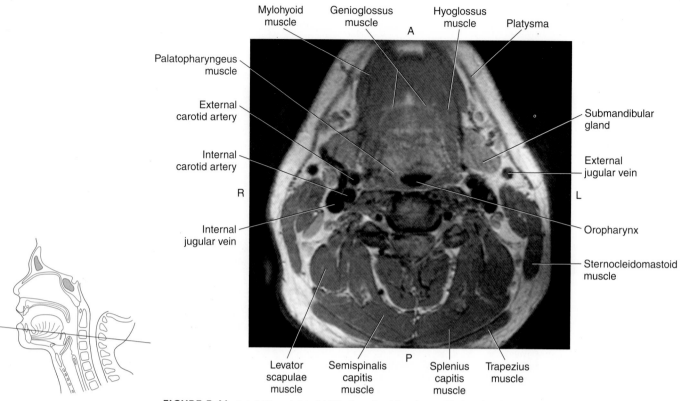

Mylohyoid muscle
Genioglossus muscle
Hyoglossus muscle
Platysma
Palatopharyngeus muscle
External carotid artery
Internal carotid artery
Internal jugular vein
Submandibular gland
External jugular vein
Oropharynx
Sternocleidomastoid muscle
Levator scapulae muscle
Semispinalis capitis muscle
Splenius capitis muscle
Trapezius muscle
A
R
L
P

FIGURE 5.41 Axial, T1-weighted MRI of neck with submandibular glands.

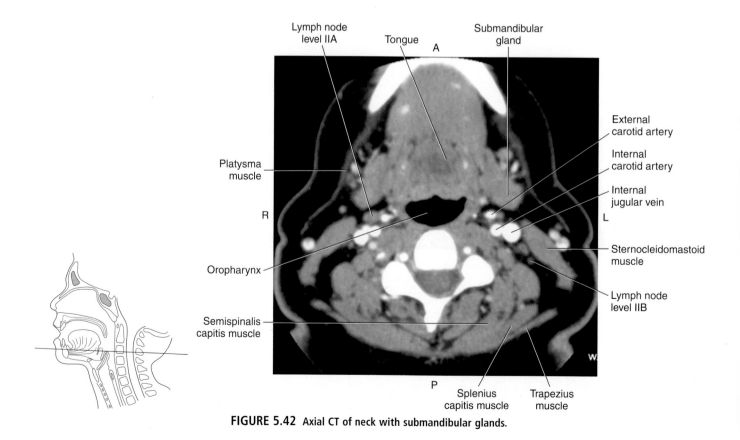

Lymph node level IIA
Tongue
Submandibular gland
Platysma muscle
External carotid artery
Internal carotid artery
Internal jugular vein
Sternocleidomastoid muscle
Lymph node level IIB
Oropharynx
Semispinalis capitis muscle
Splenius capitis muscle
Trapezius muscle
A
R
L
P

FIGURE 5.42 Axial CT of neck with submandibular glands.

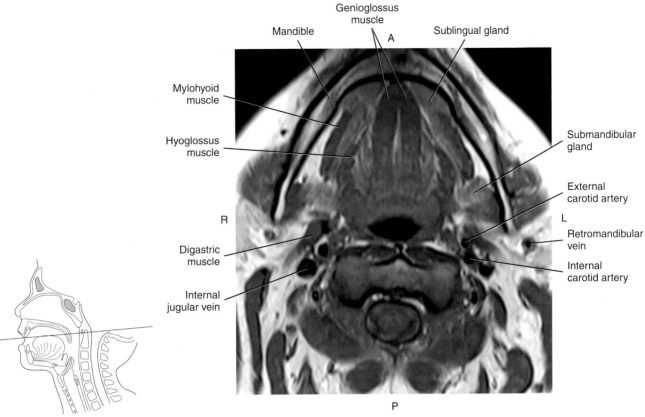

FIGURE 5.43 Axial, T1-weighted MRI of sublingual glands.

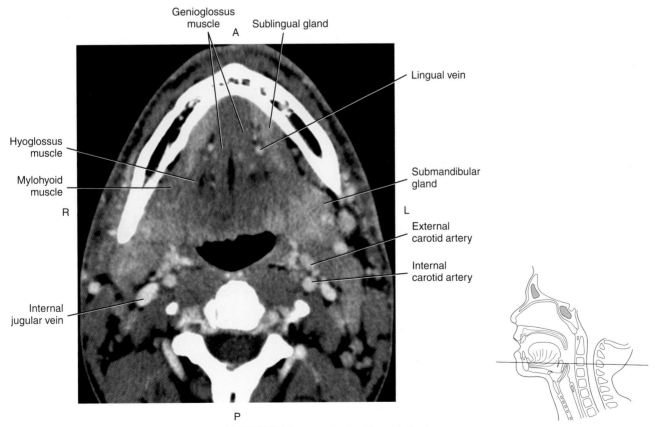

FIGURE 5.44 Axial CT of sublingual glands.

Thyroid Gland

The **thyroid gland** is an endocrine gland located at the level of the cricoid cartilage. It consists of two lobes that are joined together anteriorly by the **isthmus** (Figures 5.45 and 5.46). In the axial plane, the thyroid gland appears as a wedge-shaped structure, hugging both sides of the trachea (Figures 5.47 and 5.48). The thyroid gland excretes the hormones, thyroxine (T4), triiodothyronine (T3), and calcitonin, which affect almost every cell in the body. Thyroxine and triiodothyronine stimulate cell metabolism and are essential for normal body growth. Calcitonin lowers the blood calcium level and promotes bone formation. Also involved with metabolism of calcium and phosphorus are the parathyroid hormones (PTH), which are produced by the **parathyroid glands**. The parathyroid glands are located on the posterior surface of the thyroid lobes and are usually four in number (Figure 5.45).

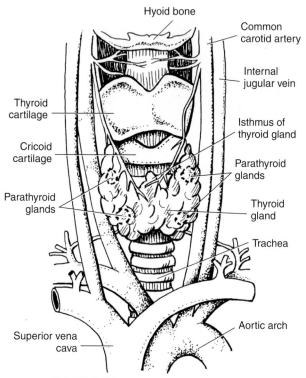

FIGURE 5.45 Anterior view of thyroid gland.

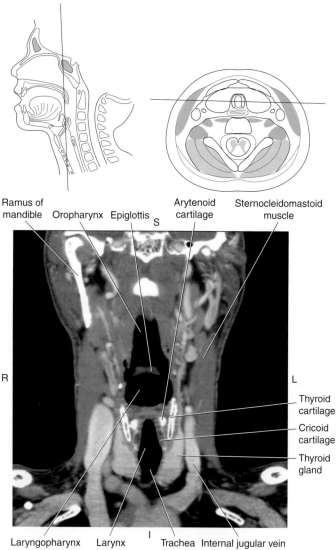

FIGURE 5.46 Coronal CT reformat of thyroid gland.

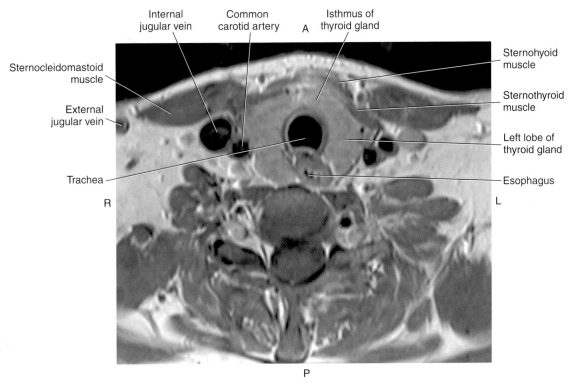

FIGURE 5.47 Axial, T1-weighted MRI of thyroid gland.

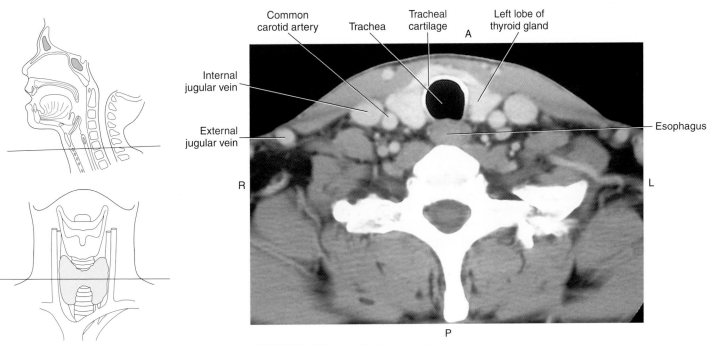

FIGURE 5.48 Axial CT of thyroid gland.

Cervical Lymph Nodes

The neck has an extensive lymphatic network containing more than one third of the body's total number of lymph nodes. Typically, as many as 75 lymph nodes are located on each side of the neck (Figures 5.49 and 5.50). **Lymph nodes** are clustered in regions throughout the vessels of the lymphatic system. The lymph vessels carry fluid from the interstitial spaces to the regional lymph nodes, which filter the lymphatic fluid of harmful foreign particles before being emptied into the venous blood supply. In the cervical region, nodes are grouped along the lower border of the jaw, in front of and behind the ears, and deep in the neck along the larger blood vessels. They drain the skin of the scalp and face, tissues of the nasal cavity, oral cavity, pharynx, trachea, upper esophagus, thyroid gland, and salivary glands. The lymph nodes of the neck can be classified or divided into seven levels or regions for ease of identification, both clinically and surgically (Table 5.1 and Figures 5.25, 5.42, and 5.49).

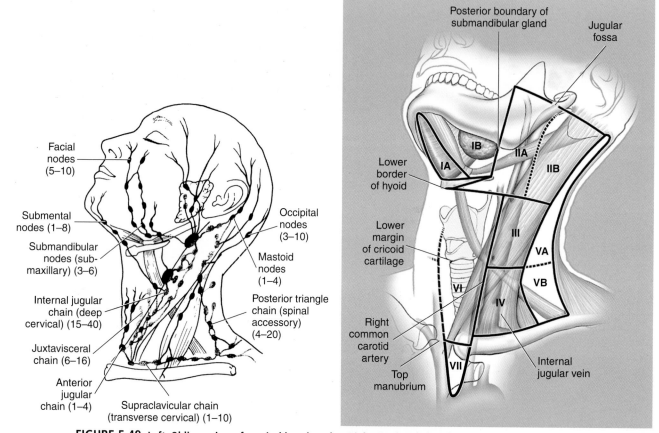

FIGURE 5.49 Left, Oblique view of cervical lymph nodes. Right, Regional classification of cervical lymph nodes.

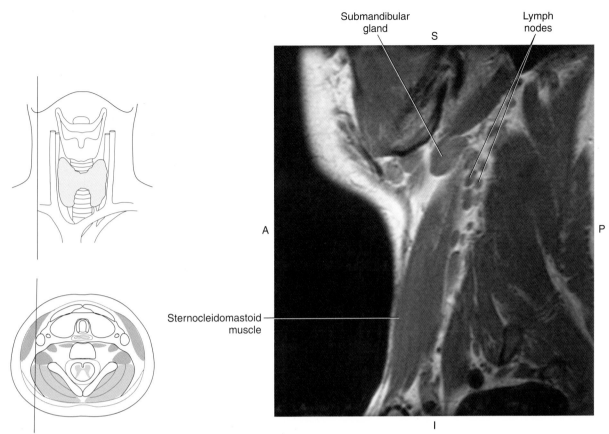

FIGURE 5.50 Sagittal, T1-weighted MRI of lymph nodes.

TABLE 5.1	Neck Lymph Nodes
Node	**Location**
Level I Submental and Submandibular Nodes	Located between the hyoid bone and the body of the mandible and in front of the posterior boundary of the submandibular gland
Level IA Submental	Midline behind the mental protuberance of the mandible
Level IB Submandibular	Midpoint between the mental protuberance of the mandible and mandibular angle
Level II Upper Internal Jugular Vein	Upper third of the internal jugular vein. Extends from the skull base to the level of the carotid bifurcation or hyoid bone. Bounded posteriorly by the sternocleidomastoid (SCM) muscle
Level IIA	A level II node that lies medial, lateral, anterior, or posterior to the internal jugular vein
Level IIB	A level II node that lies posterior to the internal jugular vein and separated by fat plane
Level III Middle Internal Jugular Vein	Extends from the carotid bifurcation or hyoid bone inferiorly to the cricoid cartilage
Level IV Lower Internal Jugular Vein	Extends superiorly from the omohyoid muscle to the clavicle inferiorly and bordered laterally by the SCM muscle
Level V Posterior Triangle Nodes	Bordered anteriorly by the SCM muscle, posteriorly by the trapezius muscle, and inferiorly by the clavicle
Level VA	Upper level V nodes. Extend inferiorly from the skull base to the cricoid cartilage
Level VB	Lower level V nodes. Extend from the bottom of the cricoid cartilage to the clavicle
Level VI Anterior Triangle Nodes, (Upper Visceral Nodes) Include Prelaryngeal, Pretracheal, and Paratracheal Nodes	Frontal compartment. Extend from the hyoid bone to the top of the manubrium. Defined laterally by carotid artery on both sides.
Level VII Superior Mediastinal Nodes	Extends from the top of the manubrium to the brachiocephalic vein, between the carotid arteries
Supraclavicular nodes	Nodes at or caudal to the clavicle and lateral to the carotid artery
Retropharyngeal nodes	Nodes behind the pharynx. Extend medial to the internal carotid artery from the base of the skull inferiorly to the hyoid bone

Fascial Planes and Spaces

The suprahyoid and infrahyoid regions of the neck can be further divided by layers of **fascia** called **fascial planes** that separate the anatomy of each region into compartments or spaces that contain distinct anatomic structures (Figure 5.51). Each compartment or space is associated with pathology specific to the anatomic structures contained within it. Knowledge of the anatomy in these compartments improves the ability to predict the spread of pathology throughout the soft tissue structures in the neck.

The **suprahyoid region** can be divided into nine main spaces: parapharyngeal, masticator, parotid, carotid, pharyngeal mucosal, retropharyngeal, prevertebral, perivertebral, and danger spaces. The **infrahyoid region** contains seven main spaces: five continuous with the suprahyoid spaces (carotid, retropharyngeal, prevertebral, perivertebral, and danger spaces) and two new spaces (posterior cervical and visceral spaces) (Figure 5.51). The fascial spaces can be identified on sequential images found in Figures 5.52 through 5.69).

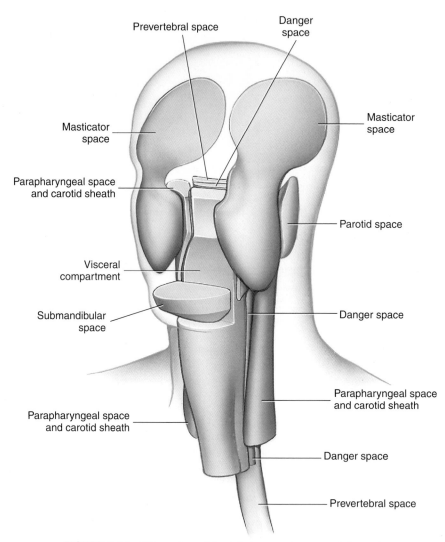

FIGURE 5.51 Oblique view of fascial planes and spaces of the neck.

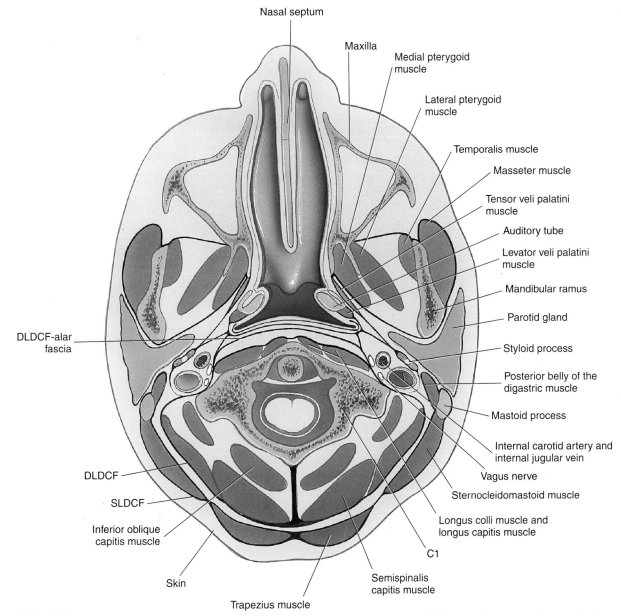

FIGURE 5.52 Axial view of neck at level of C1. DLDCF, Deep layer, deep cervical fascia; **SLDCF,** superficial layer, deep cervical fascia.

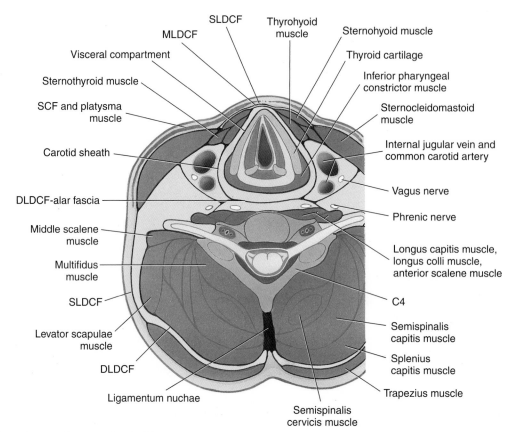

FIGURE 5.53 Axial view of neck at level of C4. DLDCF, Deep layer, deep cervical fascia; **MLDCF,** middle layer, deep cervical fascia; **SCF,** superficial cervical fascia; **SLDCF,** superficial layer, deep cervical fascia.

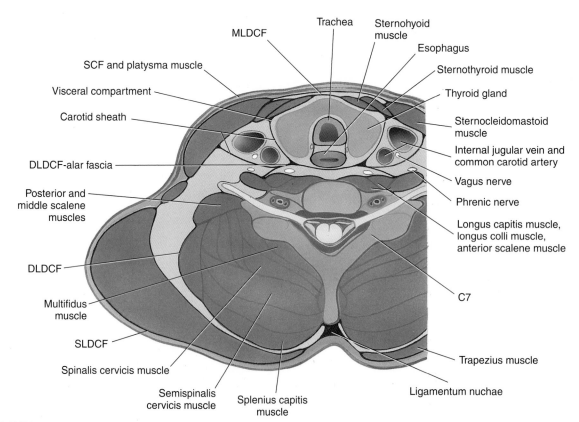

FIGURE 5.54 Axial view of neck at level of C7. DLDCF, Deep layer, deep cervical fascia; **MLDCF,** middle layer, deep cervical fascia; **SCF,** superficial cervical fascia; **SLDCF,** superficial layer, deep cervical fascia.

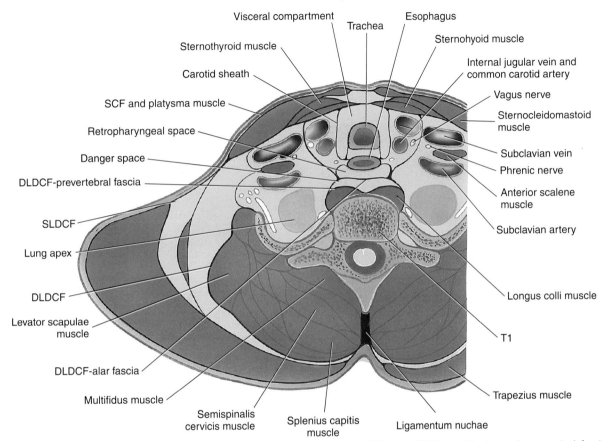

FIGURE 5.55 Axial view of neck at level of T1. DLDCF, Deep layer, deep cervical fascia; **MLDCF,** middle layer, deep cervical fascia; **SCF,** superficial cervical fascia; **SLDCF,** superficial layer, deep cervical fascia.

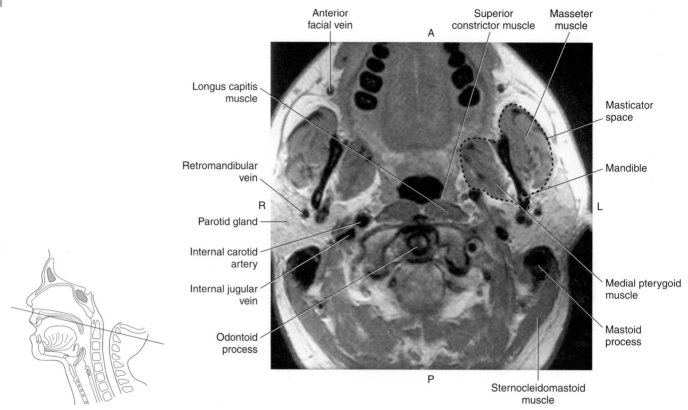

FIGURE 5.56 Axial, T1-weighted MRI of neck with parotid glands.

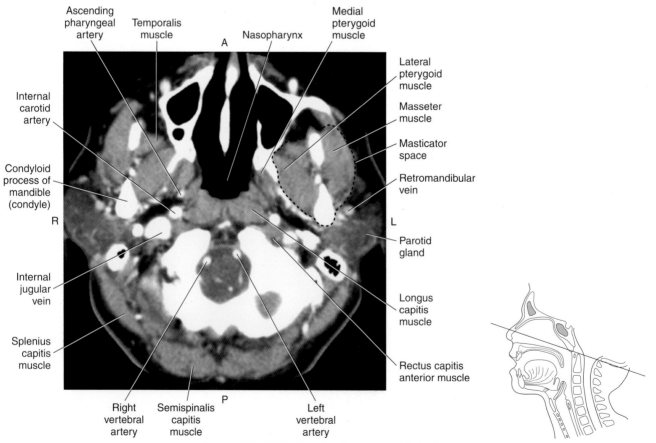

FIGURE 5.57 Axial CT of neck with parotid glands.

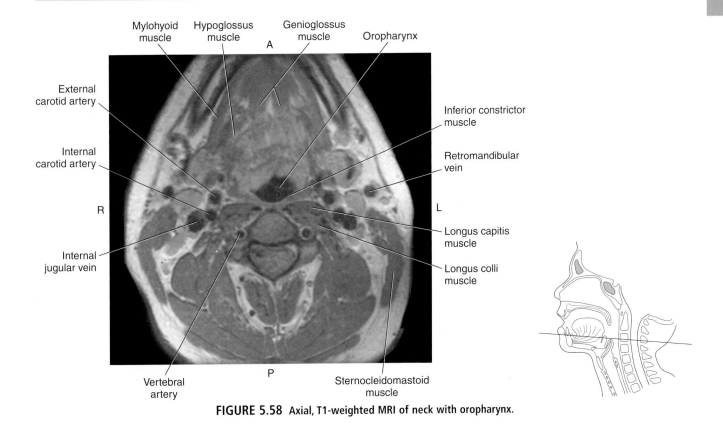

FIGURE 5.58 Axial, T1-weighted MRI of neck with oropharynx.

FIGURE 5.59 Axial CT of neck with oropharynx.

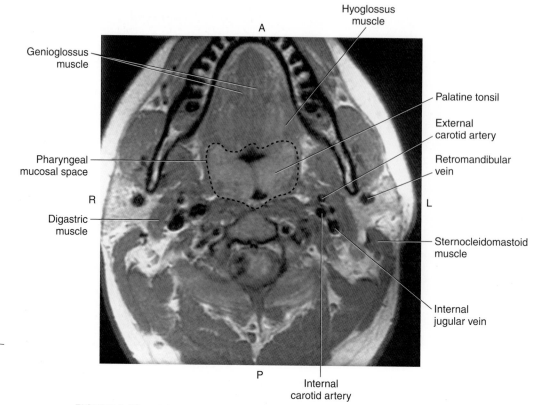

FIGURE 5.60 Axial, T1-weighted MRI of neck.

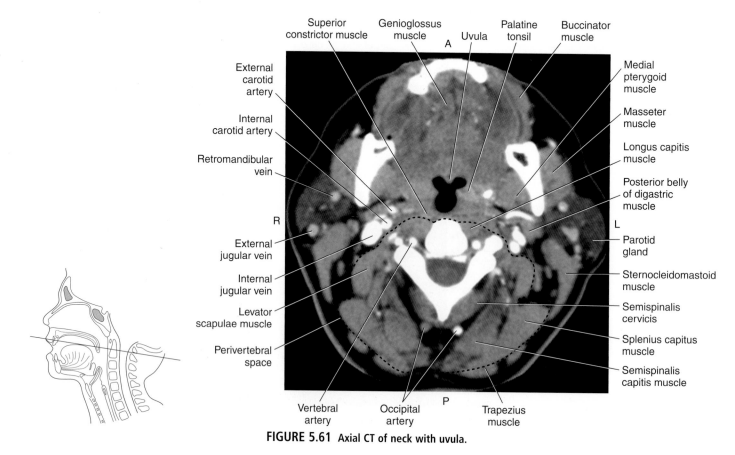

FIGURE 5.61 Axial CT of neck with uvula.

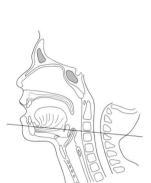

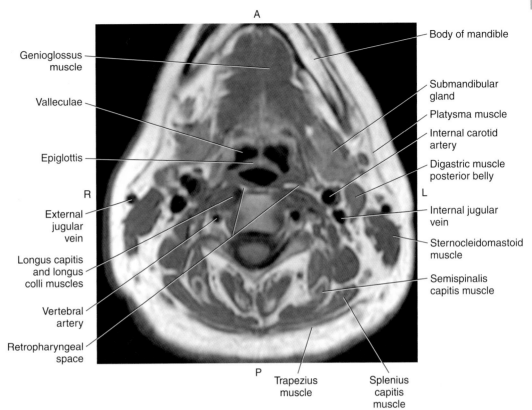

Genioglossus muscle

Valleculae

Epiglottis

R

External jugular vein

Longus capitis and longus colli muscles

Vertebral artery

Retropharyngeal space

Body of mandible

Submandibular gland

Platysma muscle

Internal carotid artery

Digastric muscle posterior belly

L

Internal jugular vein

Sternocleidomastoid muscle

Semispinalis capitis muscle

P Trapezius muscle Splenius capitis muscle

FIGURE 5.62 Axial, T1-weighted MRI of neck with epiglottis.

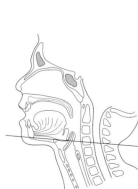

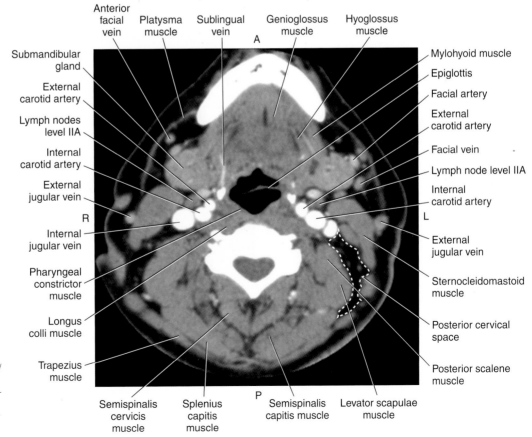

Anterior facial vein Platysma muscle Sublingual vein Genioglossus muscle Hyoglossus muscle

A

Submandibular gland

External carotid artery

Lymph nodes level IIA

Internal carotid artery

External jugular vein

R

Internal jugular vein

Pharyngeal constrictor muscle

Longus colli muscle

Trapezius muscle

Mylohyoid muscle

Epiglottis

Facial artery

External carotid artery

Facial vein

Lymph node level IIA

Internal carotid artery

L

External jugular vein

Sternocleidomastoid muscle

Posterior cervical space

Posterior scalene muscle

Semispinalis cervicis muscle Splenius capitis muscle P Semispinalis capitis muscle Levator scapulae muscle

FIGURE 5.63 Axial CT of neck with epiglottis.

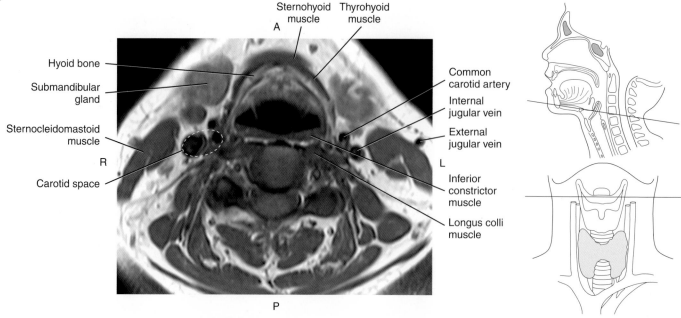

FIGURE 5.64 Axial, T1-weighted MRI of neck with hyoid bone.

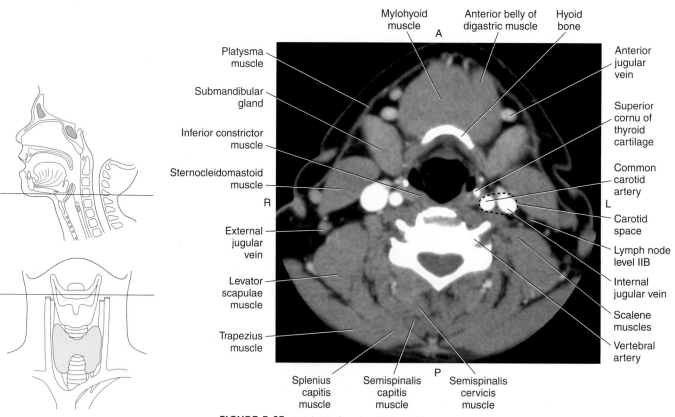

FIGURE 5.65 Axial CT of neck with hyoid bone.

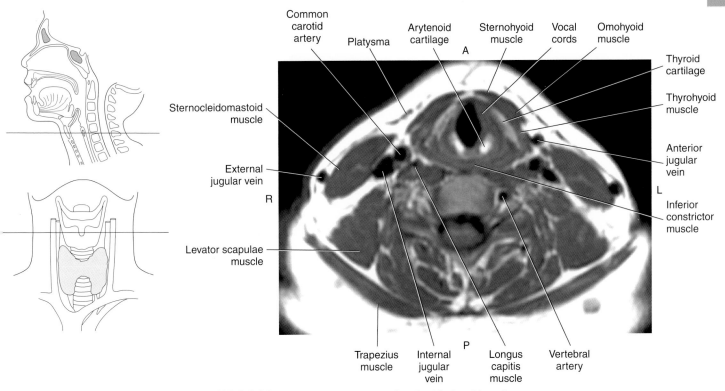

Common carotid artery
Platysma
Arytenoid cartilage
Sternohyoid muscle
Vocal cords
Omohyoid muscle
A
Thyroid cartilage
Thyrohyoid muscle
Anterior jugular vein
Inferior constrictor muscle
Sternocleidomastoid muscle
External jugular vein
R
L
Levator scapulae muscle
Trapezius muscle
Internal jugular vein
P
Longus capitis muscle
Vertebral artery

FIGURE 5.66 Axial, T1-weighted MRI of neck with thyroid cartilage.

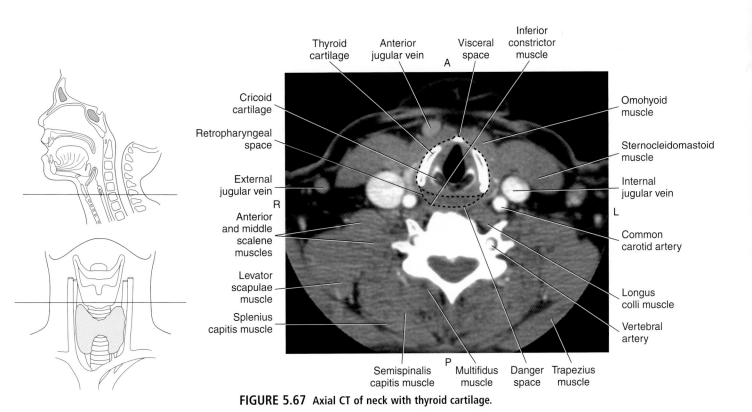

Thyroid cartilage
Anterior jugular vein
Visceral space
Inferior constrictor muscle
A
Cricoid cartilage
Omohyoid muscle
Retropharyngeal space
Sternocleidomastoid muscle
External jugular vein
Internal jugular vein
R
L
Anterior and middle scalene muscles
Common carotid artery
Levator scapulae muscle
Longus colli muscle
Splenius capitis muscle
Vertebral artery
Semispinalis capitis muscle
P
Multifidus muscle
Danger space
Trapezius muscle

FIGURE 5.67 Axial CT of neck with thyroid cartilage.

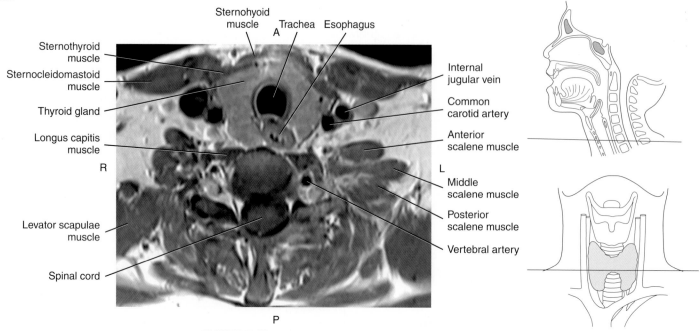

FIGURE 5.68 Axial, T1-weighted MRI of neck with thyroid gland.

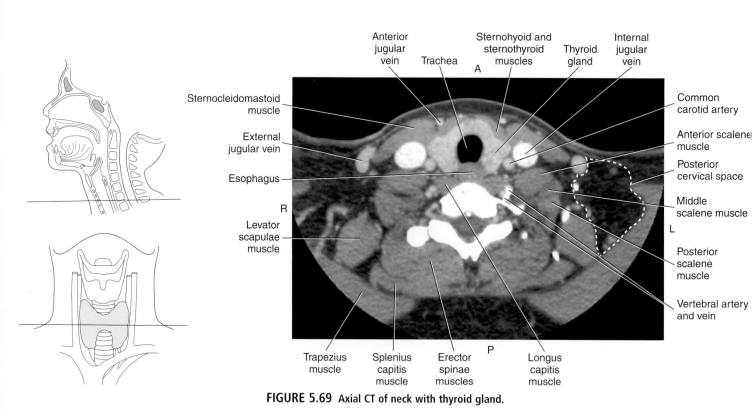

FIGURE 5.69 Axial CT of neck with thyroid gland.

MUSCLES

Numerous muscles are located within the neck. Each muscle can be difficult to identify individually because the margins seem to blend together in cross-section images. This section of the text addresses only the largest and most significant muscles of the neck region.

Pharyngeal and Tongue Muscles

The pharyngeal muscles include the circular layer of constrictors and the inner longitudinal layers (Table 5.2). There are three overlapping **constrictor muscles** (**superior, middle, inferior**) that are responsible for constricting the pharynx and inducing peristaltic waves during swallowing. The three inner longitudinal muscles include the **stylopharyngeus, palotopharyngeus,** and **salpingopharyngeus** muscles, all involved with elevating the pharynx and larynx during swallowing and speaking. The extrinsic muscles of the tongue are responsible for changing the position of the tongue and include the **genioglossus, hyoglossus, styloglossus,** and **palatoglossus muscles** (Figures 5.70 through 5.76).

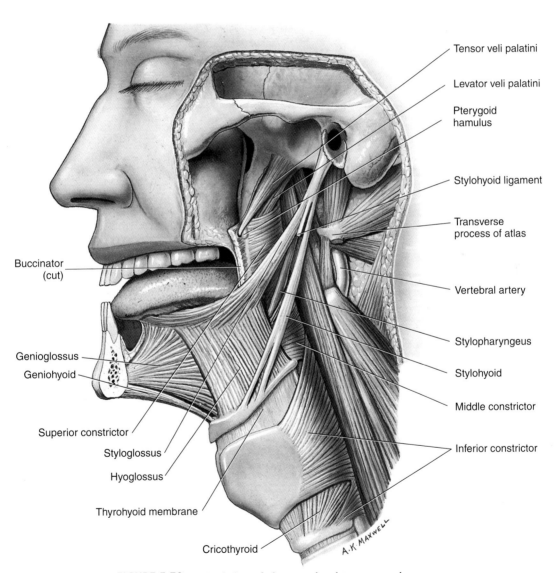

Tensor veli palatini

Levator veli palatini

Pterygoid hamulus

Stylohyoid ligament

Transverse process of atlas

Vertebral artery

Stylopharyngeus

Stylohyoid

Middle constrictor

Inferior constrictor

Buccinator (cut)

Genioglossus

Geniohyoid

Superior constrictor

Styloglossus

Hyoglossus

Thyrohyoid membrane

Cricothyroid

A.K MAXWELL

FIGURE 5.70 Sagittal view of pharyngeal and tongue muscles.

TABLE 5.2	**Pharyngeal Muscles**		
Pharyngeal Muscles	**Origin**	**Insertion**	**Action**
External (Circular) Muscles			
Superior constrictors	• Pterygoid hamulus; posterior end of mandible; side of tongue	• Pharyngeal tubercle; occipital bone; median raphe of pharynx	All constrict pharynx, induce peristaltic waves during swallowing
Middle constrictors	• Stylohyoid ligament, hyoid bone	• Median raphe of pharynx	
Inferior constrictors	• Sides of thyroid and cricoid cartilages	• Median raphe of pharynx	
Longitudinal (Internal) Muscles			
Stylopharyngeus	• Mental spine of mandible	• Posterior/superior borders of thyroid cartilage	All elevate pharynx and larynx during swallowing and speaking
Palatopharyngeus	• Hard palate; palatine aponeurosis	• Side of pharynx and esophagus, posterior border of thyroid cartilage	
Salpingopharyngeus	• Cartilaginous part of auditory tube	• Blends with palatopharyngeus muscle	
Tongue Muscles			
Genioglossus	• Mental spine of mandible	• Ventral surface of tongue; anterior hyoid bone	• Moves tongue forward
Hyoglossus	• Greater horn and body of hyoid bone	• Lateral aspect of tongue base	• Moves tongue backward
Styloglossus	• Styloid process of temporal bone	• Lateral margin of tongue	• Moves tongue upward and backward
Palatoglossus	• Oral surface of palatine aponeurosis	• Side and dorsum of tongue	• Elevates posterior tongue

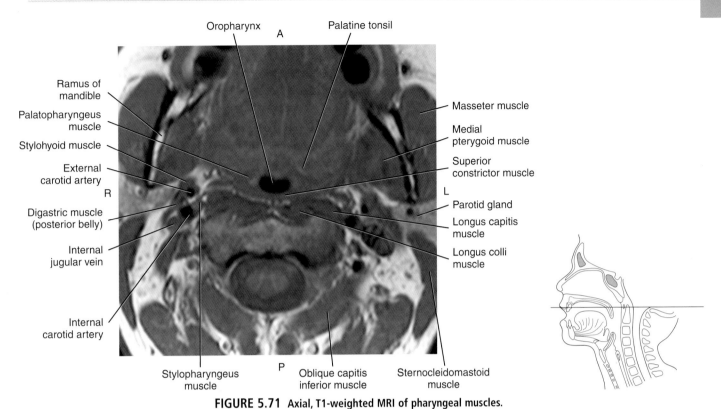

FIGURE 5.71 Axial, T1-weighted MRI of pharyngeal muscles.

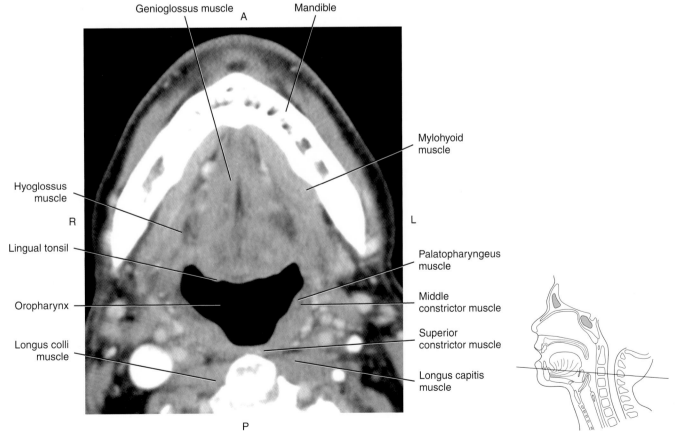

FIGURE 5.72 Axial CT of pharyngeal muscles.

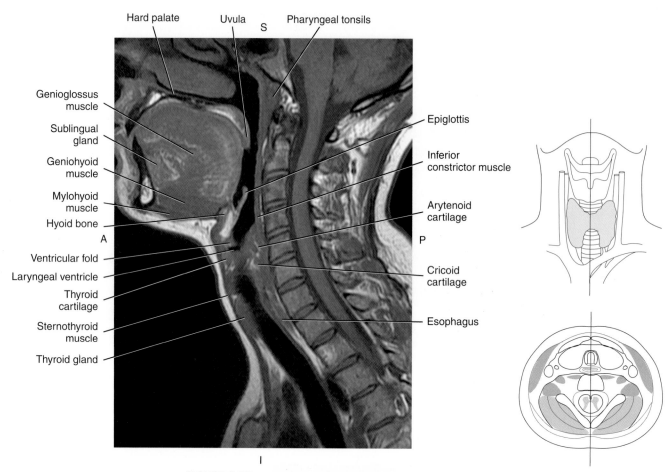

FIGURE 5.73 Sagittal, T1-weighted MRI of pharyngeal muscles.

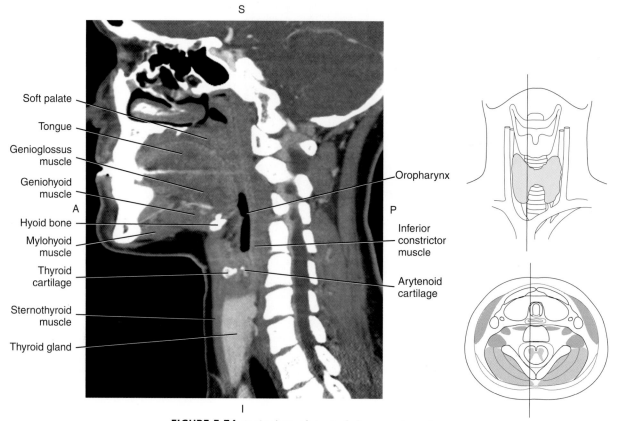

FIGURE 5.74 Sagittal CT reformat of pharyngeal muscles.

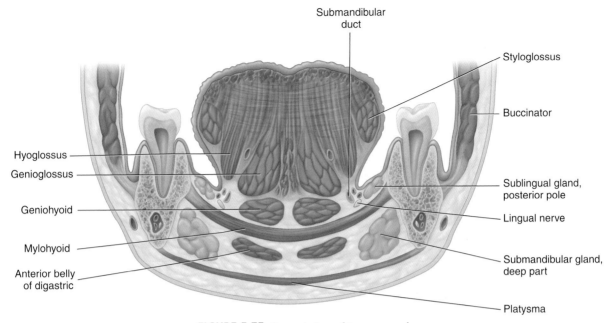

FIGURE 5.75 Coronal view of tongue muscles.

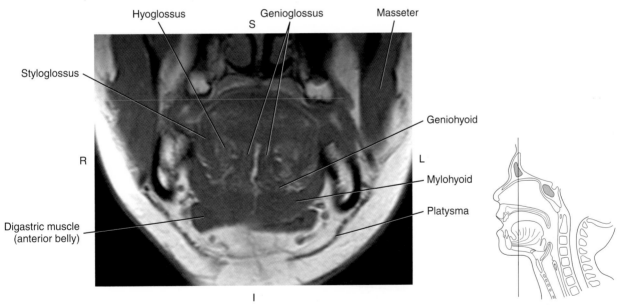

FIGURE 5.76 Coronal, T1-weighted MRI of tongue muscles.

Muscles within the Anterior Triangle

The neck is frequently divided by the **sternocleidomastoid muscle** (SCM) into two areas called the anterior and posterior triangles. Everything anteromedial to the SCM is considered part of the anterior triangle, and everything posterior to the SCM is considered part of the posterior triangle. The SCM is a broad straplike muscle that originates on the sternum and clavicle and inserts on the mastoid tip of the temporal bone. It functions to turn the head from side to side and to flex the neck (Figure 5.77) The **platysma** is the most superficial muscle found in the anterior portion of the neck. It arises from the fascia and skin overlying the pectoralis major and deltoid muscles and extends superiorly as a thin, broad muscle to the inferior portion of the mandible. It is considered a chief muscle for facial expression (Figures 5.62, 5.63, and 5.80).

Other muscles of the anterior triangle are referred to as the muscles of the throat and can be divided into the suprahyoid and infrahyoid muscle groups (Figures 5.77 and 5.78). These muscle groups are named according to their location in relation to the horseshoe-shaped hyoid bone. The **hyoid bone** lies in the anterior aspect of the neck superior to the thyroid cartilage and below the mandible; it forms a base for the tongue. The suprahyoid and infrahyoid muscles aid in the movement of the hyoid bone and larynx. The **suprahyoid muscles** (**digastric, mylohyoid, stylohyoid, geniohyoid**) connect the hyoid bone to the temporal bone and mandible and elevate the hyoid and floor of the mouth and tongue during swallowing and speaking (Figures 5.70, 5.75, 5.76, and 5.78). The **infrahyoid muscles** (**thyrohyoid, sternohyoid, sternothyroid, omohyoid**) are often called **strap muscles** because of their ribbonlike appearance (Figure 5.78). They act primarily to depress the hyoid bone and extend inferiorly to insert on the sternum, thyroid cartilage, and scapula (Table 5.3 and sequential images in Figures 5.52 through 5.69).

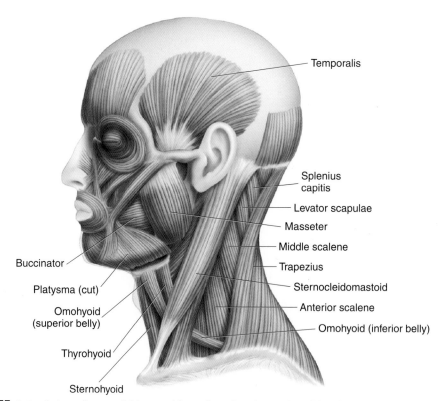

FIGURE 5.77 Lateral view of sternocleidomastoid muscle and neck muscles within the anterior and posterior triangles.

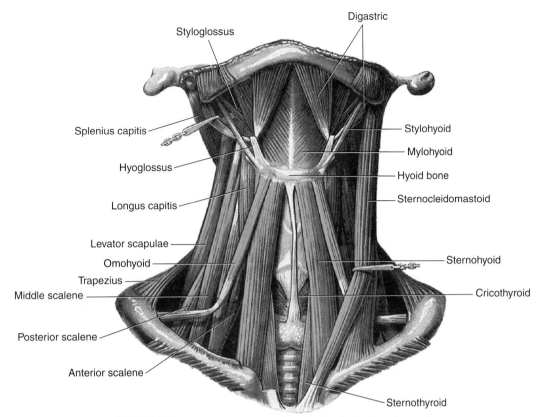

FIGURE 5.78 Anterior view of suprahyoid and infrahyoid neck muscles.

Muscles within the Posterior Triangle

The muscles of the posterior triangle include the trapezius, splenius capitis, levator scapulae, and anterior, middle, and posterior scalene muscles. The **trapezius muscle**, a superficial muscle located on the posterior portion of the neck, elevates the scapula. It originates from the occipital bone and spinous processes of C7-T12 to insert on the clavicle, acromion, and spine of the scapula (Figures 5.79 and 5.80). Located just anterior to the trapezius muscle, the **splenius capitis muscle** arises from the lower cervical and upper thoracic vertebrae to insert on the occipital bone and acts to extend the head (Figure 4.54). The **levator scapulae muscle** is located in the posterolateral portion of the neck. It arises from the transverse processes of the upper four cervical vertebrae to insert on the vertebral border of the scapula and acts to raise the scapula. The scalene muscle group (**anterior, middle, and posterior scalene muscles**) is located in the anterolateral portion of the neck. The muscles originate from the transverse processes of the cervical vertebrae to insert on the first two ribs. Together, the scalene muscles act to elevate the upper two ribs and flex the neck. The anterior and middle scalene muscles can serve as landmarks for the brachial plexus because it courses between them. (These muscles are listed in Table 5.3 and identified on Figures 5.52 through 5.69.) Two other prominent muscle groups found in the neck are the erector spinae and transversospinal, which are discussed in Chapter 4.

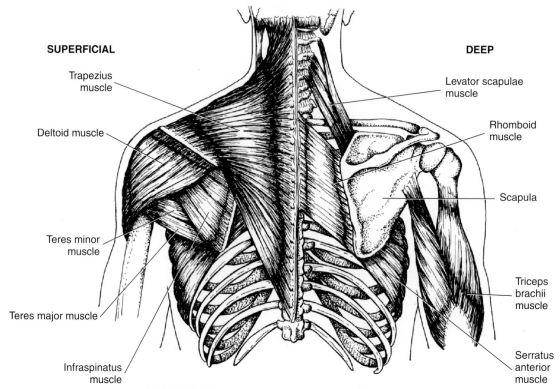

SUPERFICIAL

DEEP

Trapezius
muscle

Deltoid muscle

Teres minor
muscle

Teres major muscle

Infraspinatus
muscle

Levator scapulae
muscle

Rhomboid
muscle

Scapula

Triceps
brachii
muscle

Serratus
anterior
muscle

FIGURE 5.79 Posterior view of trapezius and levator scapulae muscles.

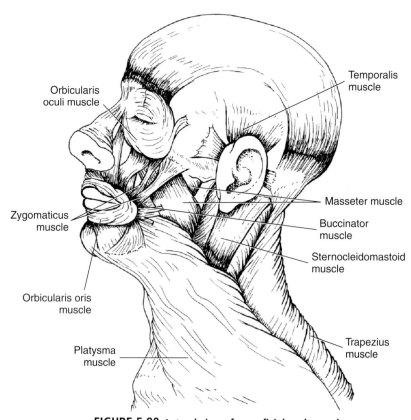

Orbicularis
oculi muscle

Zygomaticus
muscle

Orbicularis oris
muscle

Platysma
muscle

Temporalis
muscle

Masseter muscle

Buccinator
muscle

Sternocleidomastoid
muscle

Trapezius
muscle

FIGURE 5.80 Lateral view of superficial neck muscles.

TABLE 5.3	Neck Muscles		
	Origin	**Insertion**	**Action**
Front of Neck—Anterior Triangle			
Platysma	• Fascia and skin over pectoralis major and deltoid muscles	• Base of mandible and skin of lower face	• Changes facial expression
Sternocleidomastoid (SCM)			
Sternal head	• Upper manubrium	• Mastoid process, lateral half of superior nuchal line	• Flexes head and neck
Clavicular head	• Sternal end of clavicle		
Infrahyoid Muscles			
Thyrohyoid	• Thyroid cartilage	• Inferolateral border hyoid bone	• Lower hyoid bone, raise larynx
Sternohyoid	• Superior border of manubrium and medial clavicle	• Hyoid bone	
			• Lower hyoid bone
Sternothyroid	• Manubrium and medial end 1st costal cartilage	• Thyroid cartilage	• Lower larynx
Omohyoid	• Superior border of scapula	• Inferolateral border hyoid bone	• Lower hyoid bone and larynx
Suprahyoid Muscles			
Digastric	• Posterior belly—mastoid notch of temporal bone; anterior belly—lower border of mandible	• Ends as intermediate tendon between the two bellies that attach to the hyoid bone	• Jaw opener (speech muscle)
			• Elevate floor of mouth
Mylohyoid	• Body of mandible	• Mandibular symphysis and hyoid bone	• Move hyoid bone posterior and superior
Stylohyoid	• Styloid process of temporal bone	• Superior surface of hyoid bone	• Jaw opener
Geniohyoid	• Mandibular symphysis	• Body of hyoid bone	
Prevertebral Muscles			
Longus capitis	• Anterior tubercles of transverse processes C3-6	• Basilar part of occiptial bone	• Flex head
Longus colli	• Bodies of C4-T3; anterior tubercles of transverse processes C3-6	• Anterior arch C1; anterior tubercles of transverse processes C5-6, anterior bodies of C2-4	• Flex neck, rotate and bend neck laterally
Back of Neck—Posterior Triangle			
Scalene Muscles			
Anterior	• Anterior tubercles of transverse processes C3-6	• Scalene tubercle of 1st rib	• Elevates 1st rib, flexes cervical vertebrae
Middle	• Posterior tubercles of transverse processes C2-7	• 1st rib	• Elevates 1st rib, flexes cervical vertebrae
Posterior	• Posterior tubercles of transverse processes of C4-6	• 2nd rib	• Laterally flexes head; rotates head and neck
Trapezius	• Occiptial bone and spinous processes C7-T12	• Clavicle; acromion; scapular spine	• Elevates the scapula
Levator scapulae	• Transverse processes of upper 4 cervical vertebrae	• Vertebral border of the scapula	• Raises the scapula
Splenius capitis	• Lower cervical and upper thoracic vertrebrae	• Occipital bone	• Extends head
Splenius cervicis	• Spinous processes of T1-6 and ligamentum nuchae	• Posterior tubercles of transverse processes of C1-4	• Extends head

VASCULAR STRUCTURES

The extracranial or main vessels of the neck include the carotid and vertebral arteries and the jugular veins (Tables 5.4 and 5.5). These vessels are located primarily in the lateral portions of the neck (Figures 5.81 through 5.86).

Carotid Arteries

The right **common carotid artery** arises from the brachiocephalic artery posterior to the sternoclavicular joint. The left **common carotid artery** arises directly from the aortic arch (Figure 5.81). The common carotid arteries lie medial to the internal jugular vein and bifurcate into the internal and external carotid arteries at approximately the level of the thyroid cartilage (C3-C4). Located on the external surface at the bifurcation of the common carotid artery is the **carotid body,** a small neurovascular structure that acts as a chemoreceptor to sense changes in the chemical composition of blood (Figure 5.82). The

internal carotid artery ascends the neck, almost in a vertical plane, to enter the base of the skull through the carotid canal of the temporal bone. At its origin there is a dilatation called the **carotid sinus,** which contains baroreceptors that react to changes in arterial blood pressure. The internal carotid artery has no branches in the neck, but has branches in the head to supply blood to the orbit and brain. As the **external carotid artery** ascends the neck, it passes through the parotid gland to the level of the temporomandibular joint, where it bifurcates into its terminal branches to supply blood to the face and neck. These branches include the superior thyroid, lingual, facial, occipital, posterior auricular, and ascending pharyngeal arteries (Table 5.4 and Figures 5.81 through 5.85). The external carotid artery changes position in relation to the internal carotid artery as it ascends the neck. At its lower level, the external carotid artery is anterior and medial to the internal carotid artery and then becomes anterior and lateral to the internal carotid artery at its higher level (Figures 5.56 through 5.69).

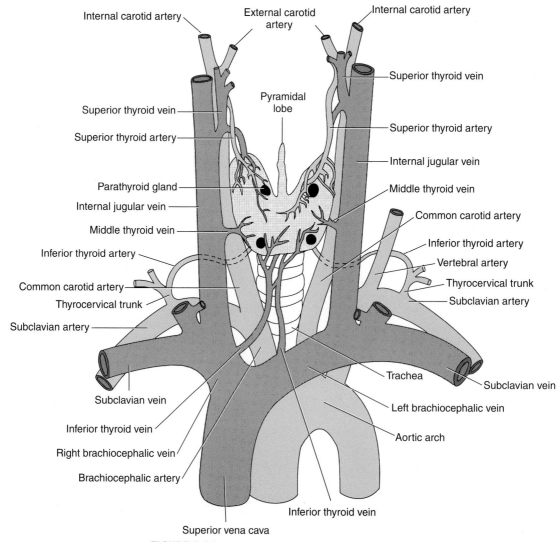

FIGURE 5.81 Anterior view of extracranial vasculature.

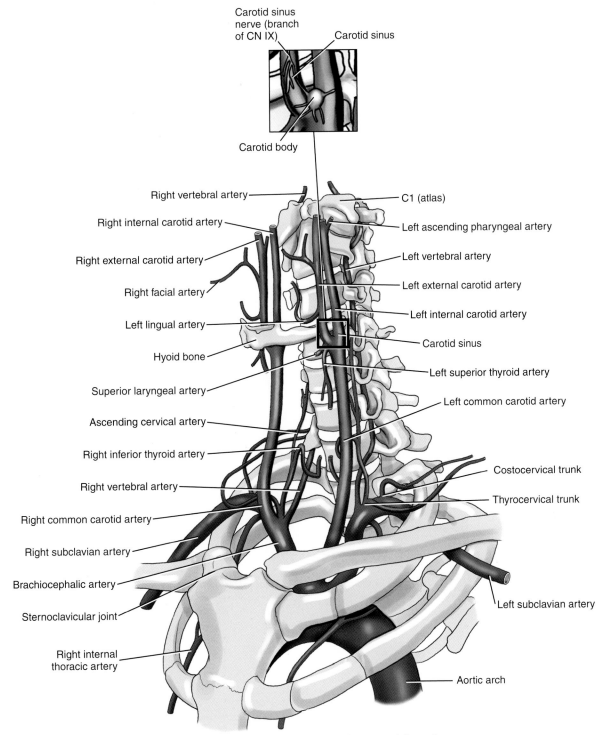

Carotid sinus nerve (branch of CN IX)

Carotid sinus

Carotid body

Right vertebral artery

Right internal carotid artery

Right external carotid artery

Right facial artery

Left lingual artery

Hyoid bone

Superior laryngeal artery

Ascending cervical artery

Right inferior thyroid artery

Right vertebral artery

Right common carotid artery

Right subclavian artery

Brachiocephalic artery

Sternoclavicular joint

Right internal thoracic artery

C1 (atlas)

Left ascending pharyngeal artery

Left vertebral artery

Left external carotid artery

Left internal carotid artery

Carotid sinus

Left superior thyroid artery

Left common carotid artery

Costocervical trunk

Thyrocervical trunk

Left subclavian artery

Aortic arch

FIGURE 5.82 Anterior oblique view of extracranial arteries.

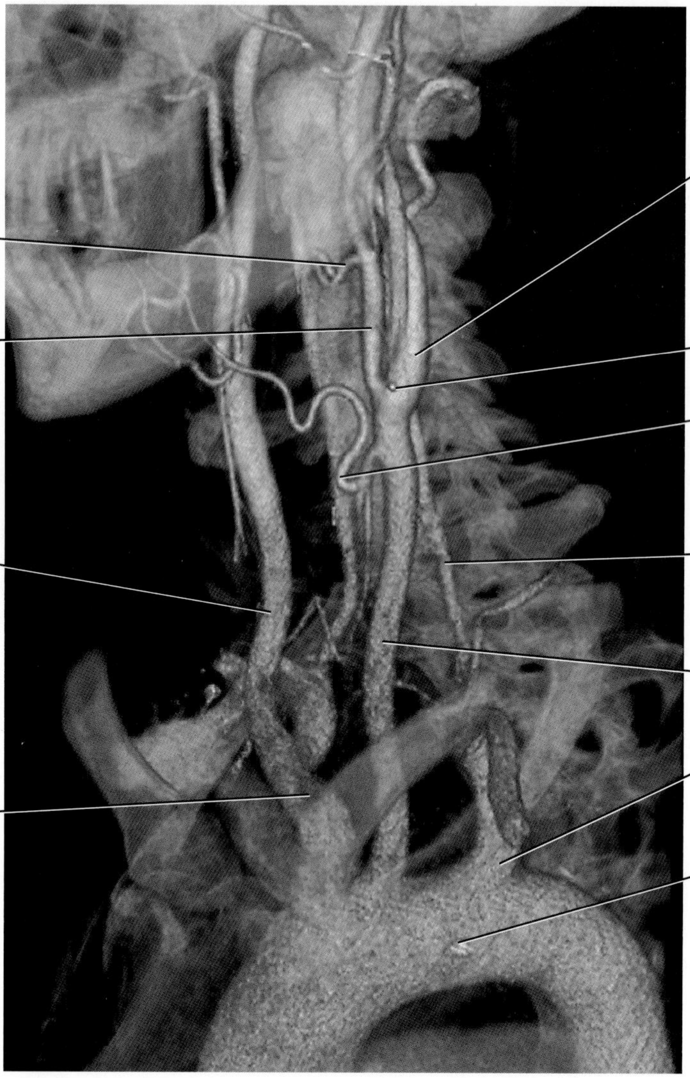

FIGURE 5.83 Anterior oblique 3D CTA of extracranial arteries.

Carotid body tumors are the most common paraganglioma of the head and neck. These tumors develop within the adventitia of the medial aspect of the carotid bifurcation. The most common presentation is as an asymptomatic palpable neck mass in the anterior triangle of the neck. As the tumor enlarges and compresses the carotid artery and the surrounding nerves, other symptoms may also be present, such as pain, tongue paresis, hoarseness, Horner syndrome, and dysphagia. They are treated with either surgery or radiotherapy.

Vertebral Arteries

The **vertebral arteries** begin as a branch of the subclavian artery and ascend the neck through the transverse foramina of C6-C1, where the arteries enter the foramen magnum and join to form the basilar artery. The vertebral and basilar arteries supply blood to the posterior aspect of the brain (Figures 5.56 through 5.69 and 5.82 through 5.85).

TABLE 5.4	Arteries of the Neck	
Arteries of the Neck	**Origin**	**Branches**
Common Carotid Artery		Internal and external carotid arteries
Left Common Carotid	Aortic arch	
Right Common Carotid	Right brachiocephalic artery	
Internal Carotid Artery	Common carotid artery	Ophthalmic, anterior and middle cerebral arteries
External Carotid Artery	Common carotid artery	Superior thyroid, lingual, facial, occipital, posterior auricular, and ascending pharyngeal arteries
Vertebral Arteries	Subclavian artery	Posterior inferior cerebellar artery

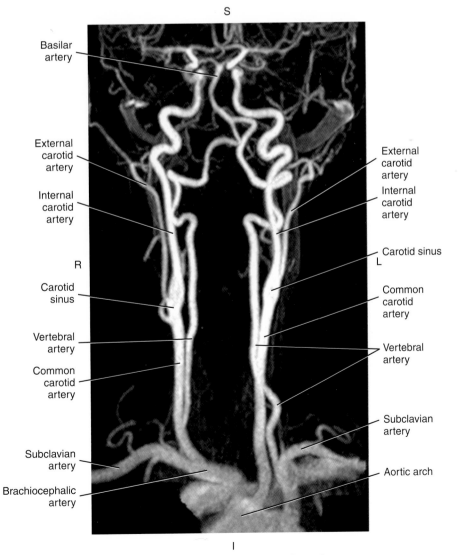

FIGURE 5.84 MRA of extracranial arteries.

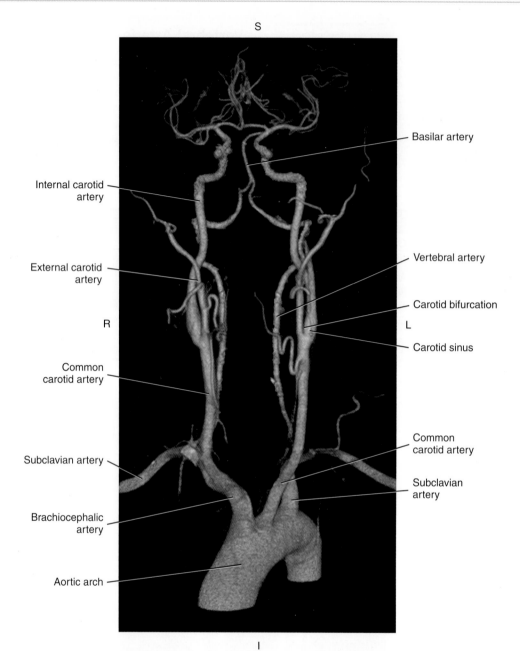

S

Basilar artery

Internal carotid artery

External carotid artery

Vertebral artery

Carotid bifurcation

R

L

Carotid sinus

Common carotid artery

Common carotid artery

Subclavian artery

Subclavian artery

Brachiocephalic artery

Aortic arch

I

FIGURE 5.85 3D CTA of intracranial and extracranial arteries.

Jugular and Vertebral Veins

The **internal jugular veins** drain blood from the brain and superficial parts of the face and neck and are typically the largest of the vascular structures of the neck (Table 5.5). The internal jugular veins commence at the jugular foramen in the posterior cranial fossa and descend the lateral portion of the neck to unite with the **subclavian vein** to form the **brachiocephalic vein** (Figures 5.81 and 5.86). The internal jugular veins typically run lateral to the common carotid artery and posterior to the internal carotid artery at the upper levels of the neck. Tributaries of the internal jugular vein include the inferior petrosal sinus, facial, lingual, pharyngeal, superior, and middle thyroid veins, and often the occipital vein. One of these tributaries, the **facial vein**, is commonly identified as it drains the anterior and lateral regions of the face (Figure 5.86).

TABLE 5.5	Veins of the Neck	
Veins of the Neck	**Termination**	**Tributaries**
Internal jugular vein	Subclavian vein	Inferior petrosal sinus, facial, lingual, pharyngeal, superior and middle thyroid, and occasionally the occipital veins
External jugular vein	Subclavian vein	Retromandibular, anterior jugular, temporal, and maxillary veins, and occasionally the occipital vein
Vertebral veins	Brachiocephalic vein	Internal and external vertebral venous plexuses and deep cervical veins

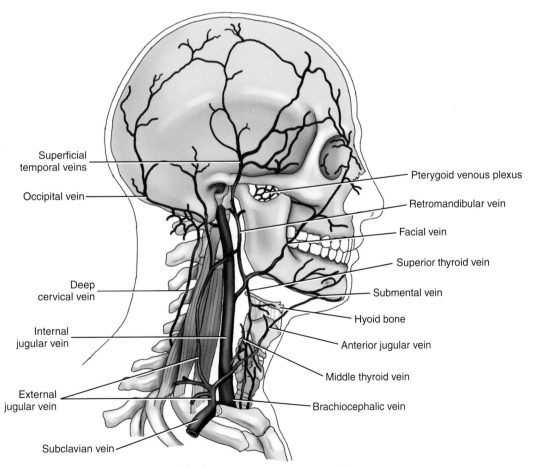

FIGURE 5.86 Lateral view of extracranial veins.

The **external jugular veins** begin near the angle of the mandible and cross the SCM just beneath the skin to empty into the subclavian vein. Tributaries of the external jugular veins include the retromandibular and anterior jugular veins and occasionally the occipital veins. Blood from the lateral region of the face is drained by the **retromandibular vein** that courses inferiorly through the parotid gland. The **anterior jugular vein** begins at approximately the level of the hyoid bone and drains blood from the lower lip. This vessel passes beneath the SCM to open into the termination of the external jugular vein. Jugular veins are identified on Figures 5.56 through 5.69.

The **vertebral veins** course within the transverse foramina of the cervical vertebrae along with the vertebral arteries to drain the cervical spinal cord and the posterior surface of the skull (Figures 4.132 and 5.53, 5.54, 5.61, and 5.69). The vertebral veins drain into the posterior aspect of the brachiocephalic vein. The vascular structures can be identified on sequential images found in Figures 5.52 through 5.69.

REFERENCES

Applegate E: *The anatomy and physiology learning system*, ed 4, St. Louis, 2010, Saunders.

Applegate E: *The sectional anatomy learning system*, ed 3, St. Louis, 2009, Saunders.

Curry RA, Tempkin BB: *Sonography: an introduction to normal structure and functional anatomy*, ed 3, St. Louis, 2010, Saunders.

Frank: *Merrill's atlas of radiographic positions and radiologic procedures*, St. Louis, ed 12, 2012, Mosby.

Haaga JR, Lanzieri CF, Gilkeson RC, et al: *CT and MR imaging of the whole body*, ed 5, Philadelphia, 2008, Mosby.

Jacob S: *Atlas of human anatomy*, Philadelphia, 2002, Churchill Livingstone.

Larsen WJ: *Anatomy: Development function clinical correlations*, Philadelphia, 2002, Saunders.

Mosby's medical, nursing, and allied health dictionary, ed 8, St. Louis, 2008, Mosby.

Ryan S, McNicholas M: *Anatomy for diagnostic imaging*, ed 3, Philadelphia, 2010, Saunders.

Sandring S: *Gray's anatomy*, ed 40, Philadelphia, 2011, Churchill Livingstone.

Seidel HM, Ball JW, Dains JE, et al: *Mosby's guide to physical examination*, ed 7, St. Louis, 2010, Mosby.

Som PM, Curtin HD: *Head and neck imaging*, ed 5, St. Louis, 2011, Mosby.

Thorax

Anyone who would attempt to operate on the heart should lose the respect of his colleagues.

Christian Albert Theodor Billroth, 1881

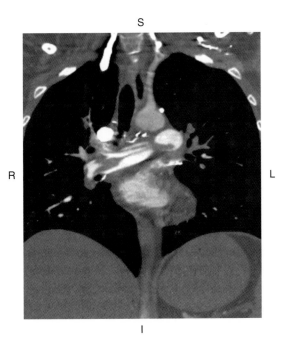

Many structures of the thorax are in constant motion. Although physiologic motion can make imaging difficult, a thorough knowledge of thoracic anatomy and physiology can improve diagnostic imaging of this area (Figure 6.1). This chapter demonstrates sectional anatomy of the following structures:

FIGURE 6.1 Coronal CT reformat of thorax with numerous pulmonary emboli.

OBJECTIVES

- Describe the structures that constitute the bony thorax.
- Define the thoracic inlet and outlet.
- Understand the function and layers of the pleura.
- Identify and describe the structures of the lungs.
- Identify the mainstem bronchi and their divisions.
- List the structures of the mediastinum and describe their anatomic relationships to each other.
- Identify the structures of the heart and explain the circulation of blood through the heart.
- Identify the great vessels and describe the distribution of their associated arteries and veins.
- Differentiate between pulmonary arteries and veins by function and location.
- Identify the coronary arteries and veins.
- List the muscles involved in respiration by function and location.

OUTLINE

BONY THORAX

The bony thorax protects the organs of the thorax and aids in respiration. It consists of the **thoracic vertebrae, sternum, ribs, and costal cartilages** (Figure 6.2). The 12 thoracic vertebrae make up the posterior boundary of the thoracic cage. The anterior boundary is created by the sternum, located midline. The sternum has three components: manubrium, body, and xiphoid process (Figures 6.3 and 6.4). The triangular-shaped **manubrium** is the most superior portion and articulates with the first two pairs of ribs and the clavicles. It articulates with the clavicle at the clavicular notch to form the **sternoclavicular (SC) joints** (Figure 6.5). A common landmark, the **jugular notch**, is located on the superior border of the manubrium at approximately the level of T2-T3. The manubrium and body of the sternum come together at an angle to form a ridge known as the **sternal angle**, which is located at approximately the level of T4-T5. The slender **body** of

the sternum has several indentations along its sides where it articulates with the cartilage of the third through seventh ribs (Figures 6.2, 6.6, and 6.7). The small **xiphoid** process is located on the inferior border of the sternum and is a site for muscle attachments (Figure 6.8).

Forming the lateral borders of the thoracic cage are the 12 pairs of **ribs**. The spaces between adjacent ribs are referred to as the **intercostal spaces**. All 12 pairs of ribs articulate posteriorly with the thoracic spine. The ribs consist of a **head, neck, tubercle,** and **body** (see Figures 6.7 and 6.8). The facets of the head of the rib articulate with the vertebral bodies at the **costovertebral joints**, whereas the facets of the tubercles articulate with the transverse processes of the vertebrae to form the **costotransverse joints** (see Figure 6.7). The first 7 pairs of ribs (true ribs) articulate anteriorly with the sternum via costal cartilage. The lower 5 pairs of ribs are considered false ribs because they do not attach directly to the sternum. The costal cartilage of the eighth, ninth, and tenth ribs attach to the costal cartilage of the seventh rib. The eleventh and twelfth ribs are considered floating because they attach only to the thoracic vertebrae and contain no neck or tubercle, only vertebral and sternal ends (see Figure 6.2).

Thoracic Apertures

There are two openings, or apertures, associated with the bony thorax. The superior aperture is formed by the first thoracic vertebra, first pair of ribs and their costal cartilages, and manubrium. This aperture, known as the **thoracic inlet**, allows for the passage of nerves, vessels, and viscera from the neck into the thoracic cavity. The inferior aperture is much larger and is made up of the twelfth thoracic vertebra, twelfth pair of ribs and costal margins, and xiphoid sternal junction. This aperture is known as the **thoracic outlet** (see Figures 6.2, 6.5, and 6.8).

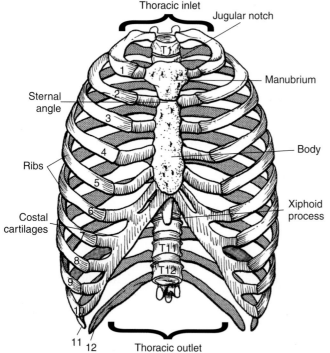

FIGURE 6.2 Anterior view of thoracic cage.

Thoracic inlet	
Jugular notch	
Manubrium	
Sternal angle	
Body	
Ribs	
Xiphoid process	
Costal cartilages	
Thoracic outlet	

Thoracic Outlet Syndrome (TOS)

A group of disorders causing pain and parasthesias in the neck, shoulder, arms or hands caused by compression of the brachial plexus and/or subclavian vessels as they pass through the thoracic outlet. The name is somewhat controversial, because the location of the pathology is technically the thoracic inlet.

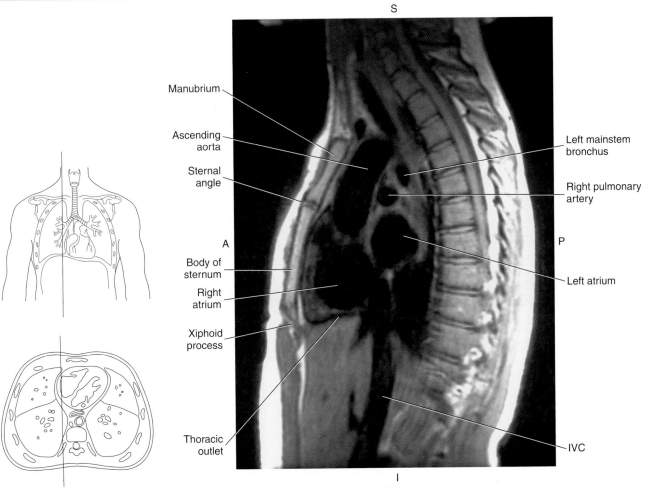

FIGURE 6.3 Sagittal, T1-weighted MRI of thoracic cage.

Labels (Figure 6.3): Manubrium, Ascending aorta, Sternal angle, Body of sternum, Right atrium, Xiphoid process, Thoracic outlet, Left mainstem bronchus, Right pulmonary artery, Left atrium, IVC

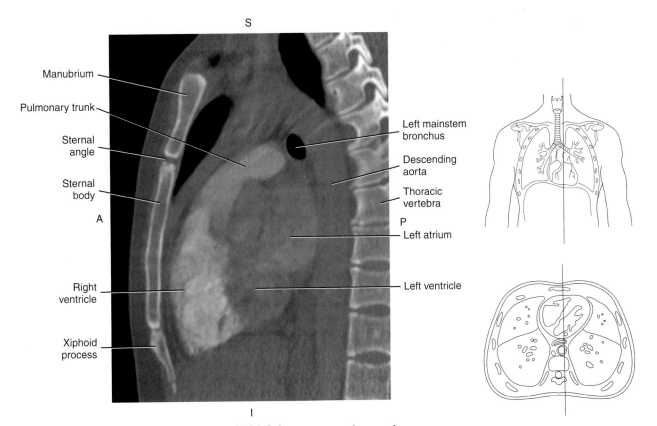

FIGURE 6.4 Sagittal CT reformat of sternum.

Labels (Figure 6.4): Manubrium, Pulmonary trunk, Sternal angle, Sternal body, Right ventricle, Xiphoid process, Left mainstem bronchus, Descending aorta, Thoracic vertebra, Left atrium, Left ventricle

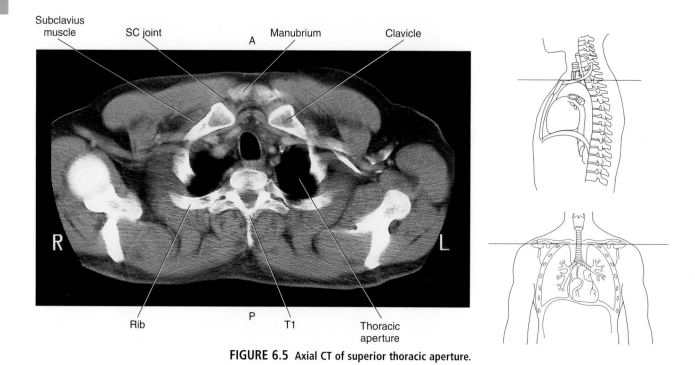

FIGURE 6.5 Axial CT of superior thoracic aperture.

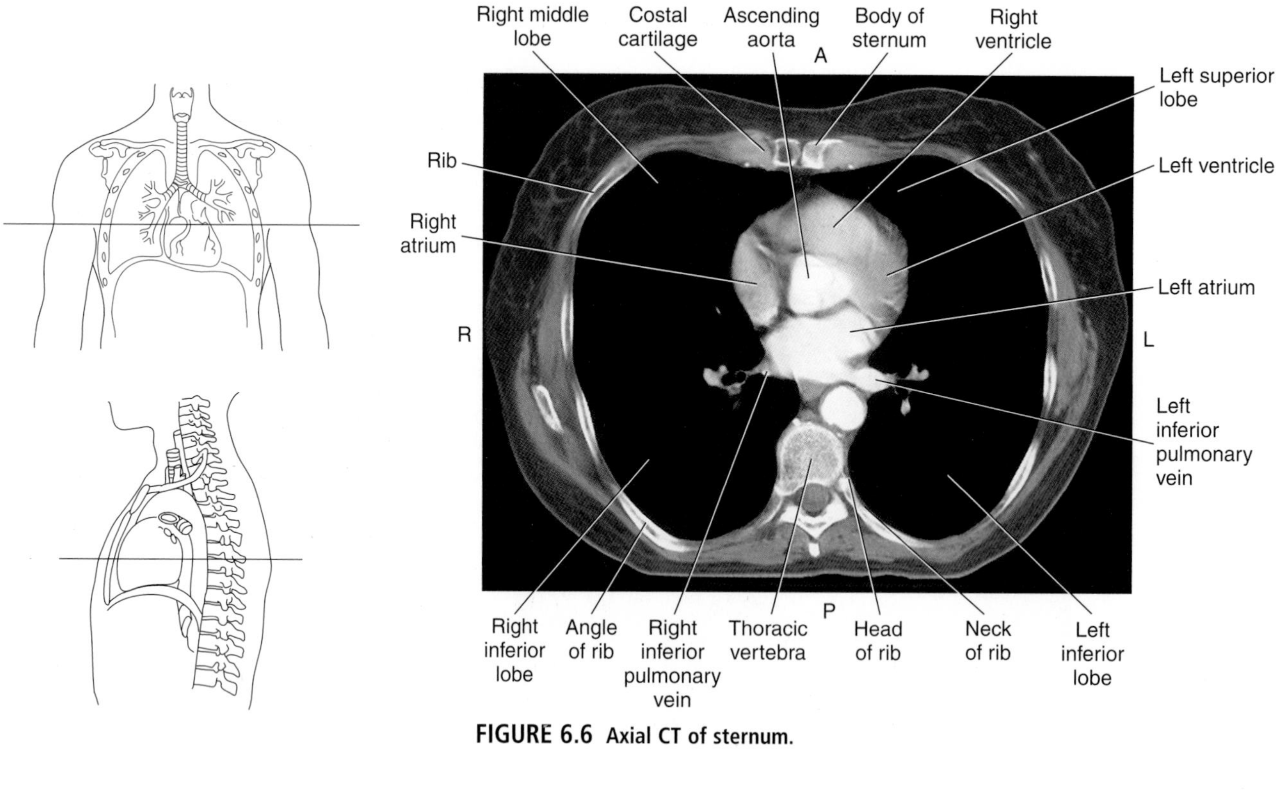

FIGURE 6.6 Axial CT of sternum.

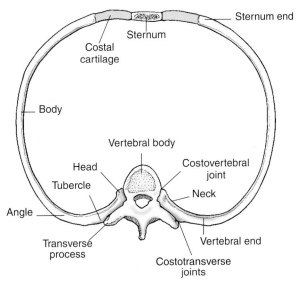

FIGURE 6.7 Axial view of costovertebral and costotransverse joints.

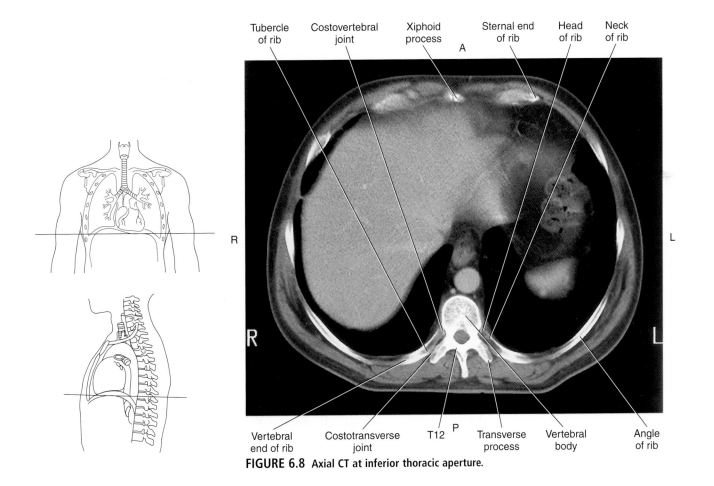

FIGURE 6.8 Axial CT at inferior thoracic aperture.

PLEURAL CAVITIES

Each lung lies within a single pleural cavity that is lined by a serous membrane, or **pleura**. The pleura can be divided into two layers. The **parietal pleura,** the outer layer, is continuous with the thoracic wall and diaphragm and moves with these structures during respiration. The **visceral pleura** is the inner layer that closely covers the outer surface of the lung and continues into the fissures to cover the individual lobes as well. Both membranes secrete a small amount of pleural fluid that provides lubrication between the surfaces during breathing. Deep pockets or recesses of the pleural cavities are the **costomediastinal** and **costodiaphragmatic recesses.** The costomediastinal recesses are located at the point where the mediastinum and costal cartilages meet anteriorly, and the costodia-phragmatic recesses are located where the diaphragm and ribs connect inferiorly. These recesses serve as expansions to provide additional pleural space where parts of the lung can glide during inspiration (Figures 6.9 and 6.10).

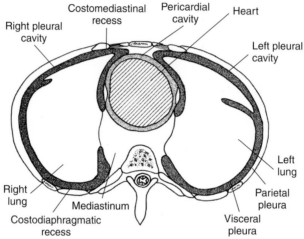

FIGURE 6.9 **Axial cross section of pleura.**

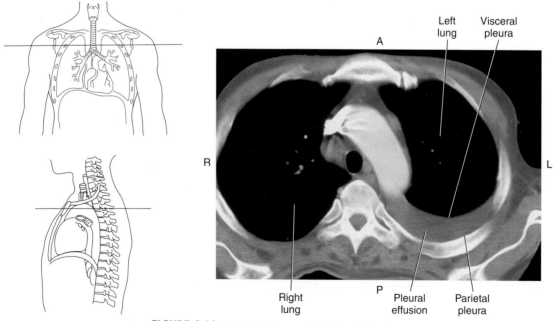

FIGURE 6.10 **Axial CT of lungs with pleural effusion.**

LUNGS

The **lungs** are the organs of respiration. They are composed of a sponge like material, the parenchyma, and are surrounded by the visceral pleura. The large conical-shaped lungs extend up to or slightly above the level of the first rib at their **apex,** and down to the dome of the diaphragm at their wide concave-shaped **bases or diaphragmatic surfaces** (Figure 6.11). Each lung has a **mediastinal or medial surface** that is apposed to the mediastinum and a **costal surface** that is apposed to the inner surface of the rib cage. Each lung also has inferior, anterior, and posterior borders. The **inferior border** extends into the costodiaphragmatic recess of the pleural cavity, and the **anterior border** of each lung extends into the costomediastinal recess of the pleural cavity (see Figure 6.9).

Two prominent angles can be identified at the medial and lateral edges of the lung bases. The **medial angle** is termed the **cardiophrenic sulcus,** and the **lateral angle** is termed the **costophrenic sulcus** (Figures 6.12 and 6.13). The lungs are divided into **lobes** by **fissures** that are lined by pleura (Figures 6.12 through 6.15). The right lung has three lobes (superior [upper], middle, and inferior

[lower]), whereas the left lung has just superior (upper) and inferior (lower) lobes (Figures 6.11 through 6.15). The inferior lobe of the right lung is separated from the middle and superior lobes by the **oblique (major) fissure,** termed oblique because of its posterosuperior to anteroinferior course (Figure 6.13). Separating the middle lobe from the superior lobe is the **horizontal (minor) fissure** (see Figures 6.11 and 6.15, A). An oblique fissure also separates the superior and inferior lobes of the left lung (see Figures 6.11 and 6.12). The left lung has a large notch on the medial surface of its superior lobe called the **cardiac notch** and a tongue-like projection off its inferoanterior surface termed the **lingula** (Figure 6.15). Each lung has an opening on the medial surface termed the **hilum.** This opening acts as a passage for mainstem bronchi, blood vessels, lymph vessels, and nerves to enter or leave the lung and is commonly referred to as the root of the lung (see Figures 6.15 through 6.17).

Cystic disease of the lung encompasses a wide variety of pathologic processes that are characterized by "holes" or abnormal air-containing spaces within the lung parenchyma.

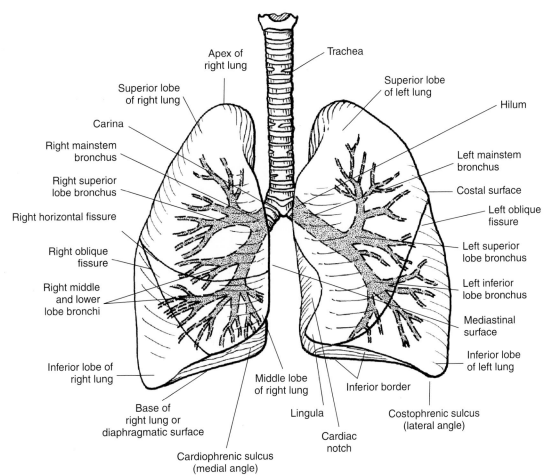

FIGURE 6.11 Anterior view of bronchial tree.

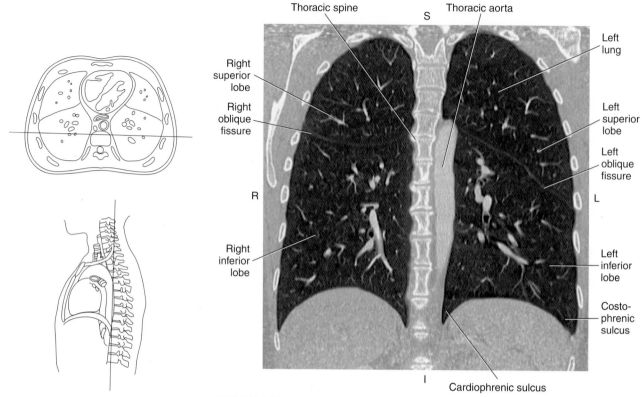

FIGURE 6.12 Coronal CT reformat of lungs.

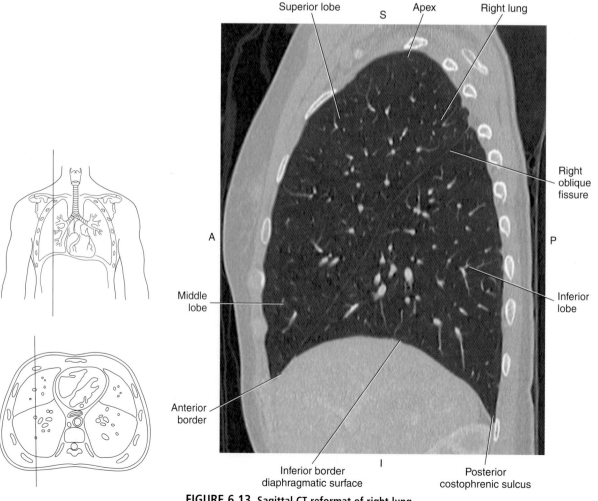

FIGURE 6.13 Sagittal CT reformat of right lung.

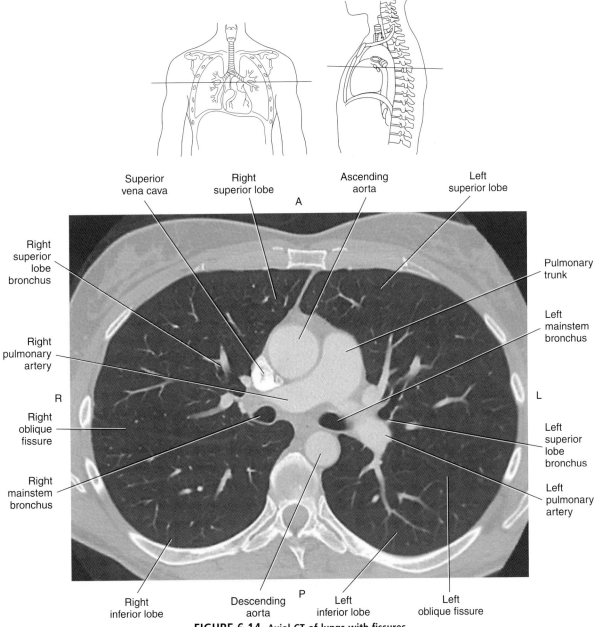

FIGURE 6.14 Axial CT of lungs with fissures.

Superior vena cava

Right superior lobe

Ascending aorta

Left superior lobe

A

Right superior lobe bronchus

Pulmonary trunk

Left mainstem bronchus

Right pulmonary artery

R

L

Right oblique fissure

Left superior lobe bronchus

Right mainstem bronchus

Left pulmonary artery

Right inferior lobe

Descending aorta

P

Left inferior lobe

Left oblique fissure

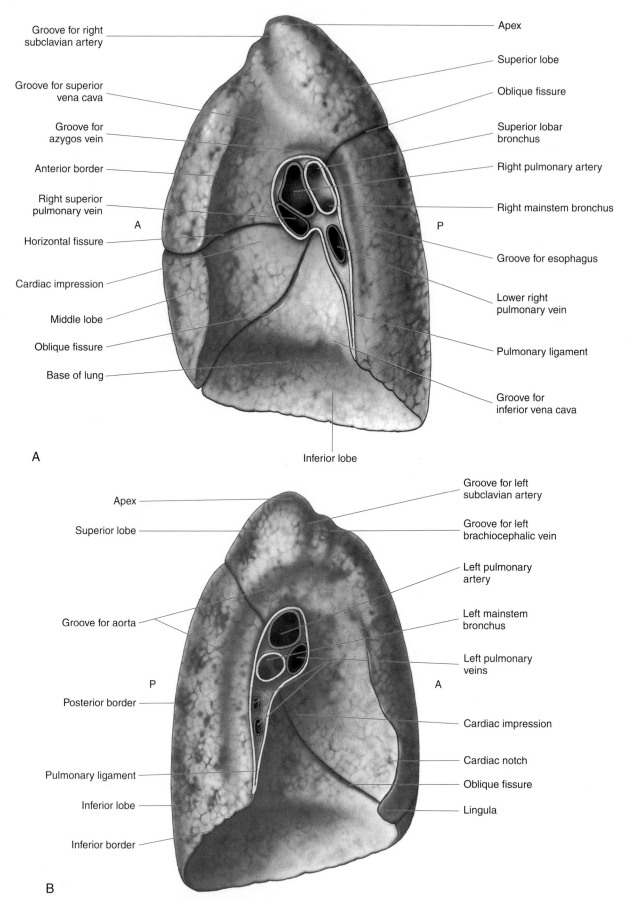

Groove for right subclavian artery

Groove for superior vena cava

Groove for azygos vein

Anterior border

Right superior pulmonary vein

Horizontal fissure

Cardiac impression

Middle lobe

Oblique fissure

Base of lung

A

Apex

Superior lobe

Oblique fissure

Superior lobar bronchus

Right pulmonary artery

Right mainstem bronchus

Groove for esophagus

Lower right pulmonary vein

Pulmonary ligament

Groove for inferior vena cava

Inferior lobe

A

Apex

Superior lobe

Groove for aorta

P

Posterior border

Pulmonary ligament

Inferior lobe

Inferior border

Groove for left subclavian artery

Groove for left brachiocephalic vein

Left pulmonary artery

Left mainstem bronchus

Left pulmonary veins

Cardiac impression

Cardiac notch

Oblique fissure

Lingula

A

B

FIGURE 6.15 Medial view of lungs. A, Right lung. **B,** Left lung.

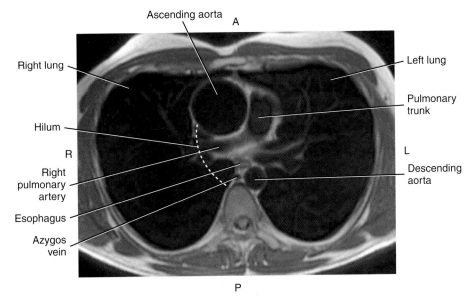

FIGURE 6.16 Axial, T1-weighted MRI of lungs at hilum.

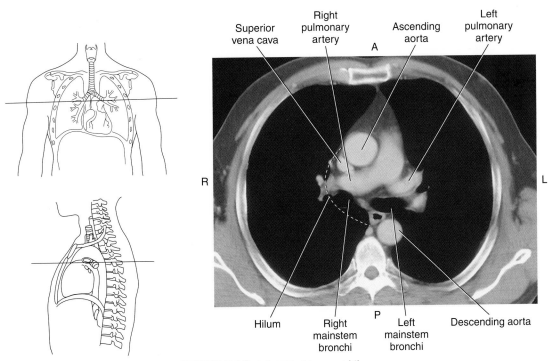

FIGURE 6.17 Axial CT of lungs at hilum.

BRONCHI

The **trachea** bifurcates into the left and right **mainstem (primary) bronchi** at approximately the level of T5. This location is commonly referred to as the **carina** (Figure 6.11). The right mainstem bronchus is wider, shorter, and more vertical in orientation then the left. At the hilum, the mainstem bronchi enter the lungs and divide into **secondary or lobar bronchi.** Secondary bronchi correspond to the lobes of the lungs, thus with three divisions on the right (superior, middle, inferior) and two divisions on the left (superior and inferior) (Figures 6.11 and 6.18 through 6.20). There is further division of the secondary bronchi into **tertiary or segmental bronchi,** which extend into each segment of the lobes (**bronchopulmonary segments**) (Figures 6.21, 6.22, and Table 6.1). There are typically 10 segments within each lung. Each bronchopulmonary segment is functionally independent and can be individually removed surgically. The bronchial tree continues to divide many times into smaller **bronchi,** then into **bronchioles.** Each bronchiole continues to divide, approximately 23 times, until it reaches the terminal end as **alveoli,** which are the functional units of the respiratory system. Gaseous exchange between alveolar air and capillary blood occurs through the walls of the alveoli.

The basic unit of pulmonary structure and function is called the **secondary pulmonary lobule.** It is the smallest component of lung tissue that is surrounded by connective tissue and it measures approximately 1-2 cm. It consists of three to five acini that contain alveoli for gas exchange with a terminal bronchiole and artery located in the center of the lobule. At the periphery of the lobule is the interstitial septa formed by connective tissue, pulmonary veins, and lymphatics (Figures 6.23 and 6.24). High-resolution CT is capable of demonstrating the secondary pulmonary lobule and can help characterize interstitial lung disease based on the type of pathology present within the lobule.

> Lung cancer remains the leading cause of cancer-related deaths in both men and women in the United States.

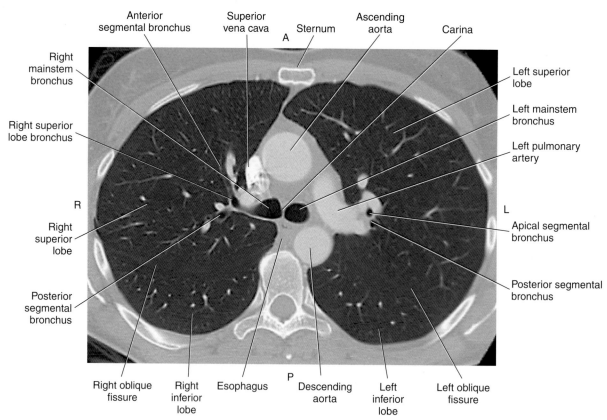

FIGURE 6.18 Axial CT of mainstem bronchi.

Anterior segmental bronchus · Superior vena cava · A · Sternum · Ascending aorta · Carina

Right mainstem bronchus

Right superior lobe bronchus

R

Right superior lobe

Posterior segmental bronchus

Right oblique fissure · Right inferior lobe · Esophagus · P · Descending aorta · Left inferior lobe · Left oblique fissure

Left superior lobe

Left mainstem bronchus

Left pulmonary artery

L

Apical segmental bronchus

Posterior segmental bronchus

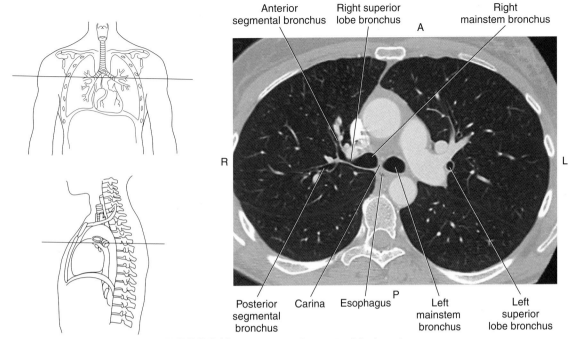

FIGURE 6.19 Axial CT of left superior lobe bronchus.

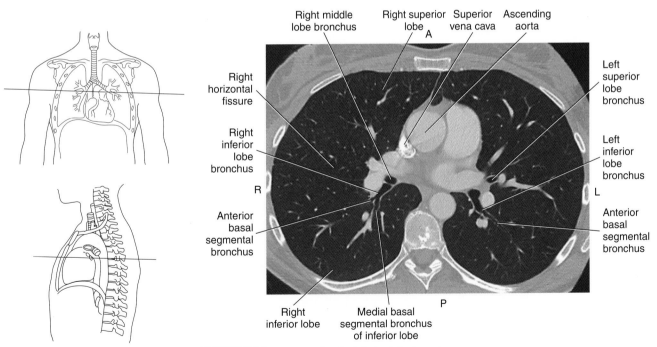

FIGURE 6.20 Axial CT of right inferior lobe bronchus.

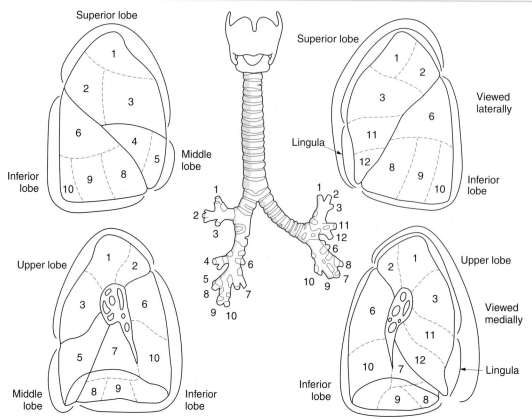

FIGURE 6.21 **Trachea and bronchopulmonary segments.** Bronchopulmonary segments: **1,** apical; **2,** posterior; **3,** anterior; **4,** lateral; **5,** medial; **6,** superior; **7,** medial basal; **8,** anterior basal; **9,** lateral basal; **10,** posterior basal; **11,** superior lingular; **12,** inferior lingular.

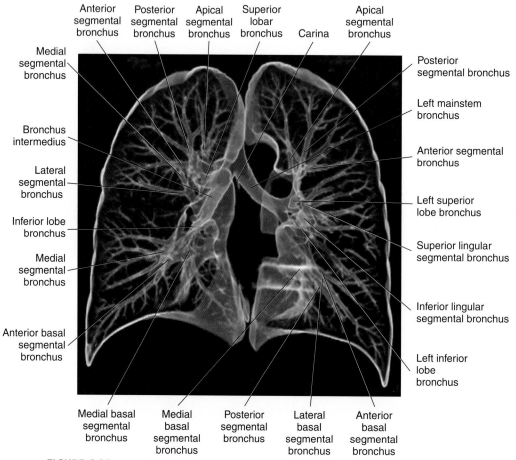

FIGURE 6.22 **Coronal CT, 3D volume-rendered image of central and peripheral airways.**

TABLE 6.1	Bronchopulmonary Segments	
Lobe	Right Lung	Left Lung
Superior lobe	Apical segment (1) Posterior segment (2) Anterior segment (3)	Apical segment (1) Posterior segment (2) Anterior segment (3) Superior lingular segment (11) Inferior lingular segment (12)
Middle lobe	Lateral segment (4) Medial segment (5)	
Inferior lobe	Superior segment (6) Medial basal segment (7) Anterior basal segment (8) Lateral basal segment (9) Posterior basal segment (10)	Superior segment (6) Medial basal segment (7) Anterior basal segment (8) Lateral basal segment (9) Posterior basal segment (10)

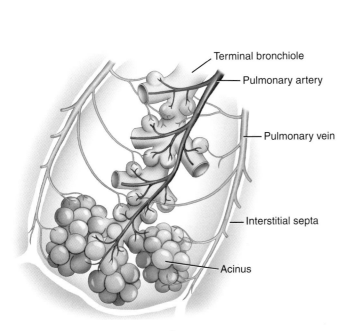

FIGURE 6.23 Axial view of secondary pulmonary lobule.

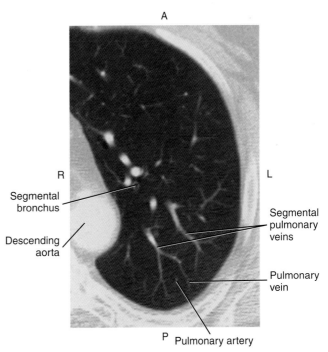

FIGURE 6.24 Axial CT of secondary pulmonary lobule.

MEDIASTINUM

The **mediastinum** is the midline region of the thoracic cavity located between the two pleural cavities of the lungs. It extends from the superior thoracic aperture to the diaphragm and is bordered anteriorly by the sternum and posteriorly by thoracic vertebrae. The mediastinum can be subdivided into compartments for descriptive purposes. The superior and inferior compartments are made by drawing an imaginary line between the sternal angle and the intervertebral disk of T4-T5. The **superior compartment** constitutes the upper portion of the mediastinum. It contains the thymus gland and acts as a conduit for structures as they enter and leave the thoracic cavity. The **inferior compartment** can be further divided into anterior, middle, and posterior compartments (Figure 6.25). The **anterior compartment** is located anterior to the pericardial sac and posterior to the sternum. The **middle compartment** is the area that contains the pericardial sac, heart, and roots of the great vessels. The **posterior compartment** is the area lying posterior to the pericardium and anterior to the inferior eight thoracic vertebrae. Structures located within the mediastinum include the thymus gland, trachea, esophagus, lymph nodes, thoracic duct, heart and great vessels, and various nerves (Table 6.2).

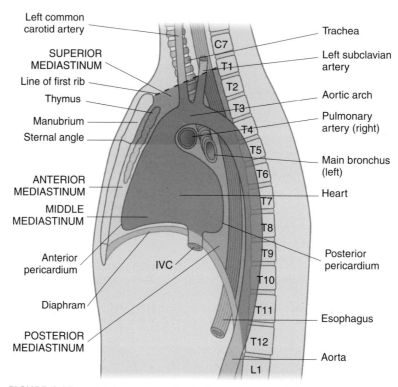

FIGURE 6.25 Sagittal view of mediastinal compartments. **IVC,** Inferior vena cava.

TABLE 6.2	Mediastinal Compartments	
Compartment	**Location**	**Structures**
Superior	Between the manubrium and T1-T4. Bounded superiorly by the thoracic inlet and inferiorly by a plane between the sterna angle and the T4-5 disk space.	Thymus, aortic arch, superior vena cava (SVC), vagus and phrenic nerves, lymph nodes, superior trachea, esophagus, and thoracic duct
Inferior	Divided into three compartments below the superior mediastinum: anterior, middle, and posterior compartments.	
Anterior	Between sternal body and pericardium	Inferior thymus, fat, lymph nodes, mediastinal branches of internal thoracic artery
Middle	Bounded by the fibrous pericardium	Pericardium, heart, ascending aorta, lower half of SVC, tracheal bifurcation and main bronchi, central pulmonary and systemic vessels, lymph nodes
Posterior	Between fibrous pericardium and lower 4th to 12th thoracic vertebral bodies	Inferior esophagus, descending thoracic aorta, azygos and hemiazygos veins, thoracic duct, lymph nodes

Thymus Gland

The **thymus gland** is a triangular-shaped bilobed gland of lymph tissue, located in the superior portion of the mediastinum just behind the manubrium (Figures 6.26 through 6.28). It is considered the primary lymphatic organ responsible for the development of cellular immunity. T-lymphocytes within the blood reach the thymus as stem cells, where they are stored while they undergo T-cell differentiation and maturation. The thymus gland produces a hormone, thymosin, that is responsible for the development and maturation of lymphocytes. The thymus gland reaches its maximum size during puberty and gradually diminishes in size in the adult.

> The thymus gland is large in children. In the newborn, it is often larger than the heart. It gradually decreases in size with increasing age and is replaced by mediastinal fat.

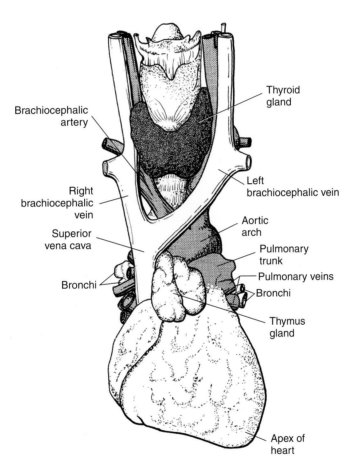

FIGURE 6.26 Anterior view of thymus gland.

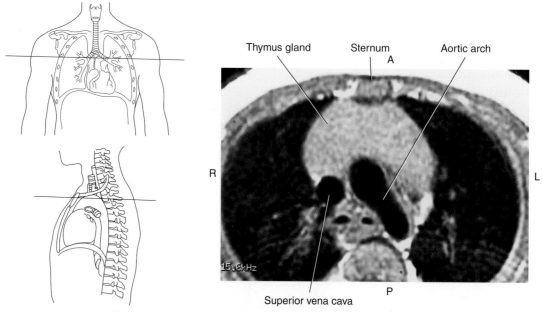

FIGURE 6.27 Axial, T1-weighted MRI of pediatric chest with thymus gland.

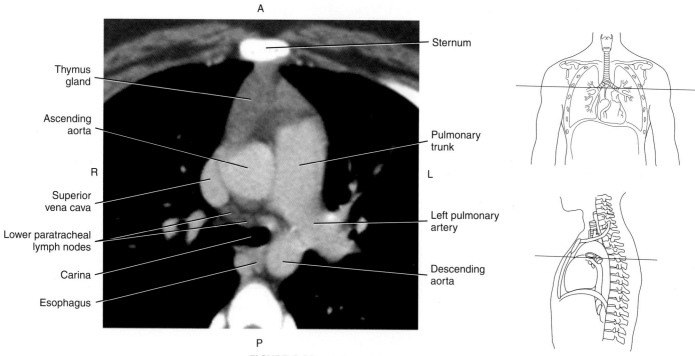

FIGURE 6.28 Axial CT of thymus gland.

Trachea and Esophagus

Throughout its course in the mediastinum, the trachea runs anterior to the esophagus. In crosssection, the trachea appears as a round air-filled structure to the point at which it bifurcates at the carina (Figures 6.11 and 6.18).

The esophagus appears as an oval-shaped structure that descends through the mediastinum to enter the abdominal cavity at the esophageal hiatus of the diaphragm. It joins the stomach at the gastroesophageal junction (Figures 6.29 and 6.30).

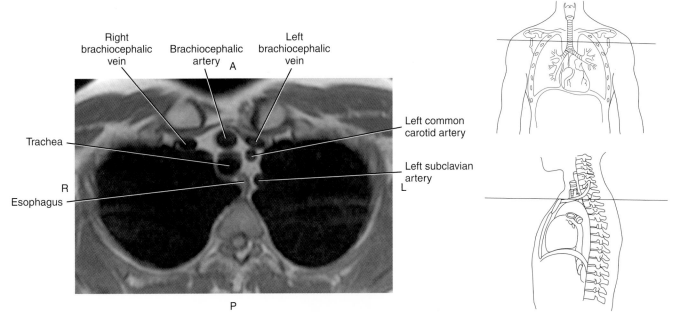

FIGURE 6.29 Axial, T1-weighted MRI of trachea and esophagus.

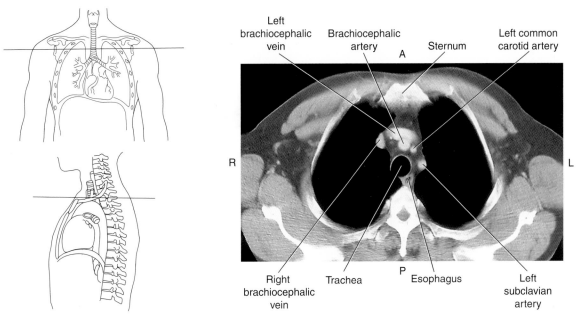

FIGURE 6.30 Axial CT of trachea and esophagus.

LYMPHATIC SYSTEM

Lymph Nodes

Lymph nodes in the mediastinum are generally clustered around the great vessels, esophagus, bronchi, and carina. Mediastinal lymph nodes are classified according to their location and are grouped into 14 regional nodal stations for use in lung cancer staging (Figure 6.31 and Table 6.3). Lymph vessels and nodes can be difficult to visualize in cross section unless they are enlarged as a result of an abnormality (Figures 6.28, 6.32, and 6.33).

> The supraclavicular lymph nodes are commonly referred to as the sentinel lymph nodes because their enlargement alerts the medical professional to the possibility of malignant disease in the thoracic and/or abdominal cavities.

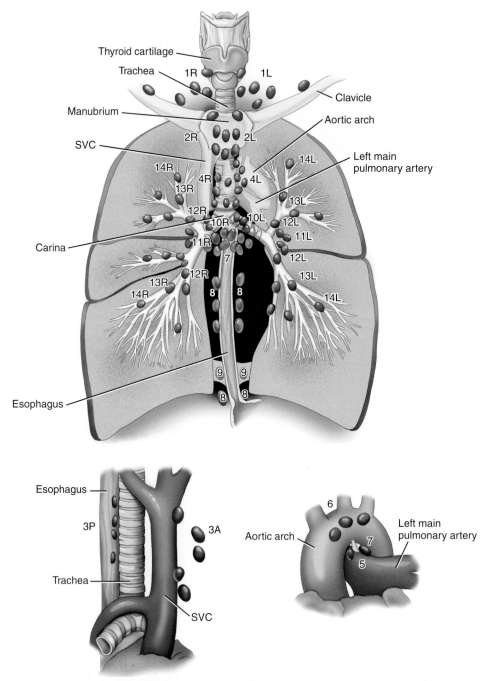

FIGURE 6.31 Coronal view with distribution of mediastinal lymph nodes. L, Left; **R,** right; **1,** highest mediastinal nodes; **2,** upper paratracheal nodes; **3,** prevascular and retrotracheal nodes; **4,** lower paratracheal (including azygos) nodes; **5,** subaortic nodes; **6,** paraaortic nodes; **7,** subcarinal; **8,** paraesophageal nodes; **9,** pulmonary ligament; **10,** hilar nodes; **11,** interlobar nodes; **12,** lobar nodes; **13,** segmental nodes; **14,** segmental nodes.

TABLE 6.3	International Association for the Study of Lung Cancer (IASLC) Lymph Node Map 2009

Supraclavicular Nodes 1

Station 1: Low Cervical, Supraclavicular and Sternal Notch; Divided into 1R and 1L by Trachea
1R—extend from lower border of cricoid cartilage to clavicles and upper margin of manubrium
1L—extend from lower border of cricoid cartilage to clavicles and upper margin of manubrium

Superior Mediastinal Nodes 2-4

Station 2: Upper Paratracheal; Divided into 2R and 2L by Lateral Border of Trachea
2R—upper border: apex of R lung to upper border of manubrium; lower border: intersection of L brachiocephalic vein with trachea
2L—upper border: apex of L lung to upper border of manubrium; lower border: superior border of aortic arch

Station 3: Prevascular (Anterior to the Vessels) and Retrotracheal (Posterior to the Esophagus)
3A—prevascular: on right side: apex of chest to level of carina & posterior sternum to anterior border of SVC. On left side: apex of chest to level of carina & posterior sternum to left carotid artery.
3P—retrotracheal: apex of chest to carina

Station 4: Lower Paratracheal; Divided into 4R and 4L by Trachea
4R—upper border: intersection of caudal margin of left brachiocephalic vein; lower border: lower border of azygos vein
4L—upper border: upper margin of aortic arch; lower border: upper margin of left main pulmonary artery

Aortic Nodes 5-6

Station 5: Subaortic; Lateral to Ligamentum Arteriosum
5—subaortic (aortopulmonary window): upper border: lower margin of aortic arch; lower border: upper rim of left main pulmonary artery

Station 6: Para-aortic; Anterior and Lateral to Ascending Aorta and Aortic Arch
6—para-aortic (ascending aorta or phrenic): upper border: upper margin of aortic arch; lower border: lower margin of aortic arch

Inferior Mediastinal Nodes 7-9

Station 7: Subcarinal; Located Caudally to Carina
7—on right: extend caudally to lower border of bronchus intermedius; on left: extend caudally to upper margin of the lower lobe bronchus

Station 8: Paraesophageal; Below Carinal Nodes, Adjacent to Wall of Esophagus
8—on right: upper border: lower margin of bronchus intermedius; lower border: interolobar region. On left: upper margin of lower lobe bronchus; lower border: interlobar region.

Station 9: Pulmonary Ligament
9—upper border: inferior pulmonary vein; lower border: diaphragm

Hilar, Lobar, and Subsegmental Nodes 10-14

Station 10: Hilar; Adjacent to Mainstem Bronchus and Hilar Vessels
10—on right: upper border: lower rim of azygos vein; lower border: interlobar region. On left: upper border: upper rim of pulmonary artery; lower border: interlobar region.

Station 11: Interlobar; between Origins of the Lobar Bronchi
11—superior: between upper lobe bronchus and bronchus intermedius on the right; inferior: between the middle and lower lobe bronchi on the right

Station 12: Lobar; Adjacent to Lobar Bronchi

Station 13: Segmental; Adjacent to Segmental Bronchi

Station 14: Subsegmental; Adjacent to Subsegmental Bronchi

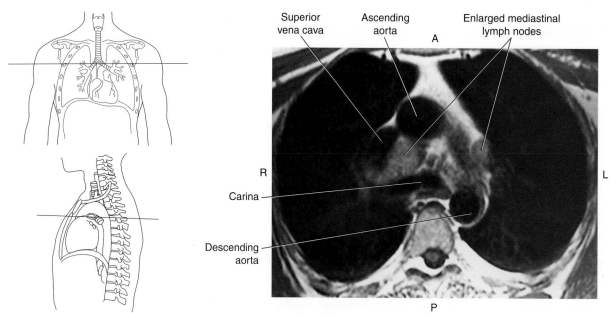

FIGURE 6.32 Axial, T1-weighted MRI of chest with enlarged lymph nodes.

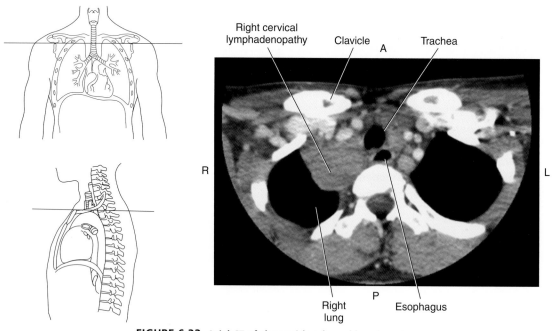

FIGURE 6.33 Axial CT of chest with enlarged lymph nodes.

Lymph Vessels

The lymphatic system consists of a network of lymphatic vessels that carry lymph fluid (excess interstitial fluid) away from the tissue and into venous circulation. Small lymph vessels (capillaries) can be found accompanying arteries and veins throughout the body. The tiny lymph vessels increase in size until they reach their terminal collecting vessels, the thoracic duct and the right lymphatic duct. The **thoracic duct** is the main vessel of the lymph system, draining all of the lymph fluid from tissues below the diaphragm and from the left side of the body above the diaphragm (Figures 6.34 through 6.36). It

begins inferior to the diaphragm at the level of L2 and passes from the abdominal cavity into the thorax through the aortic hiatus of the diaphragm. It originates in the abdomen, at the **cisterna chyli**, a dilated sac or confluence of lymph trunks into which lymph from the intestinal and lumbar lymphatic trunks open (Figure 6.34). It ascends the thorax, between the azygos vein and the descending aorta, and empties into the left subclavian vein at the level of the clavicle. The smaller **right lymphatic duct** collects lymph from the right upper side of the body and is formed by the merging of various lymphatic trunks near the right clavicle. This duct empties into the right subclavian vein (Figure 6.34).

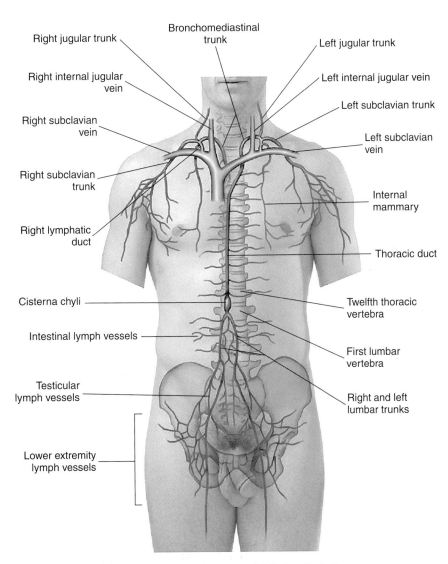

FIGURE 6.34 Anterior view of thoracic and right lymphatic ducts.

A

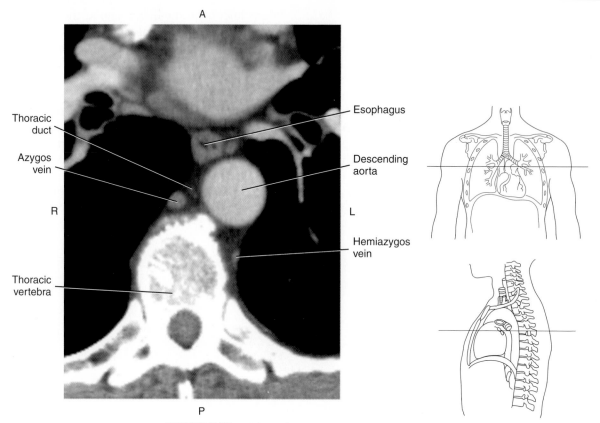

FIGURE 6.35 Axial CT of azygos vein and thoracic duct.

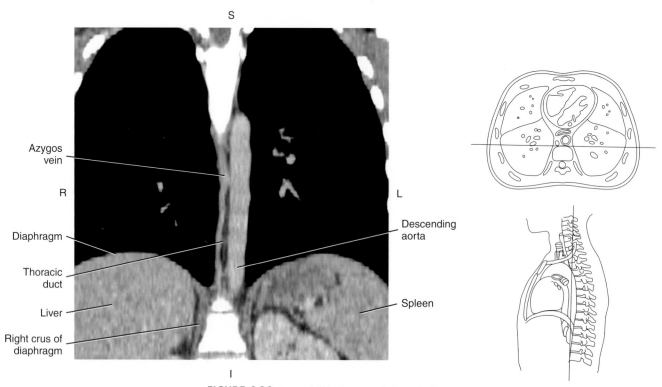

FIGURE 6.36 Coronal CT reformat of thoracic duct.

HEART AND VASCULATURE

Superficial Landmarks

The **heart** is a hollow, four-chambered muscular organ located within the middle mediastinum. It is approximately the size of a large clenched fist and is situated obliquely in the chest with one third of its mass lying to the right of the median plane and two thirds to the left. The heart can be described as being roughly trapezoid shaped (Figure 6.37). The superficial relationships of the heart include the base; apex; three surfaces (sternocostal, diaphragmatic, pulmonary); and four borders (right, inferior, left, and superior). The broad **base (posterior aspect)** is the most superior and posterior portion of the heart. It is formed by both atria, primarily the left atrium, and gives rise to the great vessels. The **apex** is formed by the left ventricle and points inferiorly, anteriorly, and to the left. It is located at the level of the fifth intercostal space, just medial to the midclavicular line. The **sterno-costal (anterior surface)** is formed primarily by the right atrium and right ventricle with a small contribution from the left ventricle. The **diaphragmatic (inferior surface)** rests on the central tendon of the diaphragm and is formed by both ventricles and a small portion of the right atrium. The **pulmonary (left surface)** is formed mainly by the left ventricle and fills the cardiac notch of the left lung. The borders of the heart represent the external surfaces of the cardiovascular silhouette in radiographic profile. The borders include the **right border,** formed by the right atrium and located between the superior and inferior venae cavae; the **left border,** formed by the apex of the heart or the left ventricle; the **superior border,** formed by the right and left atria; and the **inferior border,** which is formed primarily by the right ventricle with a small contribution from the left ventricle (Figures 6.37 through 6.39).

Carditis, an inflammation of the heart, can often lead to valvular heart disease. When infection damages or destroys the heart valves, valve leakage, heart failure, and death can ensue.

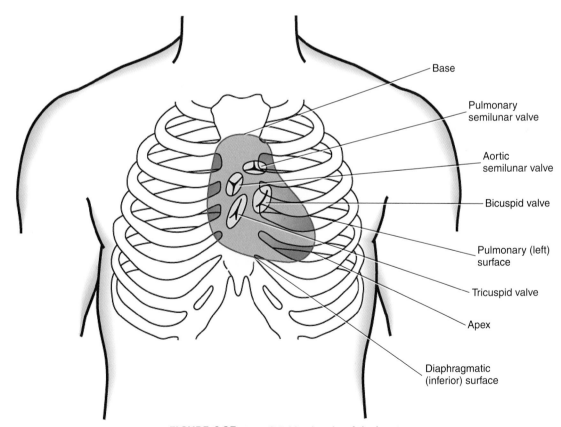

FIGURE 6.37 Superficial landmarks of the heart.

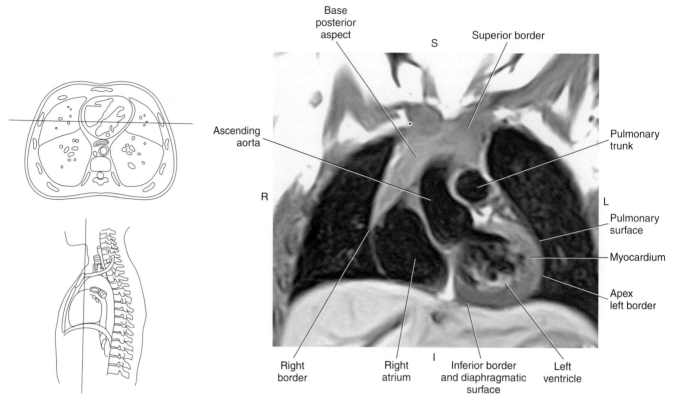

FIGURE 6.38 Coronal, T1-weighted MRI of surfaces and borders of heart.

Base posterior aspect

Superior border

S

Ascending aorta

Pulmonary trunk

R

L

Pulmonary surface

Myocardium

Apex left border

Right border

Right atrium

I

Inferior border and diaphragmatic surface

Left ventricle

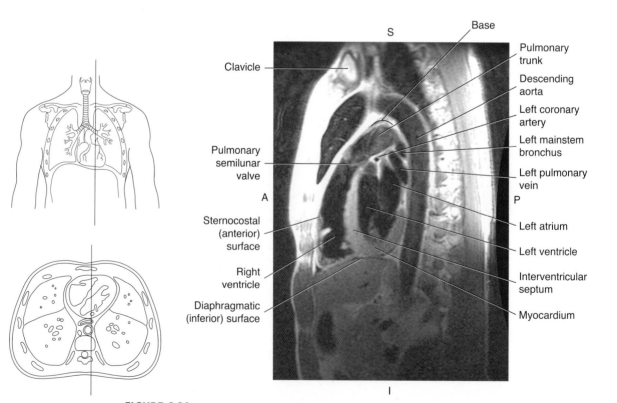

FIGURE 6.39 Sagittal, T1-weighted MRI of surfaces and borders of heart.

S

Base

Clavicle

Pulmonary trunk

Descending aorta

Left coronary artery

Pulmonary semilunar valve

Left mainstem bronchus

A

Left pulmonary vein

P

Sternocostal (anterior) surface

Left atrium

Left ventricle

Right ventricle

Interventricular septum

Diaphragmatic (inferior) surface

Myocardium

I

Pericardium

The heart is enclosed in a pericardial sac that surrounds the heart and the proximal portions of the great vessels entering and leaving the heart (Figures 6.40 through 6.42). The **fibrous pericardium** is attached to the central tendon of the diaphragm and is pierced by the inferior vena cava. The inner surface of the fibrous pericardium consists of a double-layered serous membrane termed the **serous pericardium**. The serous pericardial layers include the **parietal layer**, which lines the inner surface of the fibrous pericardium, and the **visceral layer (epicardium)**, which covers the outer surface of the heart and the roots of the great vessels. Located between the two layers is a potential space (**pericardial cavity**) containing a thin film of serous fluid that acts as a lubricant to reduce friction to the tissues caused by heart movements. During embryonic development, the heart invaginates into the serous pericardium, which creates folds called pericardial reflections. The pericardial reflections located by the great vessels result in the formation of two potential spaces: the oblique and transverse sinuses. Within the two sinuses are potential spaces called **recesses** (Figure 6.43 and Table 6.4). These spaces can be filled with fluid and may be mistaken for cystic lesions or lymphadenopathy. Located between the parietal pericardium and the heart wall is a layer of **subepicardial fat** that is typically more prominent near the inflow and outflow of the heart, the coronary vessels, and along the grooves separating the heart chambers. **Mediastinal fat** is the fat present within the thoracic cavity external to the parietal pericardium (Figures 6.40 through 6.42).

> Ten percent of the total cardiac volume of each heart-beat is required solely to supply blood to the heart muscle.

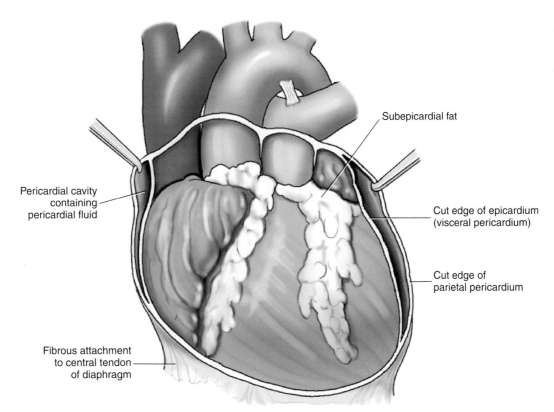

FIGURE 6.40 Anterior view of heart with pericardium.

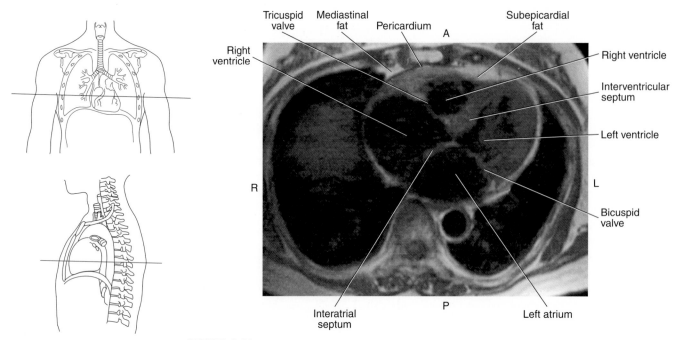

FIGURE 6.41 Axial, T1-weighted MRI of heart with pericardium.

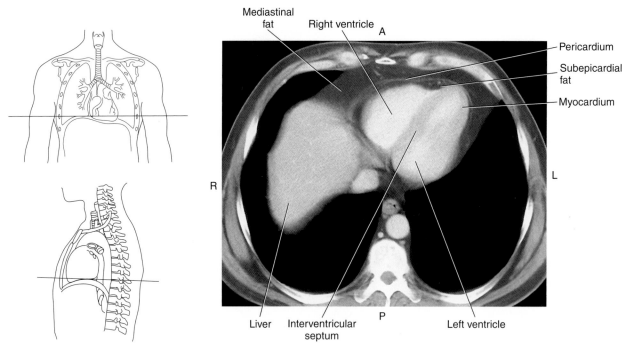

FIGURE 6.42 Axial CT of heart with pericardium.

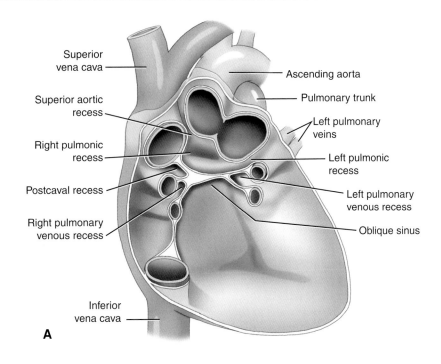

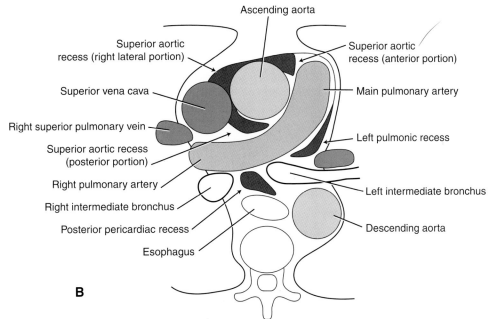

FIGURE 6.43 Pericardial sinuses and recesses. A, Anterior view of pericardial sinuses and recesses. **B,** Axial view of pericardial sinuses and recesses.

TABLE 6.4	Pericardial Sinuses and Recesses
Transverse sinus	Located posterior to ascending aorta and pulmonary trunk, extending to left atrium
Superior aortic recess	Located anterior to ascending aorta and pulmonary trunk; partially surrounds ascending aorta
Inferior aortic recess	Located between right lateral ascending aorta and right atrium; posterior to aorta and anterior to left atrium
R & L Pulmonic recesses	Right; inferior to proximal right pulmonary artery
	Left; inferior to left pulmonary artery, superior to left superior pulmonary vein
Oblique sinus	Located posterior to left atrium and inferior to the transverse sinus
Posterior pericardial recess	Extends superiorly behind the right pulmonary artery, medial to the intermediate bronchus

Heart Wall

The walls of the heart consist of three layers: (1) **epicardium**, the thin outer layer that is in contact with the pericardium; (2) **myocardium**, the thick middle layer consisting of strong cardiac muscle; and (3) **endocardium**, the thin, endothelial layer lining the inner surface (Figures 6.39, 6.42, and 6.44). The endothelial layer also lines the valves of the heart and is continuous with the inner lining of the blood vessels. The heart is divided into four chambers: the right and left atria and the right and left ventricles. The two superior collecting chambers called atria are separated by the **interatrial septum** (Figures 6.41 and 6.44). During embryonic development, an oval opening exists within the interatrial septum called the **foramen ovale**. This opening allows blood flow between the right and left atria during fetal lung development. At birth, the foramen ovale closes, leaving a small depression in the septal wall called the **fossa ovalis** in the adult heart. The two inferior pumping chambers called **ventricles** are divided by the **interventricular septum** (see Figures 6.39, 6.41, and 6.42). On the external surface of the heart are grooves that separate the chambers. The atria of the heart are separated from the ventricles by the **coronary groove** (**atrioventricular groove** or **sulcus**). The ventricles of the heart are separated by two depressions or sulci that are located on the anterior and posterior surfaces of the heart, termed the **anterior** and **posterior interventricular grooves** (Figure 6.45).

Chambers

The **right atrium** forms the right border of the heart and receives deoxygenated blood from the body via the superior and inferior venae cavae and from the coronary sinus and cardiac veins that drain the myocardium. A small muscular embryonic appendage, the **right auricle**, projects upward and toward the left, covering the root of the aorta (see Figures 6.44 and 6.45). The **right ventricle** lies on the diaphragm and comprises the largest portion of the anterior surface of the heart. It receives deoxygenated blood from the right atrium and forces it into the pulmonary trunk for conveyance to the lungs. Extending from the inferior surface of the ventricular walls are conical-shaped projections of cardiac muscle called **papillary muscles,** which anchor the cusps of the tricuspid valve to the right ventricle (see Figure 6.44). The **left atrium** lies posterior to the right atrium and is the most posterior surface of the heart. It also has an embryonic appendage, the **left auricle**, which projects to the left of the pulmonary trunk over the superior surface of the heart. The left atrium receives oxygenated blood directly from the lungs via the four pulmonary veins (two on each side). The **left ventricle** forms the apex, left border, and most of the inferior surface of the heart. It receives oxygenated blood from the left atrium and pumps it into the aorta for distribution throughout the systemic circuit. The myocardium of the left ventricle is normally three times thicker than that of the right ventricle,

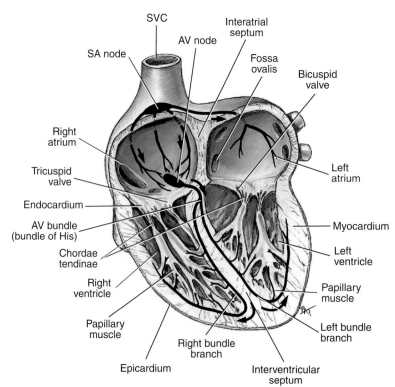

FIGURE 6.44 Coronal view of heart wall, chambers, and conduction system.

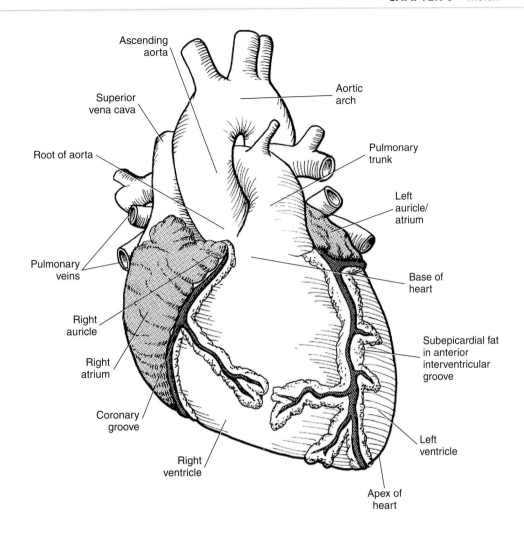

Ascending aorta

Superior vena cava

Root of aorta

Pulmonary veins

Right auricle

Right atrium

Coronary groove

Right ventricle

Aortic arch

Pulmonary trunk

Left auricle/ atrium

Base of heart

Subepicardial fat in anterior interventricular groove

Left ventricle

Apex of heart

FIGURE 6.45 Anterior view of of heart surface.

reflecting the force necessary to pump blood to the distant sites of the systemic circulation (Figures 6.46 through 6.66). Two papillary muscles project from the ventricular walls to anchor the bicuspid valve to the left ventricle (see Figures 6.44, 6.52, 6.63, 6.65, and 6.66).

To see the cardiac chambers in off-axis views refer to page 377-385.

Cardiac Conduction System

The cardiac conduction system is the electrical system that controls the heart rate by generating electrical impulses and conducting them throughout the muscles of the heart, stimulating the heart to contract and pump blood. The electrical impulses of the myocardium travel through a specific nerve pathway in the heart beginning in the **sinoatrial (SA) node**, which is a mass of specialized cardiac muscle fibers that act as the "pacemaker" of the heart. The SA node lies under the epicardium in the superior aspect of the right atrium. The electrical signal generated from the SA node travels to the right and left atrium, causing them to contract and force blood into the ventricles. The electrical signal continues to the ventricles via the **atrioventricular (AV) node**, located in the posteroinferior region of the interatrial septum near the opening of the coronary sinus, and then to the **atrioventricular (AV) bundle (bundle of His)** located along the interventricular septum. The signal continues down the bundle and into the right and left bundle branches. When the signal reaches the bundle branches, it causes the ventricles to contract and force blood to the body and lungs (see Figure 6.44).

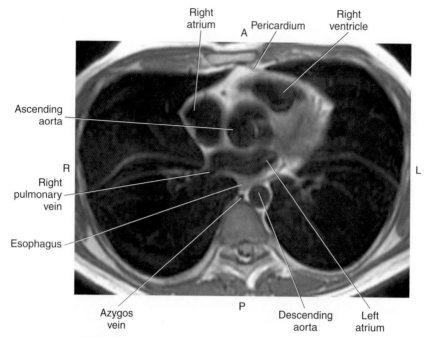

FIGURE 6.46 Axial, T1-weighted MRI of right ventricle.

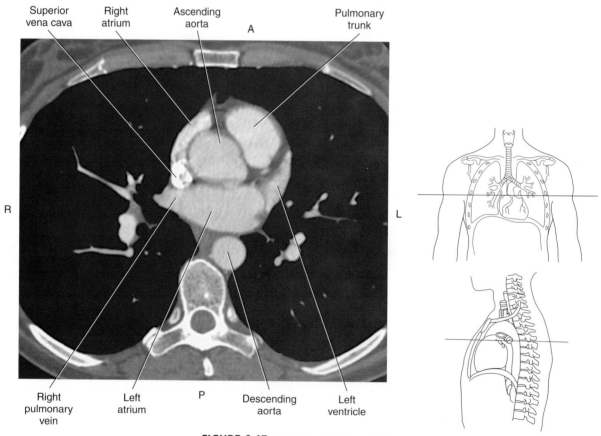

FIGURE 6.47 Axial CT of right ventricle.

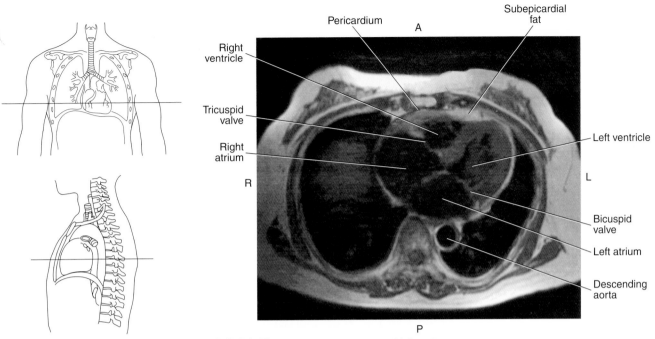

FIGURE 6.48 Axial, T1-weighted MRI of left atrium.

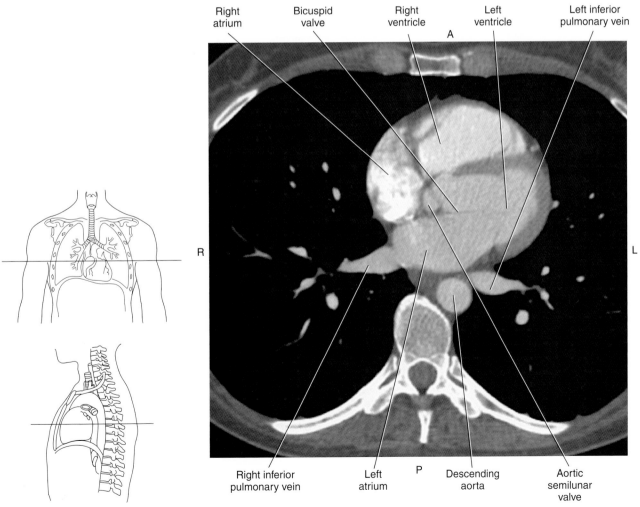

FIGURE 6.49 Axial CT of left atrium.

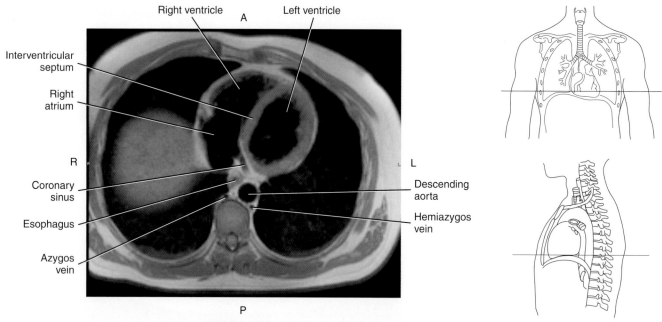

FIGURE 6.50 Axial, T1-weighted MRI of right atrium.

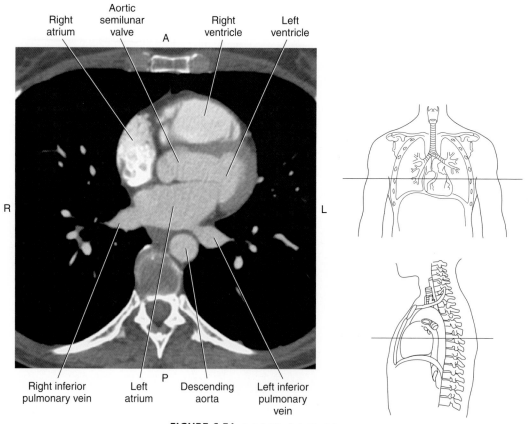

FIGURE 6.51 Axial CT of right atrium.

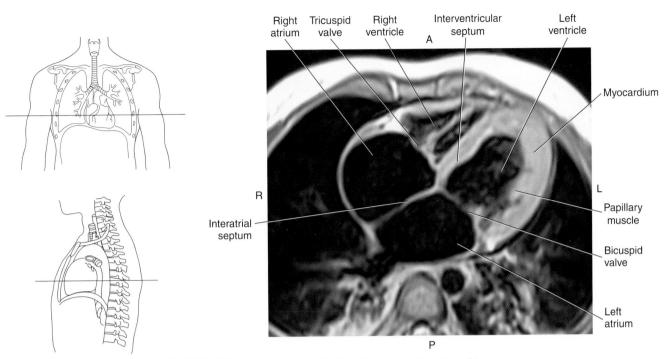

FIGURE 6.52 Axial, T1-weighted MRI with four-chamber view of heart.

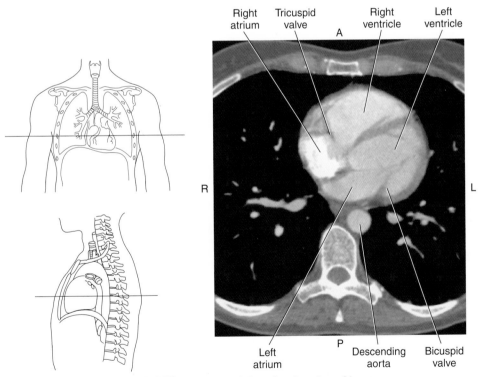

FIGURE 6.53 Axial CT with four-chamber view of heart.

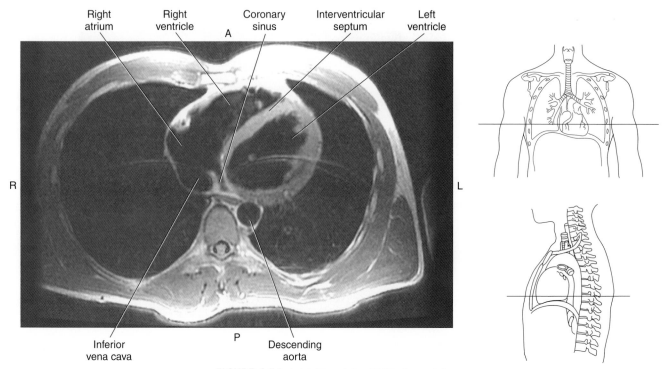

FIGURE 6.54 Axial, T1-weighted MRI of ventricles.

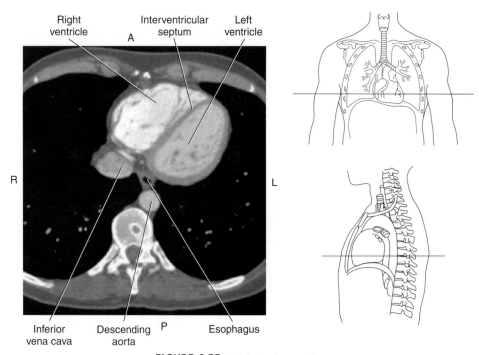

FIGURE 6.55 Axial CT of ventricles.

S

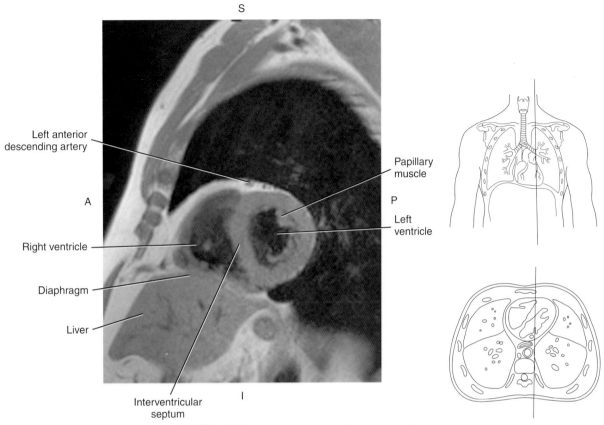

Left anterior
descending artery

A

Right ventricle

Diaphragm

Liver

Papillary
muscle

P

Left
ventricle

Interventricular
septum

I

FIGURE 6.56 Sagittal, T1-weighted MRI of ventricles.

S

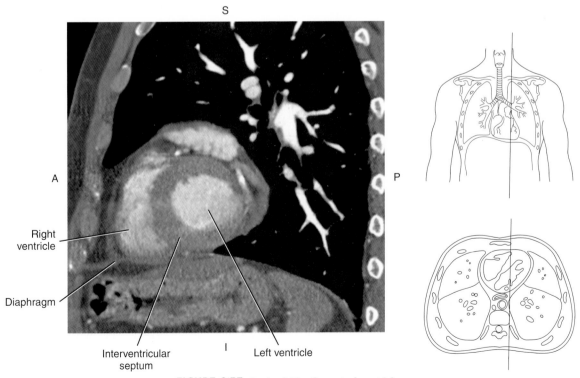

A

Right
ventricle

Diaphragm

P

Interventricular
septum

I

Left ventricle

FIGURE 6.57 Sagittal CT reformat of ventricles.

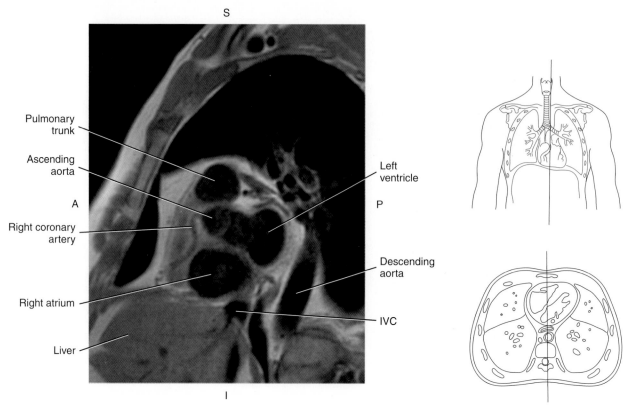

FIGURE 6.58 Sagittal, T1-weighted MRI of heart with pulmonary trunk.

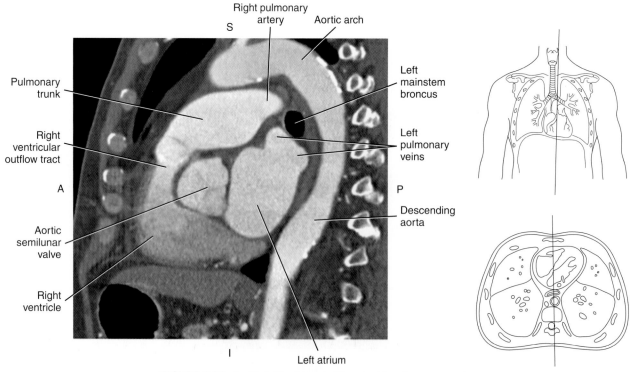

FIGURE 6.59 Sagittal CT reformat of heart with pulmonary trunk.

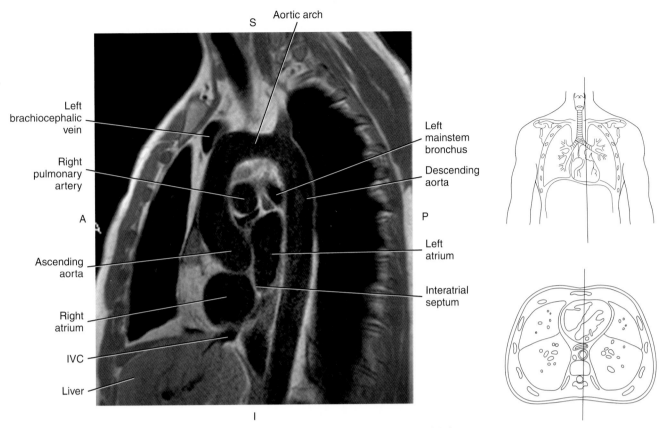

FIGURE 6.60 Sagittal, T1-weighted MRI of heart with left atrium.

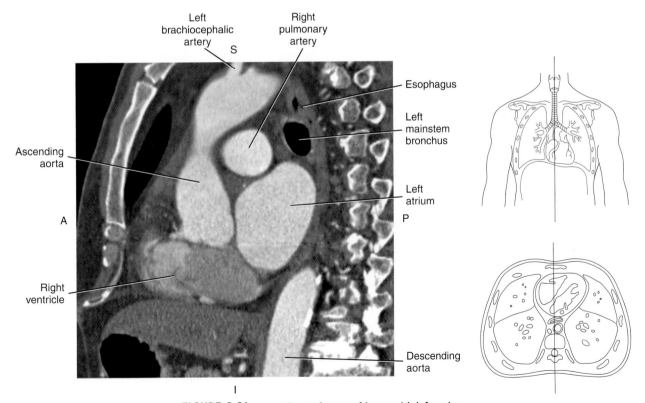

FIGURE 6.61 Sagittal CT reformat of heart with left atrium.

Cardiac Valves

Four valves are located in the heart that function to maintain one-way directional blood flow throughout the heart. The valves can be divided into two groups: atrioventricular and semilunar (see Figure 6.62).

Atrioventricular Valves. The two atrioventricular valves are found at the entrances to both ventricles and function to prevent backflow of blood between the atria and ventricles during ventricular contraction. These valves have leaflets that are attached to the papillary muscles by thin cords of fibrous tissue called **chordae tendineae**. The **right atrioventricular valve**, with three leaflets, is called the **tricuspid valve**, and the **left atrioventricular valve**, with two leaflets, is called the **bicuspid (mitral) valve** (see Figures 6.44, 6.52, 6.53, 6.63, 6.65, and 6.66).

Semilunar Valves. The semilunar valves are located at the junction where the ventricles meet the great vessels and separate the ventricles from the circulatory system. These valves are called semilunar because of their three crescent-shaped cusps and function to prevent the flow of blood back into the ventricles during ventricular relaxation. The **pulmonary semilunar valve** is located at the juncture of the right ventricle and pulmonary artery, and the **aortic semilunar valve** lies between the left ventricle and ascending aorta (see Figures 6.39, 6.62, 6.63, 6.65, and 6.66).

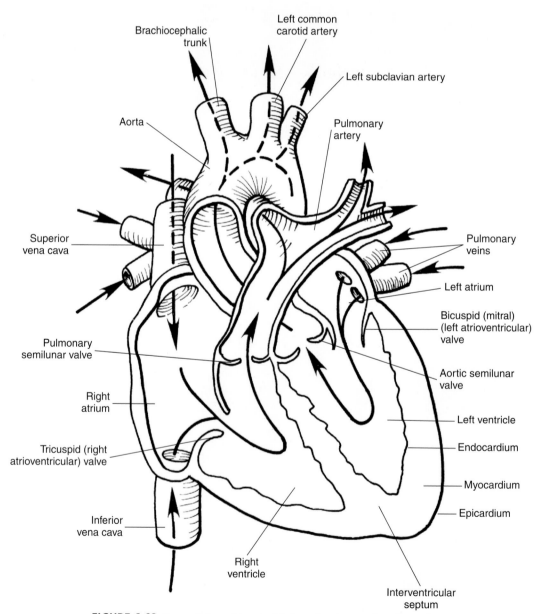

FIGURE 6.62 Coronal view of heart with four chambers and cardiac valves.

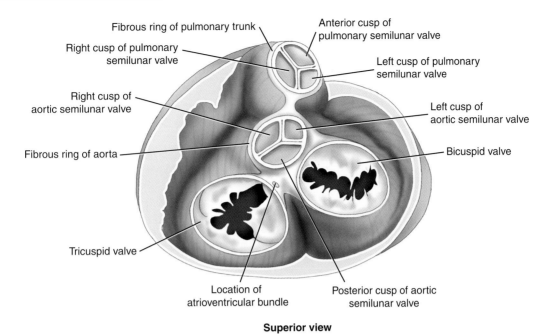

Fibrous ring of pulmonary trunk

Right cusp of pulmonary semilunar valve

Anterior cusp of pulmonary semilunar valve

Left cusp of pulmonary semilunar valve

Right cusp of aortic semilunar valve

Left cusp of aortic semilunar valve

Fibrous ring of aorta

Bicuspid valve

Tricuspid valve

Location of atrioventricular bundle

Posterior cusp of aortic semilunar valve

Superior view

FIGURE 6.63 Superior view of heart valves.

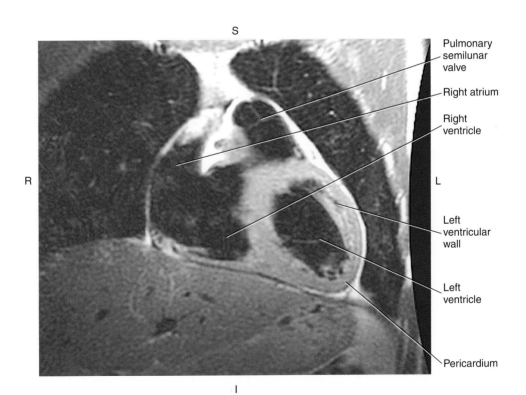

S

Pulmonary semilunar valve

Right atrium

Right ventricle

R

L

Left ventricular wall

Left ventricle

Pericardium

I

FIGURE 6.64 Coronal, T1-weighted MRI of heart.

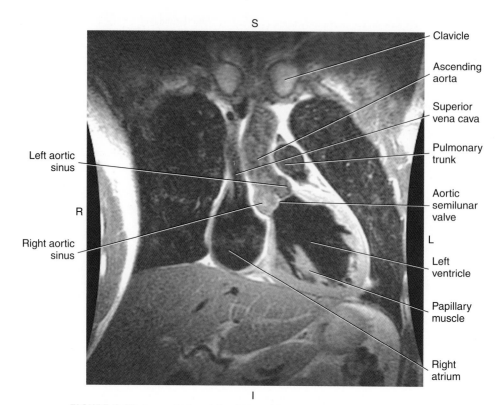

FIGURE 6.65 Coronal, T1-weighted MRI of heart with aortic semilunar valve.

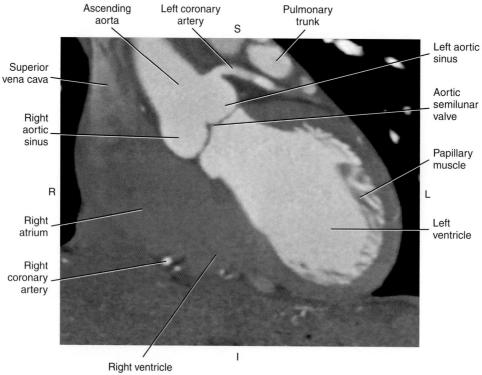

FIGURE 6.66 Coronal CT reformat of heart with aortic semilunar valve.

GREAT VESSELS

Blood travels to and from the heart through the **great vessels,** which include the aorta, pulmonary arteries and veins, and superior and inferior venae cavae (Figures 6.67 and 6.68). The **aorta** is the largest artery of the body and can be divided into the ascending aorta, aortic arch, and descending aorta. The **ascending aorta** begins at the base of the left ventricle. The origin of the ascending aorta (root) is divided into three dilations or protrusions that create spaces termed **aortic sinuses,** one left, one right, and one posterior, which correspond to the three cusps of the aortic semilunar valve. The right aortic sinus gives rise to the right coronary artery, and the left aortic sinus gives rise to the left coronary artery (Figures 6.65, 6.66, and 6.69). As no vessels arise from the posterior aortic sinus, it is considered to be noncoronary. The ascending aorta curves superiorly and posteriorly as the **aortic arch** over the right pulmonary artery and left mainstem bronchus (see Figures 6.17, 6.45, 6.59, 6.60, and 6.67). The top of the aortic arch is approximately at the level of T3 (Figures 6.70 and 6.71). The arch continues as the **descending aorta** posterior to the left bronchus and pulmonary trunk, on the left side of the vertebral body of T4 (Figures 6.72 and 6.73). The descending aorta passes slightly anterior and to the left of the vertebral

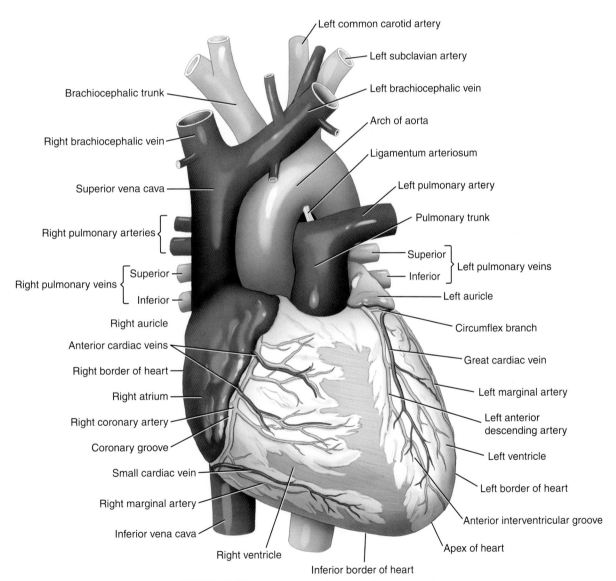

FIGURE 6.67 Anterior view of heart and great vessels.

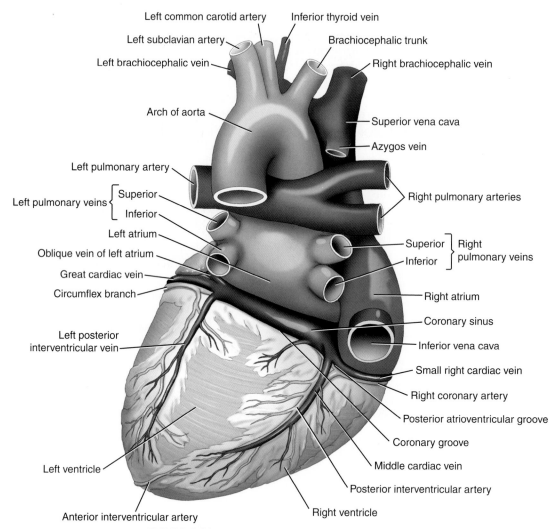

Left common carotid artery

Inferior thyroid vein

Left subclavian artery

Brachiocephalic trunk

Left brachiocephalic vein

Right brachiocephalic vein

Arch of aorta

Superior vena cava

Azygos vein

Left pulmonary artery

Left pulmonary veins { Superior / Inferior }

Right pulmonary arteries

Left atrium

Superior / Inferior } Right pulmonary veins

Oblique vein of left atrium

Great cardiac vein

Circumflex branch

Right atrium

Coronary sinus

Inferior vena cava

Left posterior interventricular vein

Small right cardiac vein

Right coronary artery

Posterior atrioventricular groove

Coronary groove

Left ventricle

Middle cardiac vein

Posterior interventricular artery

Anterior interventricular artery

Right ventricle

FIGURE 6.68 Posterior view of heart and great vessels.

column as it descends through the thoracic and abdominal cavities (Figure 6.74). In the thoracic cavity, the descending aorta is commonly called the **thoracic aorta,** and in the abdominal cavity, it is called the **abdominal aorta.** The **pulmonary trunk,** the main pulmonary artery, lies entirely within the pericardial sac. It arises from the right ventricle and ascends in front of the ascending aorta. Then it courses posteriorly and to the left, where it bifurcates at the level of the sternal angle (T4) into the right and left pulmonary arteries (Figures 6.75 through 6.78). At the origin of the pulmonary trunk are slight dilations between the wall of the pulmonary trunk and cusps of the pulmonary semilunar valves, termed **pulmonary sinuses** (see Figure 6.69). The pulmonary trunk is attached to the aortic arch by a fibrous cord called the **ligamentum arteriosum,** the remnant of an important fetal blood vessel (ductus arteriosus) that links the pulmonary and systemic circuits during fetal development (see Figures 6.67 and 6.75). The **right pulmonary artery** courses laterally, posterior to the ascending aorta and superior vena cava, and anterior to the esophagus and right mainstem

bronchus, to the hilum of the right lung. It then divides into two branches, with the lower branch supplying the middle and inferior lobes and the upper branch supplying the superior lobe (see Figures 6.75 through 6.80). The **left pulmonary artery,** shorter and smaller than the right, is also the most superior of the pulmonary vessels. It travels horizontally, arching over the left mainstem bronchus, and enters the hilum of the left lung just superior to the left mainstem bronchus (see Figures 6.15 and 6.75 through 6.82). Within the lungs, each pulmonary artery descends posterolateral to the main bronchus and divides into lobar and segmental arteries, continuing to branch out and follow along with the smallest divisions of the bronchial tree (see Figures 6.75, 6.79, and 6.80). Located inferior to the pulmonary arteries are the four **pulmonary veins,** two each (superior and inferior) extending from each lung to enter the left atrium (Figures 6.67, 6.68, 6.75, and 6.80 through 6.86). They begin as a capillary network along the walls of the alveoli, where they merge with the capillaries of the pulmonary arteries. The venous capillaries combine to form small vessels that unite

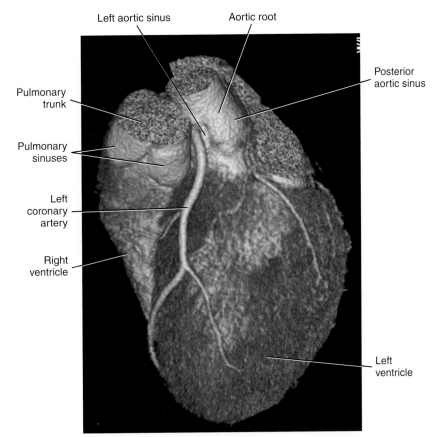

FIGURE 6.69 3D CT of pulmonary trunk and left ventricle.

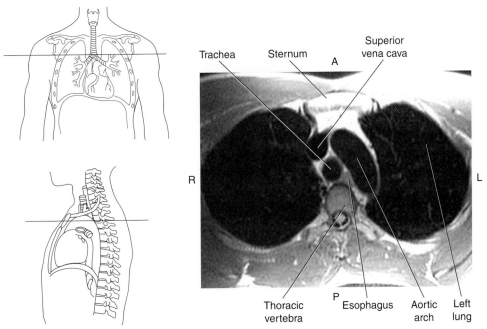

FIGURE 6.70 Axial, T1-weighted MRI of chest with aortic arch.

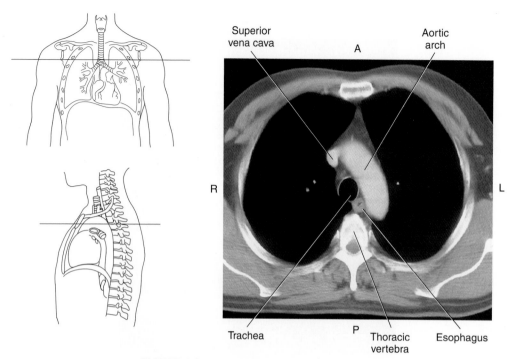

FIGURE 6.71 Axial CT of chest with aortic arch.

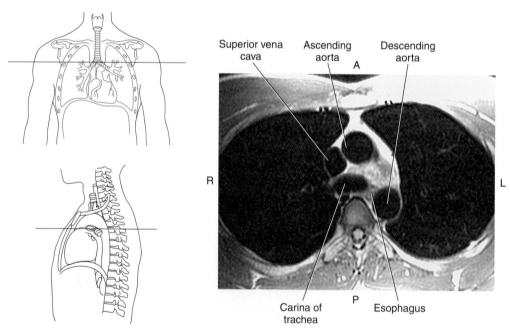

FIGURE 6.72 Axial, T1-weighted MRI of chest with ascending and descending aorta.

successively to eventually form a single trunk for each lobe: three for the right and two for the left lung. Frequently, the trunk from the middle lobe of the right lung unites with the trunk from the upper lobe, forming just two trunks on the right side prior to entering the left atrium. The **right superior pulmonary vein** collects blood from the upper lobe segments of the right lung and passes anterior and inferior to the right pulmonary artery, be-

hind the superior vena cava. The **right inferior pulmonary vein** receives blood from the lower lobes of the right lung and crosses behind the right atrium to the left atrium (see Figures 6.75 and 6.87, and 6.89). The **left superior pulmonary vein** receives blood from the left upper lobe of the left lung and courses anterior and inferior to the left main bronchus as it enters the left atrium. The **left inferior pulmonary vein** drains the inferior lobe

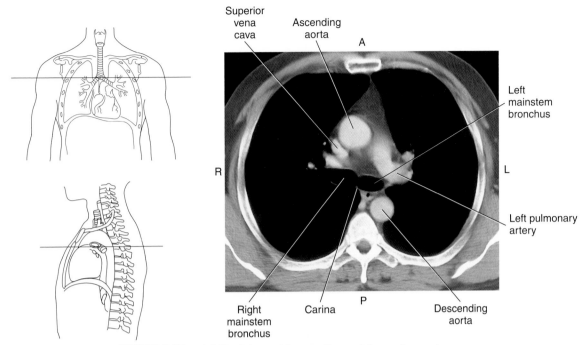

FIGURE 6.73 Axial CT of chest with ascending and descending aorta.

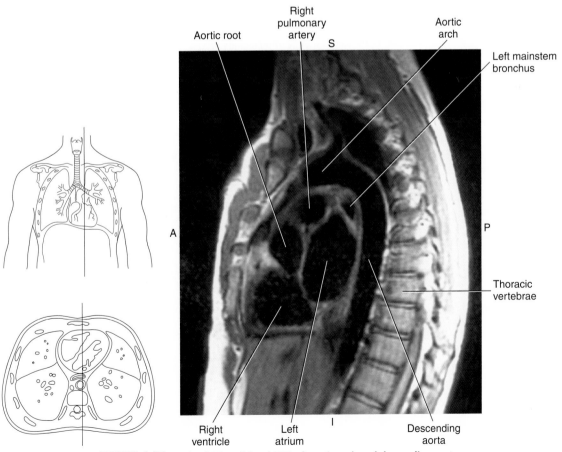

FIGURE 6.74 Sagittal, T1-weighted MRI of aortic arch and descending aorta.

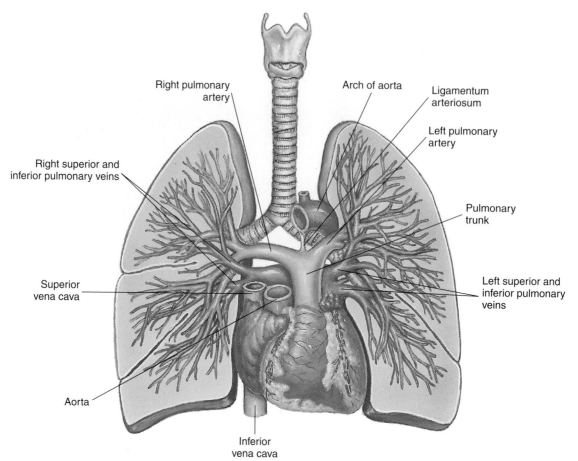

Right pulmonary artery

Arch of aorta

Ligamentum arteriosum

Left pulmonary artery

Right superior and inferior pulmonary veins

Pulmonary trunk

Superior vena cava

Left superior and inferior pulmonary veins

Aorta

Inferior vena cava

FIGURE 6.75 Anterior view of pulmonary arteries and veins.

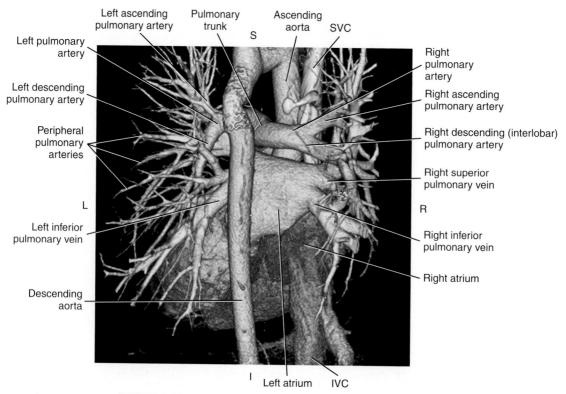

Left ascending pulmonary artery

Pulmonary trunk

Ascending aorta

SVC

S

Left pulmonary artery

Right pulmonary artery

Left descending pulmonary artery

Right ascending pulmonary artery

Peripheral pulmonary arteries

Right descending (interlobar) pulmonary artery

Right superior pulmonary vein

L

R

Left inferior pulmonary vein

Right inferior pulmonary vein

Right atrium

Descending aorta

I

Left atrium

IVC

FIGURE 6.76 3D CT of pulmonary arteries and veins, posterior view.

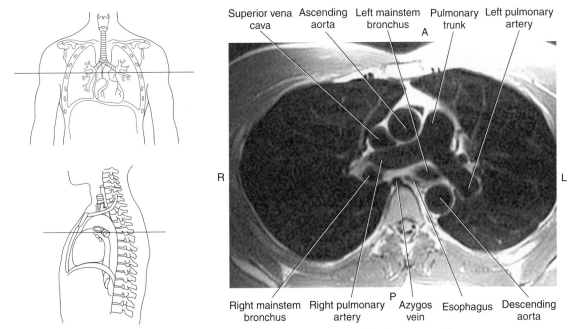

FIGURE 6.77 Axial, T1-weighted MRI of chest with pulmonary trunk.

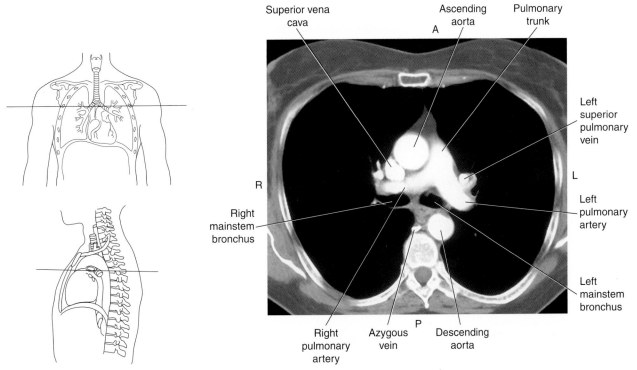

FIGURE 6.78 Axial CT of chest with pulmonary trunk.

of the left lung and passes toward the left atrium anterior to the bronchi (see Figures 6.75 and 6.90 through 6.92). The pulmonary veins course more horizontally than the pulmonary arteries and are ultimately oriented toward the left atrium. At the hilum (root) of the lungs, the pulmonary veins are anteroinferior to the pulmonary arteries. The pulmonary arteries are located anterior to the

bronchus (see Figures 6.75, 6.78, and 6.87). The superior and inferior vena cavae are the largest veins of the body. The **superior vena cava** is formed by the junction of the brachiocephalic veins, posterior to the right first costal cartilage, and carries blood from the thorax, upper limbs, head, and neck (Figure 6.26). As it travels inferiorly, it is located posterior and lateral to the ascending aorta

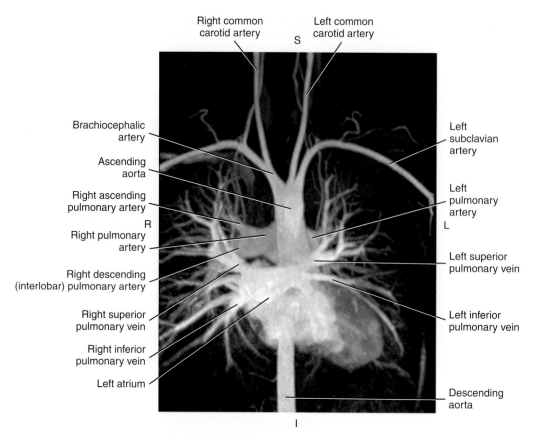

Right common carotid artery

Left common carotid artery

S

Brachiocephalic artery

Ascending aorta

Right ascending pulmonary artery

R

Right pulmonary artery

Right descending (interlobar) pulmonary artery

Right superior pulmonary vein

Right inferior pulmonary vein

Left atrium

Left subclavian artery

Left pulmonary artery

L

Left superior pulmonary vein

Left inferior pulmonary vein

Descending aorta

I

FIGURE 6.79   MRA of pulmonary vessels.

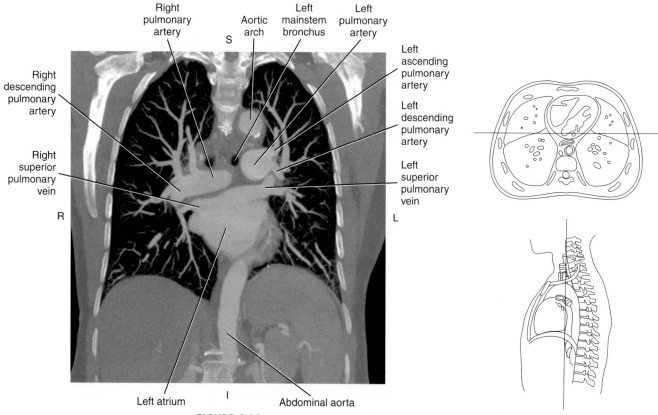

Right pulmonary artery

Aortic arch

Left mainstem bronchus

Left pulmonary artery

S

Right descending pulmonary artery

Left ascending pulmonary artery

Left descending pulmonary artery

Right superior pulmonary vein

Left superior pulmonary vein

R

L

Left atrium

I

Abdominal aorta

FIGURE 6.80   Coronal CT reformat of pulmonary vessels.

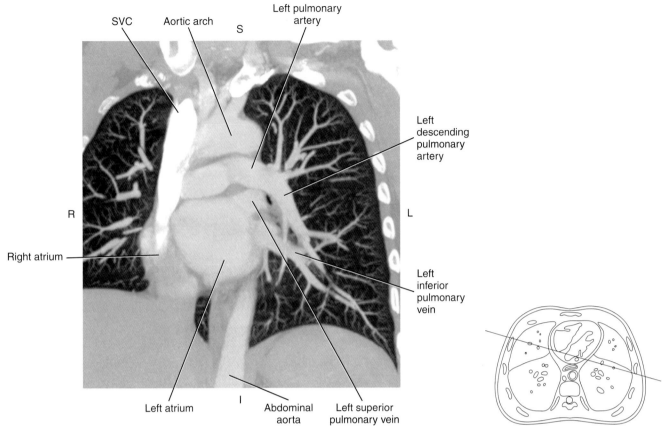

FIGURE 6.81 Coronal oblique CT reformat of left pulmonary vessels.

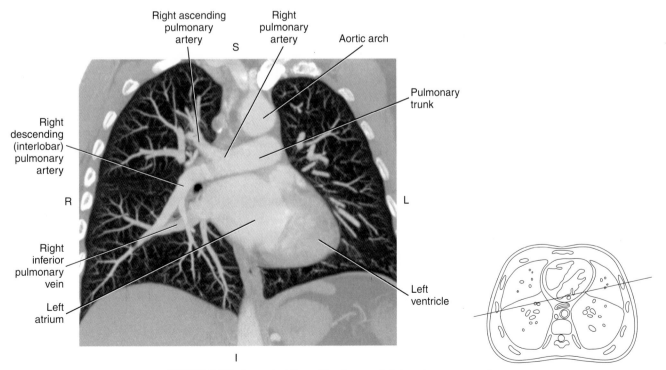

FIGURE 6.82 Coronal oblique CT reformat of right pulmonary vessels.

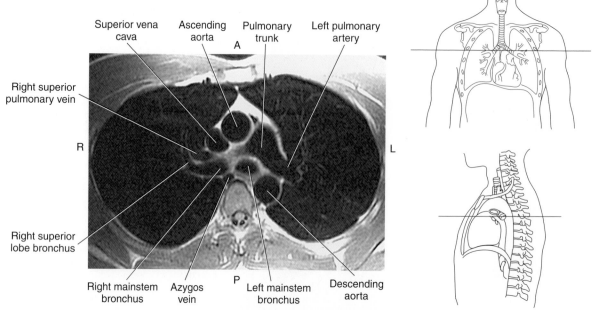

FIGURE 6.83 Axial, T1-weighted MRI of chest with right superior pulmonary vein.

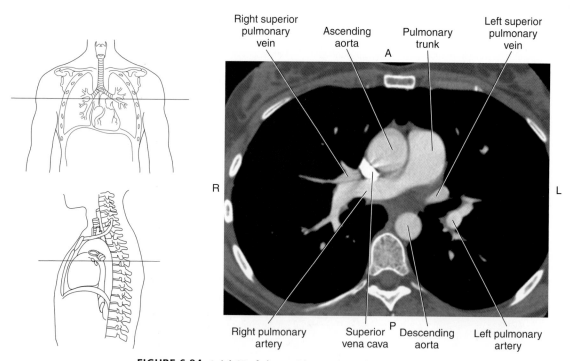

FIGURE 6.84 Axial CT of chest with superior pulmonary veins.

before entering the upper portion of the right atrium (see Figures 6.67 through 6.73). The **inferior vena cava** is formed by the junction of the common iliac veins in the pelvis and ascends the abdomen to the right of the abdominal aorta and anterior to the vertebral column. It passes through the caval hiatus of the diaphragm and almost immediately enters the inferior portion of the right atrium (Figures 6.93 and 6.94).

Obstruction of a pulmonary artery or one of its branches is known as a pulmonary embolism. This condition prevents blood flow to the alveoli and, if left in place for several hours, will result in permanent collapse of the alveoli. It is commonly caused by thrombosis from the lower extremities.

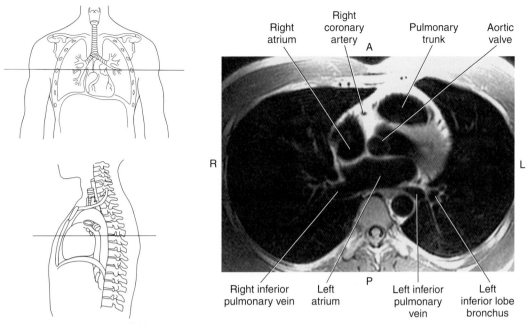

FIGURE 6.85 Axial, T1-weighted MRI of chest with inferior pulmonary veins.

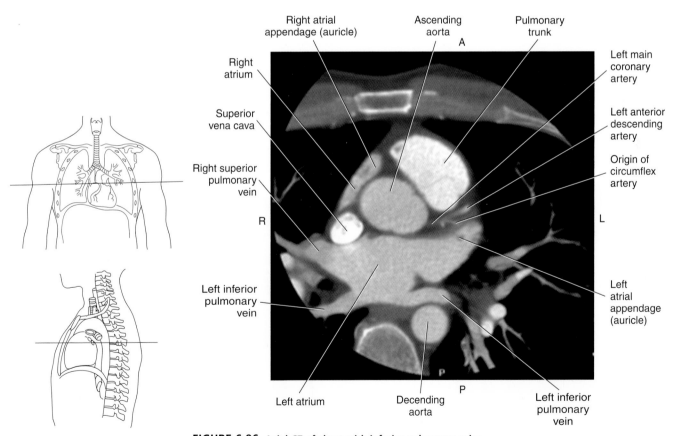

FIGURE 6.86 Axial CT of chest with inferior pulmonary veins.

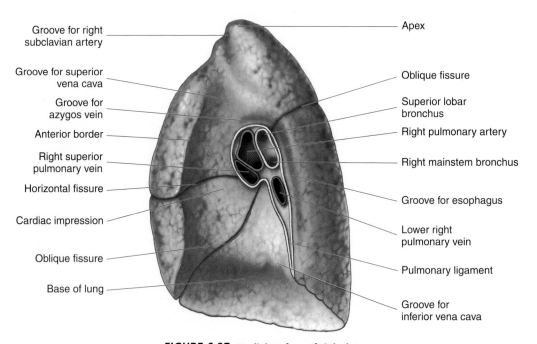

Groove for right subclavian artery

Groove for superior vena cava

Groove for azygos vein

Anterior border

Right superior pulmonary vein

Horizontal fissure

Cardiac impression

Oblique fissure

Base of lung

Apex

Oblique fissure

Superior lobar bronchus

Right pulmonary artery

Right mainstem bronchus

Groove for esophagus

Lower right pulmonary vein

Pulmonary ligament

Groove for inferior vena cava

FIGURE 6.87 Medial surface of right lung.

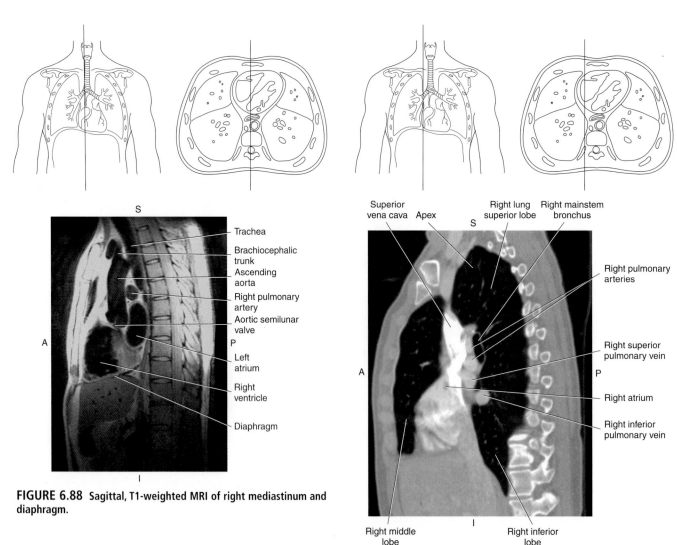

Trachea

Brachiocephalic trunk

Ascending aorta

Right pulmonary artery

Aortic semilunar valve

Left atrium

Right ventricle

Diaphragm

FIGURE 6.88 Sagittal, T1-weighted MRI of right mediastinum and diaphragm.

Superior vena cava   Apex

Right lung superior lobe

Right mainstem bronchus

Right pulmonary arteries

Right superior pulmonary vein

Right atrium

Right inferior pulmonary vein

Right middle lobe

Right inferior lobe

FIGURE 6.89 Sagittal CT reformat of right mediastinum and pulmonary vessels.

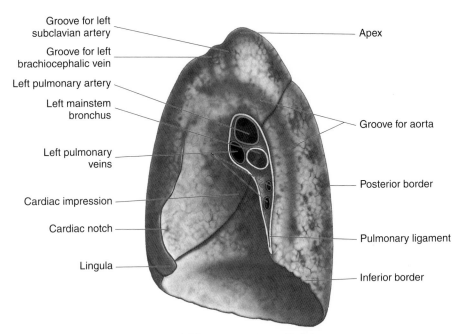

Groove for left subclavian artery
Groove for left brachiocephalic vein
Left pulmonary artery
Left mainstem bronchus
Left pulmonary veins
Cardiac impression
Cardiac notch
Lingula
Apex
Groove for aorta
Posterior border
Pulmonary ligament
Inferior border

FIGURE 6.90 Medial surface of left lung.

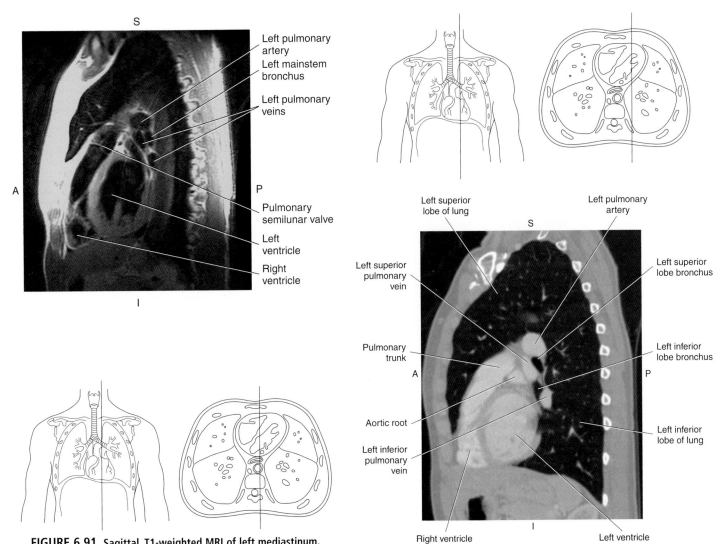

S

Left pulmonary artery
Left mainstem bronchus
Left pulmonary veins
Pulmonary semilunar valve
Left ventricle
Right ventricle

A   P

I

FIGURE 6.91 Sagittal, T1-weighted MRI of left mediastinum.

Left superior lobe of lung
Left pulmonary artery
Left superior pulmonary vein
Left superior lobe bronchus
Pulmonary trunk
Left inferior lobe bronchus
Aortic root
Left inferior pulmonary vein
Left inferior lobe of lung
Right ventricle
Left ventricle

S

A   P

I

FIGURE 6.92 Sagittal CT reformat of left mediastinum and pulmonary vessels.

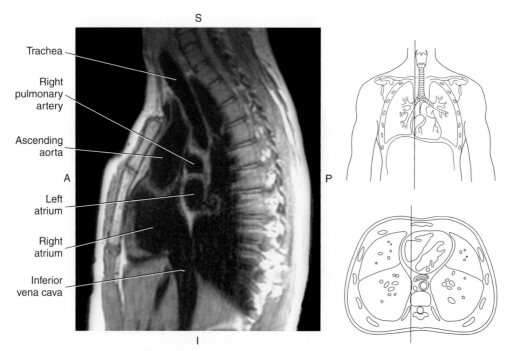

FIGURE 6.93 Sagittal, T1-weighted MRI of inferior vena cava.

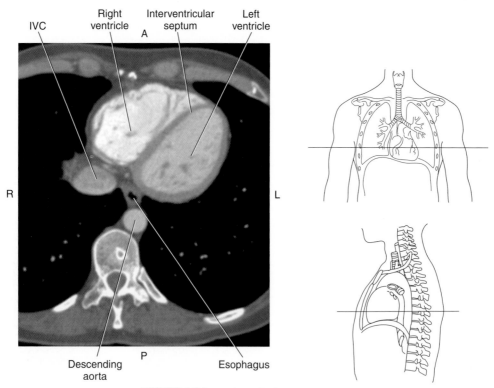

FIGURE 6.94 Axial CT of inferior vena cava.

Circulation of Blood through the Heart

Deoxygenated blood is brought to the right atrium from the peripheral tissues by the inferior and superior vena cavae. The right atrium contracts, forcing blood through the tricuspid (right atrioventricular) valve into the right ventricle. The right ventricle pumps blood through the pulmonary semilunar valve to the pulmonary arteries, which enter into the lungs. Oxygenated blood returns to the heart via the pulmonary veins, which enter the left atrium. The left atrium forces blood through the bicuspid (mitral) valve into the left ventricle, where it is then pumped through the aortic semilunar valve to the aorta (Figure 6.62).

Branches of the Aortic Arch

The three main branches of the aortic arch are the brachiocephalic trunk, left common carotid artery, and left subclavian artery (Figure 6.95). The **brachiocephalic (innominate) trunk** is the first major vessel and the largest branch arising from the aortic arch. It ascends obliquely to the upper border of the right sternoclavicular joint, where it divides into the right common carotid and right subclavian arteries (Figures 6.96 and 6.97). The **right common carotid artery** ascends the neck lateral to the trachea to the level of C4, where it divides into the right external and internal carotid arteries. The **right subclavian artery** curves posterior to the clavicle into the axillary region, where it becomes the right **axillary artery**. The **left common carotid artery** is the second vessel to branch from the aortic arch. It arises just behind the left sternoclavicular joint and ascends into the neck along the left side of the trachea to the level of C4, where it bifurcates into the left external and internal carotid arteries. The **left subclavian artery** arises from the aortic arch posterior to the left common carotid artery and arches laterally toward the axilla in a manner similar to that of the right subclavian artery, where it continues as the left axillary artery (Figures 6.95 through 6.102). The common carotid arteries supply blood to the head and neck, whereas the subclavian arteries supply blood to the upper extremities. The right and left **internal thoracic arteries** (internal mammary arteries) arise from the respective subclavian artery at the base of the neck. They run deep to the ribs, just lateral to the sternum, to supply blood to the anterior portion of the thorax (Figures 5.82, 6.97, 6.99, and 6.100).

The internal thoracic arteries create an important anastomotic pathway between the subclavian artery and external iliac vessels in the event that the descending aorta is blocked.

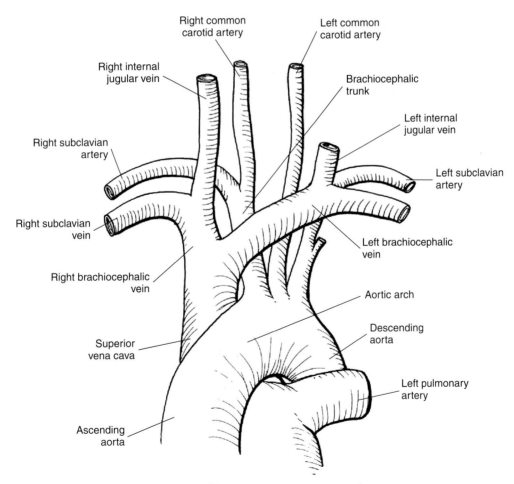

FIGURE 6.95 Anterior view of great vessels.

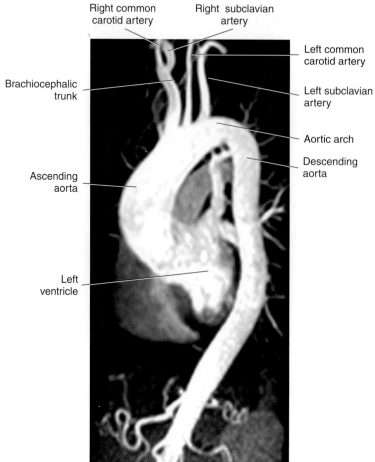

Right common
carotid artery

Right subclavian
artery

Left common
carotid artery

Brachiocephalic
trunk

Left subclavian
artery

Aortic arch

Descending
aorta

Ascending
aorta

Left
ventricle

FIGURE 6.96 MRA of aorta.

Right
common
carotid
artery

S

Left
vertebral
artery

Right
subclavian
artery

FIGURE 6.97 3D CT of aortic arch.

Internal
thoracic
artery

Left
subclavian
artery

Descending
aorta

Right
brachiocephalic
trunk

Left
common
carotid
artery

I

Aortic
arch

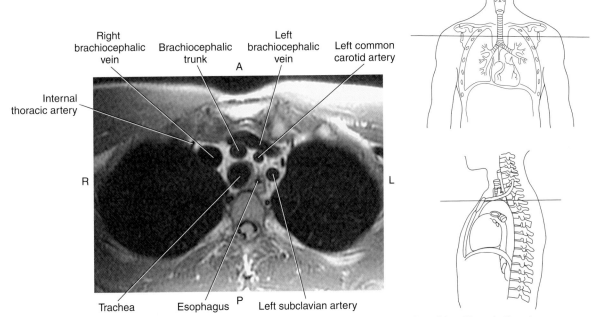

FIGURE 6.98 Axial, T1-weighted MRI of chest with branches of aortic arch and brachiocephalic veins.

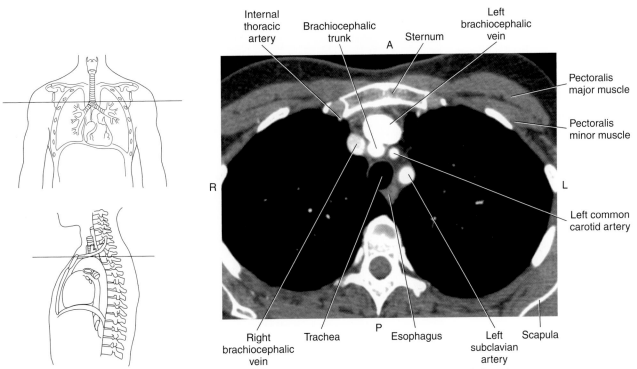

FIGURE 6.99 Axial CT of chest with branches of aortic arch and brachiocephalic veins.

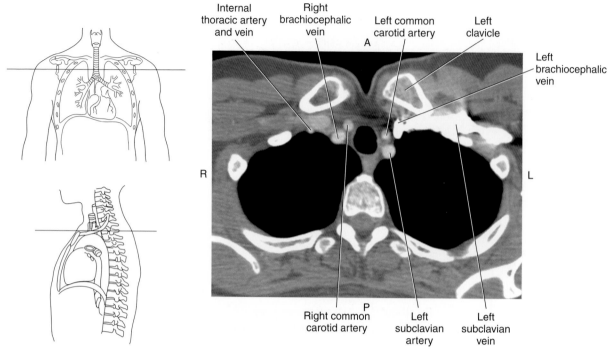

FIGURE 6.100 Axial CT with left subclavian vein.

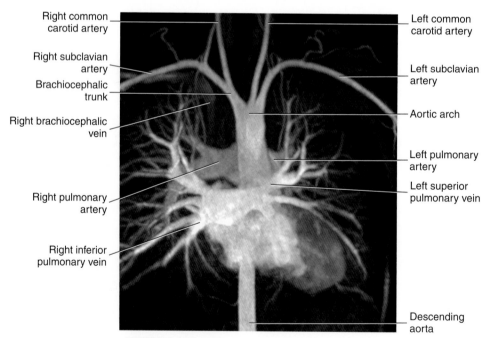

FIGURE 6.101 MRA of right brachiocephalic vein.

Tributaries of the Superior Vena Cava

The superior vena cava receives blood from the head and neck via the **internal** and **external jugular veins,** as well as from the upper extremities via the subclavian veins (see Figures 6.95, 6.101, and 6.102). The **subclavian veins** arise from the axillary veins and course posterior to the clavicles. They receive blood from the external jugular veins before uniting with the internal jugular veins behind the sternoclavicular joints, where they continue as the **brachiocephalic veins.** The left brachiocephalic vein courses across the midline, anterior to the branches of the aorta, to unite with the right brachiocephalic vein just posterior to the costal cartilage of the right first rib. The union of the two brachiocephalic veins forms the superior vena cava, which empties into the right atrium of the heart (see Figures 6.67, 6.68, 6.95, and 6.98 through 6.102).

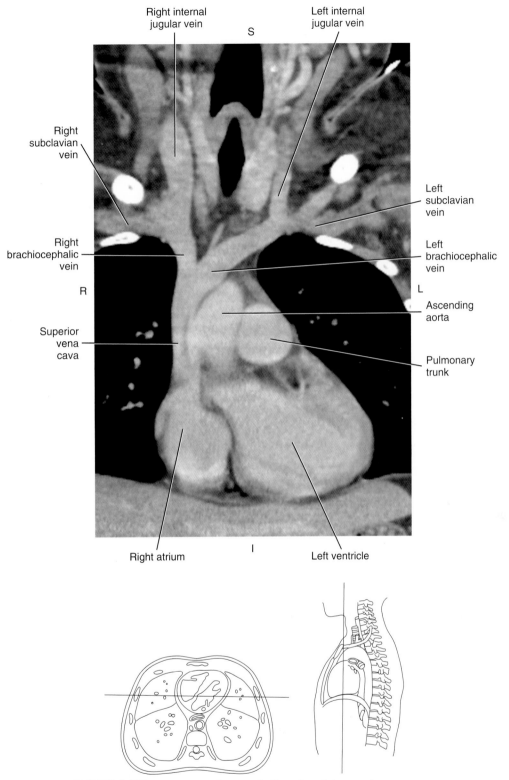

Right internal
jugular vein

Left internal
jugular vein

S

Right
subclavian
vein

Left
subclavian
vein

Right
brachiocephalic
vein

Left
brachiocephalic
vein

R

L

Ascending
aorta

Superior
vena
cava

Pulmonary
trunk

Right atrium

I

Left ventricle

FIGURE 6.102 Coronal CT reformat of tributaries of the superior vena cava.

CORONARY CIRCULATION

The cardiac muscle requires a continuous supply of oxygen and nutrients, which is supplied by **coronary circulation**. The coronary circulation consists of arteries that supply blood to the heart and cardiac veins that provide venous drainage. The vessels of the coronary circulation frequently vary in their development and distribution of blood to the heart.

Coronary Arteries

The two main coronary arteries are the first vessels to branch off the ascending aorta (Figures 6.103 and 6.104). The **right coronary artery** arises from the base or root of the aorta (right aortic sinus) and passes anteriorly between the pulmonary trunk and right atrium to descend in the coronary (atrioventricular) groove. As it reaches the diaphragmatic surface, it gives off a **right**

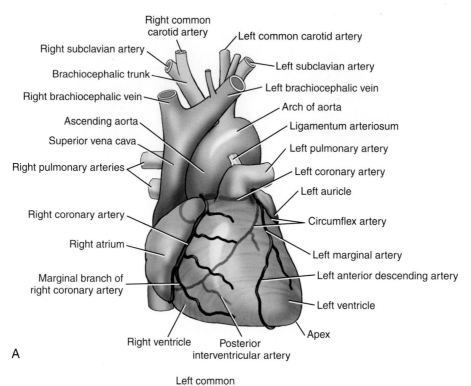

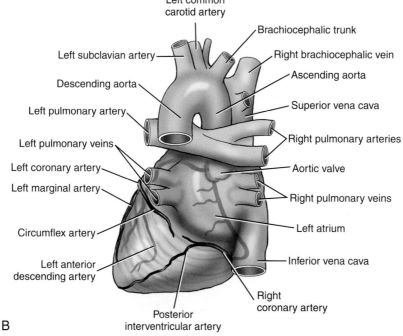

FIGURE 6.103 Heart with coronary vessels. A, Anterior view. **B,** Posterior view.

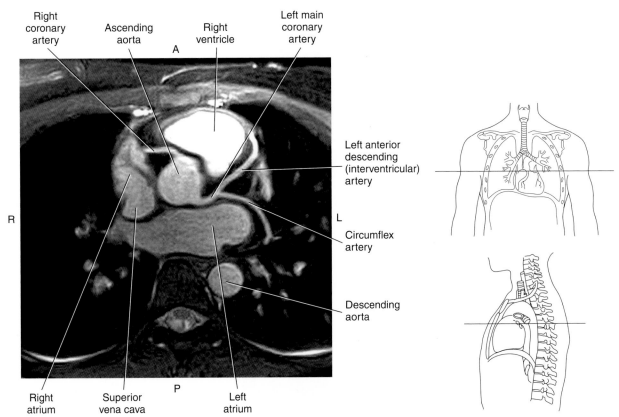

Right coronary artery — Ascending aorta — A — Right ventricle — Left main coronary artery

R

L

Left anterior descending (interventricular) artery

Circumflex artery

Descending aorta

Right atrium — Superior vena cava — P — Left atrium

FIGURE 6.104 Axial MRA of heart with right coronary artery.

marginal branch that runs toward the apex of the heart. The right coronary artery then turns to the left and enters the posterior interventricular groove, where it gives off the **posterior interventricular branch (posterior descending artery)**. The posterior interventricular branch continues to descend along the interventricular groove toward the apex, where it commonly anastomoses with the left anterior descending artery of the left coronary artery. The right coronary artery and its branches supply the right atrium, right ventricle, interventricular septum, and the sinoatrial (SA) and atrioventricular (AV) nodes. It also supplies a portion of the left atrium and ventricle (see Figures 6.104 through 6.108). The **left coronary artery** arises from the left aortic sinus and passes to the left between the pulmonary trunk and left atrium to reach the coronary groove (Figures 6.103 and 6.104). Soon after reaching the coronary groove, the left coronary

artery divides into the circumflex and left anterior descending (interventricular) arteries. The **circumflex artery** winds around the left border of the heart to the posterior surface, where it gives off the **left marginal artery**. The **left anterior descending artery (LAD)** descends in the anterior interventricular groove toward the apex of the heart, where it reaches the diaphragmatic surface to anastomose with the posterior descending artery. The left coronary artery and its branches supply the interventricular septum, including the AV bundles, and most of the left ventricle and atrium (Figures 6.105 through 6.117).

The left anterior descending artery (LAD) is also known as the "widow maker" because many men die of blockage to this artery.

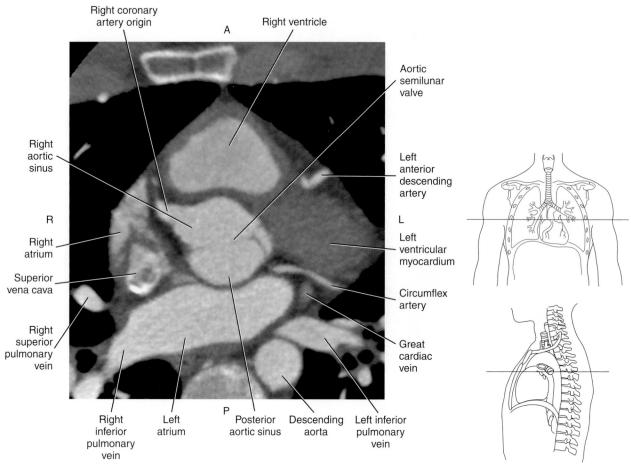

Right coronary artery origin

Right ventricle

A

Aortic semilunar valve

Right aortic sinus

R

Right atrium

Superior vena cava

Right superior pulmonary vein

Left anterior descending artery

L

Left ventricular myocardium

Circumflex artery

Great cardiac vein

Right inferior pulmonary vein

Left atrium

P

Posterior aortic sinus

Descending aorta

Left inferior pulmonary vein

FIGURE 6.105 Axial CT of heart with right coronary artery.

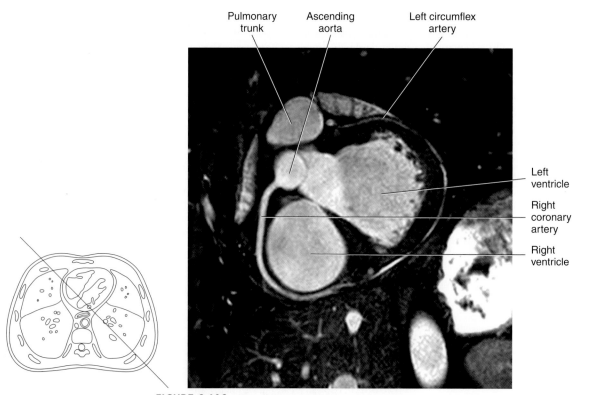

Pulmonary trunk

Ascending aorta

Left circumflex artery

Left ventricle

Right coronary artery

Right ventricle

FIGURE 6.106 MRA of heart with right coronary artery.

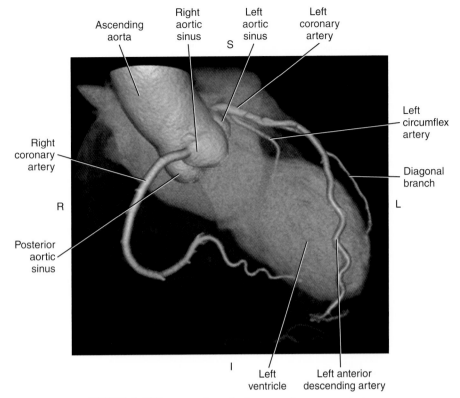

FIGURE 6.107 3D CT of aortic sinuses and coronary arteries.

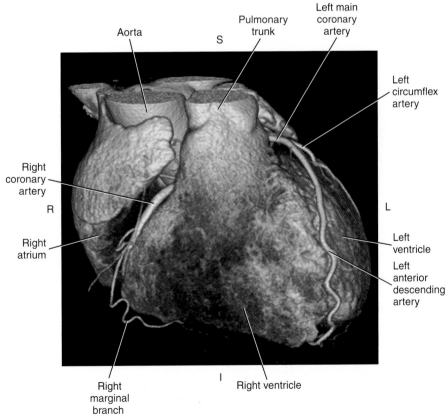

FIGURE 6.108 3D CT of right coronary artery.

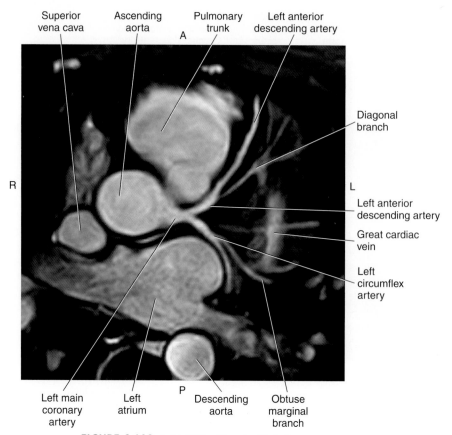

Superior vena cava

Ascending aorta

Pulmonary trunk

Left anterior descending artery

A

Diagonal branch

R

L

Left anterior descending artery

Great cardiac vein

Left circumflex artery

Left main coronary artery

Left atrium

P

Descending aorta

Obtuse marginal branch

FIGURE 6.109 Axial MRA of heart with left coronary artery.

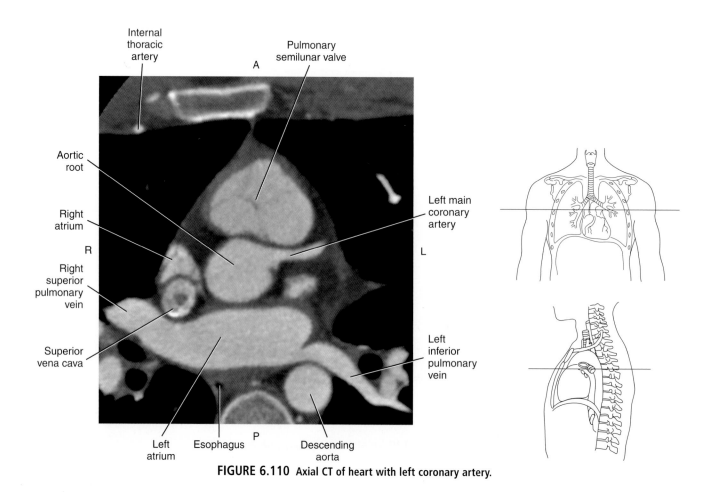

Internal thoracic artery

Pulmonary semilunar valve

A

Aortic root

Right atrium

Right superior pulmonary vein

R

Superior vena cava

Left main coronary artery

L

Left inferior pulmonary vein

Left atrium

Esophagus

P

Descending aorta

FIGURE 6.110 Axial CT of heart with left coronary artery.

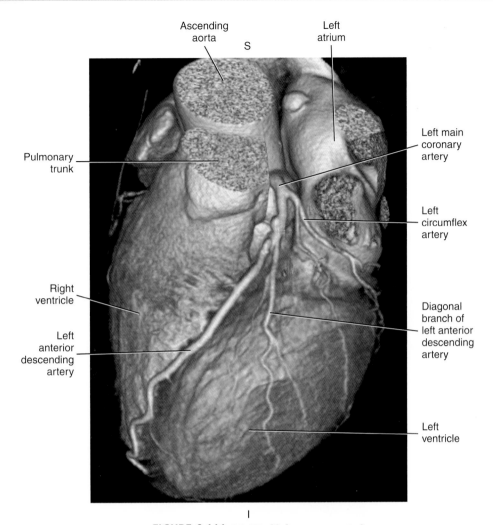

Ascending aorta

Left atrium

S

Pulmonary trunk

Left main coronary artery

Left circumflex artery

Right ventricle

Diagonal branch of left anterior descending artery

Left anterior descending artery

Left ventricle

I

FIGURE 6.111 3D CT of left coronary arteries.

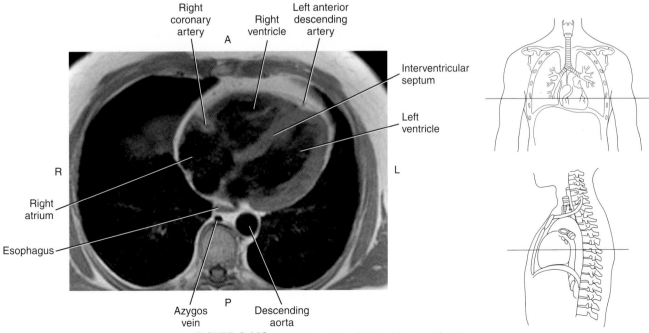

Right coronary artery

Right ventricle

Left anterior descending artery

A

Interventricular septum

Left ventricle

R

L

Right atrium

Esophagus

P

Azygos vein

Descending aorta

FIGURE 6.112 Axial, T1-weighted MRI of heart with LAD.

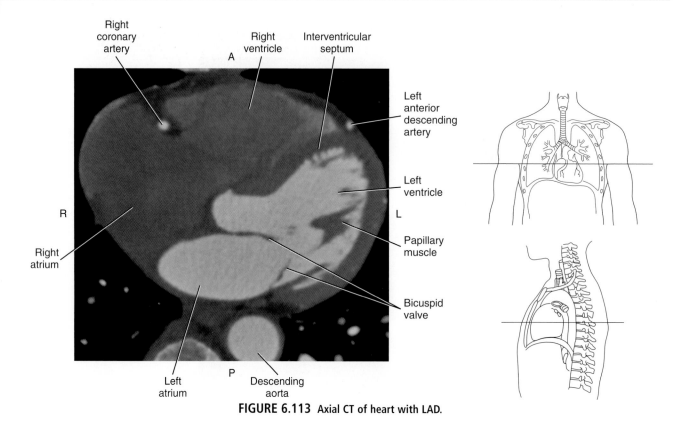

FIGURE 6.113 Axial CT of heart with LAD.

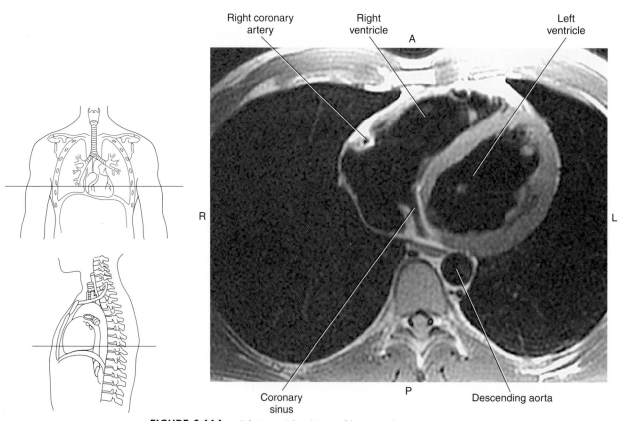

FIGURE 6.114 Axial, T1-weighted MRI of heart with coronary sinus.

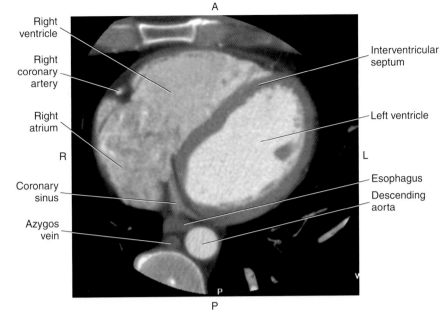

FIGURE 6.115 Axial CT of heart with coronary sinus.

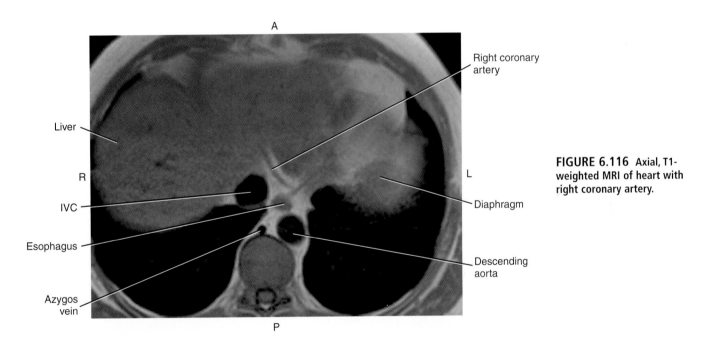

FIGURE 6.116 Axial, T1-weighted MRI of heart with right coronary artery.

FIGURE 6.117 Axial CT of heart with right coronary artery.

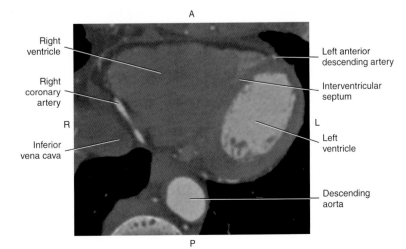

Cardiac Veins

Most of the venous return from the heart is carried by the **coronary sinus** as it runs along the posterior section of the coronary groove and terminates in the right atrium immediately to the left of the inferior vena cava. The coronary sinus is a wide venous channel situated in the posterior part of the coronary groove and is the main vein of the heart (see Figures 6.114, 6.115, 6.118, and 6.119). Its tributaries include the great, small, and middle cardiac veins, the left posterior ventricular vein, and the oblique vein of the left atrium. The **great cardiac vein**, the main tributary of the coronary sinus, arises near the apex of the heart and ascends in the anterior interventricular groove along with the anterior interventricular artery to the base of the ventricles. It receives blood from the left posterior ventricular vein and the left marginal vein before emptying into the coronary sinus. The **small (right) cardiac vein** runs in the coronary

groove between the right atrium and ventricle and joins the coronary sinus from the right side. It receives blood from the right atrium and ventricle. The **middle (posterior) cardiac vein** commences at the apex of the heart and ascends along the posterior interventricular groove to the base of the heart, where it drains into the coronary sinus near the drainage site of the small cardiac vein. It receives blood from the posterior surface of both ventricles. The **left posterior ventricular vein** carries blood from the posterior wall of the left ventricle as it runs along the diaphragmatic surface of the left ventricle to drain into either the great cardiac vein or the coronary sinus (Figure 6.119). The **oblique vein of the left atrium**, a small vessel, descends obliquely over the posterior wall of the left atrium and enters the left end of the coronary sinus. Two small **anterior cardiac veins** drain directly into the right atrium (Figure 6.118).

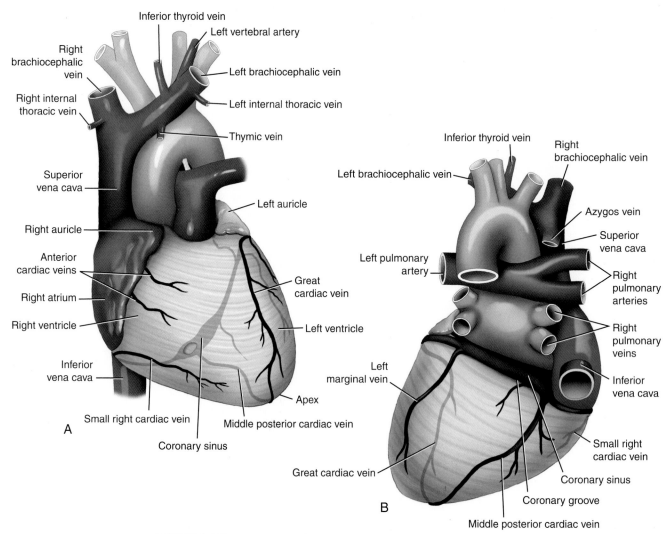

FIGURE 6.118 Heart with cardiac veins. A, Anterior view. **B,** Posterior view.

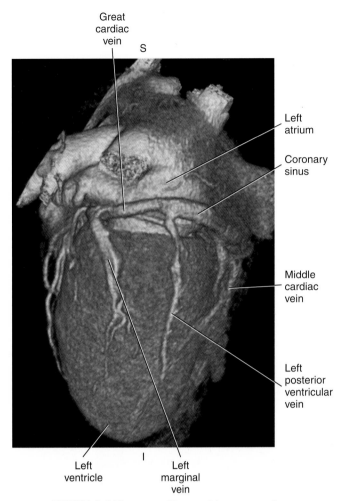

FIGURE 6.119 3D CT of heart with coronary sinus.

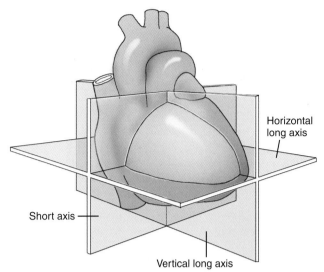

FIGURE 6.120 Off-axis planes (views) of heart.

OFF-AXIS CARDIAC IMAGING

In an effort to standardize nomenclature for tomographic imaging of the heart, the American Heart Association published a statement recommending that all cardiac imaging modalities use the same nomenclature for defining tomographic imaging planes. Their recommendation stated that "all cardiac imaging modalities should define, orient, and display the heart using the long axis of the left ventricle and selected planes oriented at 90-degree angles relative to the long axis." Their second recommendation stated, "The names for the 90-degree–oriented cardiac planes used in all imaging modalities should be vertical long axis, horizontal long axis and short axis. These correspond to the short-axis, apical two-chamber, and apical four-chamber planes traditionally used in 2D

echocardiography" (Figure 6.120). We will follow these recommendations for labeling cardiac images throughout this text. In off-axis cardiac imaging, each successive acquisition provides the landmarks for planning the next acquisition (view) and provides a logical method to obtain 90-degree viewing of the heart according to its intrinsic short and long axes. Several different methods can be used to obtain views of the cardiac planes during an examination, of which we provide an example of one method. To obtain the **vertical long axis (VLA)** view, an oblique coronal image can be positioned parallel to the interventricular septum, directly through the left atrium and ventricle (Figures 6.121 through 6.123). This plane closely approximates the right anterior oblique projection used in cineangiography and the two-chamber view used in echocardiography. The **horizontal long axis (HLA)** view can be obtained by angling an oblique coronal image to bisect the left ventricle, bicuspid valve, and left atrium (Figures 6.124 through 6.126). The HLA view demonstrates the four cardiac chambers and is comparable with the four-chamber plane used in echocardiography. The **short axis (SA)** view can be obtained by using the HLA image to prescribe an oblique plane through the right and left ventricles, oriented perpendicular to the interventricular septum (Figures 6.127 through 6.133). The right and left ventricles both have areas called the inlet and outlet depending on the flow of blood throughout the chamber. The inlets represent the flow of blood between the atria and the ventricles, while the outlets

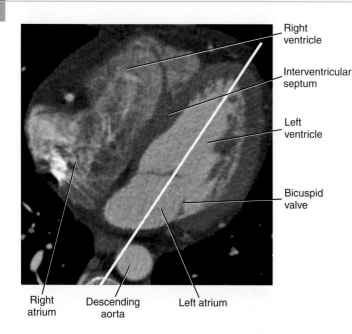

Right ventricle

Interventricular septum

Left ventricle

Bicuspid valve

Right atrium

Descending aorta

Left atrium

FIGURE 6.121 Axial CT of heart for planning vertical long axis images.

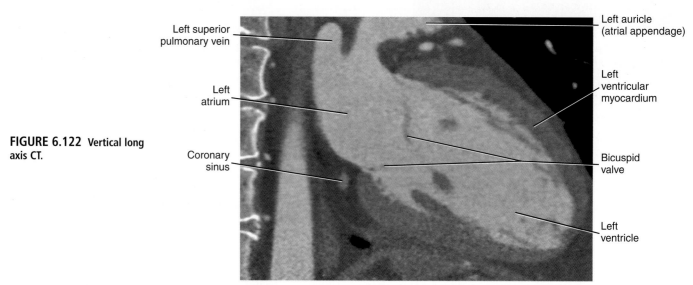

Left superior pulmonary vein

Left atrium

Coronary sinus

Left auricle (atrial appendage)

Left ventricular myocardium

Bicuspid valve

Left ventricle

FIGURE 6.122 Vertical long axis CT.

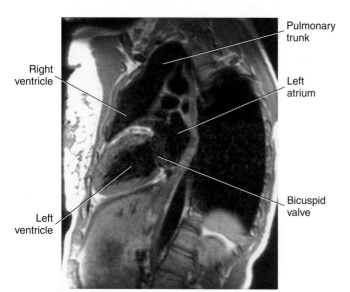

Pulmonary trunk

Left atrium

Right ventricle

Left ventricle

Bicuspid valve

FIGURE 6.123 Vertical long axis MRI.

Left atrium

S

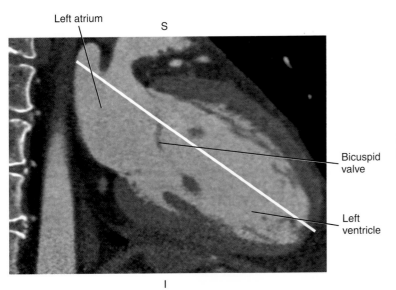

Bicuspid valve

Left ventricle

I

FIGURE 6.124 Vertical long axis CT of heart for planning horizontal long axis images.

Right ventricle

Interventricular septum

Right coronary artery

Right atrium

Left anterior descending artery

Left ventricle

Left atrium

Bicuspid valve

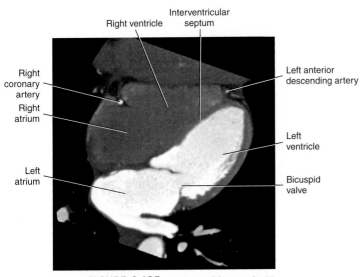

FIGURE 6.125 Horizontal long axis CT.

Right ventricle

Left ventricle

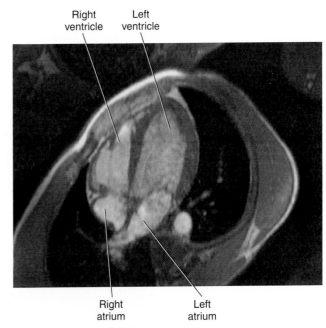

Right atrium

Left atrium

FIGURE 6.126 Horizontal long axis MRI.

Interventricular septum

Right ventricle

Right coronary artery

Right atrium

Left anterior descending artery

Left ventricle

Left atrium

Bicuspid valve

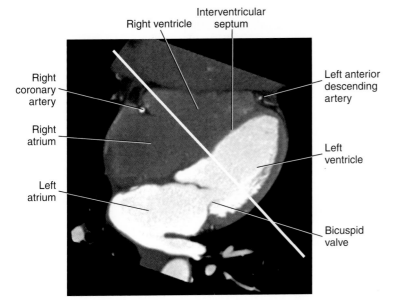

FIGURE 6.127 Horizontal long axis CT of heart for planning short axis images.

represent the flow of blood between the ventricles and the pulmonary and systemic circulations. The inlet of the right ventricle includes the tricuspid valve, and the outlet contains the pulmonary semilunar valve. The **right ventricular outflow tract (RVOT)** is used to visualize the pulmonary semilunar valve and differentiate the left ventricle from the pulmonary artery (Figures 6.134 through 6.136). The inlet of the left ventricle involves the bicuspid valve, and the outlet includes the aortic semilunar valve. Typically, the **left ventricular outflow tract (LVOT)** defines the view that provides visualization of both bicuspid and aortic semilunar valves, as well as the left atrium, left ventricle, and ascending aorta (Figures 6.137 through 6.139).

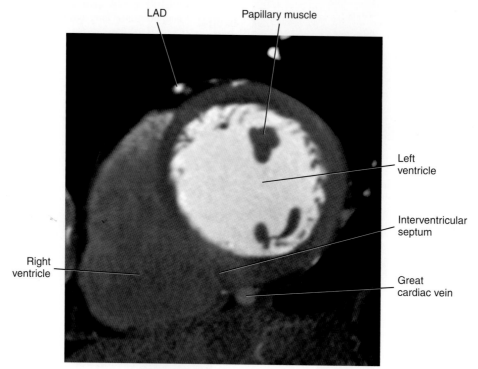

FIGURE 6.128 Short axis CT with ventricles.

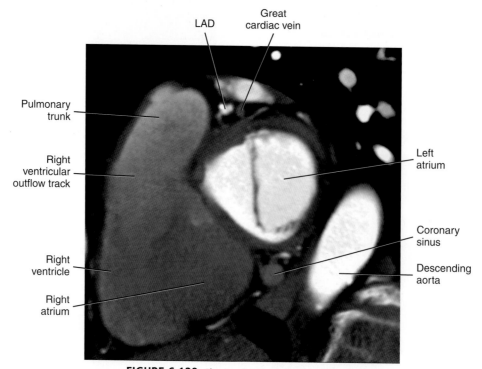

FIGURE 6.129 Short axis CT with pulmonary trunk.

S

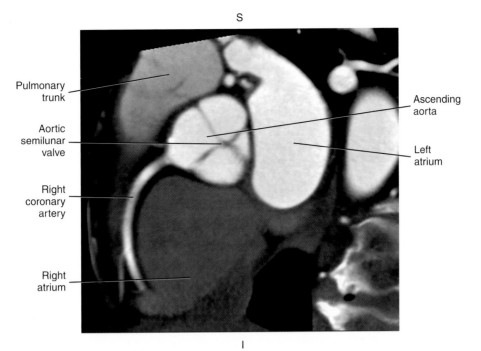

Pulmonary
trunk

Aortic
semilunar
valve

Right
coronary
artery

Right
atrium

Ascending
aorta

Left
atrium

I

FIGURE 6.130 Short axis CT with left atrium.

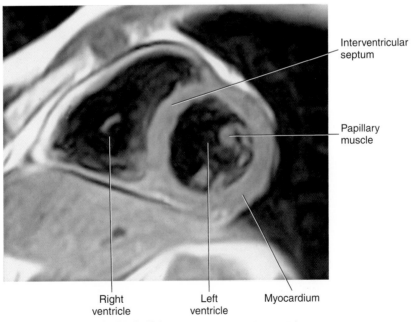

Interventricular
septum

Papillary
muscle

Right
ventricle

Left
ventricle

Myocardium

FIGURE 6.131 Short axis MRI with ventricles.

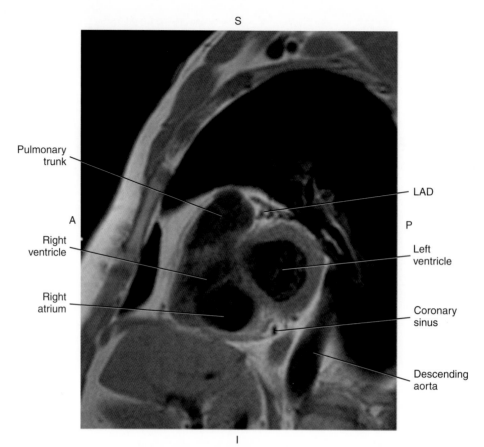

S

Pulmonary
trunk

LAD

A

P

Right
ventricle

Left
ventricle

Right
atrium

Coronary
sinus

Descending
aorta

I

FIGURE 6.132 Short axis MRI with pulmonary trunk.

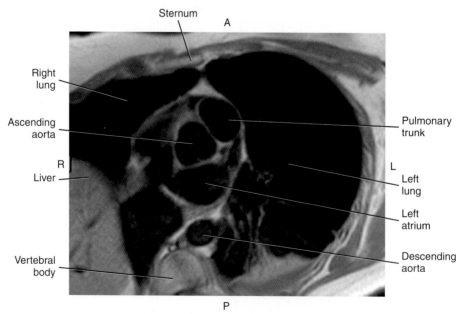

Sternum

A

Right
lung

Ascending
aorta

Pulmonary
trunk

R

L

Liver

Left
lung

Left
atrium

Vertebral
body

Descending
aorta

P

FIGURE 6.133 Short axis MRI with left atrium.

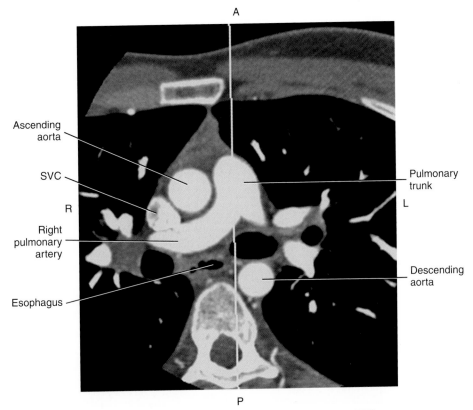

FIGURE 6.134   Axial CT of pulmonary trunk for planning RVOT images.

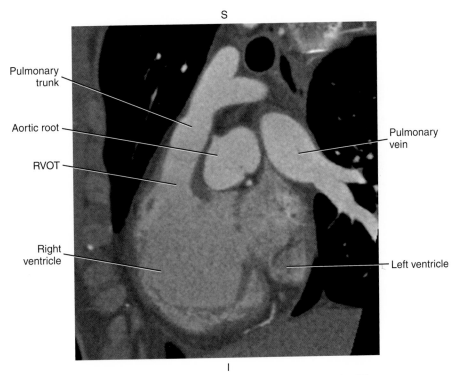

FIGURE 6.135   CT of right ventricular outflow tract (RVOT).

S

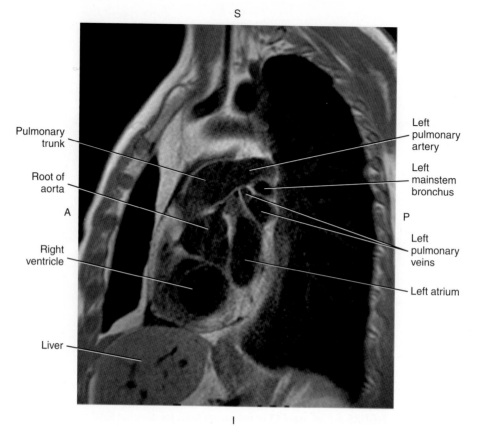

Pulmonary trunk

Root of aorta

A

Right ventricle

Liver

Left pulmonary artery

Left mainstem bronchus

P

Left pulmonary veins

Left atrium

I

FIGURE 6.136 MRI of right ventricular outflow tract (RVOT).

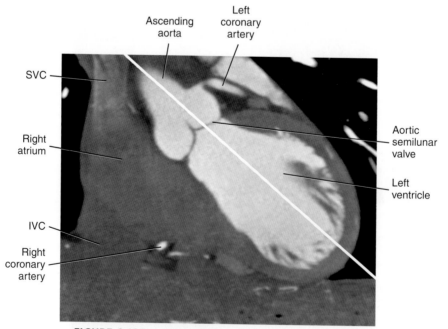

Ascending aorta

Left coronary artery

SVC

Right atrium

IVC

Right coronary artery

Aortic semilunar valve

Left ventricle

FIGURE 6.137 Coronal CT of heart for planning LVOT images.

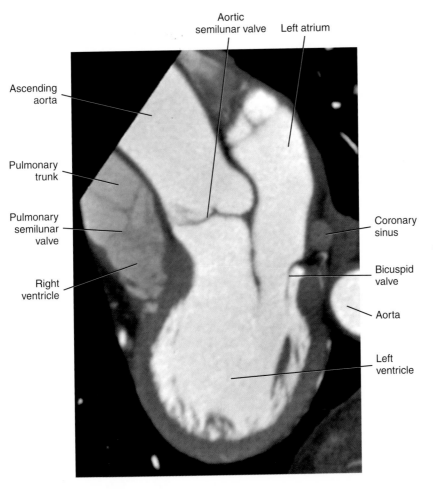

Aortic
semilunar valve

Left atrium

Ascending
aorta

Pulmonary
trunk

Pulmonary
semilunar
valve

Right
ventricle

Coronary
sinus

Bicuspid
valve

Aorta

Left
ventricle

FIGURE 6.138 CT of left ventricular outflow tract.

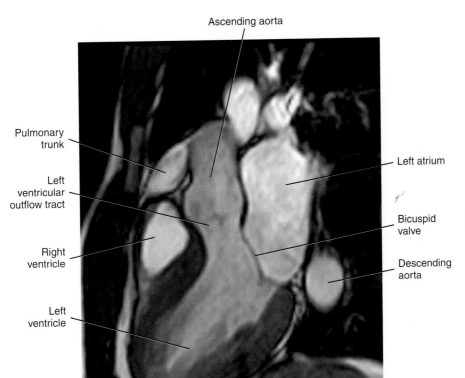

Ascending aorta

Pulmonary
trunk

Left
ventricular
outflow tract

Right
ventricle

Left
ventricle

Left atrium

Bicuspid
valve

Descending
aorta

FIGURE 6.139 MRI of left ventricular outflow tract.

AZYGOS VENOUS SYSTEM

The azygos venous system, which provides collateral circulation between the inferior and superior venae cavae, can be divided into the **azygos** and **hemiazygos veins** (Figure 6.140). Together, they drain blood from most of the posterior thoracic wall and from the bronchi, pericardium, and esophagus. The azygos vein ascends along the right side of the vertebral column, whereas the hemiazygos vein ascends along the left side. The hemiazygos vein crosses to the right behind the aorta to join the azygos vein at approximately T7-T9. The azygos vein then arches over the hilum of the right lung to empty into the posterior superior vena cava (Figures 6.141 through 6.144).

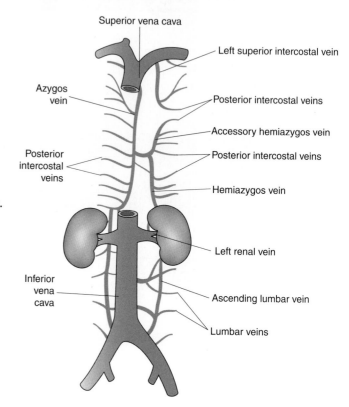

FIGURE 6.140 Anterior view of azygos venous system.

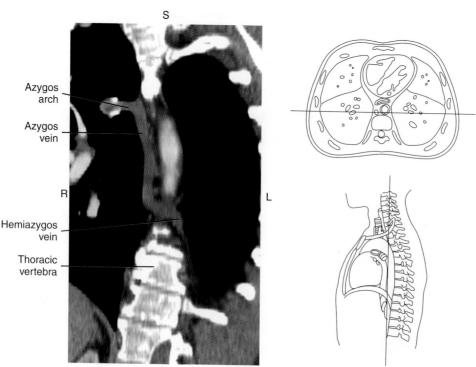

FIGURE 6.141 Coronal CT reformat of azygos vein.

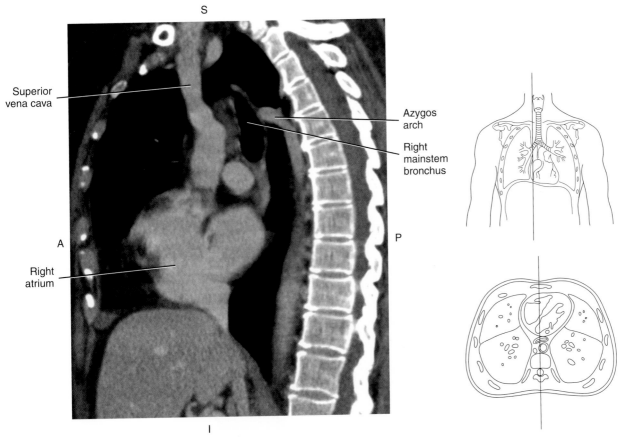

FIGURE 6.142 Sagittal CT reformat of azygos arch.

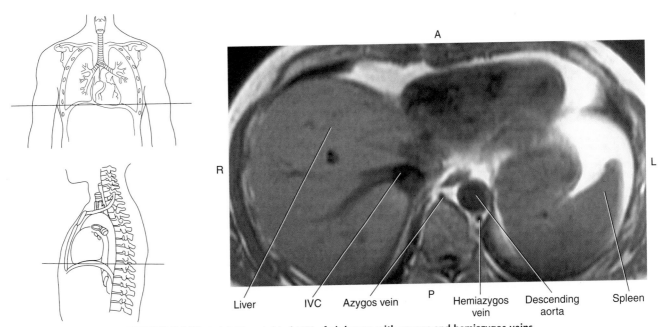

FIGURE 6.143 Axial, T1-weighted MRI of abdomen with azygos and hemiazygos veins.

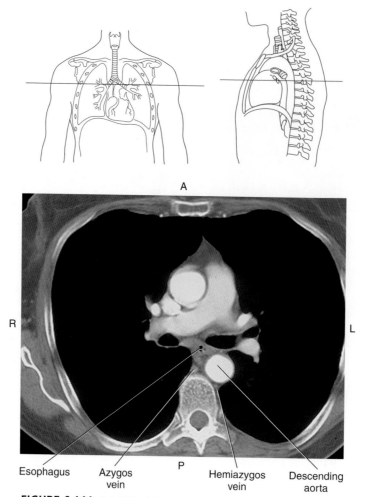

FIGURE 6.144 Axial CT of chest with azygos and hemiazygos veins.

TABLE 6.5	Muscles of the Thorax		
Muscle	**Origin**	**Insertion**	**Action**
Intercostal	Inferior border of ribs	Superior border of ribs below	Fixes intercostal spaces during respiration and aids forced inspiration by elevating ribs
Serratus posterior superior	Spinous processes and supraspinous ligaments of C7-T2	Posterior aspect of 2nd-5th ribs	Assists forced inspiration
Serratus posterior inferior	Spinous processes and supraspinous ligaments of T11-L2	Posterior aspect of 9th-12th	Assists in forced expiration
Levatores costarum	Transverse processes of C-7 and T1-T11	Rib between tubercle and angle	Elevate the ribs
Diaphragm	Xiphoid process, costal margin, fascia over the quadratus lumborum, and psoas major muscles. Vertebral bodies L1-L3	Central tendon of the diaphragm	Pushes the abdominal viscera inferiorly, increasing the volume of the thoracic cavity for inspiration

MUSCLES

Muscles Associated with Respiration

Muscles associated with respiration are the intercostal, serratus posterior superior, serratus posterior inferior, levatores costarum, and the diaphragm (Table 6.5). The spaces between the ribs, or the intercostal spaces, are filled with three layers of **intercostal muscles (external, internal, and innermost layer)** (Figures 6.145 through 6.147). These muscles act together to elevate the ribs and expand the thoracic cavity, as well as keep the intercostal spaces somewhat rigid. The **serratus posterior superior muscle** spans from C7-T2 to ribs 2 to 5 and acts to assist forced inspiration, whereas the **serratus posterior inferior muscle** spans from T11-L2 to ribs 9 to 12 and acts

to assist forced expiration (Figures 6.148 through 6.150). The **levatores costarum muscles** arise from the transverse processes of C7 and T1-T11. They extend obliquely to insert on the rib below, between the tubercle and angle (see Figure 6.148). The levatores costarum muscles act to elevate the ribs. The **diaphragm** is a large dome-shaped muscle that spans the entire thoracic outlet and separates the thoracic cavity from the abdominal cavity (Figure 6.151). It is the chief muscle of inspiration because it enlarges the thoracic cavity vertically as the domes move inferiorly and flatten. The muscle fibers of the diaphragm converge to be inserted into a **central tendon**, which is situated near the center of the diaphragm immediately below the pericardium, with which it is partially blended. The diaphragm is attached to the lumbar spine via two

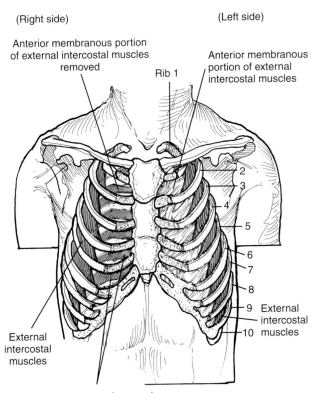

(Right side)   (Left side)

Anterior membranous portion of external intercostal muscles removed

Anterior membranous portion of external intercostal muscles

Rib 1

External intercostal muscles

Muscle fibers of external intercostal muscles in region of vertebral column (posteriorly)

External intercostal muscles

FIGURE 6.145 Anterior view of intercostal muscles.

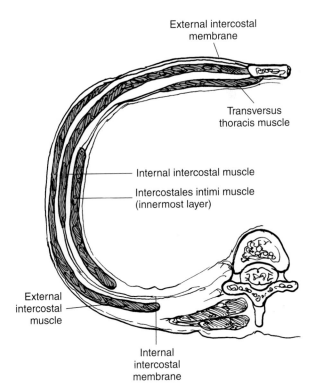

External intercostal membrane

Transversus thoracis muscle

Internal intercostal muscle

Intercostales intimi muscle (innermost layer)

External intercostal muscle

Internal intercostal membrane

FIGURE 6.146 Axial view of intercostal muscles.

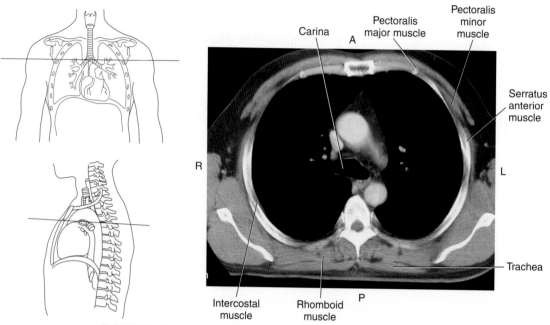

FIGURE 6.147 Axial CT of chest at level of carina with thoracic muscles.

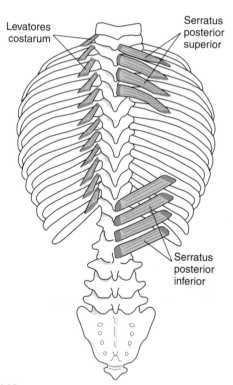

FIGURE 6.148 Posterior view of chest with posterior serratus muscles.

tendinous structures termed **crura** (see Figures 6.151 through 6.155). The right crus arises from the anterior surfaces of L1-L3, whereas the left crus arises from the corresponding parts of L1-L2 only. The left and right crura join together across the ventral aspect of the abdominal aorta to form the medial arcuate ligament. Three major openings, or hiatuses, of the diaphragm allow for the passage of vessels and organs from the thorax to the abdomen. The **aortic hiatus** allows for the passage of the descending aorta, azygos vein, and thoracic duct. The **caval hiatus** allows for the passage of the inferior vena cava and the right phrenic nerve (see Figures 6.151 and 6.152). The **esophageal hiatus** allows for the passage of the esophagus and the vagus nerve.

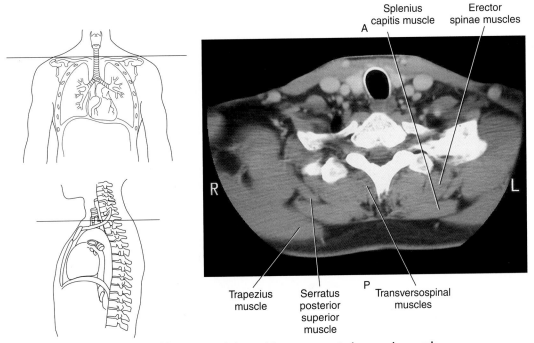

FIGURE 6.149 Axial CT of chest with serratus posterior superior muscle.

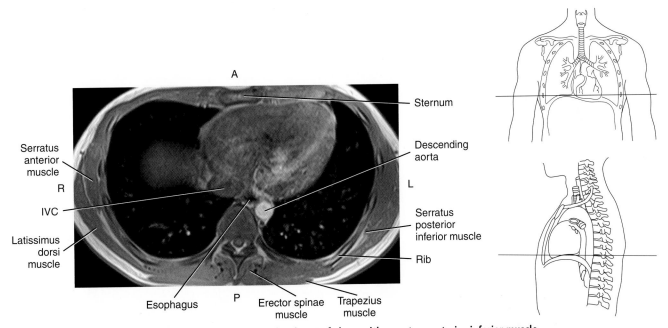

FIGURE 6.150 Axial, T1-weighted MRI of chest with serratus posterior inferior muscle.

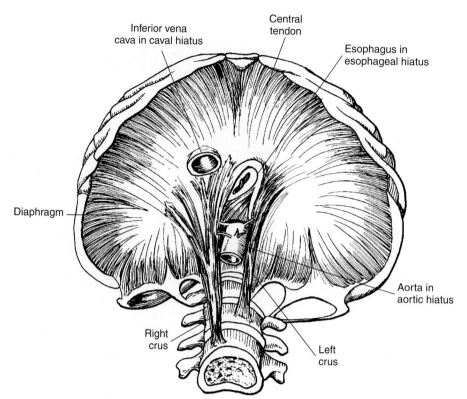

FIGURE 6.151 Inferior view of diaphragm.

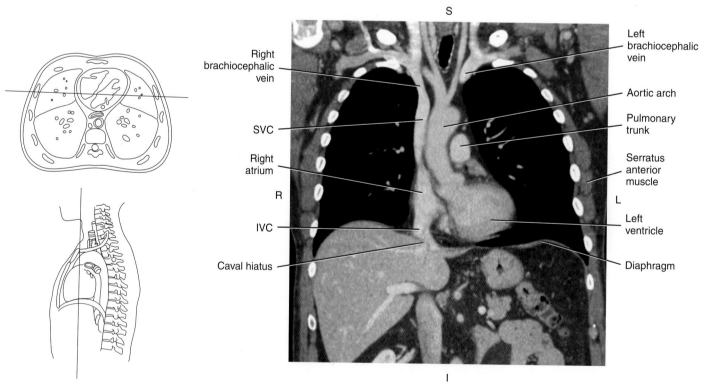

FIGURE 6.152 Coronal CT reformat of serratus anterior muscle.

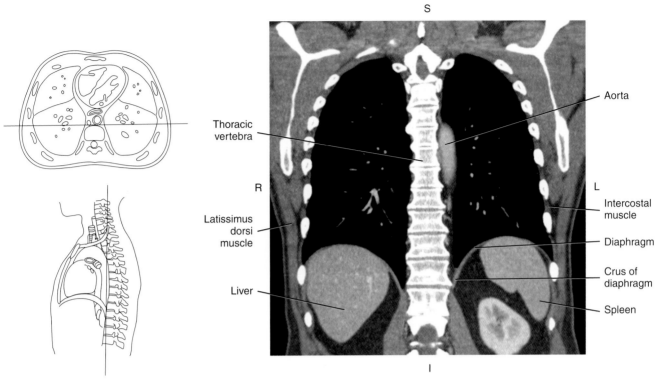

S

Thoracic
vertebra

Aorta

R

L

Latissimus
dorsi
muscle

Intercostal
muscle

Diaphragm

Crus of
diaphragm

Liver

Spleen

I

FIGURE 6.153 Coronal CT reformat of diaphragm.

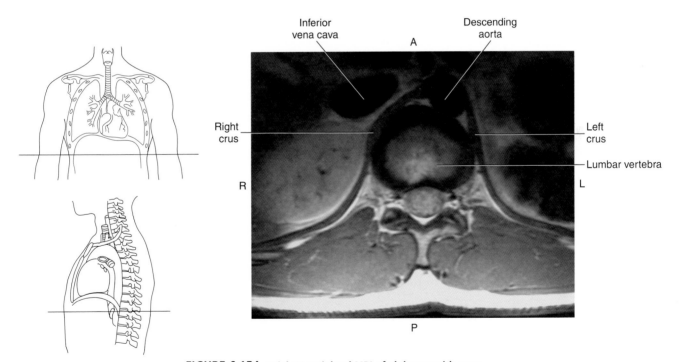

Inferior
vena cava

Descending
aorta

A

Right
crus

Left
crus

Lumbar vertebra

R

L

P

FIGURE 6.154 Axial, T1-weighted MRI of abdomen with crura.

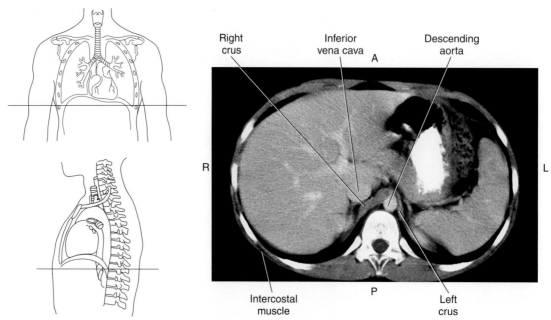

FIGURE 6.155 Axial CT of chest with crura.

Muscles Connecting the Upper Extremity to the Anterior and Lateral Thoracic Walls

Muscles of the anterior and lateral thoracic region are pectoralis major, pectoralis minor, subclavius, and serratus anterior. Muscles associated with the movement of the upper extremity, such as the pectoralis, subclavius, and serratus anterior, can also function as accessory muscles for respiration (Figure 6.156 and Table 6.6). For example, the **pectoralis muscles (major and minor)**, located on the anterior surface of the chest, primarily aid in the movement of the upper limb, but the pectoralis major muscle can also act to expand the thoracic cavity on deep inspiration (Figures 6.147 and 6.156). The **subclavius**, a small triangular-shaped muscle located between the clavicle and first rib, acts alone to stabilize the clavicle and depress the shoulder (Figure 6.5). Conjointly with the pectoralis muscles, the subclavius muscles act to raise the ribs, drawing them upward and expanding the chest, thus becoming important agents in forced inspiration. Additionally, the **serratus anterior muscles** aid in respiration. The serratus (sawlike) anterior muscle is visualized on the lateral border of the thorax. It extends from the medial border of the scapula to the lateral surface of the first rib through eighth ribs. The primary action of the serratus anterior muscle is to laterally rotate and protract the scapula. It can, however assist in raising the ribs for inspiration (Figures 6. 152 and 6.156; see also Chapter 9).

FIGURE 6.156 Anterior view of muscles associated with thorax.

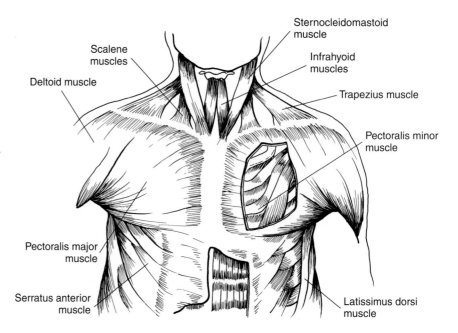

TABLE 6.6	Muscles of the Anterior and Lateral Wall of the Thorax		
Muscle	**Origin**	**Insertion**	**Action**
Pectoralis major	Clavicular head—medial half of clavicle Sternal head—lateral manubrium and sternum, six upper costal cartilages	Bicipital groove of humerus and deltoid tuberosity	Flexes, adducts, and medially rotates arm, and accessory for inspiration
Pectoralis minor	Anterior surface of 3rd-5th ribs	Coracoid process of the scapula	Elevates ribs of scapula, protracts scapula, and assists serratus anterior
Subclavius	First rib and cartilage	Inferior surface of the clavicle	Depresses the shoulder and assists pectoralis in inspiration
Serratus anterior	Angles of superior 8th or 9th ribs	Medial border of scapula	Laterally rotates and protracts scapula

BREAST

The female **breast**, or **mammary gland**, lies within the subcutaneous tissue overlying the pectoralis major muscle. Typically, the breast extends laterally from the sternum to the axilla, and inferiorly from the second to the seventh ribs. For examination purposes, the breast can be divided into **four quadrants** (upper inner, upper outer, lower outer, lower inner) and the **tail of Spence** (Figures 6.157 and 6.158). The breast consists of three layers of tissue: subcutaneous layer, mammary layer, and retromammary layer (Figure 6.158). The **subcutaneous layer** contains the skin and all of the subcutaneous fat. The **mammary layer** consists of glandular tissue, excretory (lactiferous) ducts, and connective tissues. The **glandular tissue** consists of 15 to 20 lobes arranged radially around a centrally located nipple. The glandular lobes are embedded in connective tissue and fat, which give the breast its size and shape. **Excretory (lactiferous) ducts** extend from each lobe to the nipple, where they terminate as small openings. Cords of connective tissue coursing throughout the mammary layer, from the dermis to

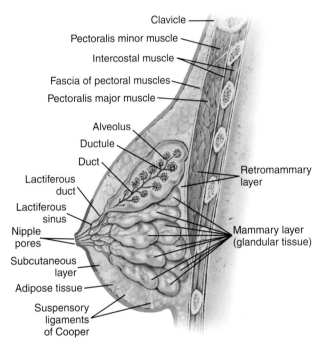

FIGURE 6.158 Sagittal view of female breast.

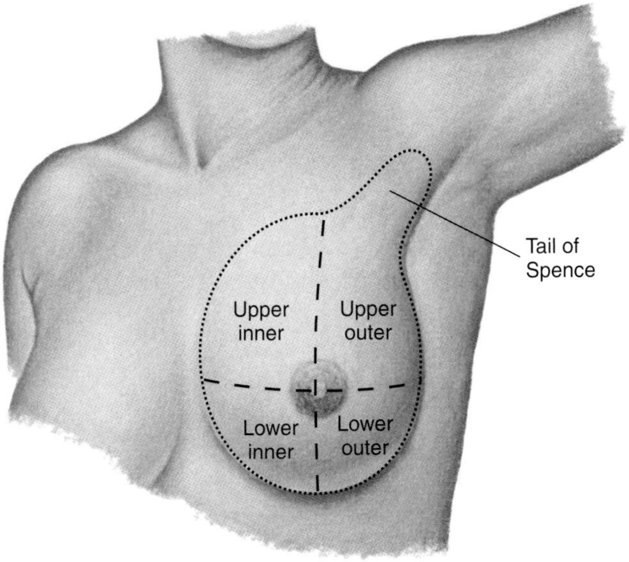

the thoracic fascia, are known as the **suspensory ligaments** of the breast or **Cooper's ligaments**. These ligaments provide support for the breasts. The **retromammary layer** contains muscle, deep connective tissue, and retromammary fat (Figures 6.159 and 6.160).

Axillary lymph nodes drain the lymphatics from the breast, arm, and integument of the back. They are frequently clustered around the axillary vessels, the lower border of the pectoralis major muscle, and the lower margin of the posterior wall.

FIGURE 6.157 Anterior view of left breast.

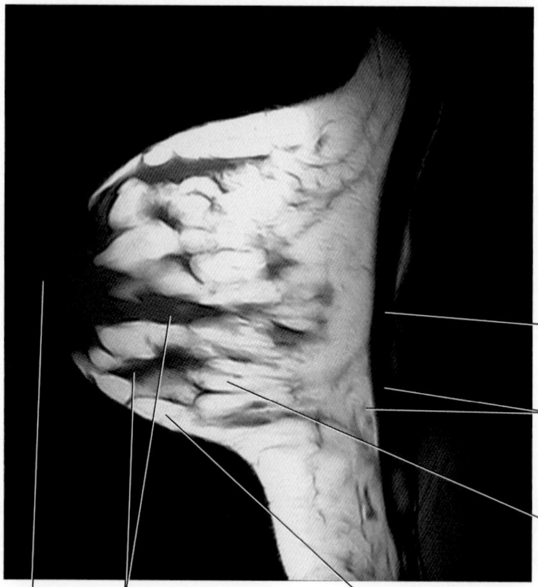

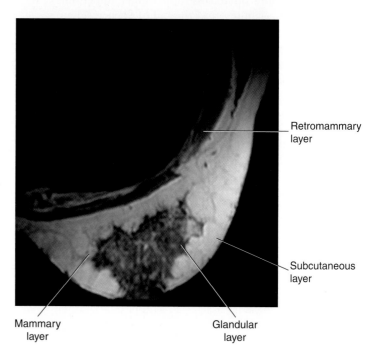

FIGURE 6.159 Sagittal, T1-weighted MRI of female breast.

S

A   P

Pectoralis major
muscle

Retromammary
layer

Mammary
layer

I

Nipple   Glandular   Subcutaneous
layer

FIGURE 6.160 Axial, T1-weighted MRI of female breast.

Retromammary
layer

Subcutaneous
layer

Mammary
layer   Glandular
layer

REFERENCES

Applegate E: *The anatomy and physiology learning system,* ed 4, Philadelphia, 2010, Saunders.

Applegate E: *The sectional anatomy learning system,* ed 3, Philadelphia, 2009, Saunders.

Frank: *Merrill's atlas of radiographic positions and radiologic procedures,* ed 12, St. Louis, 2011, Mosby.

Cerqueira MD, Weissman NJ, Dilsizian V, et al: *Standardized myocardial segmentation and nomenclature for tomographic imaging of the heart: a statement for healthcare professionals from the Cardiac Imaging Committee of the Council on Clinical Cardiology of the American Heart Association,* Circulation *105:*539, 2002.

Sandring S: *Gray's anatomy,* ed 40, Philadelphia, 2009, Churchill Livingstone.

Haaga JR, Lanzieri CF, Gilkeson RC, et al: *CT and MRI imaging of the whole body,* ed 5, Philadelphia, 2008, Mosby.

Jacob S: *Atlas of human anatomy,* Philadelphia, 2002, Churchill Livingstone.

Larsen WJ: *Anatomy: development function clinical correlations,* Philadelphia, 2002, Saunders.

Manning WJ, Pennel DJ: *Cardiovascular magnetic resonance,* ed 2, Philadelphia, 2010, Saunders.

Mosby's medical, nursing, and allied health dictionary, ed 7, St. Louis, 2006, Mosby.

Seidel HM, Ball JW, Dains JE, et al: *Mosby's guide to physical examination,* ed 7, St. Louis, 2011, Mosby.

Som PM, Curtin HD: *Head and neck imaging,* ed 5, St. Louis, 2012, Mosby.

Abdomen

A man's liver is his carburetor.

Anonymous

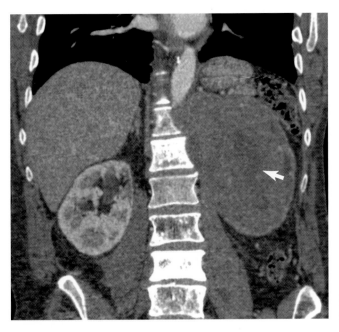

FIGURE 7.1 Coronal CT reformat of abdomen with large heterogeneous left renal mass.

The abdominal cavity houses many critical structures that have a large array of functions. It is for this reason that cross-sectional imaging of the abdomen is so essential in visualizing these various organs and body systems (Figure 7.1).

OBJECTIVES

- List the structures of the abdominal cavity and differentiate among those that are contained within the peritoneum and those that are contained within the retroperitoneum.
- Describe the peritoneal and retroperitoneal spaces.
- Describe the lobes, segments, and vasculature of the liver.
- Define the structures of the biliary system.
- State the functions and location of the pancreas and spleen.

- Identify the structures of the urinary system.
- List and identify the structures of the stomach and intestines.
- Identify the branches of the abdominal aorta and the structures they supply.
- Identify the tributaries of the inferior vena cava and the structures they drain.
- List the muscles of the abdomen and describe their functions.

OUTLINE

ABDOMINAL CAVITY

The abdominal cavity is the region located between the diaphragm and sacral promontory (Figure 7.2). The abdominal and pelvic cavities are commonly divided into four quadrants or nine distinct regions (see Chapter 1). Contents of the abdominal cavity include the liver, gallbladder and biliary system, pancreas, spleen, adrenal glands, kidneys, ureters, stomach, intestines, and vascular structures.

Peritoneum

The walls of the abdominal cavity are lined by a thin serous membrane called the **peritoneum**. This membrane is divided into two layers: the **parietal peritoneum**, which lines the abdominal walls, and the **visceral peritoneum**, which covers the organs (Figures 7.3). The two layers of peritoneum are separated by a film of serous fluid for lubrication to allow organs to move against each other without friction. The peritoneum forms a cavity that encloses the following organs of the abdomen: liver (except for the bare area), gallbladder, spleen, stomach, ovaries, and majority of intestines (Figures 7.4 and 7.5). In males, the **peritoneal cavity** is a closed cavity, but in females it communicates with the exterior through the uterine tubes, uterus, and vagina (Figure 7.6, A and B). The peritoneal cavity includes the **greater sac** and **lesser sac** (**omental bursae**). The greater sac is located between the inner surface of the anterior abdominal wall and the outer surface of the abdominal viscera. It is bounded by the parietal and visceral peritoneum, and communicates with the lesser sac through the **epiploic foramen (of Winslow)** (Figure 7.3). The lesser sac is located primarily between the posterior surface of the stomach and the posterior abdominal wall (Figures 7.3 and 7.7 through 7.9).

Numerous folds of peritoneum extend between organs, serving to hold them in position and at the same time enclose the vessels and nerves proceeding to each part. These folds or double layers of peritoneum are termed mesentery, omenta, and peritoneal ligaments. The **mesentery** is a double layer of peritoneum, which encloses the intestine and attaches it to the abdominal wall. An **omentum** is a mesentery or double layer of peritoneum that is attached to the stomach. The normal omentum is usually imperceptible on routine scans, visible

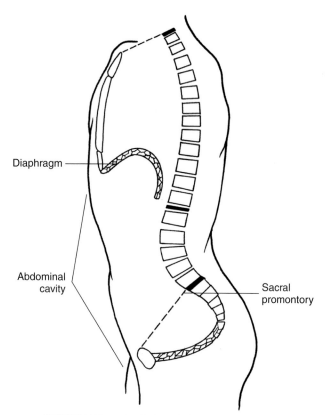

FIGURE 7.2 Sagittal view of the abdominal cavity.

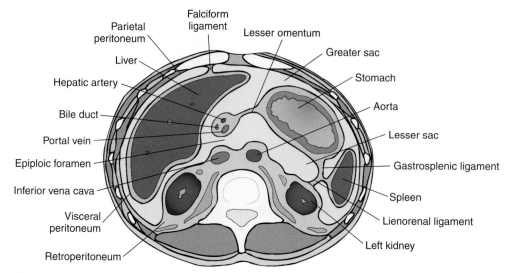

FIGURE 7.3 Axial view of abdomen with greater and lesser sac, falciform, gastrosplenic, and lienorenal ligaments.

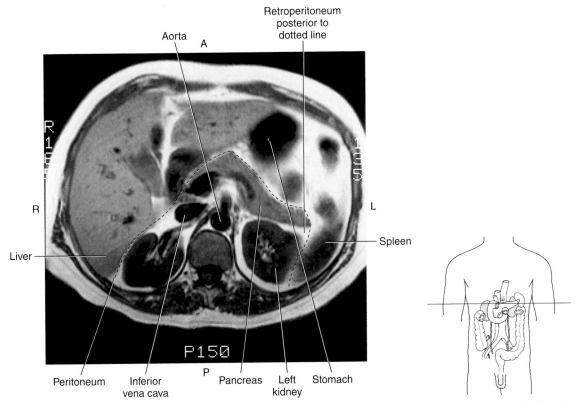

FIGURE 7.4 Axial, T1-weighted MRI of peritoneal and retroperitoneal structures (separated by dotted line).

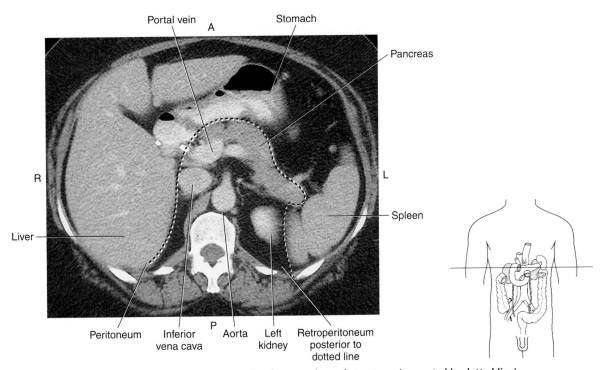

FIGURE 7.5 Axial CT of peritoneal and retroperitoneal structures (separated by dotted line).

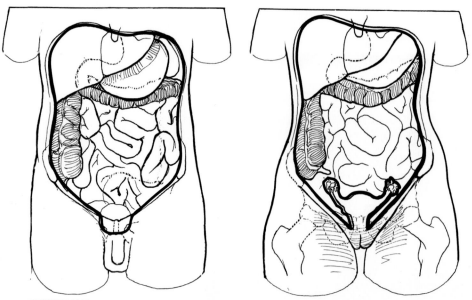

FIGURE 7.6 Anterior view of peritoneum. A, Male peritoneum. B, Female peritoneum.

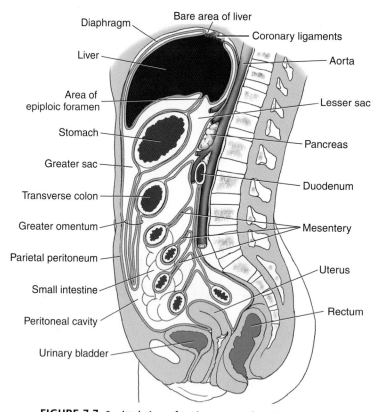

FIGURE 7.7 Sagittal view of peritoneum and peritoneal cavity.

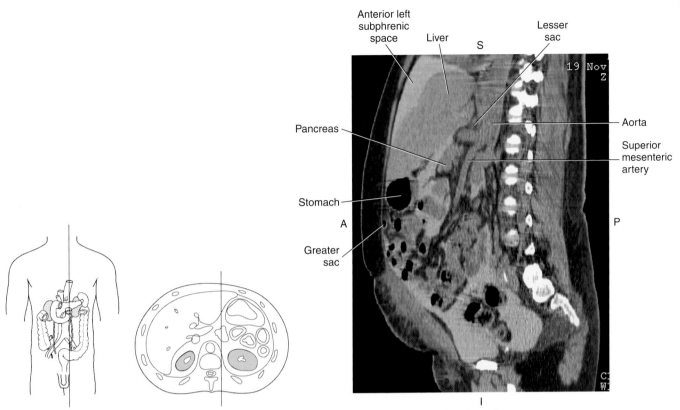

FIGURE 7.8 Sagittal CT reformat of abdomen with lesser sac and peritoneal spaces.

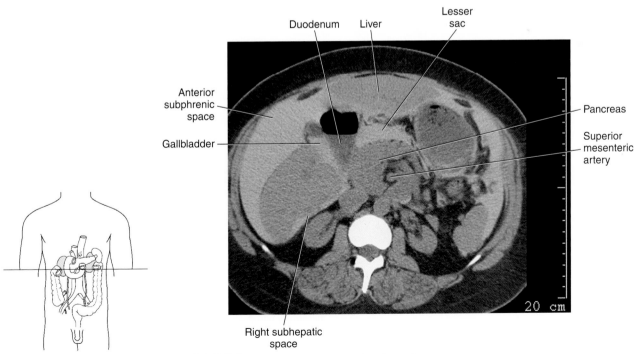

FIGURE 7.9 Axial CT of abdomen and peritoneal spaces.

only when fluid is present (Figures 7.8, 7.9, 7.12, and 7.13). The **greater omentum** is a fat-laden fold of peritoneum that drapes down from the greater curvature of the stomach and connects the stomach with the spleen, and transverse colon, whereas the **lesser omentum** attaches the duodenum and lesser curvature of the stomach to the liver (Figures 7.10 through 7.13).

Numerous **peritoneal ligaments** serve to connect an organ with another organ or abdominal wall. These peritoneal ligaments are not ligaments in the classic sense but are distinct regions of mesentery connecting the structures for which they are named. Three regions of the greater omentum that are characterized as peritoneal ligaments include **gastrocolic, gastrosplenic, and gastrophrenic**. These ligaments attach the greater omentum to the transverse colon, hilum of the spleen, greater curvature and fundus of the stomach, diaphragm, and esophagus (Figures 7.3, and 7.10 through 7.12). Ligaments of the lesser omentum include the **hepatogastric** and **hepatoduodenal**, which serve to connect the stomach and duodenum to the liver (Figure 7.10). Ligaments associated specifically with the liver are the

round ligament (ligamentum teres), falciform ligament, and coronary ligaments. The **round ligament** is a remnant of the left umbilical vein and runs within the free inferior margin of the falciform ligament to the umbilicus. The **falciform ligament** extends from the liver to the anterior abdominal wall and diaphragm, and forms a plane that divides the liver anatomically into right and left lobes. The falciform ligament provides the structural support that attaches the upper surfaces of the liver to the diaphragm and upper abdominal wall. (Figures 7.14 and 7.15). The **coronary ligaments** surround the superior pole of the liver and attach the liver to the diaphragm, forming the margins of the bare area (Figures 7.7 and 7.16). Additional peritoneal ligaments are described in Table 7.1.

> Inflammation of the peritoneal cavity is termed peritonitis. Acute peritonitis is most commonly caused by the leakage of infection through a perforation in the bowel.

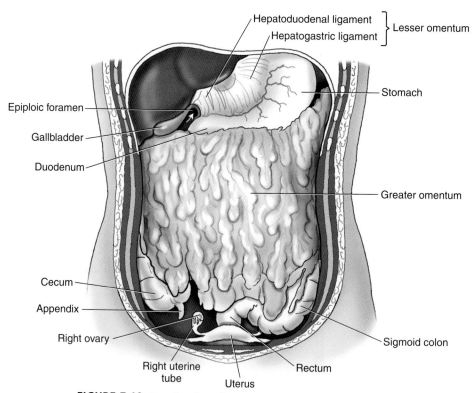

FIGURE 7.10 Anterior view of mesentery and peritoneal ligaments.

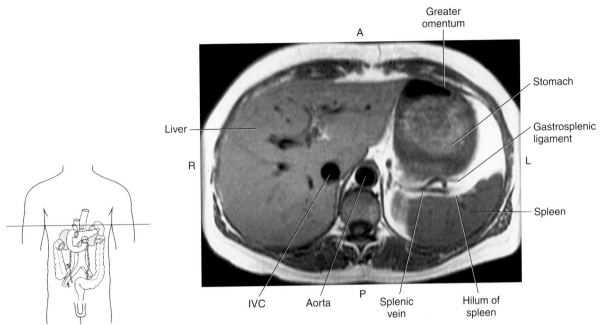

FIGURE 7.11 Axial, T1-weighted MRI of abdomen with greater omentum and gastrosplenic ligament.

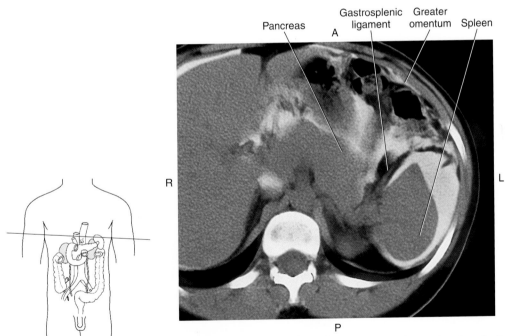

FIGURE 7.12 Axial CT of abdomen with blood accumulation demonstrating the greater omentum and gastrosplenic ligament.

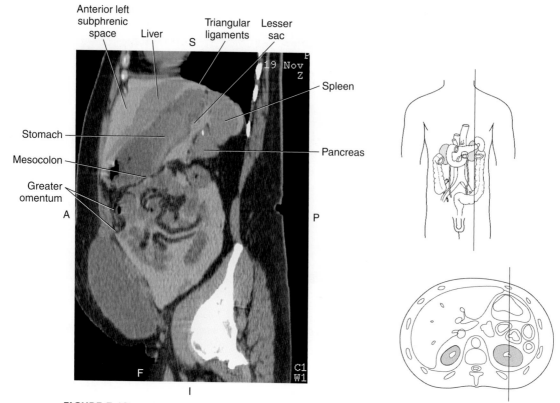

FIGURE 7.13 Sagittal CT reformat of abdomen with greater omentum and peritoneal spaces.

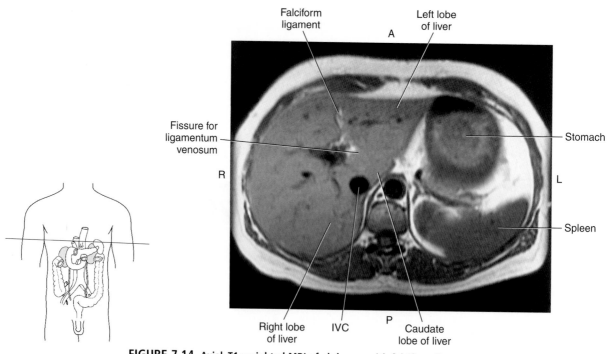

FIGURE 7.14 Axial, T1-weighted MRI of abdomen with falciform ligament.

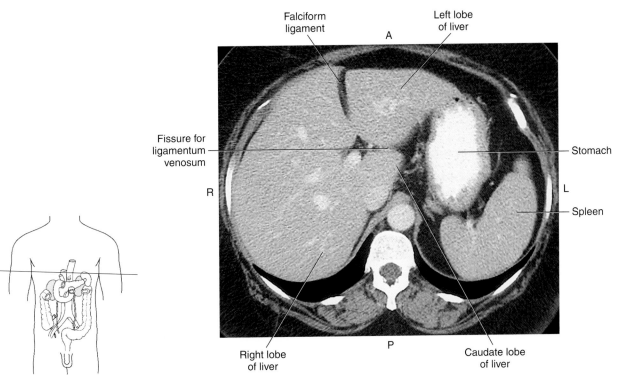

FIGURE 7.15 Axial CT of abdomen with falciform ligament.

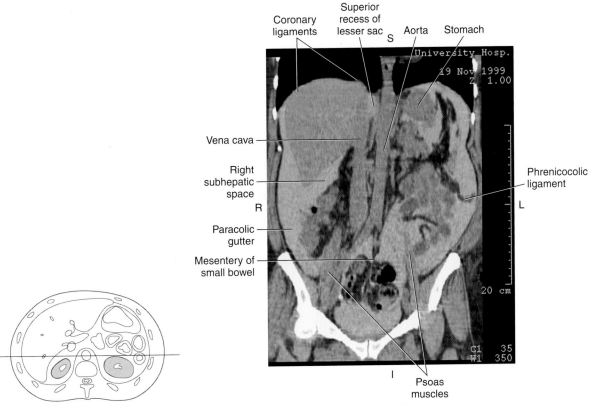

FIGURE 7.16 Coronal CT reformat of liver and coronary ligaments.

TABLE 7.1	Peritoneal Ligaments
Ligaments	**Location**
Gastrocolic ligament	Apron portion of the greater omentum attached to the transverse colon
Gastrosplenic ligament (gastrolienal ligament)	The left portion of the greater omentum that connects the hilum of the spleen to the greater curvature and fundus of the stomach
Splenorenal (lienorenal) ligament	Connects the spleen and kidney
Gastrophrenic ligament	Superior portion of greater omentum attached to the diaphragm and posterior aspect of the fundus and esophagus
Hepatorenal ligament	Connects the liver and kidney
Hepatoesophageal ligament	Connects the liver and esophagus
Hepatogastric ligament	Connects the liver to the lesser curvature of the stomach
Hepatoduodenal ligament	Connects the superior region of the duodenum to the liver
Falciform ligament	Extends from the liver to the anterior abdominal wall and diaphragm
Round ligament (ligamentum teres)	Remnant of the left umbilical vein, lying in the free edge of the falciform ligament
Coronary ligaments	Reflections of the peritoneum that surround the bare area of the liver
Triangular (left and right)	Where the layers of the coronary ligament meet to the left and right, respectively
Phrenocolic ligament	Attaches the left flexure of the colon to the diaphragm.

Peritoneal Spaces

The peritoneal cavity contains potential spaces resulting from folds of peritoneum that extend from the viscera to the abdominal wall. These spaces can be divided into the **supracolic** and **infracolic compartments** (Figure 7.17). The supracolic compartment is located above the transverse colon and contains the right and left **subphrenic spaces** and right and left **subhepatic spaces**. The subphrenic spaces are located between the diaphragm and the anterior portion of the liver. They are divided into right and left compartments by the falciform ligament (Figures 7.18 and 7.19). The subhepatic spaces are located posterior and inferior between the liver and the abdominal viscera. The right subhepatic space, located between the liver and kidney, contains **Morison's pouch**, which is the deepest point of the abdominal cavity in a supine patient and a common site for collection of fluid (Figures 7.20 and 7.21).

Below the transverse colon is the **infracolic compartment**, which consists of the right and left **infracolic spaces** and the **paracolic gutters**. The right and left infracolic spaces are divided by the mesentery of the small intestine. The right and left paracolic gutters are trough-like spaces located lateral to the ascending and descending colon (Figures 7.17 and 7.22, and Table 7.2). The deeper right gutter is a common site for free fluid collection.

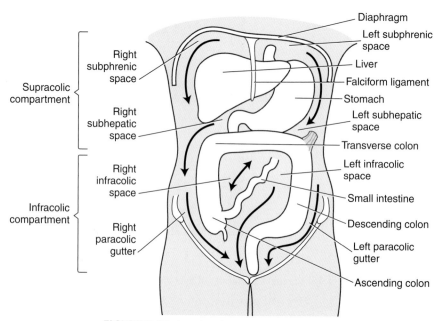

FIGURE 7.17 Anterior view of peritoneal spaces.

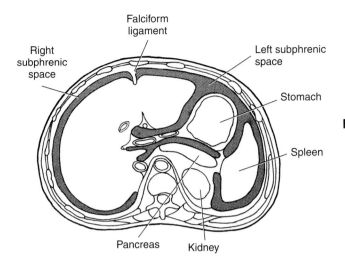

FIGURE 7.18 Axial view of subphrenic spaces.

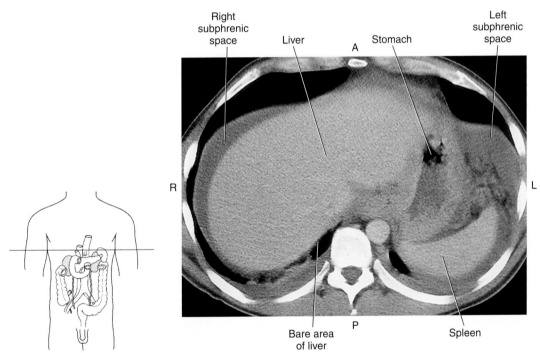

FIGURE 7.19 Axial CT of abdomen with subphrenic spaces.

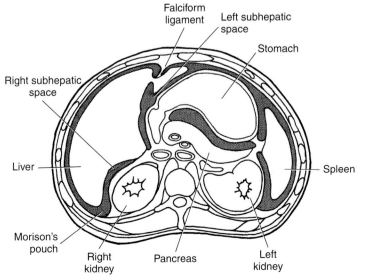

FIGURE 7.20 Axial view of subhepatic spaces and Morison's pouch.

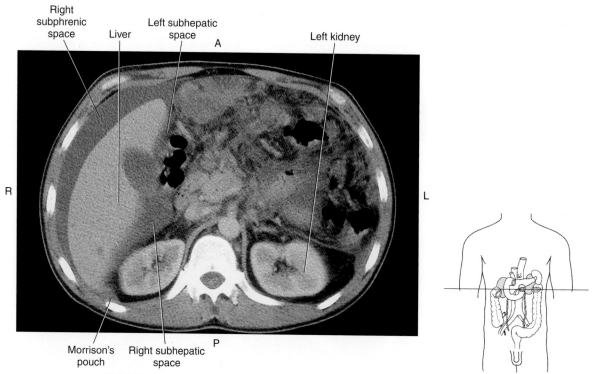

FIGURE 7.21 Axial CT of abdomen with subhepatic spaces and Morison's pouch.

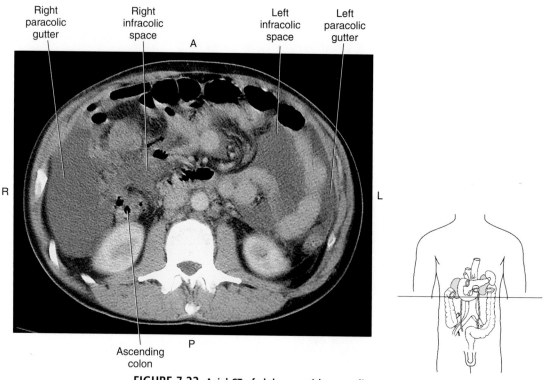

FIGURE 7.22 Axial CT of abdomen with paracolic gutters.

TABLE 7.2	Peritoneal and Retroperitoneal Spaces	
Space	**Location**	
<u>Peritoneal Spaces</u>		
Supracolic Compartment	Above Transverse Colon	
Subphrenic Space	Between diaphragm and anterior liver	
Right	Right and left spaces divided by falciform ligament	
Left		
Subhepatic Space	Posterior and inferior to liver	
Right	Between right lobe of liver and kidney; contains Morison's pouch	
Left	Between left lobe of liver and kidney; includes lesser omentum	
Infracolic Compartment	Below Transverse Colon	
Infracolic Spaces		
Right and Left	Divided by mesentery of small intestine	
Paracolic Gutters		
Right	Between ascending colon and right abdominal wall	
Left	Between descending colon and left abdominal wall	
<u>Retroperitoneal Spaces</u>		
Pararenal Spaces		
Anterior	Between renal (Gerota's) fascia and posterior surface of peritoneum	
Posterior	Between renal (Gerota's) fascia and muscles of posterior abdominal wall	
Perirenal Space		
Right	Around kidney and adrenal glands; completely enclosed by renal (Gerota's) fascia	
Left		

Retroperitoneum

Structures located posterior to the peritoneum, yet lined by it anteriorly, are considered to be in the **retroperitoneum** and include abdominal and pelvic structures, such as the kidneys, ureters, adrenal glands, pancreas, duodenum, aorta, inferior vena cava, bladder, uterus, and prostate gland. In addition, the ascending and descending colon and most of the duodenum are situated in the retroperitoneum (Figures 7.3 through 7.5).

Retroperitoneal Spaces

The retroperitoneum can be divided into compartments or spaces that include the anterior and posterior pararenal spaces and left and right perirenal spaces (Figure 7.23).

The **anterior pararenal space** is located between the anterior surface of the **renal fascia (Gerota's fascia)** and the posterior position of the peritoneum. It contains the retroperitoneal portions of the ascending and descending colon, the pancreas, and the duodenum. The **posterior pararenal space** is located between the posterior renal fascia and the muscles of the posterior abdominal wall. There are no solid organs located in this space, just fat and vessels (Figures 7.24 and 7.25). The left and right **perirenal spaces** are the areas located directly around the kidneys and are completely enclosed by renal fascia. The perirenal spaces contain the kidneys, adrenal glands, lymph nodes, blood vessels, and perirenal fat. The perirenal fat separates the adrenal glands from the kidneys and provides cushioning for the kidney (Figure 7.26 and Table 7.2).

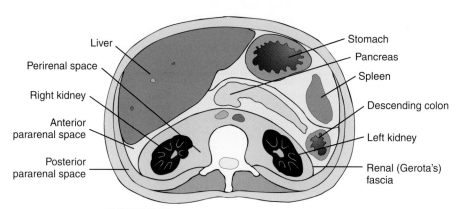

FIGURE 7.23 Axial view of retroperitoneal spaces.

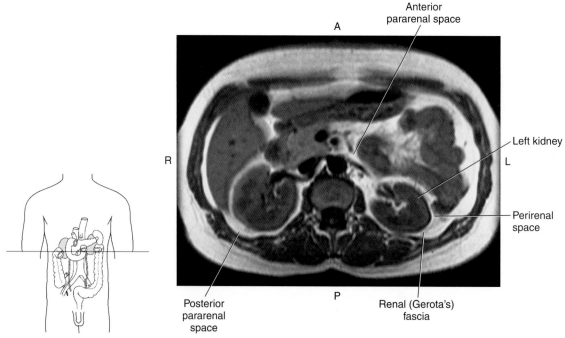

FIGURE 7.24 Axial, T1-weighted MRI of abdomen with kidneys and pararenal spaces.

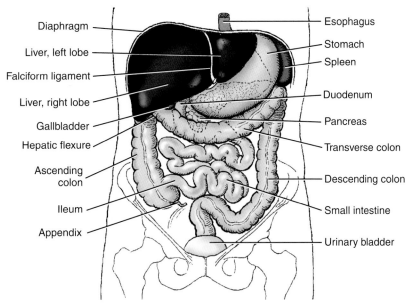

FIGURE 7.29 Anterior view of abdominal viscera.

Surface Anatomy

The liver can be divided into lobes according to surface anatomy or into segments according to vascular supply. The four lobes commonly used for reference based on surface anatomy are the left, right, caudate, and quadrate. The **left lobe** is the most anterior of the liver lobes, extending across the midline. The **right lobe** is the largest of the four lobes and is separated from the left lobe by the interlobar fissure. The smallest lobe is the **caudate lobe**, which is located on the inferior and posterior liver surface, sandwiched between the IVC and the **ligamentum venosum**. The **quadrate lobe** is located on the anteroinferior surface of the left lobe between the gallbladder and the round ligament. The hilum of the liver, **porta hepatis**, is located on the inferomedial border of the liver. It is the central location for vessels to enter and exit the liver (Figures 7.27 through 7.34).

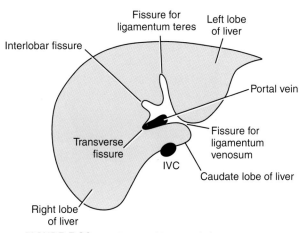

FIGURE 7.30 Axial view of liver with fissures.

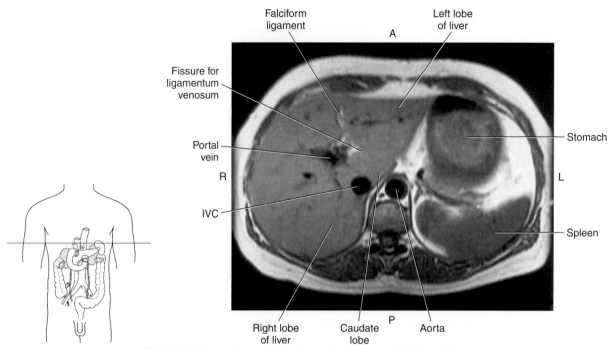

FIGURE 7.31 Axial, T1-weighted MRI of abdomen with lobes of liver.

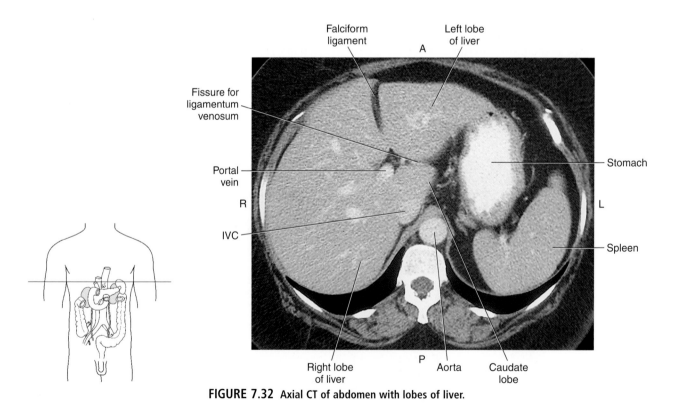

FIGURE 7.32 Axial CT of abdomen with lobes of liver.

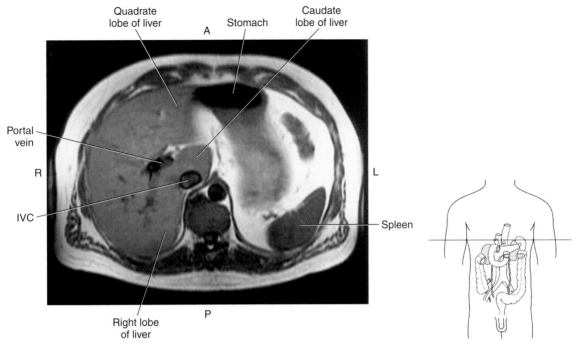

FIGURE 7.33 Axial, T1-weighted MRI of liver with quadrate lobe.

Within the liver there are several main grooves or fissures that are useful in defining the lobes and boundaries of the hepatic segments. The **fissure for the round ligament** divides the left hepatic lobe into medial and lateral segments. The **fissure for the ligamentum venosum** separates the caudate lobe from the left lobe, and the **transverse fissure (portal)** contains the horizontal portions of the right and left portal veins. The **interlobar fissure (main lobar fissure)**, an imaginary line drawn through the gallbladder fossa and the middle hepatic vein to the inferior vena cava, divides the right from the left lobes of the liver (Figure 7.30).

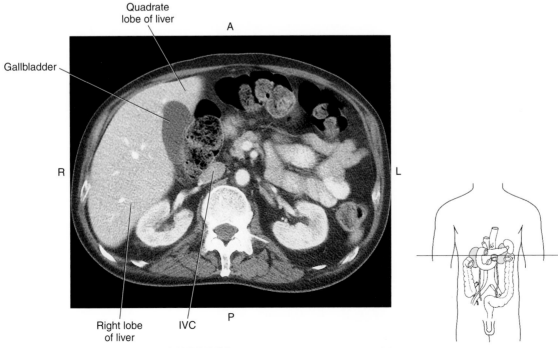

FIGURE 7.34 Axial CT of liver with quadrate lobe.

Segmental Anatomy

Current practice favors division of the liver into eight segments, according to its vascular supply, which can aid in surgical resection. According to the French anatomist Couinaud, the liver can be divided into segments based on the branching of the portal and hepatic veins. The three main hepatic veins divide the liver longitudinally into four sections (Figure 7.35). The middle hepatic vein divides the liver into right and left lobes. The right lobe is divided into anterior and posterior sections by the right hepatic vein, and the left lobe is divided into medial and lateral sections by the left hepatic vein. Each section is then subdivided transversely by the right and left portal veins, creating eight segments. Each segment can be considered functionally independent with its own branch of the hepatic artery, portal vein, and bile duct and is drained by a branch of the hepatic veins (Figures 7.36 through 7.49).

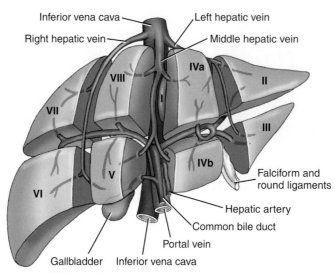

FIGURE 7.35 Anterior view of segmentation of liver.

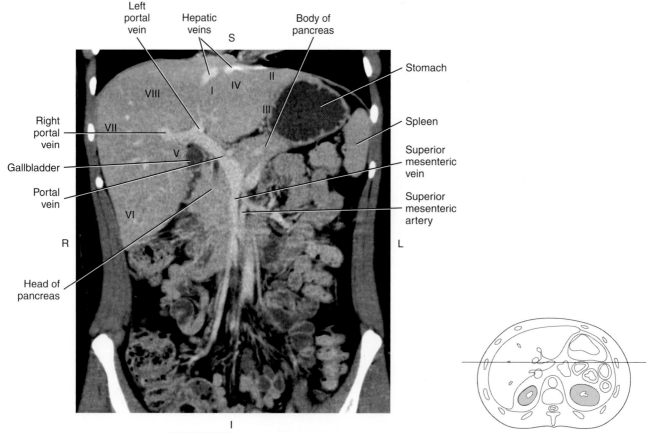

FIGURE 7.36 Coronal CT reformat of liver segments and portal vein.

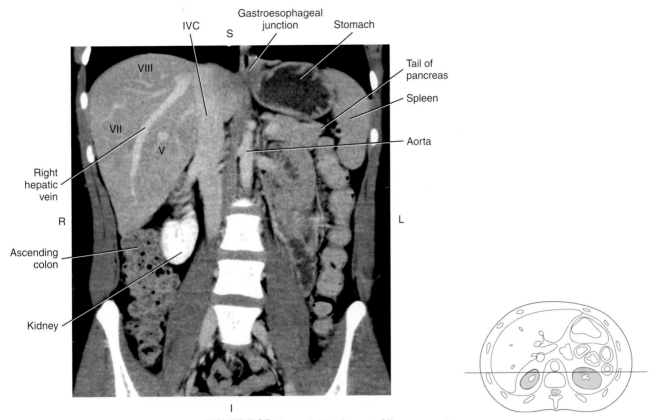

FIGURE 7.37 Coronal CT reformat of liver segments.

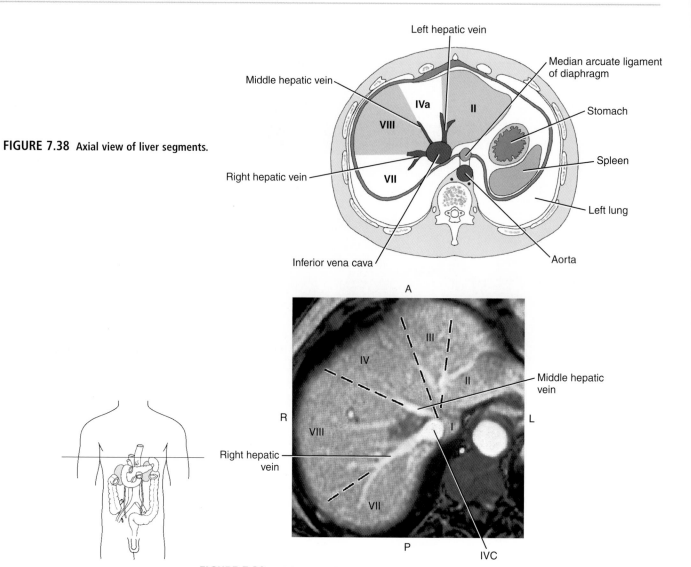

FIGURE 7.38 Axial view of liver segments.

FIGURE 7.39 Axial, T1-weighted MRI of liver segments.

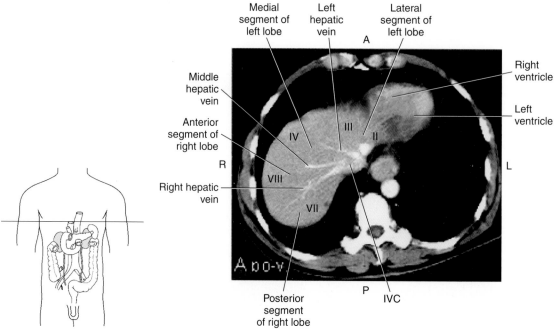

FIGURE 7.40 Axial CT of liver segments.

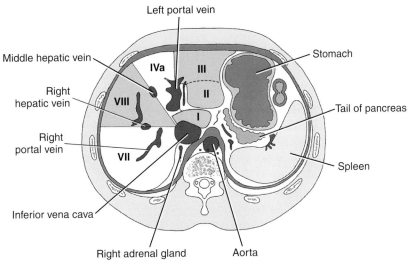

FIGURE 7.41 Axial view of liver segments.

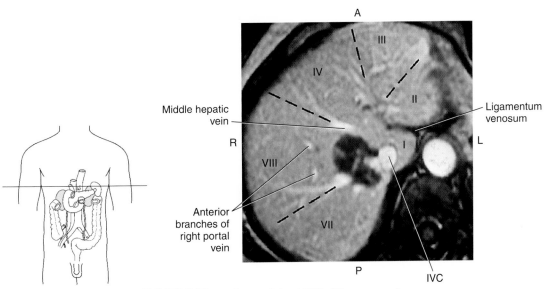

FIGURE 7.42 Axial, T1-weighted MRI of liver segments.

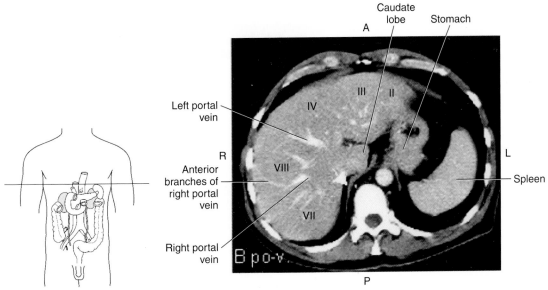

FIGURE 7.43 Axial CT of liver segments.

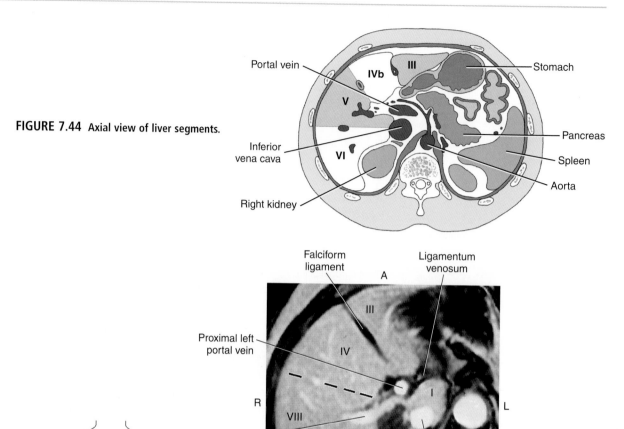

Portal vein

IVb

III

Stomach

V

Inferior
vena cava

VI

Pancreas

Spleen

Aorta

Right kidney

FIGURE 7.44 Axial view of liver segments.

Falciform
ligament

Ligamentum
venosum

A

III

Proximal left
portal vein

IV

I

R

L

VIII

Portal
vein

VII

Posterior
branches of
right portal
vein

P

IVC

FIGURE 7.45 Axial, T1-weighted MRI of liver segments.

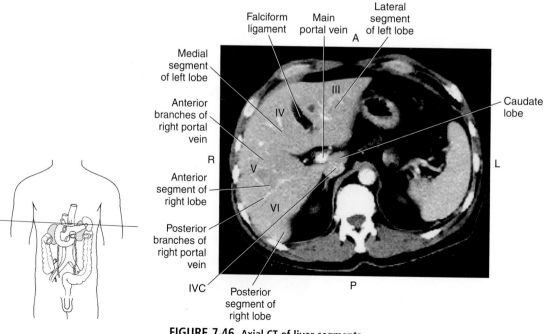

Falciform
ligament

Main
portal vein

Lateral
segment
of left lobe

A

Medial
segment
of left lobe

III

Anterior
branches of
right portal
vein

IV

Caudate
lobe

R

L

V

Anterior
segment of
right lobe

VI

Posterior
branches of
right portal
vein

IVC

Posterior
segment of
right lobe

P

FIGURE 7.46 Axial CT of liver segments.

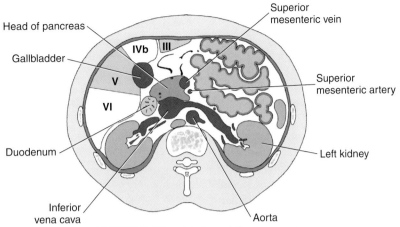

FIGURE 7.47 Axial view of liver segments.

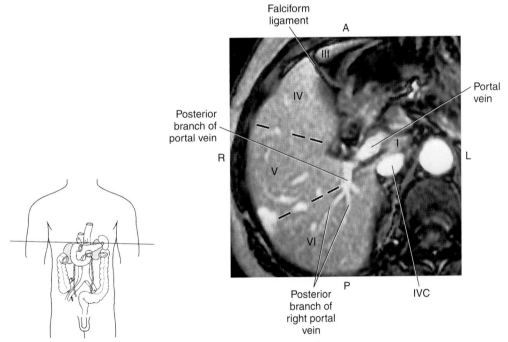

FIGURE 7.48 Axial, T1-weighted MRI of liver segments.

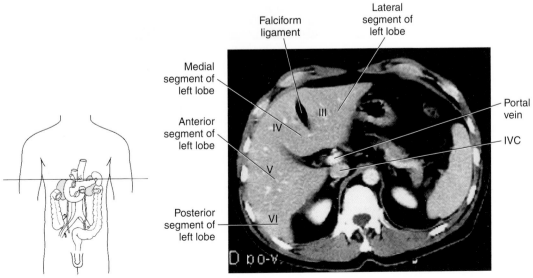

FIGURE 7.49 Axial CT of liver segments.

Portal Hepatic System

The liver receives nutrient-rich blood from the gastrointestinal tract via the **portal hepatic system** (Figures 7.35 and 7.50). The major vessel of this system is the **portal vein**, which is formed in the retroperitoneum by the union of the superior mesenteric and splenic veins, posterior to the neck of the pancreas (Figures 7.50 through 7.55). It passes obliquely to the right, posterior to the hepatic artery within the lesser omentum, and enters the liver at the porta hepatis (Figures 7.28, 7.56 and 7.57). At the **porta hepatis**, the portal vein branches into **right** and **left main portal veins** that then follow the course of the right and left hepatic arteries. The right portal vein first sends branches to the caudate lobe and then divides into anterior and posterior branches that subdivide into superior and inferior branches to supply the right lobe of the liver. The left portal vein initially courses to the left, then turns medially toward the ligamentum teres. It branches to supply the lateral segments (segments II and III) of the left lobe and the superior and inferior sections of segment IV (Figures 7.35 and 7.41 through 7.49).

Portal hypertension is caused by obstruction of blood flow in the portal hepatic system. This condition can lead to splenomegaly and ascites.

FIGURE 7.50 Anterior view of portal hepatic system.

Right hepatic vein
Middle hepatic vein
Liver
Left main portal vein
Right main portal vein
Portal vein
Superior mesenteric vein
Ascending colon
Ileum

Inferior vena cava
Left hepatic vein
Spleen
Splenic vein
Inferior mesenteric vein
Descending colon
Rectum

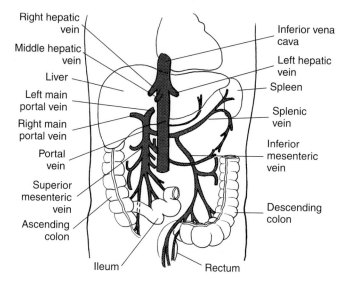

FIGURE 7.51 CT MIP of portal vein.

Right hepatic vein
Left portal vein
IVC
S
Middle hepatic vein
Right portal vein
Portal vein
R
Superior mesenteric vein
Splenic vein
L
I

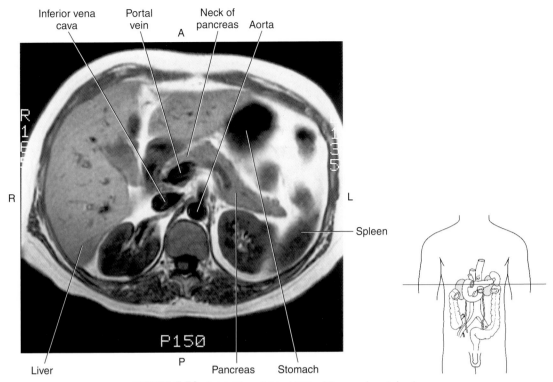

FIGURE 7.52 Axial, T1-weighted MRI of liver and portal vein.

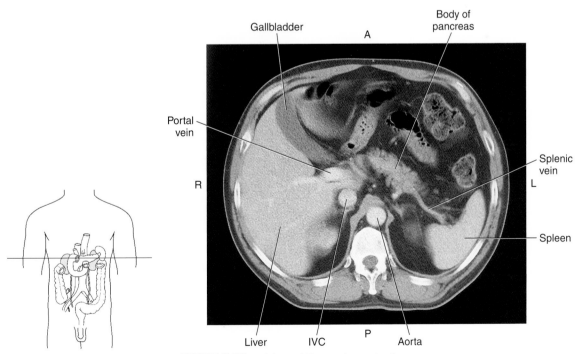

FIGURE 7.53 Axial CT of liver and portal vein.

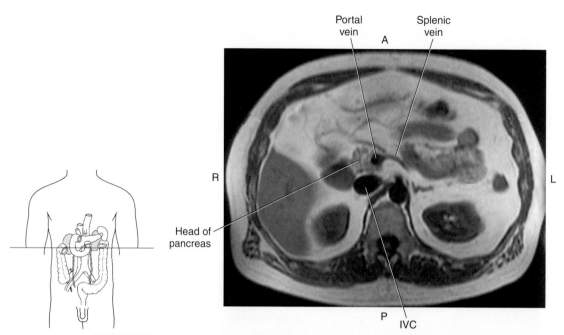

FIGURE 7.54 Axial, T1-weighted MRI of abdomen with portal and splenic veins.

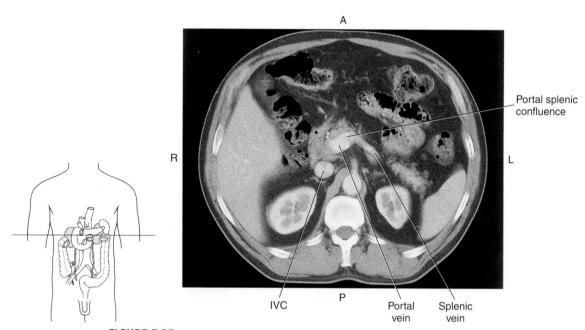

FIGURE 7.55 Axial CT of abdomen with portal and splenic veins.

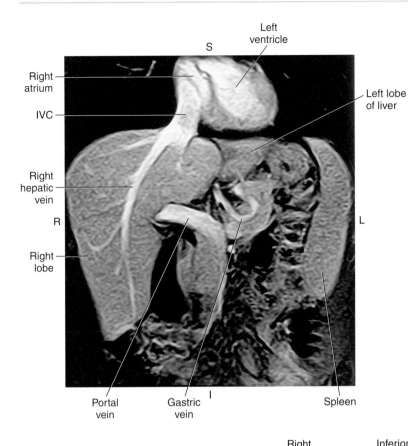

Left ventricle

Right atrium

Left lobe of liver

IVC

Right hepatic vein

Right lobe

S

R

L

I

Portal vein

Gastric vein

Spleen

FIGURE 7.56 Coronal MR venogram of portal system.

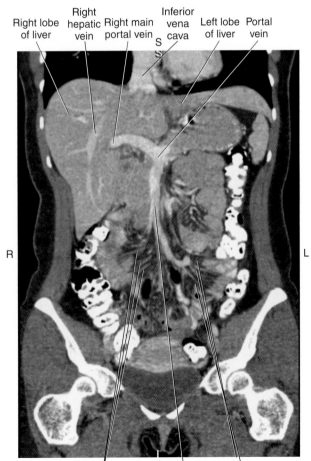

Right lobe of liver

Right hepatic vein

Right main portal vein

Inferior vena cava

Left lobe of liver

Portal vein

S

R

L

I

Ileal branches of superior mesenteric vein

Superior mesenteric vein

Jejunal branches of superior mesenteric vein

FIGURE 7.57 Coronal CT reformat of portal system.

Vasculature

The liver is unusual in that it has a dual blood supply, receiving arterial blood (20%-25%) from the common hepatic artery and nutrient-rich venous blood (75%-80%) from the portal vein. The **common hepatic artery** usually arises as one of the three branches off the celiac artery, coursing to the right to enter the lesser omentum anterior to the portal vein (Figures 7.58 through 7.61). It branches into the right gastric and gastroduodenal arteries just above the duodenum and continues in the hepatoduodenal ligament as the **proper hepatic artery**. While within or just before entering the porta hepatis,

the proper hepatic artery divides into left and right hepatic arteries, which continue to branch and supply the lobes of the liver.

The **right hepatic artery** is larger than the left and supplies the majority of the right lobe of the liver. It passes posterior to the uncinate process of the pancreas and runs along the posterior wall of the bile duct into the right hepatic lobe. The **left hepatic artery** is located between the lesser curvature of the stomach and approaches the liver in the lesser omentum and branches to supply the caudate, quadrate, and medial and lateral segments of the left lobe of the liver (Figure 7.62). The venous drainage of the liver

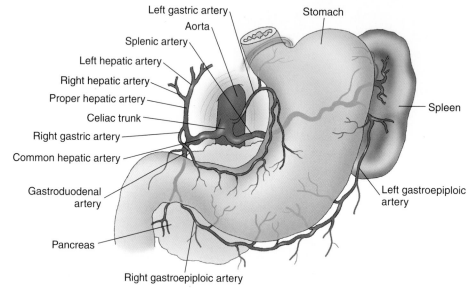

FIGURE 7.58 Anterior view of celiac trunk and hepatic artery.

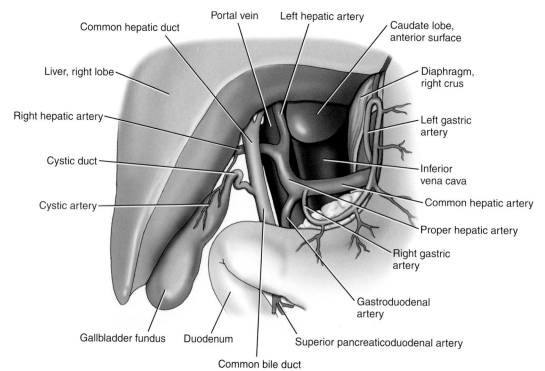

FIGURE 7.59 Anterior view of hepatic artery, CBD, and portal vein.

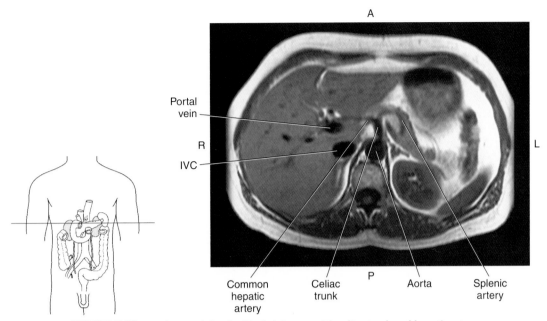

FIGURE 7.60 Axial, T1-weighted MRI of abdomen with celiac trunk and hepatic artery.

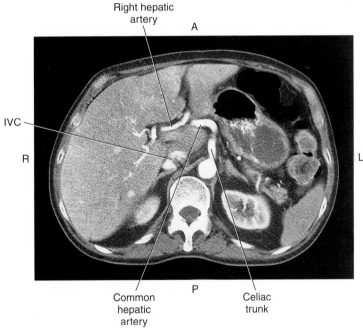

FIGURE 7.61 Axial CT of abdomen with celiac trunk and hepatic artery.

occurs via the small interlobar and intersegmental hepatic vessels that merge into the three major hepatic veins, emptying directly into the IVC, just below the diaphragm (Figures 7.50 and 7.63). The **right hepatic vein**, the largest, lies between the right anterior and posterior hepatic segments, drains segments V, VI, and VII, and enters the IVC at the right lateral aspect. The **middle hepatic vein** lies in the interlobar fissure, drains segments IV, V, and VIII, then enters the IVC at the anterior or right anterior surface. The smallest hepatic vein, the **left hepatic vein**, courses between the medial and lateral segments of the left lobe, drains segments II and III, then enters the left anterior surface of the IVC (Figures 7.35 through 7.49, 7.64, and 7.65). Frequently, the middle and left hepatic veins converge to form a common trunk before emptying into the IVC just below the diaphragm. The **IVC** lies in a groove along the posterior wall of the liver and ascends into the thoracic cavity through the **caval hiatus** of the diaphragm and enters the right atrium of the heart (Figures 7.64 through 7.67).

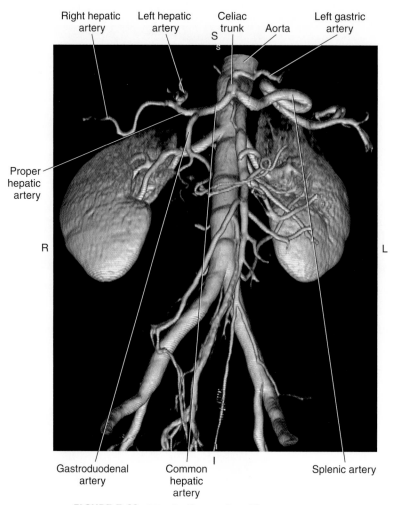

Right hepatic artery

Left hepatic artery

Celiac trunk

Aorta

Left gastric artery

Proper hepatic artery

Gastroduodenal artery

Common hepatic artery

Splenic artery

FIGURE 7.62 CTA of celiac trunk and hepatic artery.

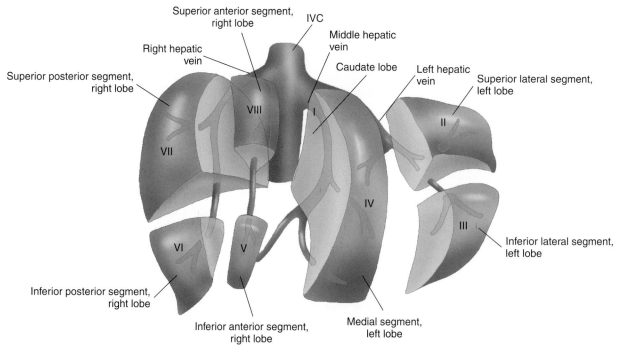

Superior anterior segment, right lobe

IVC

Middle hepatic vein

Right hepatic vein

Caudate lobe

Superior posterior segment, right lobe

Left hepatic vein

Superior lateral segment, left lobe

VIII

I

II

VII

IV

Inferior lateral segment, left lobe

III

VI

V

Inferior posterior segment, right lobe

Inferior anterior segment, right lobe

Medial segment, left lobe

FIGURE 7.63 Couinaud's segmentation of the liver with hepatic veins.

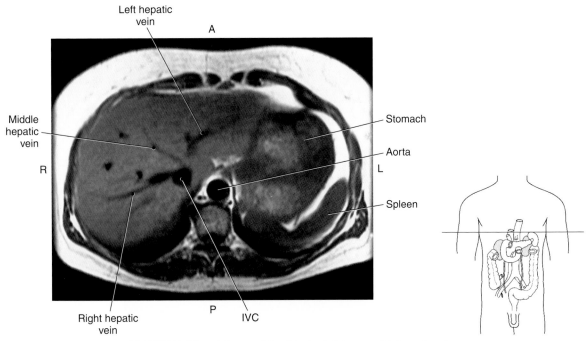

FIGURE 7.64 Axial, T1-weighted MRI of abdomen with hepatic veins.

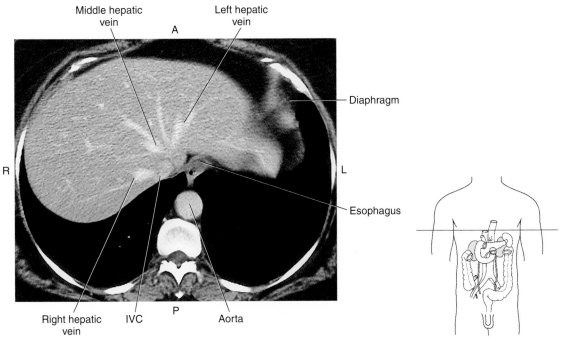

FIGURE 7.65 Axial CT of liver with hepatic veins.

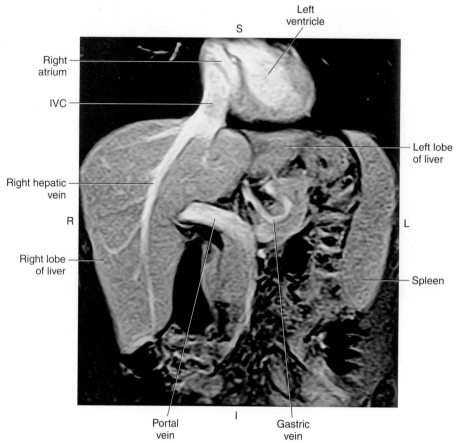

FIGURE 7.66 MRV with hepatic and portal veins.

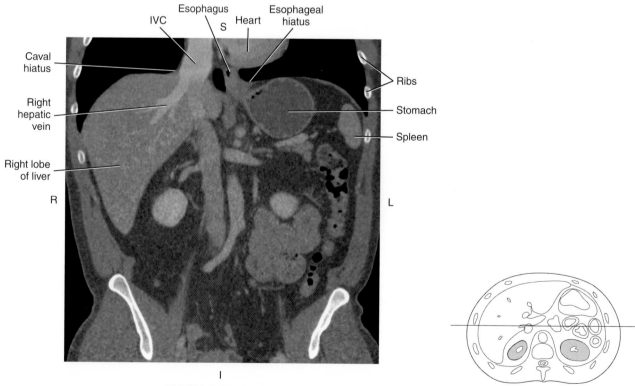

FIGURE 7.67 Coronal CT reformat of right hepatic vein and IVC.

GALLBLADDER AND BILIARY SYSTEM

The **biliary system** is composed of the gallbladder and bile ducts (both intrahepatic and extrahepatic), which serve to drain the liver of bile and store it until it is transported to the duodenum to aid in digestion (Figure 7.68). The hollow pear-shaped **gallbladder** is located in the **gallbladder fossa** on the anteroinferior portion of the right lobe of the liver, closely associated with the interlobar fissure. It functions as the reservoir for storing and concentrating bile before it is transported to the duodenum. The gallbladder can be divided into a fundus, body, and neck (Figures 7.69 through 7.74). The **fundus** is the rounded distal portion of the gallbladder

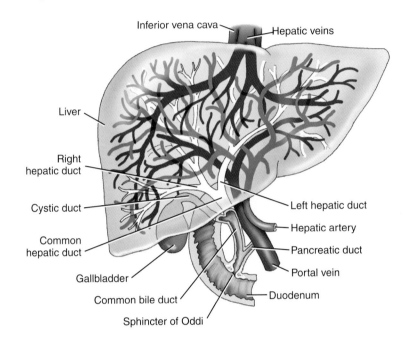

Inferior vena cava — Hepatic veins
Liver
Right hepatic duct
Cystic duct
Common hepatic duct
Gallbladder
Common bile duct
Sphincter of Oddi
Left hepatic duct
Hepatic artery
Pancreatic duct
Portal vein
Duodenum

FIGURE 7.68 Anterior view of intrahepatic biliary system.

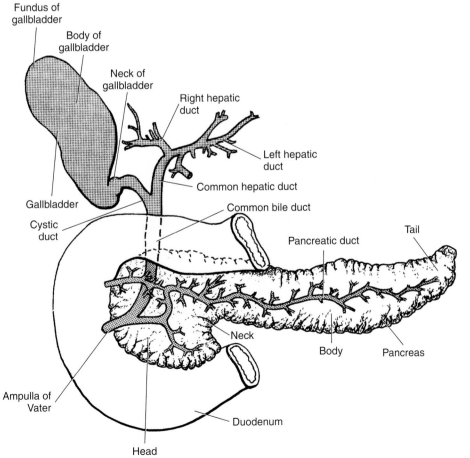

Fundus of gallbladder
Body of gallbladder
Neck of gallbladder
Right hepatic duct
Left hepatic duct
Common hepatic duct
Gallbladder
Cystic duct
Common bile duct
Pancreatic duct
Tail
Neck
Body
Pancreas
Ampulla of Vater
Duodenum
Head

FIGURE 7.69 Anterior view of extra-hepatic biliary system.

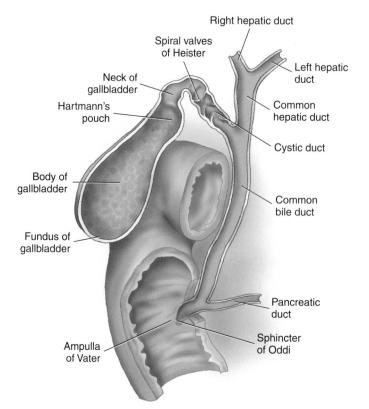

FIGURE 7.70 Gallbladder and biliary system.

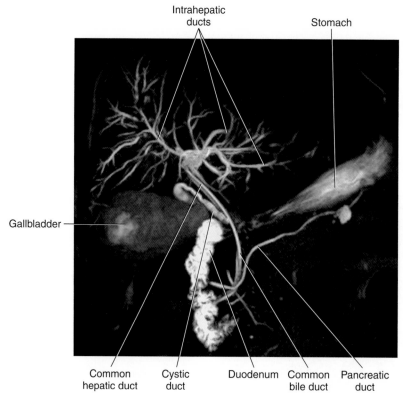

FIGURE 7.71 MR cholangiopancreatogram (MRCP) of biliary system.

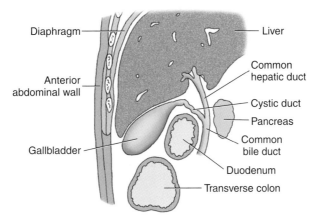

FIGURE 7.72 Sagittal view of liver and gallbladder.

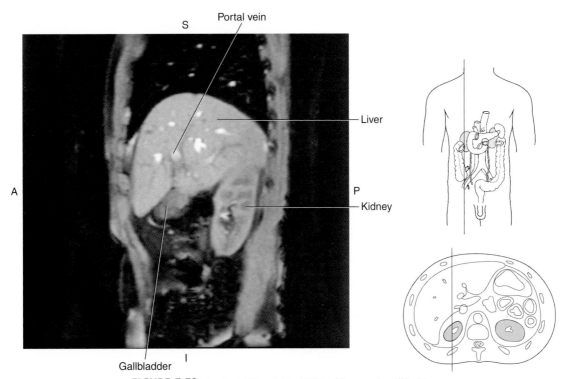

FIGURE 7.73 Sagittal, T2-weighted MRI of liver and gallbladder.

sac that is frequently in contact with the anterior abdominal wall. The widest portion, the **body**, gently tapers superiorly into the neck. The narrow **neck** lies to the right of the porta hepatis and continues as the **cystic duct**. The neck contains circular muscles that create spiral folds within the mucosa called the **spiral valves of Heister** (Figure 7.70). These valves are particularly prominent at the bend formed by the neck and cystic duct, a common area for gallbladder impaction during acute or chronic cholecystitis. The gallbladder has a muscular wall that contracts when stimulated by cholecystokinin, forcing bile through the extrahepatic biliary system into the duodenum. Bile, formed within the liver, is collected for transport to the gallbladder by

the intrahepatic bile ducts. The **intrahepatic bile ducts** run beside the hepatic arteries and portal veins throughout the liver parenchyma. The intrahepatic ducts merge into successively larger ducts as they follow a course from the periphery to the central portion of the liver, eventually forming the **right** and **left hepatic** ducts (Figures 7.68 through 7.71). The right and left hepatic ducts unite at the porta hepatis to form the proximal portion of the **common hepatic duct** (CHD), which marks the beginning of the **extrahepatic biliary system** (Figure 7.69). The CHD is located anterior to the portal vein and lateral to the hepatic artery in its caudal descent from the porta hepatis. As the CHD descends in the free border of the lesser omentum, it is joined from the right

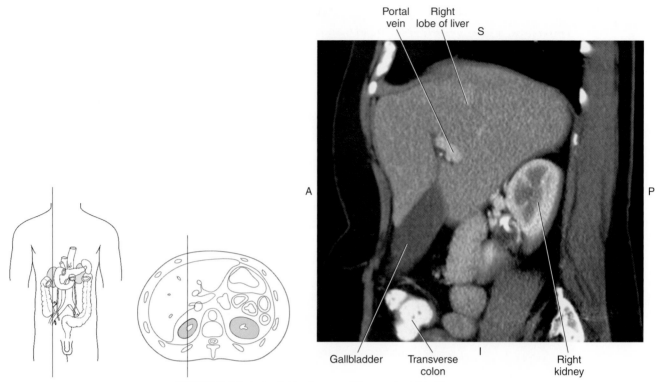

FIGURE 7.74 Sagittal CT reformat of liver and gallbladder.

by the cystic duct to form the **common bile duct** (CBD). The CBD continues a caudal descent along with the hepatic artery and portal vein within the hepatoduodenal ligament (Figure 7.68). It curves slightly to the right, away from the portal vein, then courses posterior and medial to the first part of the duodenum behind the head of the pancreas (Figures 7.71, 7.72, and 7.75 through 7.79). The CBD follows a groove on the posterior surface of the pancreatic head, then pierces the medial wall of the second part of the duodenum along with the **main pancreatic duct (duct of Wirsung)** through the **ampulla of Vater** (Figure 7.69). The ends of both ducts are surrounded by the circular muscle fibers of the **sphincter of Oddi** (Figure 7.70).

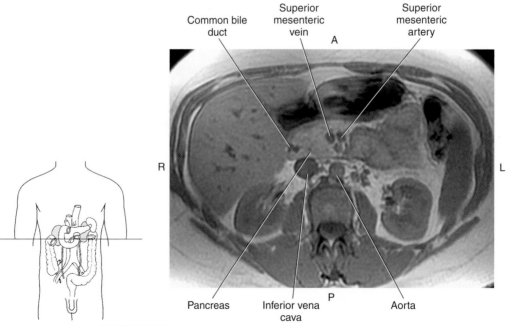

FIGURE 7.75 Axial, T1-weighted MRI of abdomen and CBD.

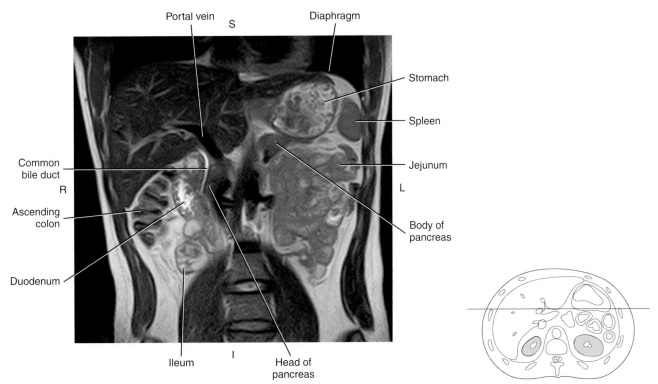

FIGURE 7.76 Coronal, T2-weighted MRI of abdomen and CBD.

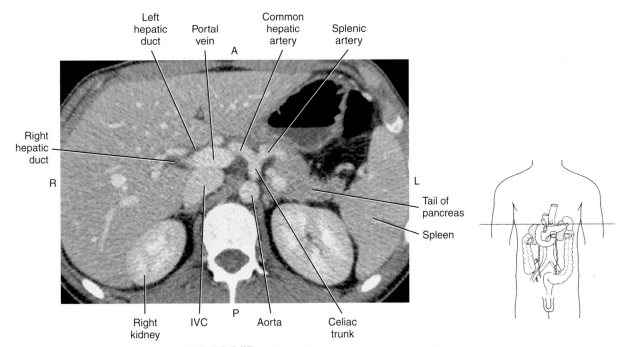

FIGURE 7.77 Axial CT of abdomen with hepatic ducts.

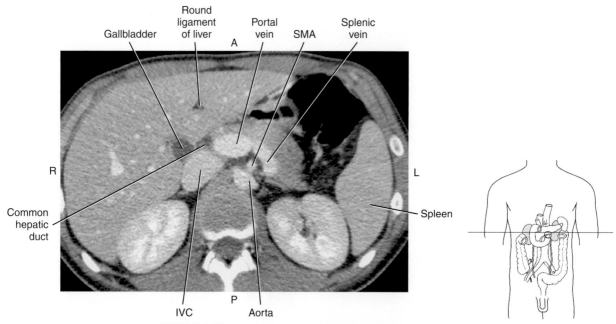

FIGURE 7.78 Axial CT of abdomen with common hepatic duct.

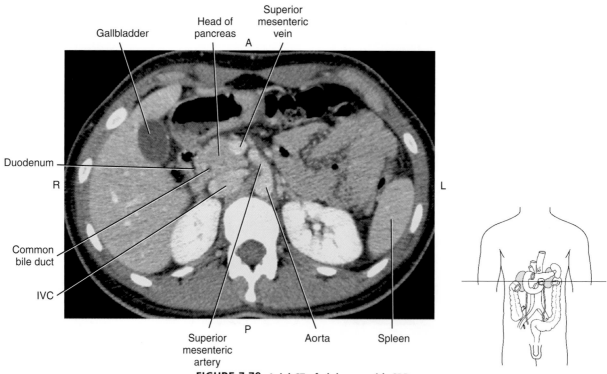

FIGURE 7.79 Axial CT of abdomen with CBD.

PANCREAS

The **pancreas** is a long, narrow retroperitoneal organ that lies posterior to the stomach and extends transversely at an oblique angle between the duodenum and splenic hilum. The pancreas can be divided into the head, uncinate process, neck, body, and tail (Figure 7.80). The broad, flat **head** of the pancreas lies inferior and to the right of the body and tail, nestled in the curve of the second portion of the duodenum at approximately the level of L2-L3. The head is anterior to the IVC and renal veins (Figure 7.81). Two vessels can be commonly seen running through the head: the common bile duct in the right posterior aspect and the gastroduodenal artery in the anterior aspect (Figures 7.82 and 7.83). The **uncinate process** is a medial and posterior extension of the head, lying between the superior mesenteric vein and inferior vena cava (Figures 7.80 and 7.81). The **neck**, the constricted portion of the gland, is located between the pancreatic head and body. Located just posterior to the neck is the **portal splenic confluence**, where the portal vein is formed by the merging of the superior mesenteric and splenic veins (Figures 7.55 and 7.80). The **body** is the largest and most anterior portion of the pancreas, extending transversely to the left, anterior to the aorta and superior mesenteric artery (Figures 7.84 and 7.85). The splenic vein runs along the posterior surface of the body on its route to the portal splenic confluence. The body tapers superiorly and posteriorly into the **pancreatic tail**. The tail extends into the left anterior pararenal space, anterior to the left kidney, to end at the splenic hilum (Figures 7.80, and 7.84 through 7.86). The

pancreas has both an endocrine (insulin, glucagon) and exocrine (digestive enzymes) function. It delivers its endocrine hormones into the draining venous system and its enzymes into the small intestines. The endocrine hormones help control plasma glucose concentration. Insulin's chief role is to regulate cellular absorption and utilization of glucose, thereby affecting carbohydrate, protein, and lipid metabolism in body tissues. Glucagon, acting in opposition to insulin, tends to raise plasma sugar levels by increasing the rate of glycogen breakdown and glucose synthesis in the liver. Pancreatic enzymes include amylase for the digestion of starch, lipase for the digestion of lipids, peptidases for protein digestion, and sodium bicarbonate to neutralize gastric acid. The pancreatic enzymes are carried to the duodenum via a system of ducts. The **main pancreatic duct** (**duct of Wirsung**) begins in the tail and runs the length of the gland to the **ampulla of Vater**, where it empties, together with the common bile duct, into the duodenum through the sphincter of Oddi (Figures 7.69 and 7.86). The arterial supply of the pancreas comes from branches of the celiac and superior mesenteric arteries. Venous blood drains from the pancreas into the portal vein via the superior mesenteric or splenic vein. The pancreas is unencapsulated and has a distinct lobulated appearance, making identification easy in cross-section.

Acute pancreatitis can lead to the leakage of powerful digestive enzymes. Pancreatic necrosis results when the enzymes "digest" the surrounding tissue.

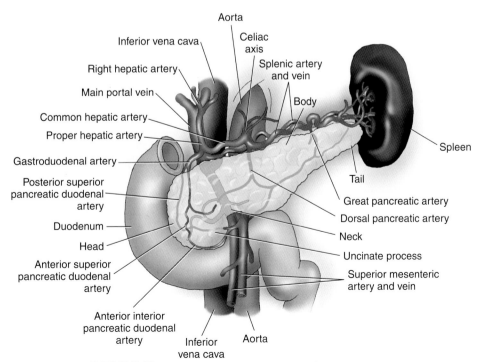

FIGURE 7.80 Anterior view of pancreas and adjacent structures.

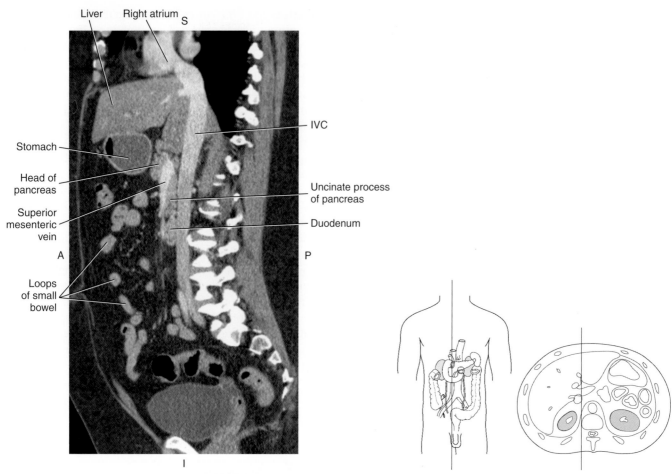

FIGURE 7.81 Sagittal CT reformat of pancreas and IVC.

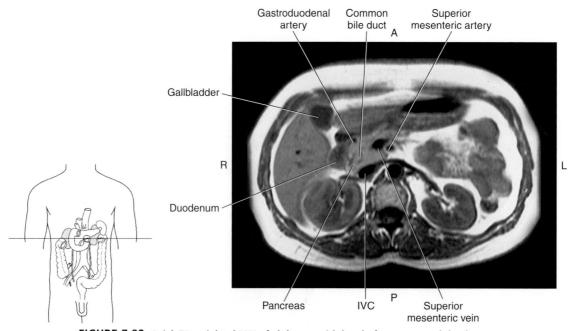

FIGURE 7.82 Axial, T1-weighted MRI of abdomen with head of pancreas and duodenum.

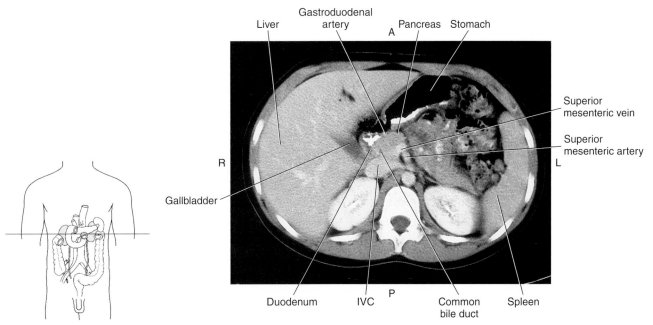

FIGURE 7.83 Axial CT of abdomen with head of pancreas and duodenum.

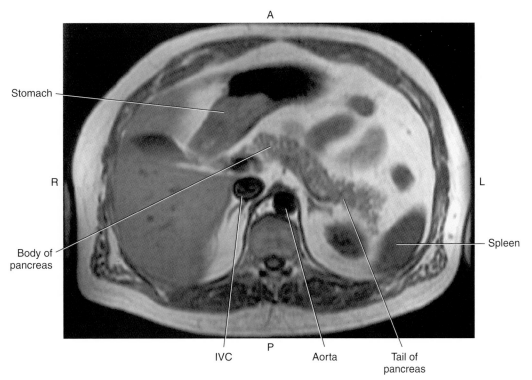

FIGURE 7.84 Axial, T1-weighted MRI of pancreas.

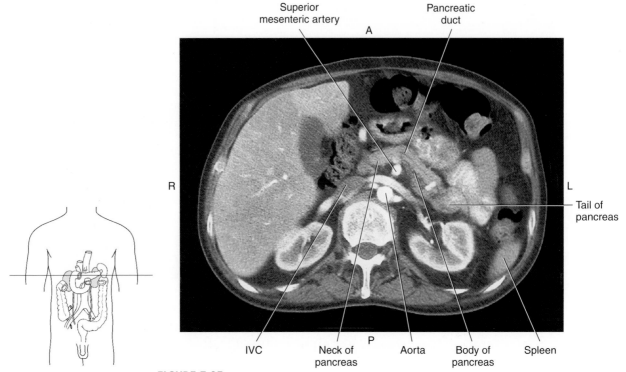

FIGURE 7.85 Axial CT of pancreas and pancreatic duct.

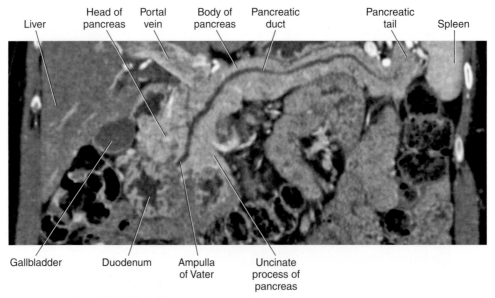

FIGURE 7.86 Coronal CT curved-reformat of pancreatic duct.

SPLEEN

The **spleen** is the largest lymph organ in the body composed of lymphoid tissue. The cellular components of the spleen create a highly vascular, spongy parenchyma called **red** and **white pulp**. The red pulp contains large quantities of blood, and the white pulp contains lymphoid tissue and white blood cells. The spleen is an intraperitoneal organ that is covered entirely with peritoneum except at its small bare area at the splenic hilum. It is located posterior to the stomach in the left upper quadrant of the abdomen, protected by the ninth through eleventh ribs (Figures 7.66, 7.67, and 7.87 through 7.89). The spleen is bordered on its medial side by the left kidney, splenic flexure of the colon, and pancreatic tail. The posterior border of the spleen is in contact with the diaphragm, pleura, left lung, and ribs. The spleen is attached to the greater curvature of the stomach and the left kidney by the **gastrosplenic** and **lienorenal ligaments**, respectively (Figure 7.87). The spleen receives its arterial blood from the splenic artery and is drained via the splenic vein. The splenic artery and vein enter and exit the spleen at the splenic hilum between the gastric and renal depressions (Figures 7.88 and 7.89). The spleen is a highly vascular organ that functions to produce white blood cells, filter abnormal blood cells from the blood, store iron from red blood cells, and initiate the immune response. Normal splenic parenchyma is homogeneous; however, immediately after intravenous contrast injection, the spleen can have a heterogeneous appearance on early arterial phase images (Figure 7.89).

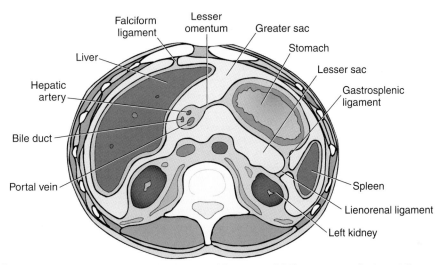

FIGURE 7.87 Axial view of the abdomen with greater and lesser sac, falciform, gastrosplenic, and lienorenal ligaments.

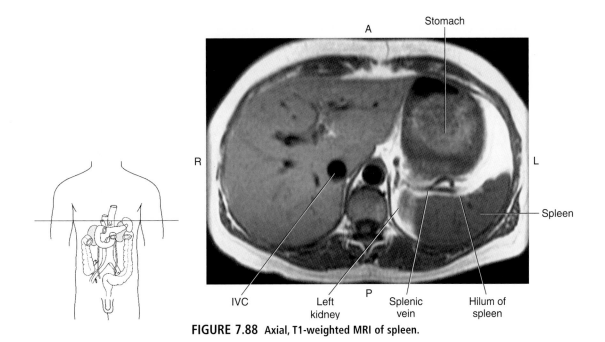

FIGURE 7.88 Axial, T1-weighted MRI of spleen.

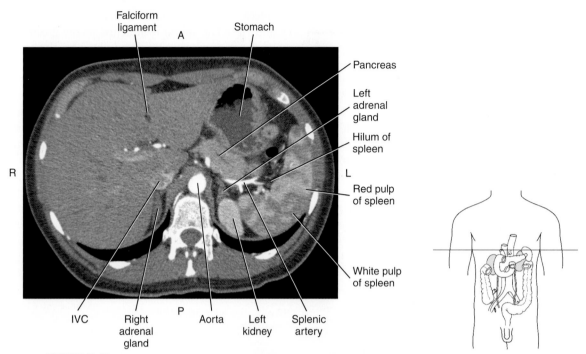

FIGURE 7.89 Axial CT of spleen, early arterial phase demonstrating heterogenous contrast enhancement.

ADRENAL GLANDS

The paired **adrenal (suprarenal) glands** are retroperitoneal organs located superior to each kidney (Figures 7.90 and 7.91). They are separated from the superior surface of the kidneys by **perirenal fat** and are enclosed, along with the kidneys, by **renal fascia (Gerota's fascia)** (Figures 7.26 and 7.92). The **right adrenal gland** is located just posterior to the IVC, medial to the posterior segment of the right hepatic lobe, and lateral to the right crus of the diaphragm. It is generally lower and more medial than the left adrenal gland and commonly appears as an inverted V in cross-section

(Figures 7.93 through 7.95). The **left adrenal gland** lies anteromedial to the upper pole of the left kidney. It is located in a triangle formed by the aorta, pancreatic tail, and left kidney (Figure 7.96). It commonly appears as a triangular or Y-shaped configuration (Figures 7.97 and 7.98). The posterior surfaces of both the right and left glands border the **crus** of the diaphragm. Each adrenal gland has an outer cortex and an inner medulla, which function independently (Figure 7.90). The **adrenal cortex** produces more than two dozen steroids, collectively called adrenocortical steroids or just corticosteroids. The corticosteroids are

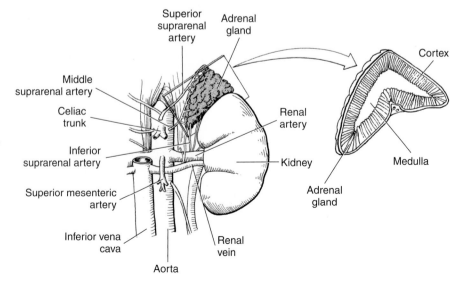

FIGURE 7.90 Anterior view of adrenal glands.

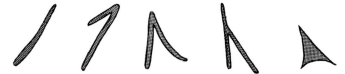

FIGURE 7.91 Axial view with common configurations of adrenal glands.

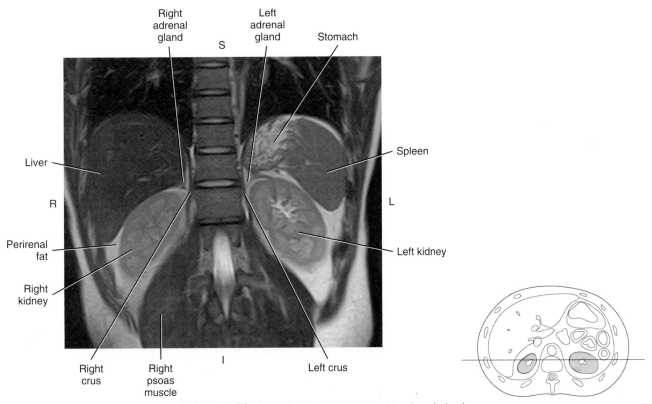

FIGURE 7.92 Coronal, T2-weighted MRI with adrenal glands.

broken into three main categories: glucocorticoids, which affect glucose metabolism; mineralocorticoids, which regulate sodium and potassium levels; and androgens and estrogens, which are responsible for promoting normal development of bone and reproductive organs. The adrenal medulla produces the hormones epinephrine and norepinephrine, which accelerate metabolism and increase energy and are responsible for the body's "fight or flight" response. The adrenal glands receive arterial blood from the superior, middle, and inferior suprarenal arteries. The drainage of the right gland is via a short suprarenal vein that empties directly into the IVC. The left gland is drained by the left suprarenal vein, which empties into the left renal vein.

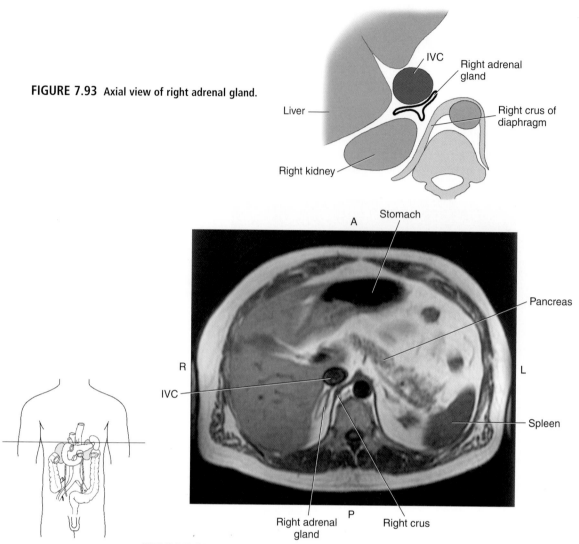

FIGURE 7.93 Axial view of right adrenal gland.

FIGURE 7.94 Axial, T1-weighted MRI of right adrenal gland.

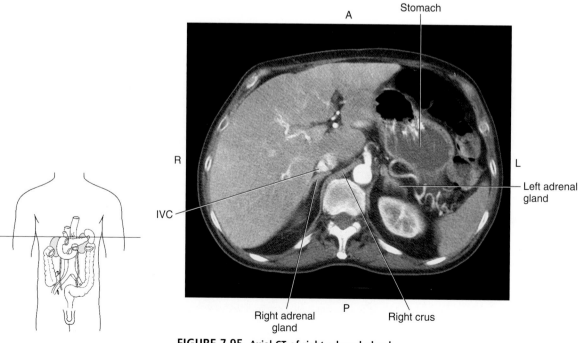

FIGURE 7.95 Axial CT of right adrenal gland.

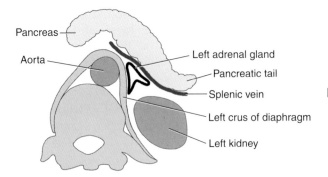

FIGURE 7.96 Axial view of left adrenal gland.

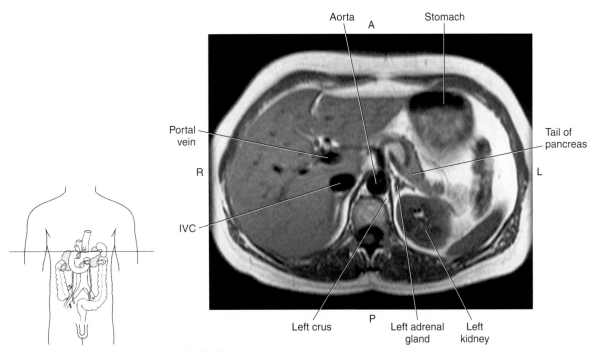

FIGURE 7.97 Axial, T1-weighted MRI of left adrenal gland.

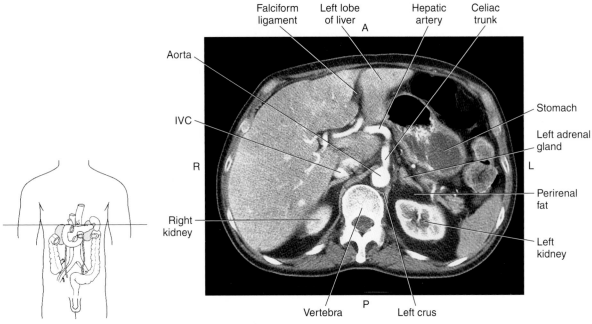

FIGURE 7.98 Axial CT of left adrenal gland.

URINARY SYSTEM

The structures of the urinary system include the kidneys, ureters, bladder, and urethra. Those that are located within the abdomen are the kidneys and ureters (Figure 7.99). The bladder and urethra are located in the pelvis and are discussed in Chapter 8. The **kidneys** are retroperitoneal bean-shaped organs that lie against the posterior abdominal wall on either side of the vertebral column (Figures 7.98 and 7.100). They lie at an oblique orientation, with the upper poles more medial and posterior than the lower poles. They are located on each side of the spine between T12 and L4 and are embedded in **perirenal fat** (Figure 7.101). The right kidney is usually slightly lower due to displacement by the liver (Figures 7.102 and 7.103). Each kidney is composed of an outer cortex and an inner medulla. The **renal cortex** comprises the outer one third of the renal tissue and has extensions between the renal pyramids of the medulla. The cortex contains the functional subunit of the kidney, the **nephron,** which consists of the **glomerulus** and **convoluted tubules** and is responsible for filtration of urine (Figure 7.104). The **renal medulla** consists of segments called **renal pyramids** that radiate from the renal

sinus to the outer surface of the kidney. The striated-appearing pyramids contain the **loops of Henle** and collecting tubules and function as the beginning of the collecting system. Arising from the renal papilla are the cup-shaped minor calyces (Figure 7.104). Each kidney has 7 to 14 **minor calyces** that merge into 2 or 3 **major calyces.** The major calyces join to form the **renal pelvis,** which is the largest dilated portion of the collecting system and is continuous with the ureters (Figure 7.104). The fat-filled cavity surrounding the renal pelvis is called the renal sinus.

Surrounding the kidneys and perirenal fat is another protective layer called the **renal fascia (Gerota's fascia).** The renal fascia functions to anchor the kidneys to surrounding structures in an attempt to prevent bumps and jolts to the body from injuring the kidneys. In addition, the renal fascia acts as a barrier, limiting the spread of infection that may arise from the kidneys. The medial indentation in the kidney is called the **hilum;** it allows the renal artery and vein and ureters to enter and exit the kidney (Figures 7.99, and 7.105 through 7.108). The kidneys can be divided into five segments according to their vascular supply: **apical, anterosuperior (upper anterior), anteroinferior (middle inferior), inferior,** and

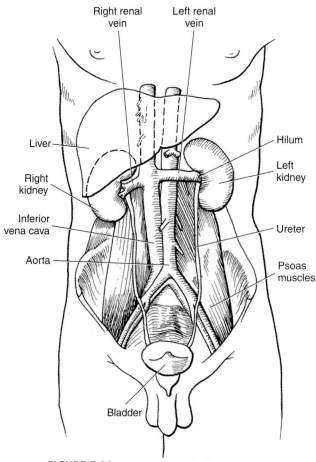

FIGURE 7.99 Anterior view of urinary system.

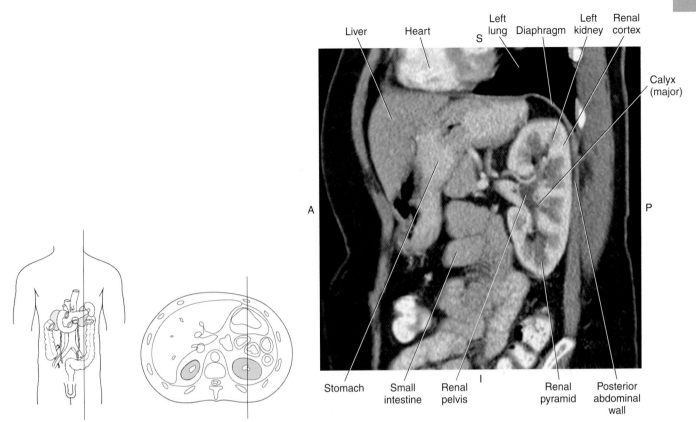

FIGURE 7.100 Sagittal CT reformat of left kidney.

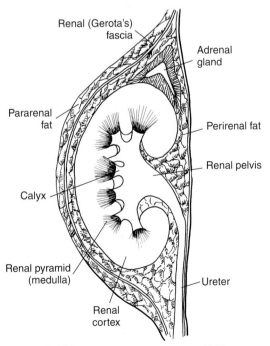

FIGURE 7.101 Coronal midsection view of kidney.

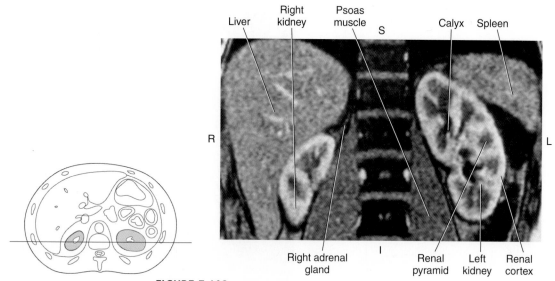

FIGURE 7.102 Coronal, T1-weighted MRI of kidneys.

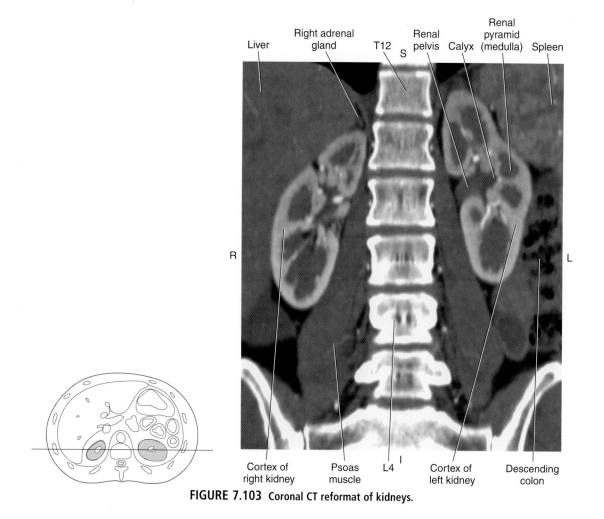

FIGURE 7.103 Coronal CT reformat of kidneys.

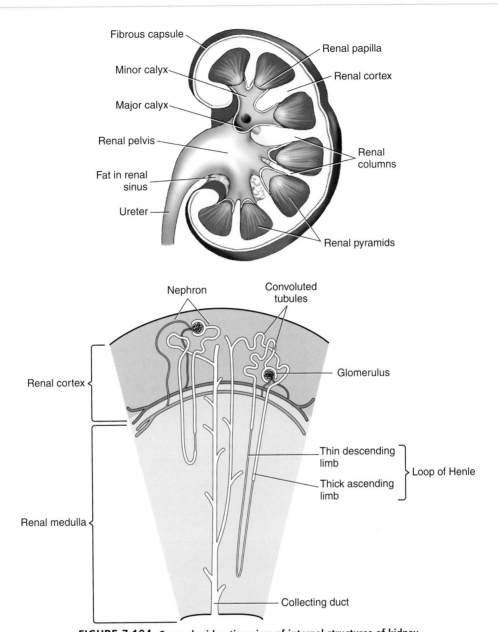

FIGURE 7.104 Coronal midsection view of internal structures of kidney.

posterior (Figure 7.109). The segmental classification helps with surgical planning for partial nephrectomies. The **ureters** are paired muscular tubes that transport urine to the urinary bladder. Each ureter originates at the renal pelvis and descends anteriorly and medially toward the psoas muscles, just anterior to the transverse processes of the lumbar spine (Figures 7.108 through 7.110). The ureters then enter the posterior wall of the bladder at an oblique angle (Figure 7.111). The primary functions of the urinary system are to filter blood, produce and excrete urine, and help maintain normal body physiology.

Renal agenesis is the failure of kidney formation during fetal development resulting in the absence of one or both kidneys. Unilateral renal agenesis may be asymptomatic and is often incidentally diagnosed by abdominal CT or ultrasound. Bilateral renal agenesis is invariably fatal.

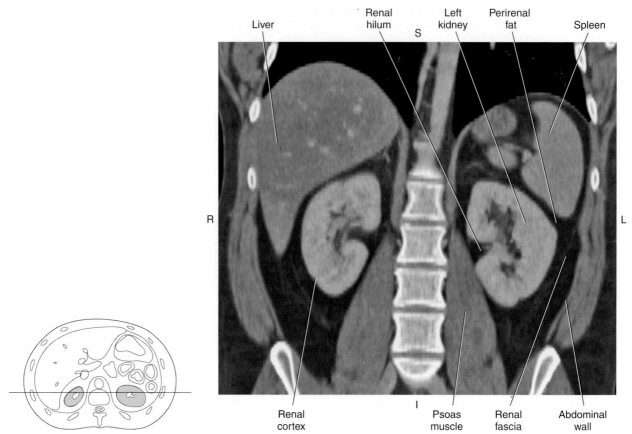

FIGURE 7.105 Coronal CT reformat of kidneys in nephrogram phase.

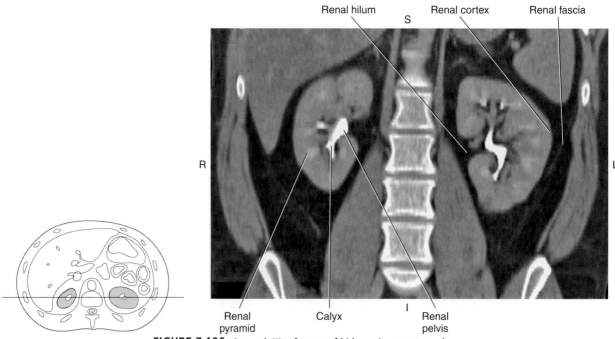

FIGURE 7.106 Coronal CT reformat of kidneys in excretory phase.

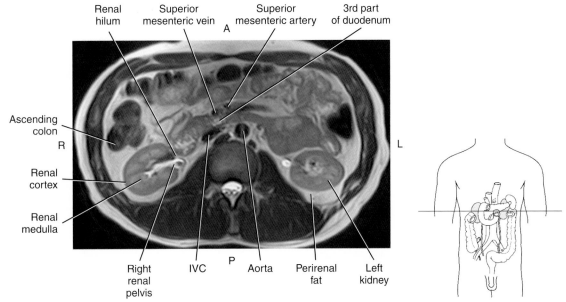

FIGURE 7.107 Axial, T1-weighted MRI of kidney.

Labels (clockwise): Renal hilum, Superior mesenteric vein, Superior mesenteric artery, 3rd part of duodenum, A, L, Ascending colon, R, Renal cortex, Renal medulla, Right renal pelvis, IVC, P, Aorta, Perirenal fat, Left kidney

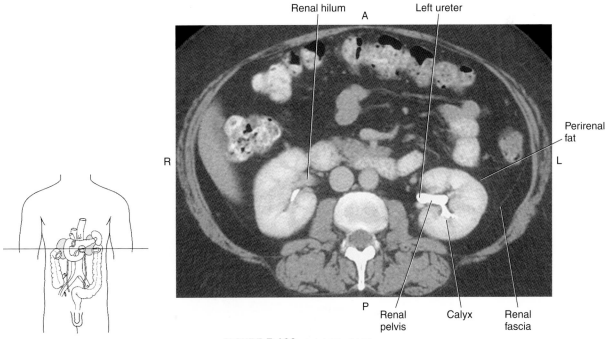

FIGURE 7.108 Axial CT of kidney.

Labels: Renal hilum, A, Left ureter, Perirenal fat, R, L, P, Renal pelvis, Calyx, Renal fascia

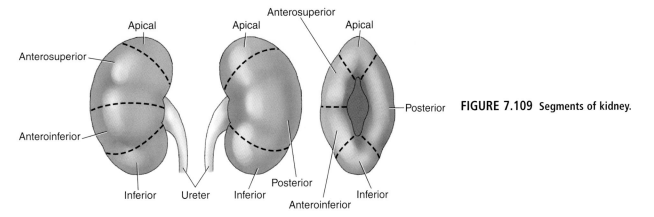

FIGURE 7.109 Segments of kidney.

Labels: Apical, Apical, Anterosuperior, Apical, Anterosuperior, Posterior, Anteroinferior, Inferior, Ureter, Inferior, Posterior, Anteroinferior, Inferior

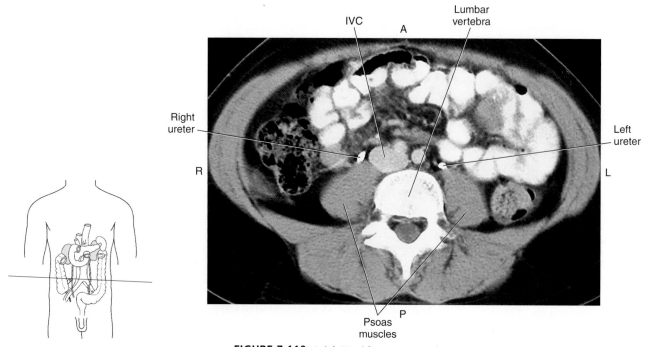

FIGURE 7.110 Axial CT with ureters.

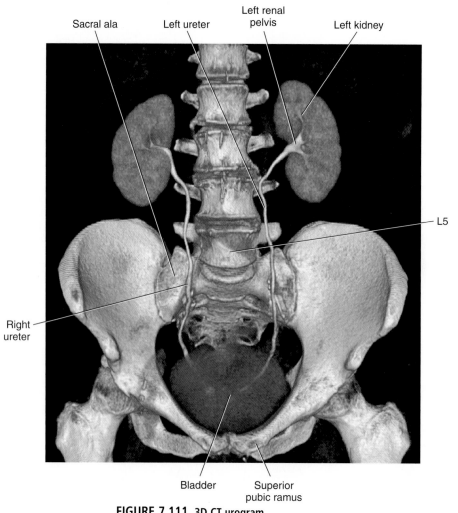

FIGURE 7.111 3D CT urogram.

STOMACH

The **stomach** is the dilated portion of the digestive system that acts as a food reservoir and is responsible for the early stages of digestion. It has four major functions: (1) storage of food, (2) mechanical breakdown of food, (3) dissolution of chemical bonds via acids and enzymes, and (4) production of intrinsic factor. The stomach is located under the left dome of the diaphragm, with the superior portion joining the esophagus at the **cardiac orifice** (cardiac sphincter), creating the **gastroesophageal junction** (Figures 7.112 through 7.115). The stomach has two borders called the **lesser** and **greater curvatures.** Between the two curvatures is the largest portion of the stomach, termed the **body** (Figures 7.116 through 7.118). On the superior surface of the body is a rounded surface called the **fundus** (Figures 7.114 and 7.115). The inferior portion (**pyloric antrum**) empties into the duodenum through the **pyloric sphincter** (Figures 7.118 and 7.119). The anterior surface is in contact with the diaphragm, anterior abdominal wall, and left lobe of the liver. Located posterior to the stomach is the gastric portion of the spleen, the left adrenal gland and kidney, and the body and tail of the pancreas. When empty, the inner surface of the stomach creates prominent folds called **rugae,** which allow the stomach to expand with the ingestion of food (Figures 7.112 and 7.115). The stomach is one of the most vascular organs within the body. The arterial blood is supplied by branches of the gastric, splenic, and gastroduodenal arteries (Figure 7.58). Venous drainage corresponds to the arterial supply. The gastric veins usually drain directly into the portal vein or into the superior mesenteric vein.

The average adult produces 2 to 3 liters per day of gastric juices, which contain mucus, hydrochloric acid, intrinsic factor, and the digestive enzymes pepsinogen and lipase. The stomach can hold up to 3 liters of food, which is mixed with digestive juices to form chyme.

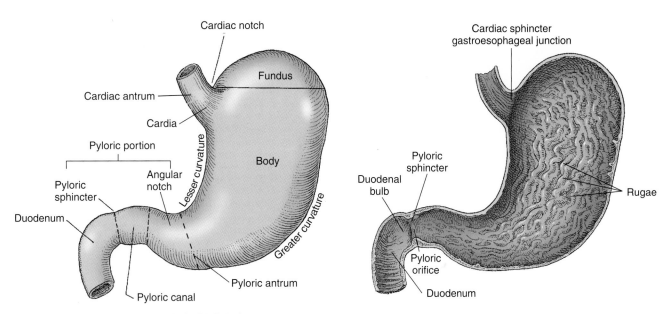

FIGURE 7.112 Stomach. Left, Anterior surface. Right, Internal surface.

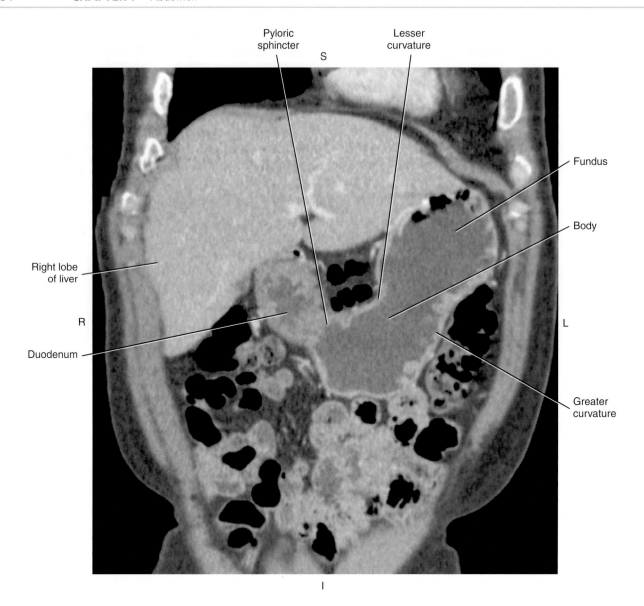

Pyloric sphincter

Lesser curvature

S

Fundus

Body

Right lobe of liver

R

L

Duodenum

Greater curvature

I

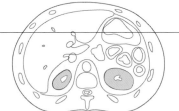

FIGURE 7.113 Coronal CT reformat of stomach.

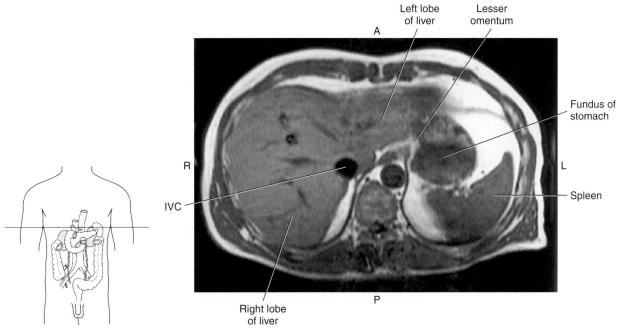

FIGURE 7.114 Axial, T1-weighted MRI of stomach.

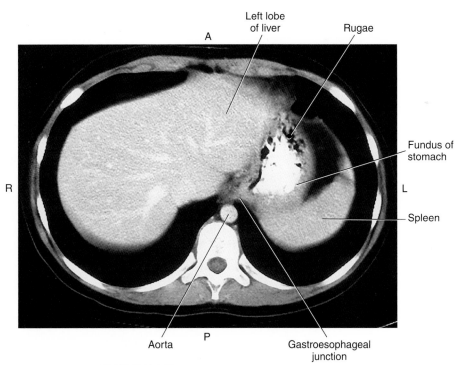

FIGURE 7.115 Axial CT of gastroesophageal junction.

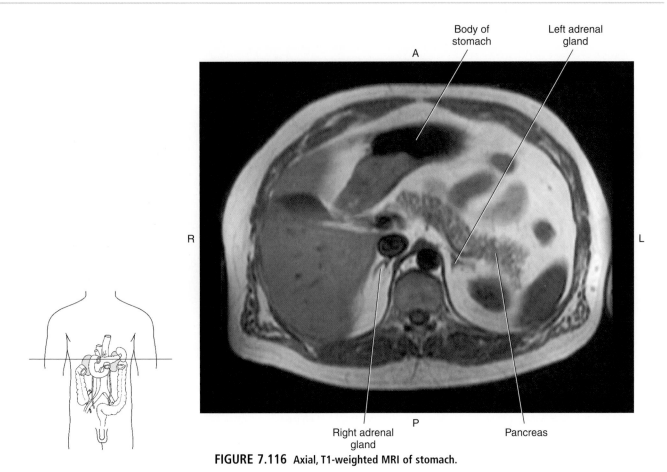

FIGURE 7.116 Axial, T1-weighted MRI of stomach.

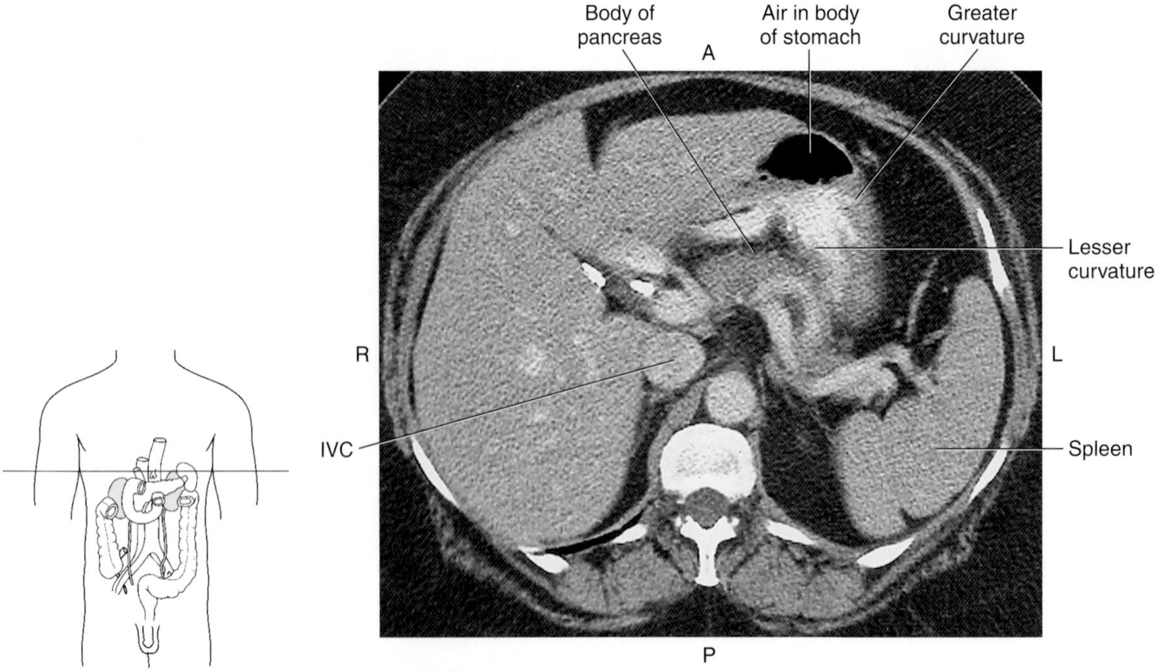

FIGURE 7.117 Axial CT of stomach.

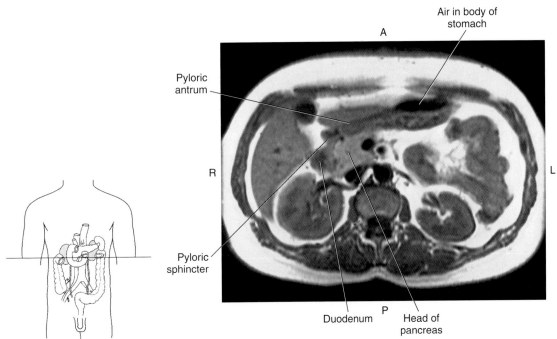

FIGURE 7.118 Axial, T1-weighted MRI of pyloric antrum and pyloric sphincter.

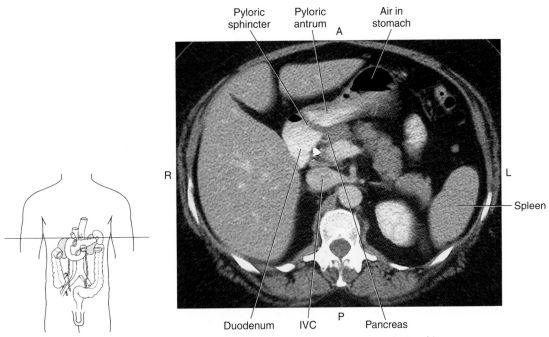

FIGURE 7.119 Axial CT of stomach with pyloric antrum and pyloric sphincter.

INTESTINES

The **small intestine (small bowel)** is located between the pylorus and ileocecal valve and consists of loops of bowel averaging 6 to 7 meters in length. It can be subdivided into the duodenum, jejunum, and the ileum (Figures 7.120 and 7.121). The proximal portion of the small intestine is the **duodenum**, which begins at the gastric pylorus and curves around the head of the pancreas, forming the letter C (Figures 7.118 through 7.122). The duodenum is mostly retroperitoneal, making it less mobile than the rest of the small intestine. Although quite short, the duodenum is divided into four portions. The **first (superior) portion** is formed by the first 2 inches of the duodenum, the conical-shaped **duodenal bulb**. It is the most common site for peptic ulcer formation. The **second (descending) portion** is formed by the next 4 inches of duodenum that descends along the right side of the vertebral column; it contains the ampulla of Vater and receives pancreatic and biliary drainage. The **third (horizontal) portion** is about 10 cm long and runs horizontally in front of the third lumbar vertebra. In its horizontal course from right to left, the third portion of the duodenum runs anterior to the IVC, aorta, and inferior mesenteric artery, and posterior to the superior mesenteric artery (Figures 7.123 and 7.124). The **fourth (ascending) portion** is about 2.5cm in length and ascends on the left side of the aorta to the level of the L2 vertebra, where it meets up with the jejunum at the **duodenojejunal flexure**. The duodenojejunal

flexure is fixed in place by the **ligament of Treitz**, a suspensory ligament created from the connective tissue around the celiac axis and left crus of the diaphragm (Figure 7.122). This location marks the entry of the small bowel into the peritoneal cavity. The remainder of the small intestine, the jejunum and ileum, is suspended from the posterior abdominal wall by a fan-shaped mesentery. The **jejunum** is approximately 2.5 meters long and occupies the left upper abdomen or umbilical region of the abdomen (Figures 7.120 through 7.124). This section of small bowel is where the bulk of chemical digestion and nutrient absorption occurs. The jejunum contains numerous circular folds that give it a feathery appearance on barium or computed tomography (CT) examinations. The lower three-fifths of the small intestine, the **ileum**, is the longest portion of the small intestine, averaging 3.5 meters long and located in the right lower abdomen (Figures 7.120, 7.121, and 7.124 through 7.126). It is in the ileum that intrinsic factor from the stomach combines with vitamin B_{12} for absorption in the terminal ileum. Vitamin B_{12} is essential for normal red blood cell (RBC) formation and nervous system function. The loops of ileum terminate at the **ileocecal valve**, a sphincter that controls the flow of material from the ileum into the cecum of the large intestine (Figures 7.120, 7.121, and 7.127). The mesentery serves as a route for blood vessels, lymphatics, and nerves to reach the small intestine. The segments of the small intestine receive blood from branches of the superior mesenteric artery and are drained by branches of the superior mesenteric vein.

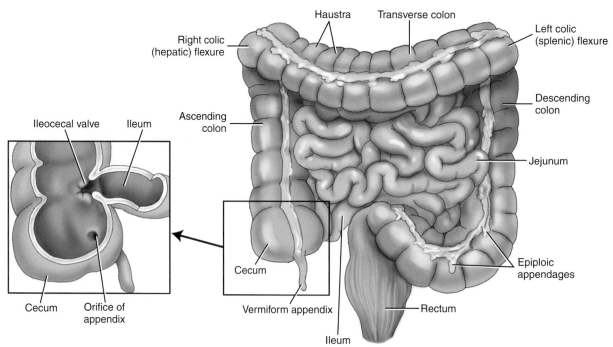

FIGURE 7.120 Anterior view of small bowel.

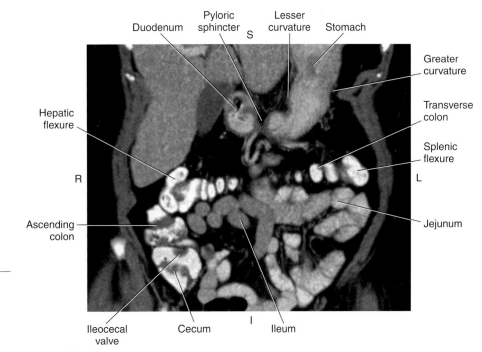

FIGURE 7.121 Coronal CT reformat of small bowel.

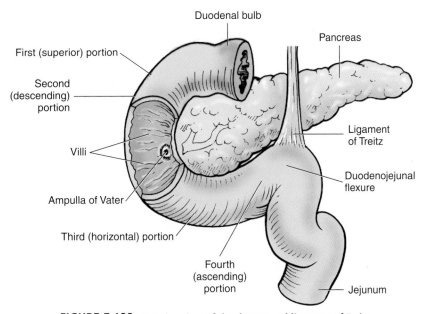

FIGURE 7.122 Anterior view of duodenum and ligament of Treitz.

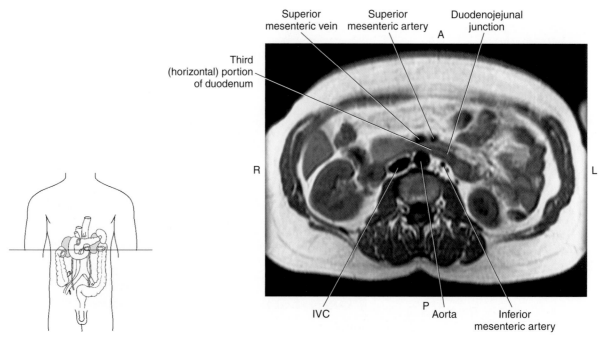

FIGURE 7.123 Axial, T1-weighted MRI at duodenojejunal junction.

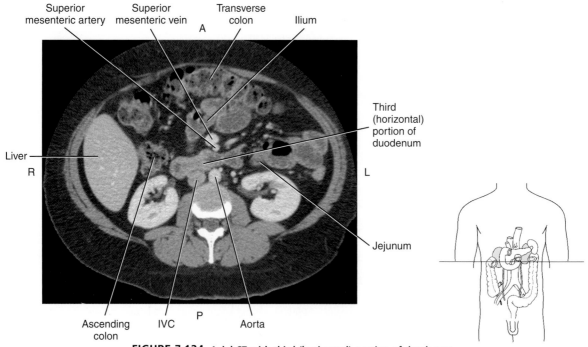

FIGURE 7.124 Axial CT with third (horizontal) portion of duodenum.

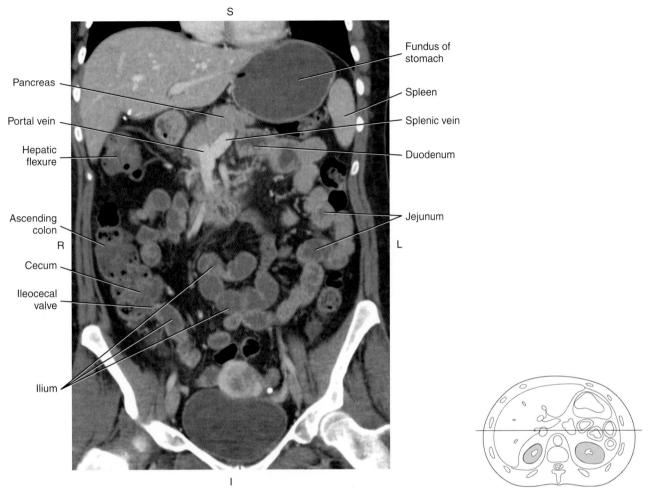

FIGURE 7.125 Coronal CT reformat of small bowel and ileocecal valve.

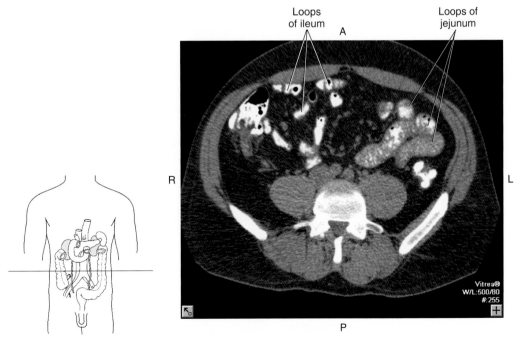

FIGURE 7.126 Axial CT with ileum.

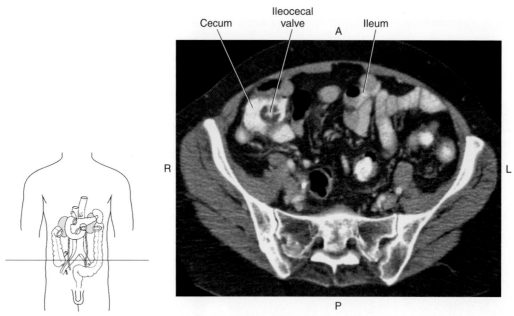

Cecum   Ileocecal valve   Ileum   A

R   L

P

FIGURE 7.127 Axial CT with ileocecal valve.

The **large intestine (large bowel)** lies inferior to the stomach and liver and almost completely frames the small intestine (Figures 7.120 and 7.128). The large intestine has a larger diameter and thinner walls than the small intestine and is approximately 1.5 meters long, starting at the ileocecal junction and ending at the anus. The outer, longitudinal muscle of the large intestine forms three thickened bands called **taenia coli,** which gather the cecum and colon into a series of pouchlike folds called **haustra.** On the outer surface of the large intestine are small fat-filled sacs of omentum called the **epiploic appendages.** The three main divisions of the large intestine are the cecum, colon, and rectum (Figure 7.128). The **cecum** is a pouchlike section of the proximal portion of the large intestine located at the ileocecal valve. The slender **vermiform appendix** attaches to the posteromedial surface of the cecum (Figures 7.128 through 7.130). The **colon** is the longest portion of the

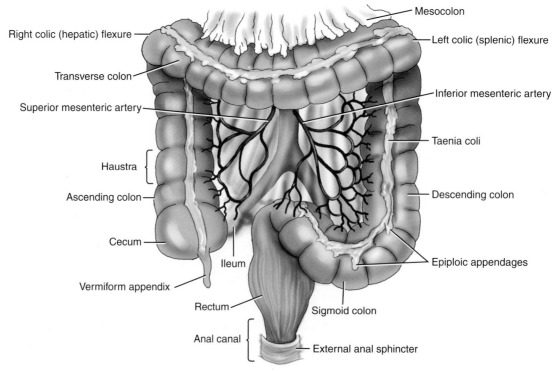

Right colic (hepatic) flexure

Transverse colon

Superior mesenteric artery

Haustra

Ascending colon

Cecum

Vermiform appendix

Ileum

Rectum

Anal canal

Mesocolon

Left colic (splenic) flexure

Inferior mesenteric artery

Taenia coli

Descending colon

Epiploic appendages

Sigmoid colon

External anal sphincter

FIGURE 7.128 Anterior view of large intestine.

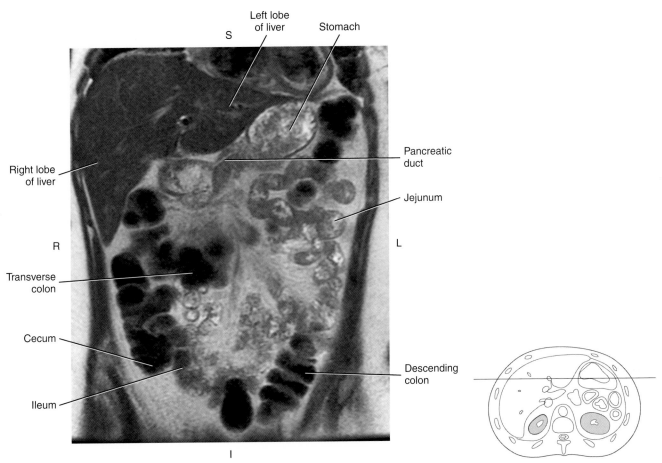

FIGURE 7.129 Coronal, T2-weighted MRI of cecum.

large intestine and can be subdivided into four distinct portions: ascending, transverse, descending, and sigmoid (Figures 7.131 and 7.132). The **ascending colon** is retroperitoneal and commences at the cecum, ascending the right lateral wall of the abdomen to the level of the liver. It then curves sharply to the left, creating the hepatic flexure (Figures 7.128, 7.133, and 7.134). The **hepatic flexure** marks the beginning of the transverse colon. The **transverse colon** travels horizontally across the anterior abdomen toward the spleen, where it bends sharply downward, creating the **splenic flexure** and the beginning of the descending colon (Figures 7.135 and 7.136). The transverse colon is located within the peritoneal cavity and is the largest and most mobile portion of the large intestine, making its position quite variable in the patient. The **descending colon** is retroperitoneal and continues inferiorly along the left lateral abdominal wall to the iliac fossa, where it curves to become the S-shaped sigmoid colon

posterior to the bladder (Figure 7.128). The **sigmoid colon** joins the rectum, which is the terminal portion of the colon (Figures 7.137 and 7.138). The rectum is considered a pelvic organ and is covered in greater detail in Chapter 8. The superior and inferior mesenteric arteries and veins supply and drain blood from the large intestine. The major functions of the large intestine include reabsorption of water and the storage and elimination of fecal material.

When the epiploic appendages become inflamed due to torsion or ischemia it results in a condition called epiploic appendagitis. The condition commonly presents with acute lower quadrant pain, which can simulate appendicitis or diverticulitis. Epiploic appendagitis can occur at any age but is more common in the 3rd through 5th decades. Treatment is somewhat controversial but conservative therapy is generally favored since it is typically a self-limiting condition.

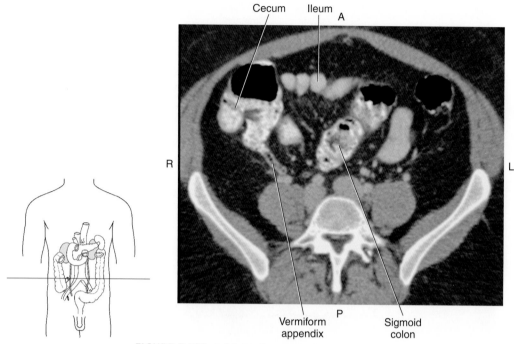

FIGURE 7.130 Axial CT of cecum and appendix.

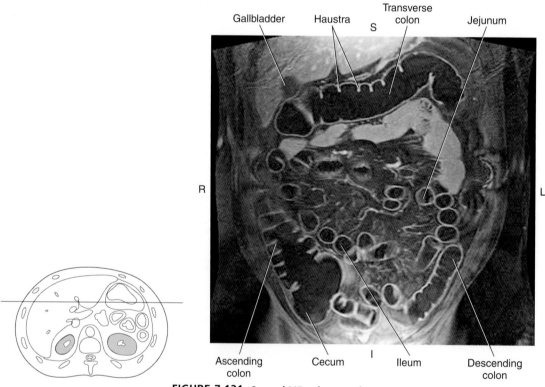

FIGURE 7.131 Coronal MR colonography.

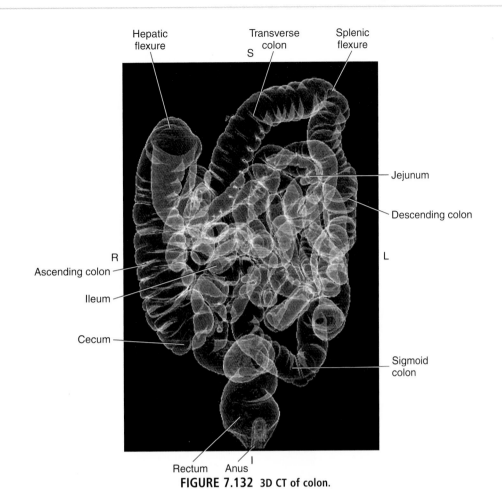

FIGURE 7.132 3D CT of colon.

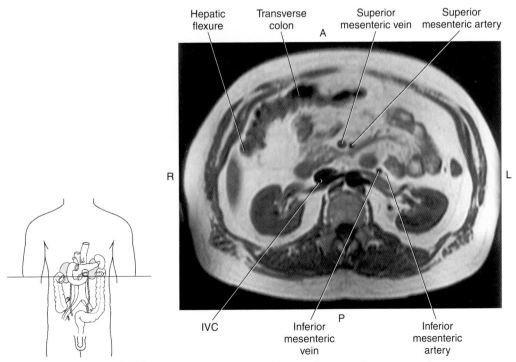

FIGURE 7.133 Axial, T1-weighted MRI of hepatic flexure and transverse colon.

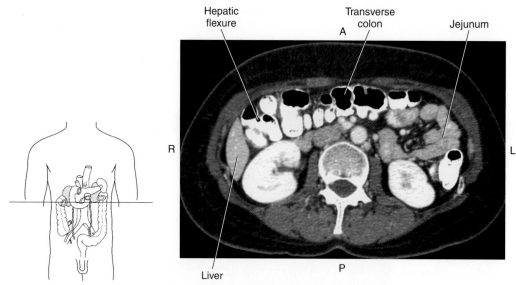

FIGURE 7.134 Axial CT of hepatic flexure and transverse colon.

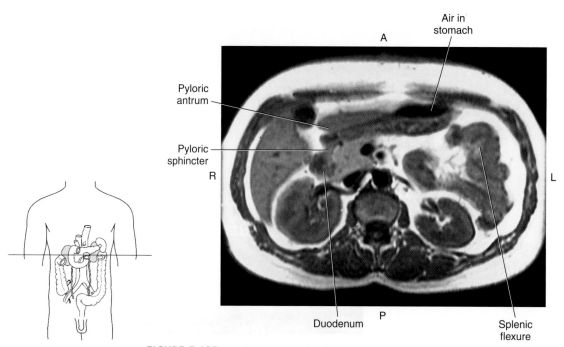

FIGURE 7.135 Axial, T1-weighted MRI of splenic flexure.

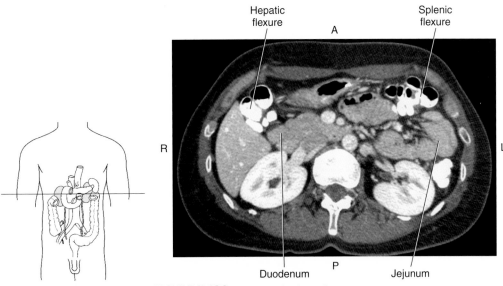

FIGURE 7.136 Axial CT of splenic flexure.

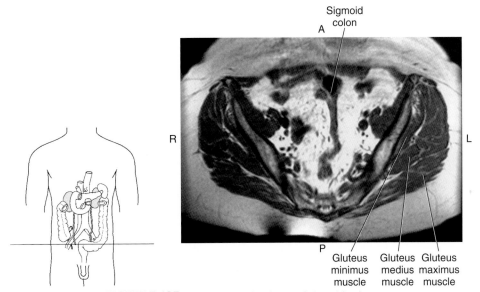

FIGURE 7.137 Axial, T1-weighted MRI of sigmoid colon.

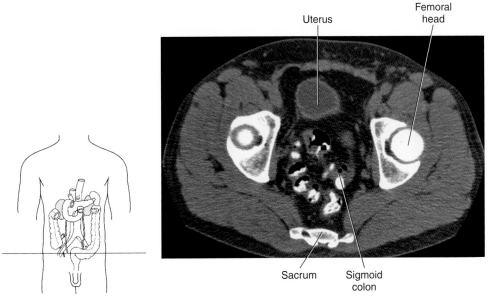

FIGURE 7.138 Axial CT of sigmoid colon.

ABDOMINAL AORTA AND BRANCHES

The **abdominal aorta** is a retroperitoneal structure beginning, as an extension of the thoracic aorta, at the aortic hiatus of the diaphragm. The abdominal aorta gradually diminishes in diameter as it descends the abdomen just left of the midline next to the vertebral bodies. It delivers blood to all the abdominopelvic organs and structures. At approximately the level of L4, the abdominal aorta bifurcates into the right and left **common iliac** arteries. The branches of the abdominal aorta can be divided into the paired branches, including the inferior phrenic, lumbar, suprarenal, renal, and gonadal arteries; and unpaired branches, which include the celiac trunk, splenic, superior mesenteric, and inferior mesenteric arteries (Figures 7.139 through 7.142). Each of these branches has a typical configuration that is described within this text; however, many normal variations of these vessels may occur.

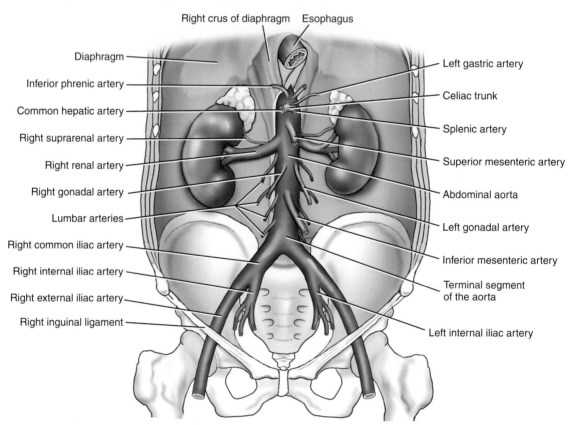

FIGURE 7.139 Anterior view of abdominal aorta.

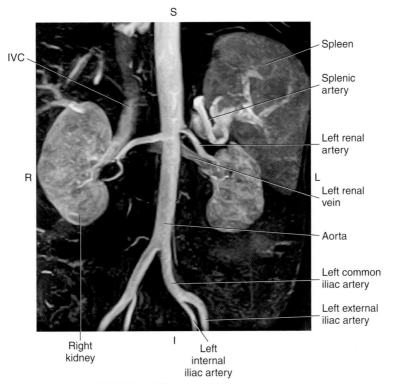

S

IVC

Spleen

Splenic
artery

Left renal
artery

R

L

Left renal
vein

Aorta

Left common
iliac artery

Left external
iliac artery

Right
kidney

I

Left
internal
iliac artery

FIGURE 7.140 MRA of abdominal aorta.

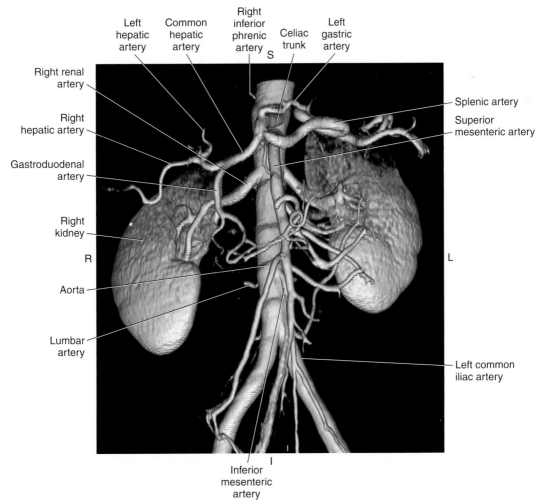

Left
hepatic
artery

Common
hepatic
artery

Right
inferior
phrenic
artery

S

Celiac
trunk

Left
gastric
artery

Right renal
artery

Splenic artery

Superior
mesenteric artery

Right
hepatic artery

Gastroduodenal
artery

Right
kidney

R

L

Aorta

Lumbar
artery

Left common
iliac artery

I

Inferior
mesenteric
artery

FIGURE 7.141 CD CTA of abdominal aorta.

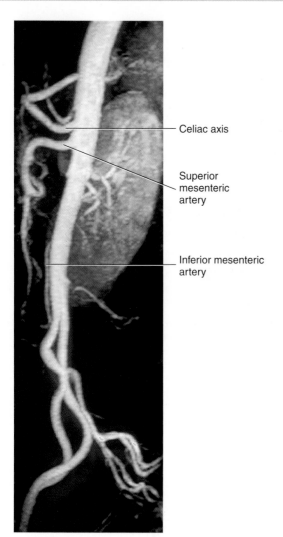

FIGURE 7.142 Sagittal MRA of abdominal aorta.

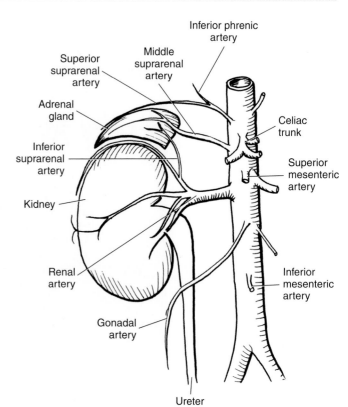

FIGURE 7.143 **Anterior view of paired branches of the abdominal aorta.**

Paired Branches

Inferior Phrenic Arteries The paired **inferior phrenic arteries** are the first to branch from the lateral surface of the abdominal aorta just as it descends through the aortic hiatus. The **right inferior phrenic artery** passes upward on the right side behind the IVC, and the **left inferior phrenic artery** passes behind the stomach and the abdominal part of the esophagus (Figures 7.139, 7.141, and 7.143). The inferior phrenic arteries extend to supply the inferior surface of the diaphragm.

Lumbar Arteries Four pairs of **lumbar arteries** arise from the posterior wall of the abdominal aorta at the level of L1-L4 (Figures 7.139 and 7.141). The lumbar arteries supply the posterior abdominal wall, lumbar vertebrae, and the inferior end of the spinal cord.

Suprarenal Arteries The **middle suprarenal arteries** exit the lateral walls of the aorta near the base of the superior mesenteric artery. These arteries course laterally and slightly superiorly to supply the adrenal glands. The **superior suprarenal** arteries are branches of the inferior

phrenic arteries, and the **inferior suprarenal arteries** extend from the renal arteries (Figures 7.90 and 7.143).

Renal Arteries The two large **renal arteries** arise from the lateral walls of the aorta just below the superior mesenteric artery. Each vessel travels horizontally to the hilum of the corresponding kidney (Figures 7.139 through 7.141). Because of the position of the aorta on the left side of the vertebral column, the right renal artery is slightly longer than the left renal artery. The right renal artery passes posterior to the IVC and right renal vein on its course to the right kidney (Figure 7.144). Typically, the left kidney is higher than the right kidney, which means the left renal artery is generally slightly superior to the right (Figure 7.145). As each renal artery reaches the renal hilum, it typically divides into anterior and posterior branches from which five segmental arteries—**apical, upper, middle, lower, and posterior**—arise (Figures 7.146 through 7.148). Each segmental artery further divides into interlobar arteries, one for each pyramid and adjoining cortex. As the interlobar arteries curve over the renal pyramids they become the arcuate arteries from which the interlobular arteries arise to supply the renal cortex (Figure 7.146).

 Renal artery stenosis causes renal ischemia and can result in secondary hypertension.

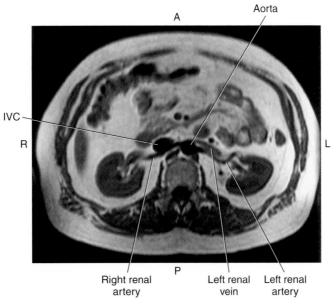

FIGURE 7.144 Axial, T1-weighted MRI of abdomen with renal arteries and veins.

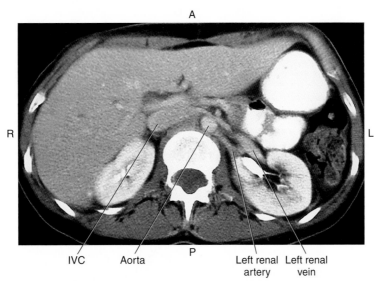

FIGURE 7.145 Axial CT of abdomen with renal arteries and veins.

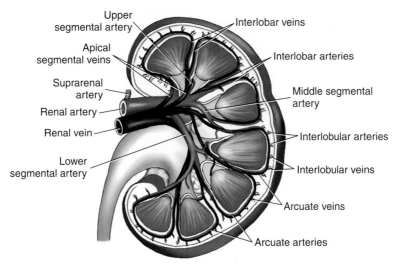

FIGURE 7.146 Anterior view of renal vasculature.

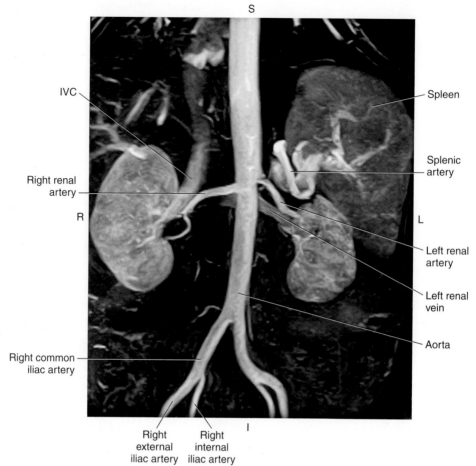

FIGURE 7.147 MRA of renal arteries.

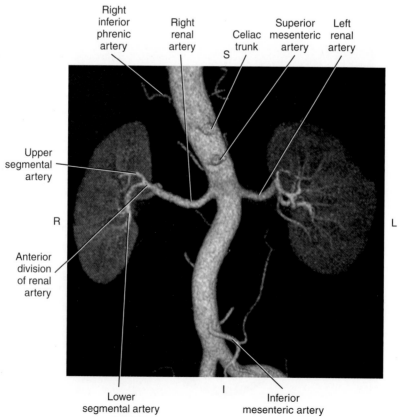

FIGURE 7.148 CTA of renal arteries.

Gonadal Arteries The **gonadal arteries** originate from the anterior wall of the aorta just inferior to the renal arteries. They descend along the psoas muscles to reach their respective organs (Figures 7.139, 7.149, and 7.150).

In the male, the gonadal arteries are termed the **testicular arteries,** which supply the testes and scrotum, whereas the gonadal arteries in the female are termed the **ovarian arteries,** which supply the ovaries, uterine tubes, and uterus.

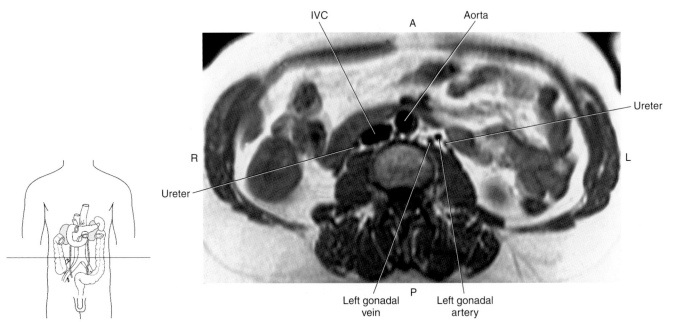

FIGURE 7.149 Axial, T1-weighted MRI of abdomen and gonadal arteries and veins.

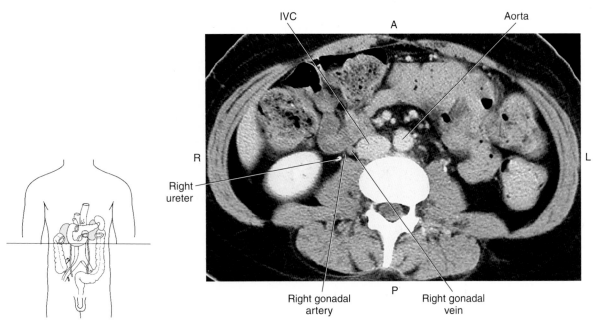

FIGURE 7.150 Axial CT of abdomen and gonadal arteries and veins.

Unpaired Branches

Celiac Trunk The **celiac trunk** is a very short vessel that leaves the anterior wall of the aorta just after the aorta passes through the diaphragm. The short celiac trunk divides into three branches: left gastric, common hepatic, and splenic arteries (Figures 7.151 through 7.153). Variations of the celiac trunk are not rare; occasionally, the hepatic artery will branch from the superior mesenteric artery.

The **left gastric artery** courses superiorly and leftward within the lesser omentum to supply the cardiac region of the stomach, then passes along the lesser curvature toward the pylorus, giving off esophageal and gastric branches to supply the abdominal esophagus and adjacent anterior and posterior walls of the body of the stomach. The left gastric artery continues toward the right to anastomose with the right gastric artery, which is a branch of the hepatic artery (Figures 7.151, and 7.154 through 7.157).

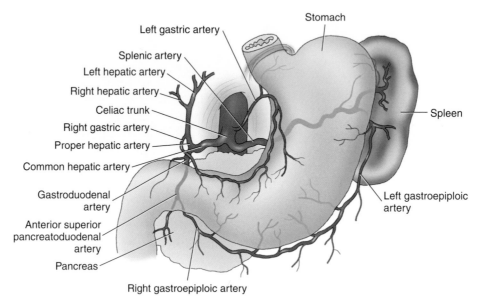

FIGURE 7.151 Anterior view of celiac trunk and branches.

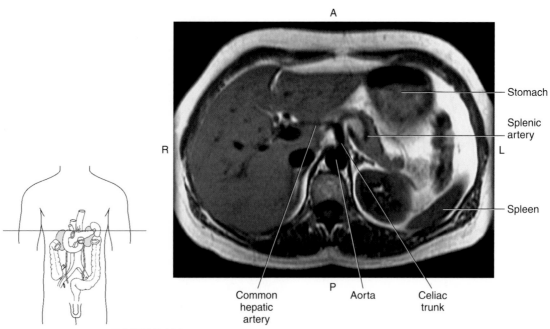

FIGURE 7.152 Axial, T1-weighted MRI of abdomen with celiac trunk.

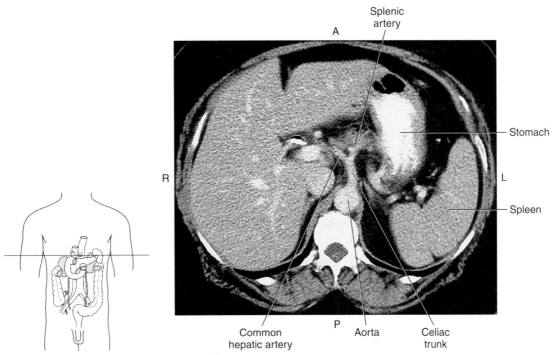

FIGURE 7.153 Axial CT of abdomen with celiac trunk.

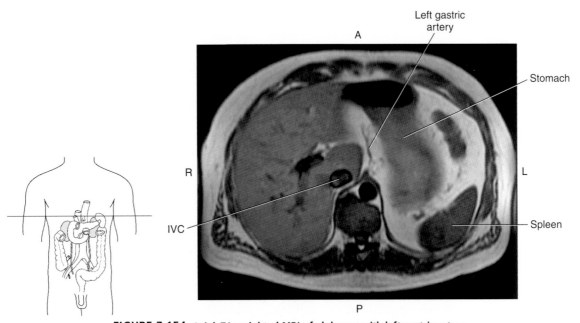

FIGURE 7.154 Axial, T1-weighted MRI of abdomen with left gastric artery.

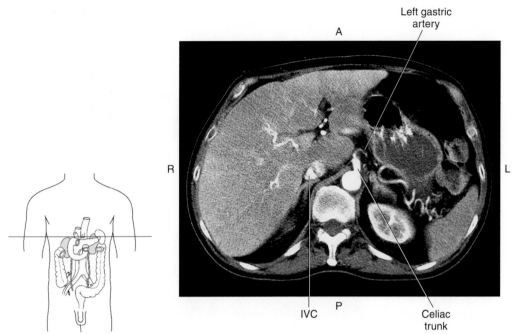

FIGURE 7.155 Axial CT of abdomen with left gastric artery.

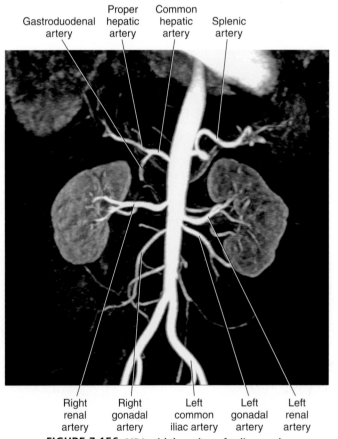

FIGURE 7.156 MRA with branches of celiac trunk.

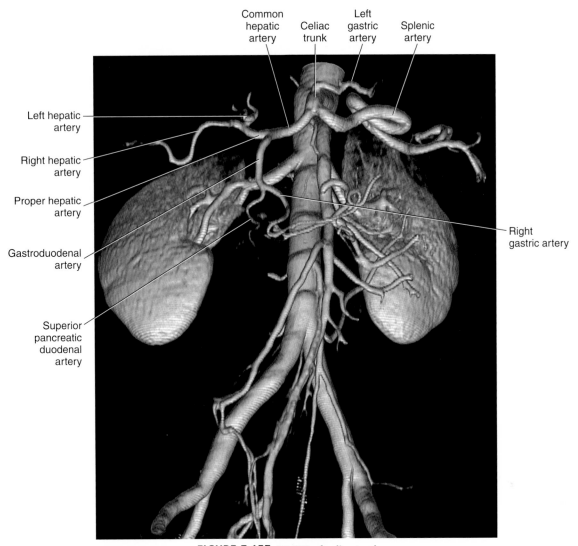

Common
hepatic
artery

Celiac
trunk

Left
gastric
artery

Splenic
artery

Left hepatic
artery

Right hepatic
artery

Proper hepatic
artery

Gastroduodenal
artery

Superior
pancreatic
duodenal
artery

Right
gastric artery

FIGURE 7.157 3D CTA of celiac trunk.

The **common hepatic artery** crosses to the right toward the superior aspect of the duodenum and divides into the **hepatic artery proper** and the **gastroduodenal artery** (Figures 7.151 through 7.153, 7.156, and 7.157). The hepatic artery proper ascends obliquely to the right in the hepatoduodenal ligament, adjacent to the portal vein and CBD, and divides near the porta hepatis into the **right** and **left hepatic** branches, and usually gives off the **right gastric artery** (Figures 7.151, 7.156, and 7.157). The right hepatic branch dispatches the **cystic artery** to the gallbladder and divides into the anterior and posterior segmental arteries to supply the segments of the right and caudate lobes of the liver. The left branch also gives off an artery to the caudate lobe, as well as medial and lateral segmental arteries to supply the segments of the left lobe and the intermediate branch to the quadrate lobe. The **right gastric artery**, which can also come from the common hepatic or gastroduodenal

arteries, supplies the lower part of the lesser curvature of the stomach and anastomoses with the left gastric artery within the lesser curvature of the stomach (Figures 7.151 and 7.157). The **gastroduodenal artery** descends behind the pylorus to give off many branches, including the **anterior and posterior superior pancreaticoduodenal arteries**, which supply the superior part of the duodenum and head of the pancreas, and the **right gastroepiploic (gastro-omental) artery**. The right gastroepiploic artery passes through the greater omentum, anastomoses with the left gastroepiploic artery on the inferior surface of the greater curvature, and dispatches numerous gastric branches to the anterior and posterior walls of the pyloric and body portions of the stomach (Figures 7.151, and 7.156 through 7.158).

The **splenic (lienal) artery** is the largest branch of the celiac trunk and passes to the left behind the stomach and along the upper border of the pancreas, within

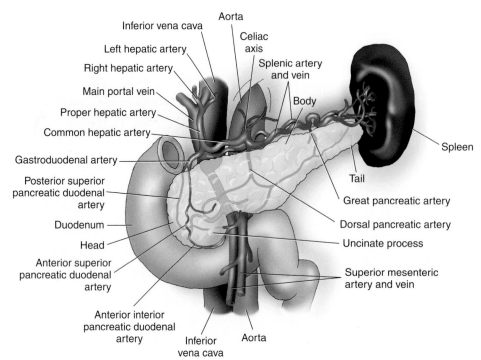

FIGURE 7.158 Anterior view of hepatic artery, CBD, and portal vein.

the splenorenal ligament, to the hilum of the spleen. At the point where the splenic artery courses near the border of the pancreas, it gives off numerous **pancreatic branches** including the **dorsal, great,** and **caudal pancreatic arteries** that supply the body and tail of the pancreas (Figure 7.159). Just before the splenic artery terminates into numerous splenic branches, it gives rise to the **left gastroepiploic (gastro-omental) artery,** which gives off epiploic and gastric branches to the greater omentum and anterior and posterior walls of the fundus of the stomach (Figures 7.151, and 7.156 through 7.161).

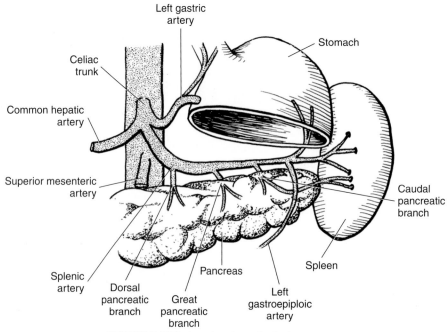

FIGURE 7.159 Anterior view of splenic artery.

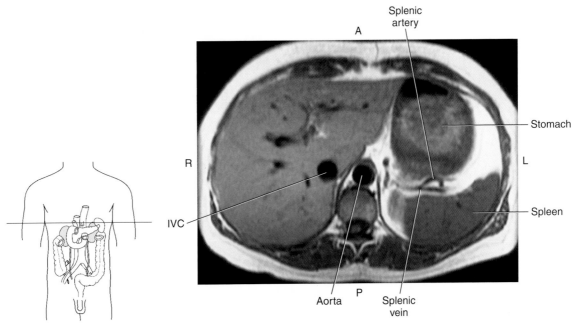

FIGURE 7.160 Axial, T1-weighted MRI of splenic artery.

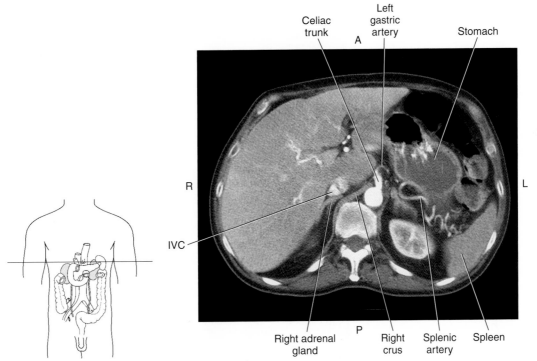

FIGURE 7.161 Axial CT of splenic artery.

Superior Mesenteric Artery The large **superior mesenteric artery (SMA)** emerges just below the celiac trunk at approximately the level of L1 (Figures 7.139, 7.162, and 7.163). It descends behind the body of the pancreas, then over the horizontal portion of the duodenum to course in the mesentery to the ileum (Figures 7.162, 7.164, and 7.167). The artery supplies the head of the pancreas and the majority of the small and large intestines. Branches of the superior mesenteric artery include the inferior pancreaticoduodenal artery, jejunal arteries, ileal arteries, middle colic artery, right colic artery, and ileocolic artery

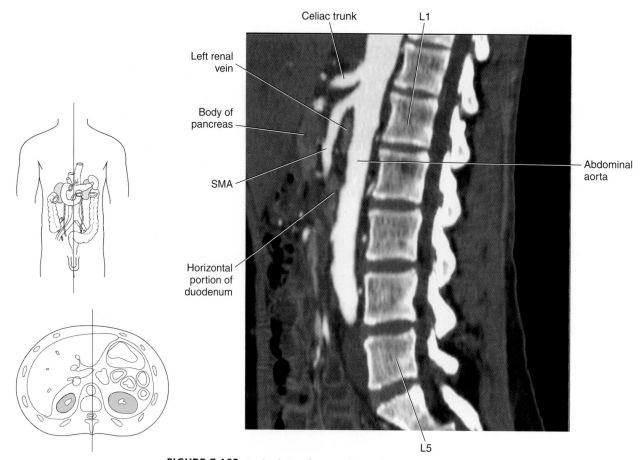

FIGURE 7.162 Sagittal CT reformat of superior mesenteric artery.

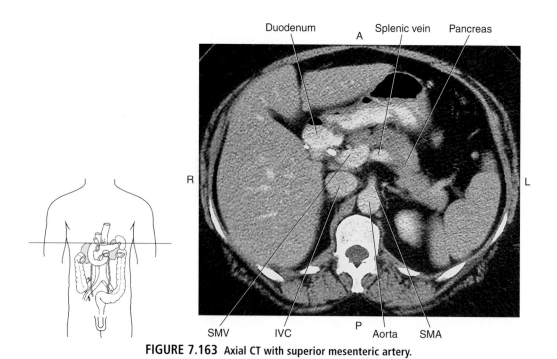

FIGURE 7.163 Axial CT with superior mesenteric artery.

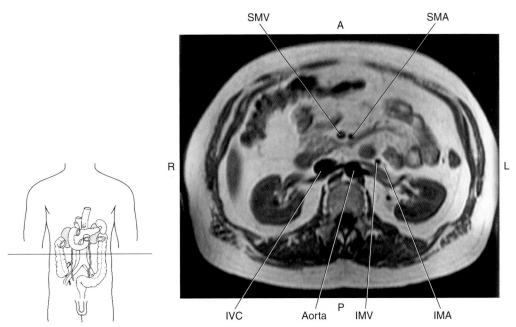

FIGURE 7.164 Axial, T1-weighted MRI of superior mesenteric vessels.

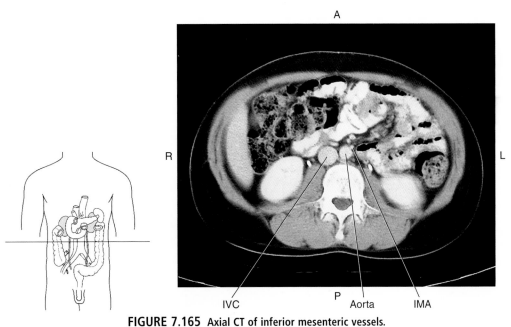

FIGURE 7.165 Axial CT of inferior mesenteric vessels.

(Figure 7.166). The **inferior pancreaticoduodenal artery** extends to the head of the pancreas and duodenum, then divides into the posterior ramus anastomosing with the posterior superior pancreaticoduodenal artery and the anterior ramus, which anastomoses with the anterior superior pancreaticoduodenal artery. The **jejunal** and **ileal arteries** extend to supply the jejunum and ileum,

except the end segment near the cecum. The **middle colic artery** reaches the transverse colon, and the **right colic artery** passes to the ascending colon. The **ileocolic artery** courses behind the peritoneum across the right ureter into the right iliac fossa and divides to supply a portion of the ascending colon, cecum, vermiform appendix, and terminal portion of the ileum (Figures 7.166 and 7.168).

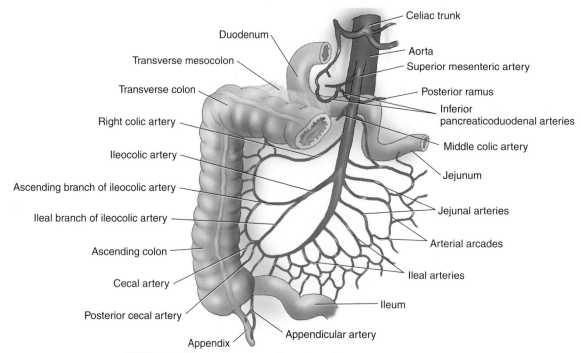

FIGURE 7.166 Anterior view of branches of superior mesenteric artery.

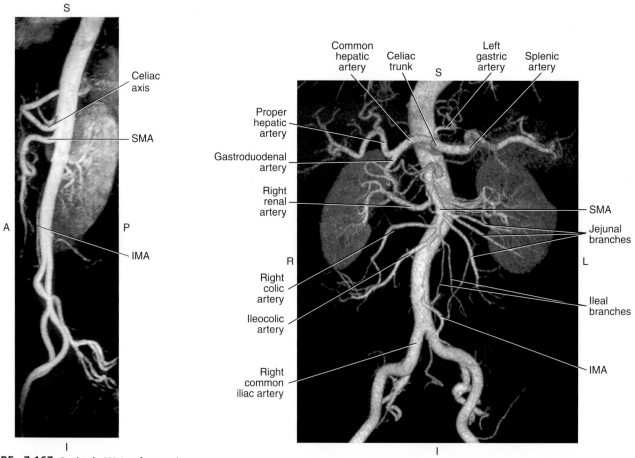

FIGURE 7.167 Sagittal MRA of superior mesenteric artery.

FIGURE 7.168 3D CTA of superior and inferior mesenteric arteries.

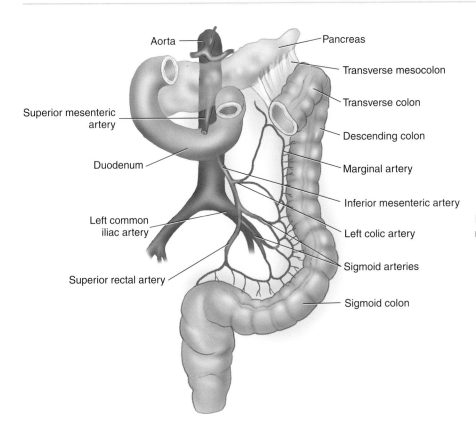

FIGURE 7.169 Anterior view of inferior mesenteric artery.

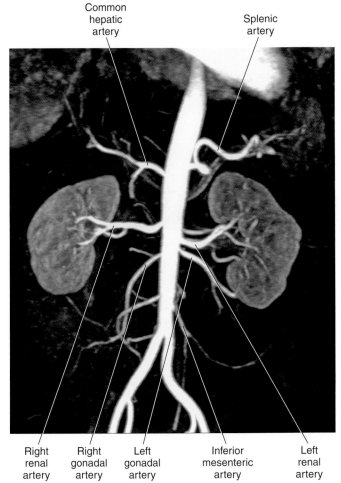

FIGURE 7.170 MRA of inferior mesenteric artery (IMA).

Inferior Mesenteric Artery The inferior mesenteric artery (**IMA**) arises 3 to 4cm above the bifurcation of the aorta at approximately the level of L3-L4. It descends in front of the abdominal aorta and then to the left, where it gives off the left colic artery, sigmoid arteries, and the superior rectal arteries (Figures 7.164, 7.165, and 7.169). The **left colic artery** is a retroperitoneal structure that passes along the posterior body wall on the anterior surface of the left psoas and quadratus lumborum muscles. It bifurcates into ascending and descending branches that supply the walls of the left third of the transverse colon and the entire descending colon. The **sigmoid branches** (2 or 3) course within the mesentery to supply branches to the terminal descending colon and to the sigmoid colon. The **superior rectal artery** crosses the common iliac artery and vein as it descends to branch and supply the rectum (Figures 7.169 through 7.171).

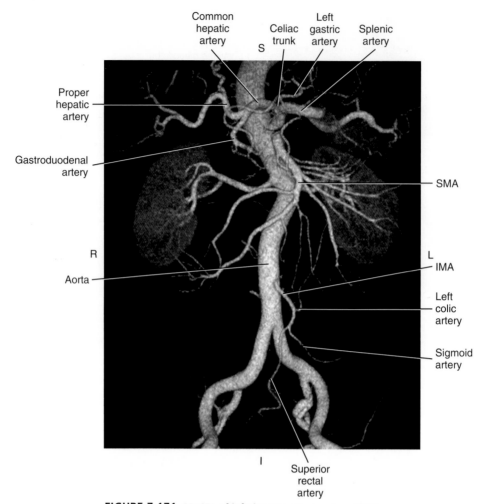

FIGURE 7.171 3D CTA of inferior mesenteric artery (IMA).

INFERIOR VENA CAVA AND TRIBUTARIES

The **inferior vena cava** (**IVC**) is the largest vein of the body (Figure 7.172). It carries blood to the heart from the lower limbs, pelvic organs and the abdominal viscera, and abdominal wall. The IVC is formed by the union of the common iliac veins at approximately the level of L5. It courses superiorly through the retroperitoneum along the anterior aspect of the vertebral column and to the right of the aorta (Figures 7.164 and 7.165). As the IVC ascends the abdominal cavity, it passes the posterior surface of the liver and pierces the diaphragm at the caval hiatus to enter the right atrium of the heart. The IVC receives many tributaries, including the inferior phrenic, lumbar, right gonadal, renal, right suprarenal, and hepatic veins, throughout its course in the abdomen (Figure 7.172).

Inferior Phrenic Veins

The inferior phrenic veins extend from the inferior surface of the diaphragm. The **left inferior phrenic vein** is often doubled and drains into either the left suprarenal vein, left renal vein, or the IVC. The **right inferior phrenic vein** drains directly into the IVC (Figure 7.172).

Lumbar Veins

The **lumbar veins** consist of four pairs of vessels that collect blood from the posterior abdominal wall from the level of L1-L4 (Figures 7.173 through 7.175). They receive veins from the vertebral plexuses and then travel horizontally along the transverse processes deep to the psoas muscles. The lumbar veins on the left are typically longer than those on the right because they must cross over the vertebral column to drain into the IVC. The arrangement of these veins varies, with some entering the lateral walls of the IVC and others emptying into the common iliac vein or are united on each side by a vertical connecting vein termed the **ascending lumbar vein**. Typically, the right ascending lumbar vein continues as the azygos vein and the left ascending lumbar vein continues as the hemiazygos vein. Additionally, a diminutive median sacral vein may accompany the median sacral artery. It typically drains into the left common iliac vein but may also drain into the junction of the common iliac veins (Figures 7.172 and 7.173).

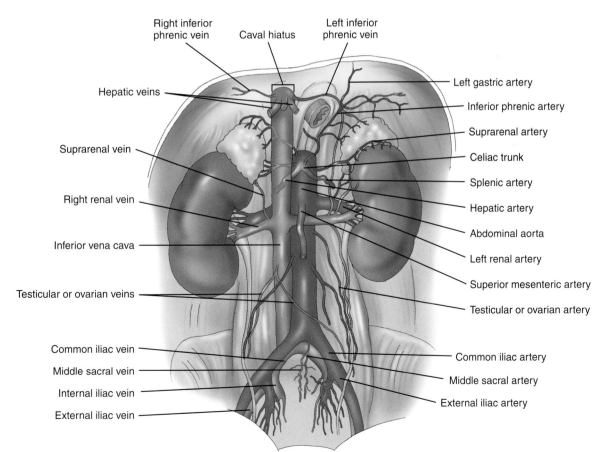

Right inferior phrenic vein
Caval hiatus
Left inferior phrenic vein
Hepatic veins
Left gastric artery
Inferior phrenic artery
Suprarenal artery
Suprarenal vein
Celiac trunk
Splenic artery
Right renal vein
Hepatic artery
Abdominal aorta
Inferior vena cava
Left renal artery
Superior mesenteric artery
Testicular or ovarian veins
Testicular or ovarian artery
Common iliac vein
Common iliac artery
Middle sacral vein
Middle sacral artery
Internal iliac vein
External iliac artery
External iliac vein

FIGURE 7.172 Anterior view of abdominal aorta and IVC.

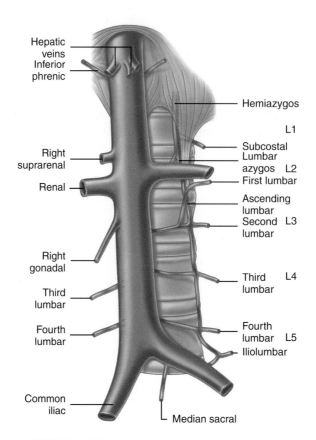

Hepatic veins
Inferior phrenic
Hemiazygos
L1
Subcostal
Lumbar
Right suprarenal
azygos   L2
First lumbar
Renal
Ascending lumbar
Second   L3
lumbar
Right gonadal
Third   L4
lumbar
Third lumbar
Fourth lumbar
Fourth lumbar   L5
Iliolumbar
Common iliac
Median sacral

FIGURE 7.173 Anterior view of IVC and lumbar veins.

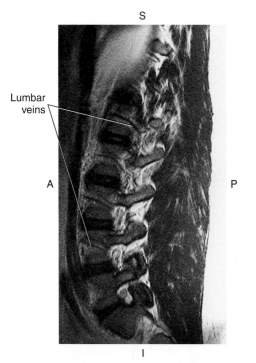

S

Lumbar veins

A   P

I

FIGURE 7.174 Sagittal, T1-weighted MRI with lumbar veins.

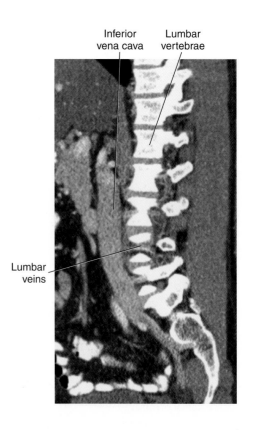

Inferior vena cava   Lumbar vertebrae

Lumbar veins

FIGURE 7.175 Sagittal CT reformat with lumbar veins. SMA, Superior mesenteric artery.

Gonadal Veins

The gonadal veins, ovarian in females and testicular in males, ascend the abdomen along the psoas muscle, anterior to the ureters. The **right gonadal vein** enters the anterolateral wall of the IVC just below the opening for the right renal vein, whereas the **left gonadal vein** typically empties directly into the left renal vein (Figures 7.149, 7.150, 7.172, and 7.173).

Renal Veins

Blood leaves the kidney by way of **interlobular veins** that carry blood from the renal cortex to the **arcuate veins**, which carry blood from the medulla to the interlobar veins. The **interlobar veins** drain into the segmental veins. The five segmental veins correspond to the respective segmental arteries and merge to form the renal vein (Figure 7.146). The **renal veins** pass anterior to the renal arteries to empty into the IVC at about the level of L2. The **left renal vein** passes posterior to the superior mesenteric artery and anterior to the aorta on its route from the left kidney to enter the left lateral wall of the IVC. It receives the left gonadal vein, left inferior phrenic vein, and generally the left suprarenal vein. The shorter **right renal vein** is typically lower than the left renal vein as it travels its short course to enter the right lateral wall of the IVC (Figures 7.172, 7.173, 7.176, and 7.177).

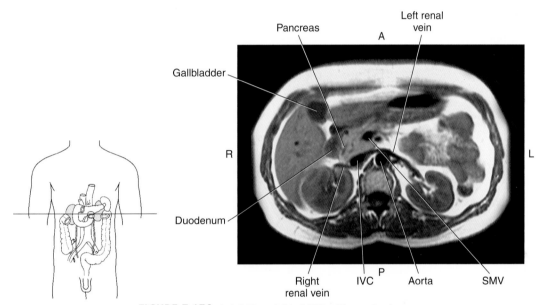

FIGURE 7.176 Axial, T1-weighted MRI with renal veins.

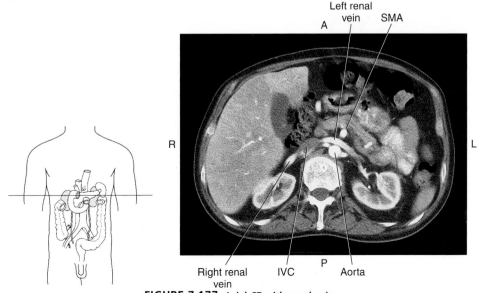

FIGURE 7.177 Axial CT with renal veins.

Suprarenal Veins

The **right suprarenal vein** courses from the medial side of the right suprarenal gland to empty directly into the IVC. The **left suprarenal vein** courses from the inferior pole of the left suprarenal gland to empty directly into the left renal vein or left inferior phrenic vein (Figures 7.172 and 7.173).

Hepatic Veins

The three short **hepatic veins** (**right, middle, left**) begin as smaller vessels that collect blood from the liver parenchyma. The hepatic veins course from the inferior aspect of the liver to the superior aspect of the liver, where they empty into the IVC just below the diaphragm. In general, the right and left hepatic veins drain the right and left lobes of the liver, respectively; whereas, the middle hepatic vein drains the medial segment of the left lobe and the anterior portions of the right lobe (see Liver section, Figures 7. 63 through 7.68, and 7.172).

LYMPH NODES

Many lymph nodes exist within the abdominal cavity. **Abdominal lymph nodes** occur in chains along the main branches of the arteries of the intestine and abdominal aorta. Most abdominal lymph nodes appear as small oblong soft tissue masses oriented parallel to their accompanying vessels and may be difficult to visualize in cross-section unless they are enlarged as a result of an abnormality. Typically, lymph nodes are considered enlarged if their short axis diameter is greater than 1cm. Abdominal nodal groups surround the aorta and IVC and organs of the abdomen. Lymph from the abdominal cavity empties into the **lumbar trunks**, which drain lymph from the legs, lower abdominal wall, and the pelvic organs; and the **intestinal trunks**, which drain organs located within the abdominal cavity. These trunks then join the **thoracic duct** and ultimately enter the venous system (See chapter 6, Figures 6.34 through 6.36, and 7.178 through 7.180).

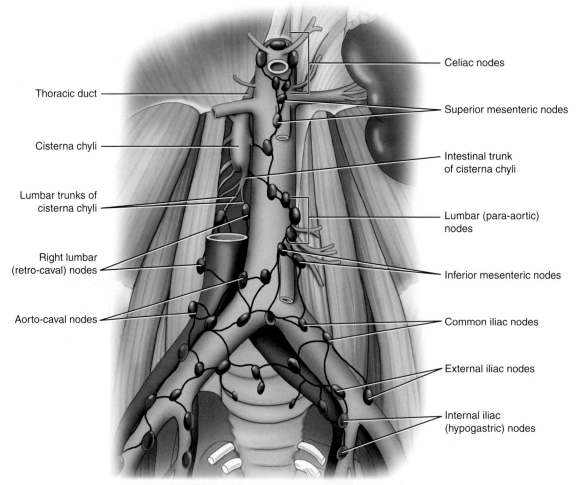

FIGURE 7.178 Anterior view of lymphatic system.

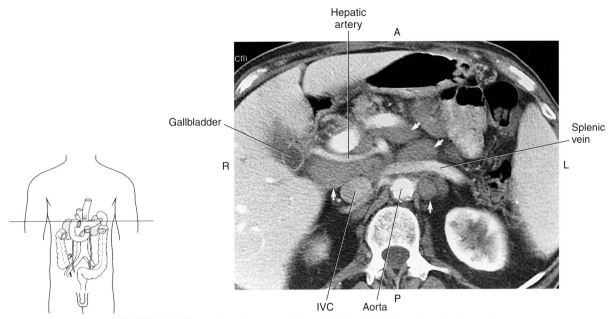

FIGURE 7.179 Axial CT of upper abdomen with enlarged lymph nodes (arrows).

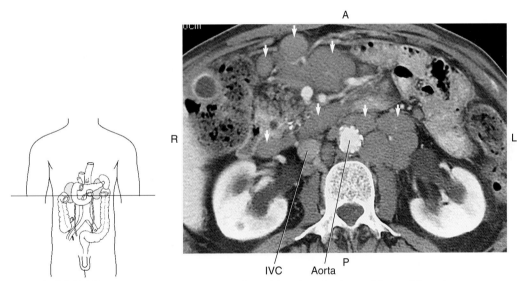

FIGURE 7.180 Axial CT of abdomen with enlarged lymph nodes (arrows) in small bowel mesentery.

MUSCLES OF THE ABDOMINAL WALL

The **abdominal wall** is formed superiorly by the **diaphragm** and is inferiorly continuous with the pelvic cavity at the pelvic inlet. Posteriorly, the abdominal wall is formed by the five lumbar vertebrae, the twelfth pair of ribs, the upper portion of the pelvis, quadratus lumborum muscles, and psoas muscles (Figure 7.181). The **quadratus lumborum muscle** forms a large portion of the posterior abdominal wall. It extends from the iliac crest to the inferior border of the twelfth rib and transverse processes of the lumbar vertebrae to aid in lateral flexion of the vertebral column. The large **psoas muscles** extend along the lateral surfaces of the lumbar vertebrae to insert on the lesser trochanter of the femur and act to flex the thigh and trunk (Figures 7.182 through 7.184). Anteriorly, the abdominal wall is formed by the lower portion of the thoracic cage and by layers of muscles that include the rectus abdominis, external oblique, internal oblique, and transversus abdominis (Figures 7.185 and 7.186). The paired **rectus abdominis muscles**, visualized on the anterior surface of the abdomen and pelvis, originate from the pubic symphysis and extend vertically to the xiphoid process and costal cartilage of the fifth, sixth, and seventh ribs. They function to flex the lumbar vertebrae and support the abdomen (Figures 7.182 and 7.184). The anterior surface of the rectus abdominis muscle is crossed by three tendinous intersections that course transversely, forming individual muscle bellies that can contract separately (Figures 7.185 and 7.186). A longitudinal band of fibers that forms a central anterior attachment for the muscle layers of the abdomen is the **linea alba**, which extends from the xiphoid process of the sternum to the pubic symphysis. The linea alba is formed, at the midline, by the interlacing of fibers from the rectus abdominis and oblique muscles (Figures 7.184, 7.185, and 7.186). The **external** and **internal oblique** muscles are located on the outer lateral portion of the abdomen and extend from the cartilages of the lower ribs to the level of the iliac crest (Figures 7.182, 7.184, 7.186, and 7.187). The oblique muscles work together to flex and rotate the vertebral column and compress the abdominal viscera. The external oblique is the most extensive of the three broad abdominal muscles and contains a triangular opening, the superficial inguinal

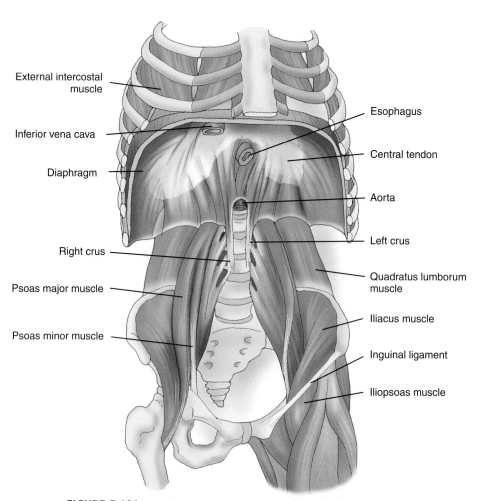

FIGURE 7.181 Anterior view of psoas and quadratus lumborum muscles.

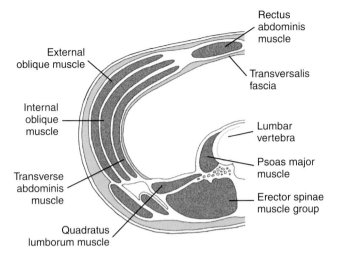

External oblique muscle

Internal oblique muscle

Transverse abdominis muscle

Quadratus lumborum muscle

Rectus abdominis muscle

Transversalis fascia

Lumbar vertebra

Psoas major muscle

Erector spinae muscle group

FIGURE 7.182 Axial view of the abdominal wall.

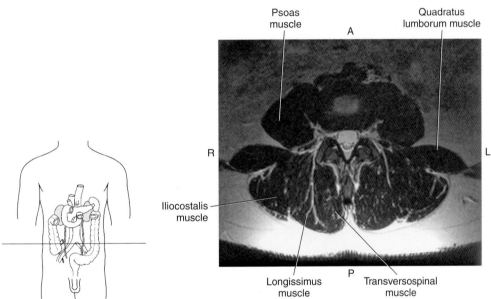

Psoas muscle

Quadratus lumborum muscle

Iliocostalis muscle

Longissimus muscle

Transversospinal muscle

FIGURE 7.183 Axial, T2-weighted MRI of psoas and quadratus lumborum muscles.

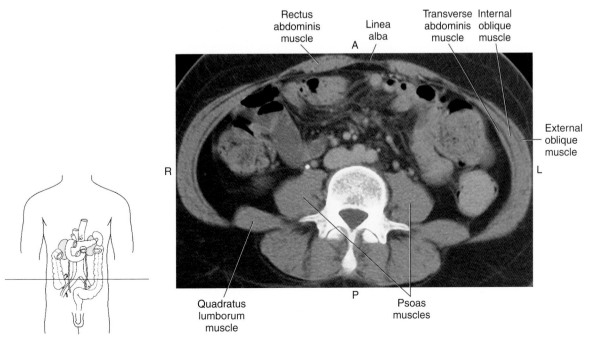

Rectus abdominis muscle

Linea alba

Transverse abdominis muscle

Internal oblique muscle

External oblique muscle

Quadratus lumborum muscle

Psoas muscles

FIGURE 7.184 Axial CT of psoas and quadratus lumborum muscles.

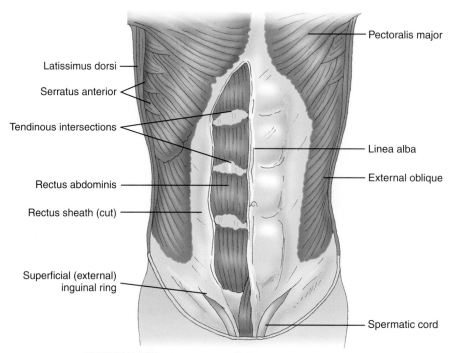

FIGURE 7.185 Anterior view of muscles of abdominal wall.

Labels for Figure 7.185:
- Pectoralis major
- Latissimus dorsi
- Serratus anterior
- Tendinous intersections
- Linea alba
- External oblique
- Rectus abdominis
- Rectus sheath (cut)
- Superficial (external) inguinal ring
- Spermatic cord

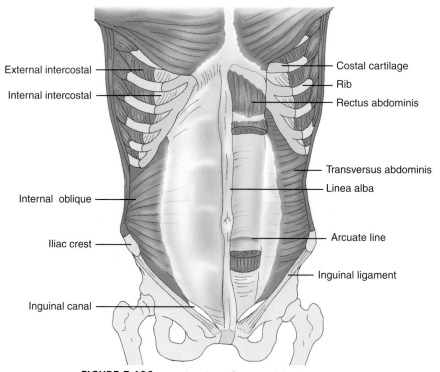

FIGURE 7.186 Anterior view of rectus abdominis muscle.

Labels for Figure 7.186:
- External intercostal
- Internal intercostal
- Costal cartilage
- Rib
- Rectus abdominis
- Transversus abdominis
- Linea alba
- Internal oblique
- Arcuate line
- Iliac crest
- Inguinal ligament
- Inguinal canal

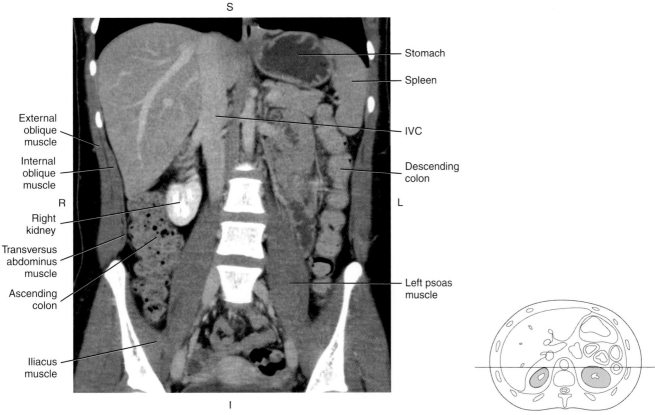

FIGURE 7.187 Coronal CT reformat of psoas muscles.

ring, that allows for the passage of the spermatic cord or round ligament of the uterus (Figure 7.185). The **inguinal ligament** is a fibrous band formed by the thickened inferior border of the aponeurosis of the external oblique muscle. It extends from the anterior superior iliac spine to the pubic tubercle and gives rise to the lowermost fibers of the internal oblique and transversus abdominis muscles (Figure 7.186). The transversus abdominis muscle lies deep to the internal oblique muscles. Its fibers extend transversely across the abdomen to provide maximum support for the abdominal viscera. The **transversus abdominis** muscle extends from the lower six costal cartilages, lumbar fascia, iliac crest, and inguinal ligament to insert into the xiphoid process, linea alba, and pubic symphysis (Figures 7.182, 7.184, 7.186, and 7.187, and Table 7.3).

TABLE 7.3	Abdominal Muscles		
Muscle	**Origin**	**Insertion**	**Function**
Rectus abdominis	Pubic bone near symphysis	Costal cartilage of fifth, sixth, seventh ribs; xiphoid process of sternum	Flexes trunk
External oblique	Lower eight ribs	Linea alba and iliac crest	Compresses abdominal viscera, flexes and rotates spine
Internal oblique	Iliac crest, lumbodorsal fascia, and inguinal ligament	Lower three ribs	Compresses abdominal viscera, flexes and rotates spine
Transversus abdominis	Lower six ribs, iliac crest, and lumbodorsal fascia	Pubic bone and linea alba	Compresses abdominal viscera
Quadratus lumborum	Iliac crest	Twelfth rib and transverse processes of lumbar vertebrae	Flexes spine laterally

Pelvis

"These, gentlemen, are the tuberosities of the ischia, on which man was designed to sit and survey the works of creation.

Oliver Wendell Holmes (1809-1894),
Life and Letters of Oliver Wendell Holmes, vol. I, Chapter VII

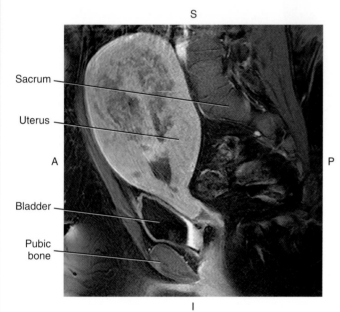

The pelvis provides structural support for the body and encloses the male and female reproductive organs. Because of its role as a support mechanism for the body, the pelvis has a large amount of musculoskeletal anatomy, which, together with the differences in male and female anatomy, makes this area challenging to learn (Figure 8.1).

FIGURE 8.1 Sagittal, T1-weighted contrast-enhanced MRI of the pelvis demonstrating endometrial carcinoma.

OBJECTIVES

- Identify the structures of the bony pelvis.
- Define the pelvic inlet and outlet.
- Describe the perineum.
- Describe the function and location of the pelvic muscles.
- Differentiate between the pelvic and urogenital diaphragms.
- Describe the location of the bladder in relation to the reproductive organs and the course of the male and female urethras.
- Describe the location and function of the male and female reproductive organs.
- Identify the major arteries and veins that are located within the pelvis.
- Describe the location of the pelvic lymph nodes.

OUTLINE

BONY PELVIS

Sacrum, Coccyx, and Os Coxae

The bony pelvis is formed by the sacrum, coccyx, and two os coxae or innominate bones (Figures 8.2 and 8.3). The **sacrum** is a triangular-shaped bone formed by the fusion of five vertebral segments. The first sacral segment has a prominent ridge located on the anterior surface of the body termed the **sacral promontory**, which acts as a bony landmark separating the abdominal cavity from the pelvic cavity. The transverse processes of the five sacral segments combine to form the **lateral mass (ala)**, which articulates with the os coxae at the **sacroiliac joints** (Figures 8.3 through 8.5). The lateral mass contains **sacral foramina** that allow for the passage of sacral nerves (Figures 8.6 and 8.7). Articulating with the fifth sacral segment is the **coccyx**, which consists of three to five small fused bony segments (Figure 8.8).

The **os coxae** are made up of three bones: ilium, pubis, and ischium (Figure 8.9).

Ilium. The ilium, the largest and most superior portion, consists of a body and a large winglike projection called the **ala** (Figures 8.9 through 8.11). The concave, anterior surface of the ala is termed the **iliac fossa**, which is separated from the body by the **arcuate line**. This arch-shaped line, which is located on the anterior surface of the ilium, forms part of the pelvic brim (Figures 8.11 and 8.12). The superior ridge of the ala is termed the **iliac crest**; it slopes down to give rise to the **superior** and

inferior iliac spines on both the anterior and posterior surfaces (Figures 8.9 through 8.11). The **body of the ilium** creates the upper portion of the **acetabulum**, which is a deep fossa that articulates with the head of the femur (Figures 8.13 and 8.14).

Pubis. The pubis, or pubic bone, forms the lower anterior portion of the acetabulum and consists of a body and superior and inferior pubic rami (Figure 8.9). The **bodies** of the two pubic bones meet at the midline to form the **pubic symphysis** (Figure 8.15). The **superior pubic ramus** projects inferiorly and medially from the acetabulum to the midline of the body (Figure 8.16). Located on the upper surface of the superior pubic ramus is a ridge termed the **pectineal line**, which is continuous with the arcuate line of the ilium, forming the pelvic brim (Figure 8.12). The **inferior pubic ramus** projects inferiorly and laterally from the body to join the ischium at an indistinct point; therefore, the two together are often referred to as the ischiopubic ramus (Figures 8.11 and 8.17).

Ischium. The ischium, the inferior portion of the os coxae, like the pubis, is composed of a body and two rami. The **body** of the ischium forms the lower posterior portion of the acetabulum (Figures 8.9, 8.11, 8.13, and 8.14). The **superior ischial ramus** extends posteriorly and inferiorly to a roughened, enlarged area termed the **ischial tuberosity** (Figures 8.9, 8.10, and 8.17). From the ischial tuberosity, the **inferior ischial ramus** extends anteriorly and medially to join the inferior pubic ramus. The **ischial spine** projects from the

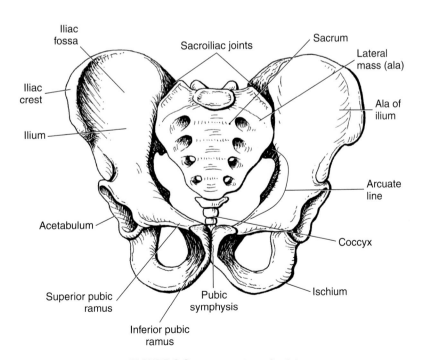

FIGURE 8.2 Anterior view of pelvis.

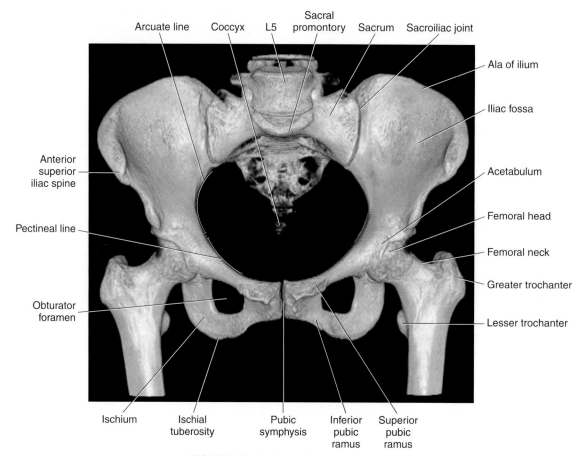

FIGURE 8.3 3D CT of pelvis, anterior view.

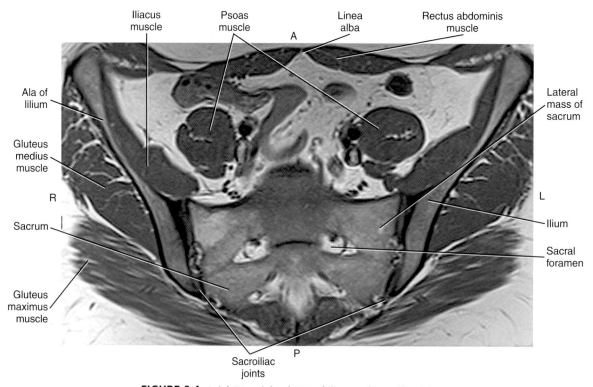

FIGURE 8.4 Axial, T1-weighted MRI of ilium and sacroiliac joints.

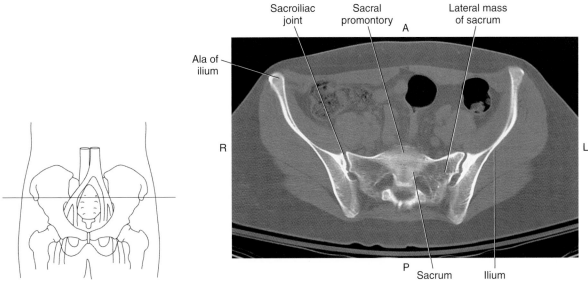

FIGURE 8.5 Axial CT of sacroiliac joints.

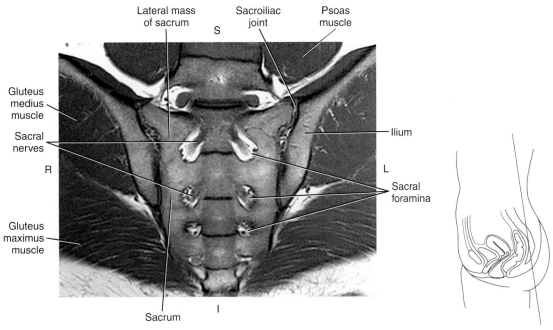

FIGURE 8.6 Coronal, T1-weighted MRI of sacroiliac joints.

superior ischial ramus between two prominent notches on the posterior surface of the os coxae (Figures 8.9 through 8.11, and 8.16). The **greater sciatic notch** extends from the posterior inferior iliac spine to the ischial spine, and the **lesser sciatic notch** extends from the ischial spine to the ischial tuberosity (Figures 8.9 and 8.10). The two notches are spanned by ligaments that create foramina for the passage of nerves and vessels. The union of the pubic rami and ischium surrounds a large opening termed the **obturator foramen**, which is enclosed by the obturator muscles (Figures 8.3 and 8.11).

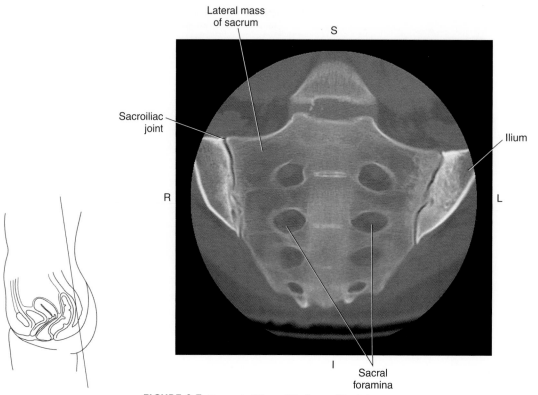

FIGURE 8.7 Coronal oblique CT of sacroiliac joints.

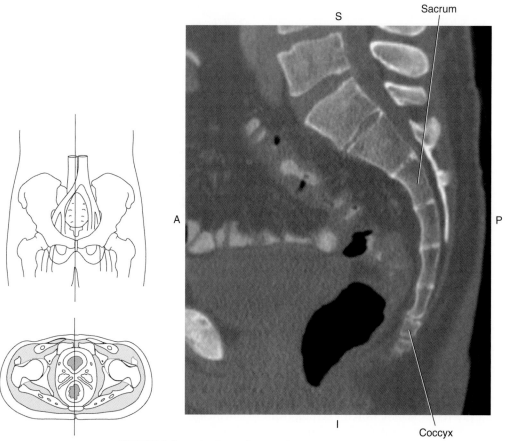

FIGURE 8.8 Sagittal CT reformat of sacrum and coccyx.

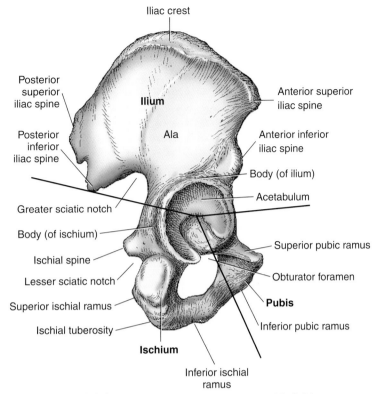

Iliac crest

Posterior superior iliac spine

Ilium

Ala

Anterior superior iliac spine

Posterior inferior iliac spine

Anterior inferior iliac spine

Body (of ilium)

Acetabulum

Greater sciatic notch

Body (of ischium)

Superior pubic ramus

Ischial spine

Obturator foramen

Lesser sciatic notch

Pubis

Superior ischial ramus

Ischial tuberosity

Inferior pubic ramus

Ischium

Inferior ischial ramus

FIGURE 8.9 Lateral aspect of right os coxae with divisions.

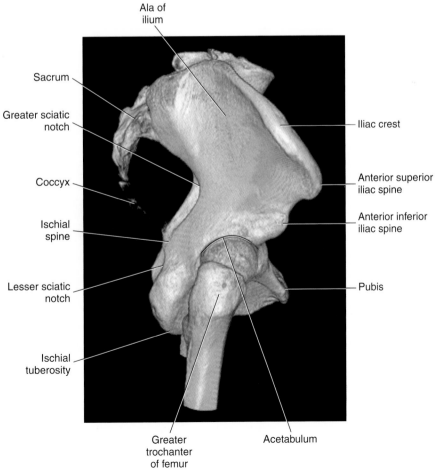

Ala of ilium

Sacrum

Greater sciatic notch

Iliac crest

Coccyx

Anterior superior iliac spine

Ischial spine

Anterior inferior iliac spine

Lesser sciatic notch

Pubis

Ischial tuberosity

Greater trochanter of femur

Acetabulum

FIGURE 8.10 3D CT of os coxae, lateral view.

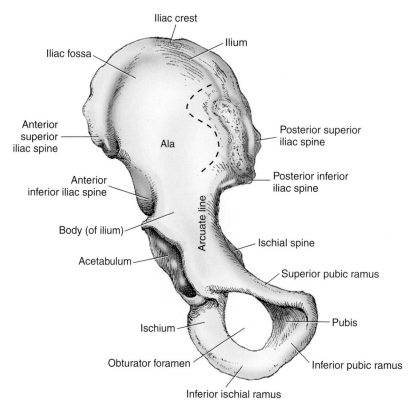

FIGURE 8.11 Anterior aspect of right os coxae.

Iliac crest

Ilium

Iliac fossa

Anterior superior iliac spine

Ala

Posterior superior iliac spine

Posterior inferior iliac spine

Anterior inferior iliac spine

Arcuate line

Body (of ilium)

Ischial spine

Acetabulum

Superior pubic ramus

Ischium

Pubis

Obturator foramen

Inferior pubic ramus

Inferior ischial ramus

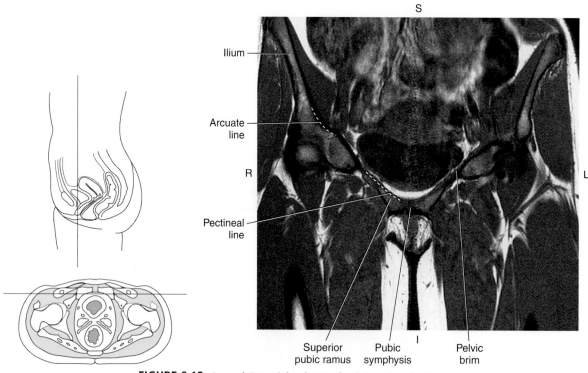

FIGURE 8.12 Coronal, T1-weighted MRI of pelvis with pelvic brim.

Ilium

Arcuate line

Pectineal line

Superior pubic ramus

Pubic symphysis

Pelvic brim

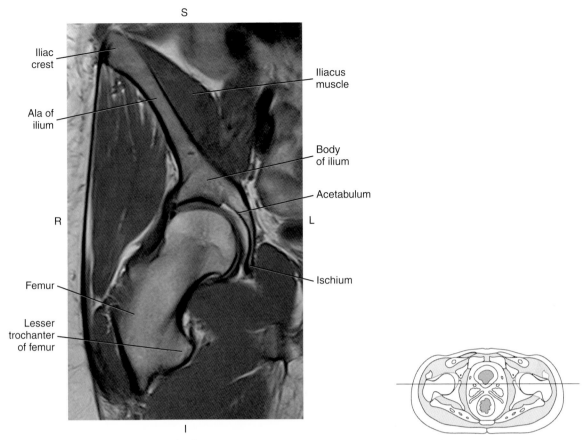

FIGURE 8.13 Coronal, T1-weighted MRI of right hip and acetabulum.

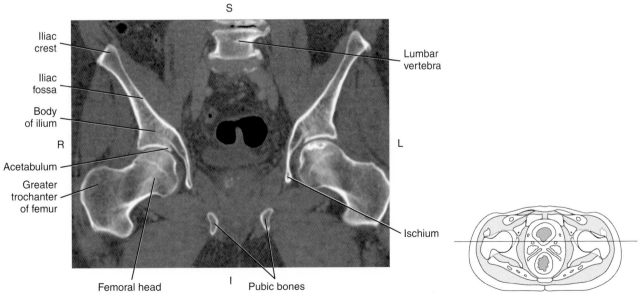

FIGURE 8.14 Coronal CT reformat of pelvis with acetabulum.

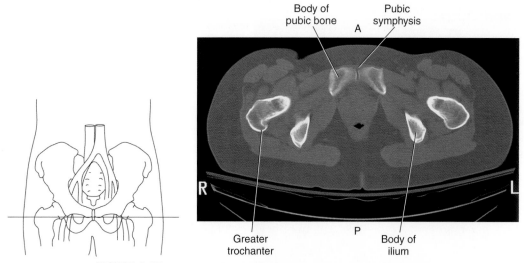

FIGURE 8.15 Axial CT with pubic symphysis and superior pubic ramus.

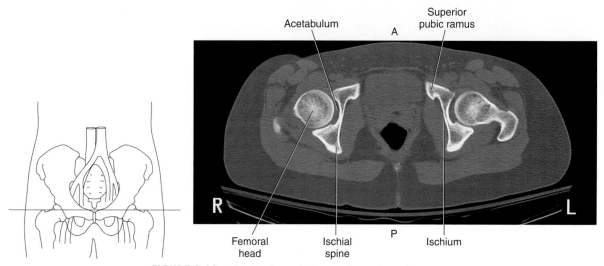

FIGURE 8.16 Axial CT of acetabulum and superior pubic ramus.

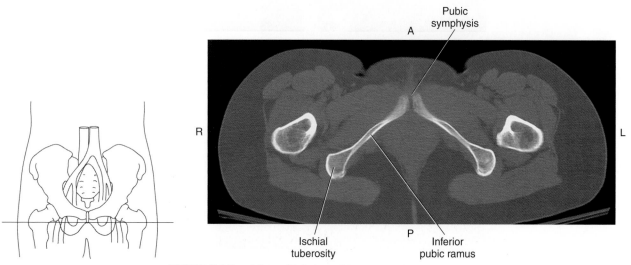

FIGURE 8.17 Axial CT of inferior pubic ramus and ischial tuberosity.

Pelvic Inlet and Outlet

The pelvis is divided into the false or greater pelvis and the true or lesser pelvis by an oblique plane that extends from the upper anterior margin of the sacrum, along the arcuate line, to the upper margin of the pubic symphysis. The boundary line of this plane is called the **pelvic brim**, which delineates the boundaries of the abdominal and pelvic cavities (Figures 8.18 and 8.19). The region above the brim is called the **false pelvis**, and the region below the brim is called the **true pelvis**, which can be subdivided by the pelvic diaphragm into the main pelvic cavity and the perineum. The **superior aperture** or **inlet** of the true pelvis is measured in the anteroposterior direction from the sacral promontory to the superior margin or crest of the pubic bone. The **pelvic outlet** or **inferior aperture** is an opening bounded by the inferior edges of the pelvis and is measured from the tip of the coccyx to the inferior margin of the pubic symphysis in the anteroposterior direction and between the ischial spines in the horizontal direction (Figures 8.18 through 8.20).

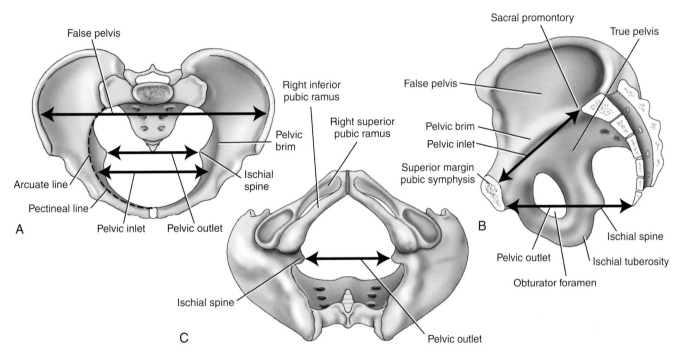

FIGURE 8.18 Divisions of the pelvis. A, Superior view. **B,** Lateral view. **C,** Inferior view.

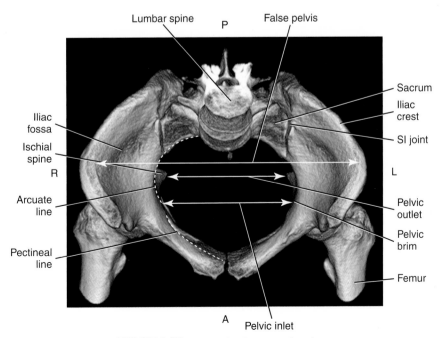

FIGURE 8.19 3D CT of pelvis, superior view.

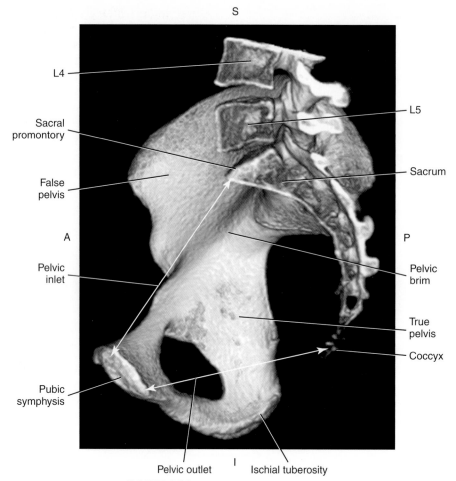

S

L4

Sacral
promontory

False
pelvis

A

Pelvic
inlet

Pubic
symphysis

L5

Sacrum

P

Pelvic
brim

True
pelvis

Coccyx

Pelvic outlet   I   Ischial tuberosity

FIGURE 8.20 3D CT of pelvis, lateral view.

MUSCLES

Multiple muscles are visualized in the pelvis. For ease of description, the major pelvic muscles have been divided into functional groups: extrapelvic, pelvic wall, and pelvic diaphragm.

Extrapelvic Muscles

Several of the muscles visualized in the pelvis are actually abdominal muscles, such as the rectus abdominis, psoas, and internal and external oblique muscles. The **rectus abdominis muscles**, visualized on the anterior surface of the abdomen and pelvis, originate from the symphysis pubis and extend to the xiphoid process and the costal cartilage of the fifth, sixth, and seventh ribs. They function to flex the lumbar vertebrae and support the abdomen. The **psoas muscles** extend along the lateral surfaces of the lumbar vertebrae and act to flex the thigh or trunk. The **external** and **internal oblique muscles** are located on the outer lateral portion of the abdomen and span primarily between the cartilages of the lower ribs to the level of the iliac crest. The oblique muscles work together to flex and rotate the vertebral column and compress the abdominal viscera. An inferior band of fibrous connective tissue from the external oblique

muscle folds back on itself to form the **inguinal ligament**, which extends between the anterior superior iliac spine and the pubic bone. Just superior to the inguinal ligament is the **inguinal canal**, a short (4 cm), diagonal tunnel passing through the lower anterior pelvic wall. It has openings at the outer portion called the superficial inguinal ring and the inner portion called the deep inguinal ring. The inguinal canal transmits the spermatic cord in males and the round ligament in females, (see Chapter 7, Figures 7.181 through 7.187).

Many of the muscles visualized in the pelvis are considered to be muscles of the hip. The largest of this group are the **gluteus muscles** (maximus, medius, minimus), which function together to abduct, rotate, and extend the thigh. The largest and most superficial is the **gluteus maximus muscle**, which makes up the bulk of the buttocks. The **gluteus medius** and **minimus muscles** are smaller in size, respectively, and are deep to the gluteus maximus muscle (Figures 8.21 through 8.24; also see Chapter 10).

 Indirect inguinal hernias are protrusions of the intestine at the inguinal ring. They account for approximately 80% of all hernias.

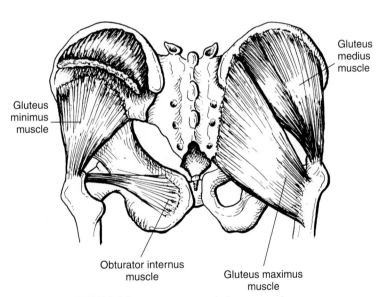

FIGURE 8.21 Posterior view of gluteus muscle group.

Gluteus medius muscle

Gluteus minimus muscle

Obturator internus muscle

Gluteus maximus muscle

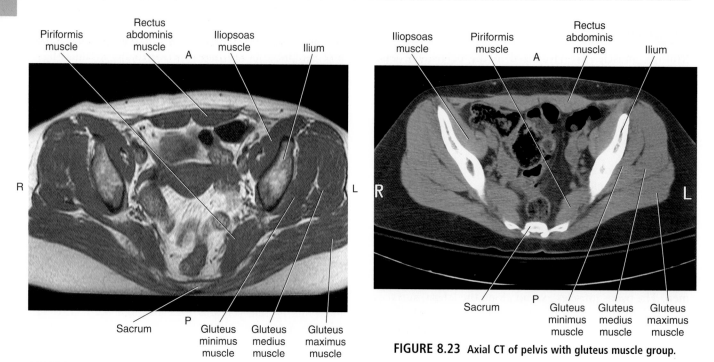

FIGURE 8.22 Axial, T1-weighted MRI of pelvis with gluteus muscle group.

FIGURE 8.23 Axial CT of pelvis with gluteus muscle group.

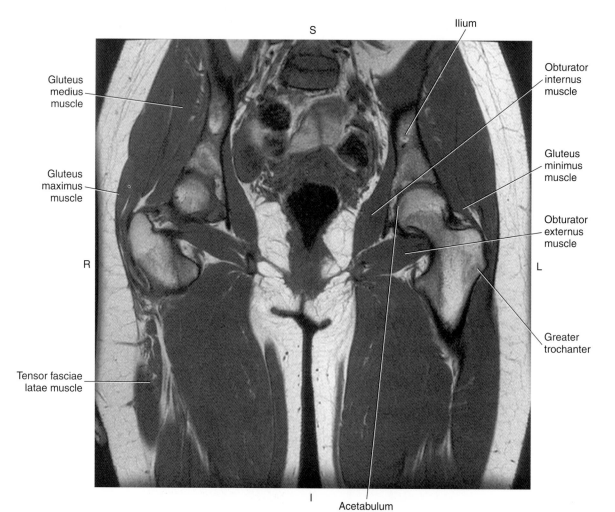

FIGURE 8.24 Coronal, T1-weighted MRI of pelvis with gluteus muscle group.

Pelvic Wall Muscles

The muscles of the pelvic wall include the piriformis, obturator internus and externus, and iliacus muscles. The **piriformis muscle**, which acts to rotate the thigh laterally, originates from the ilium and the sacrum and passes through the greater sciatic notch to insert on the greater trochanter of the femur. Also functioning to rotate the thigh laterally is the **obturator internus muscle**. This fan-shaped muscle extends from the pubic bone and obturator foramen to pass through the lesser sciatic notch and attaches to the greater trochanter of the femur. Inserting

on the greater trochanter just below the obturator internus muscle is the **obturator externus muscle**. This strong muscle originates on the obturator foramen, aiding in adduction and rotation of the thigh. Extending from the iliac crest and sacrum is the triangular-shaped **iliacus muscle**. As the iliacus muscle spans the iliac fossa, it is joined by the psoas muscle to form the **iliopsoas muscle**, which extends to insert on the lesser trochanter of the femur. The iliopsoas muscle is the most important muscle for flexing the leg, which makes walking possible (Figures 8.21 through 8.30, and Table 8.1; also see Chapter 10).

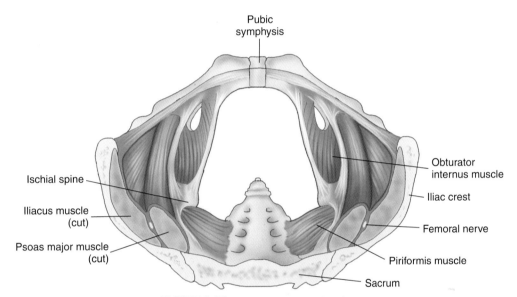

FIGURE 8.25 Pelvic cavity, superior view.

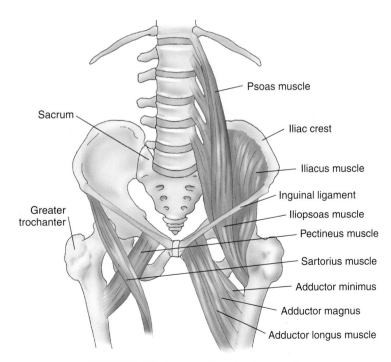

FIGURE 8.26 Anterior view of pelvic muscles.

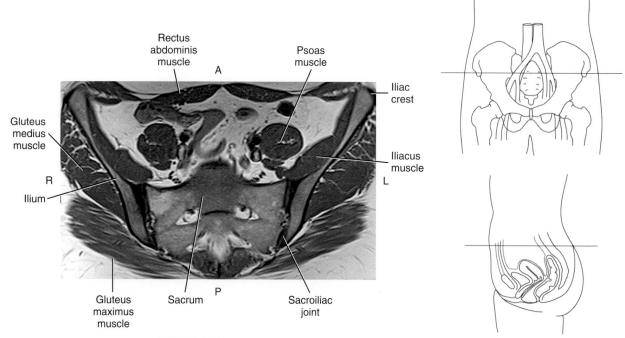

FIGURE 8.27 Axial, T1-weighted MRI of ilium and sacroiliac joints.

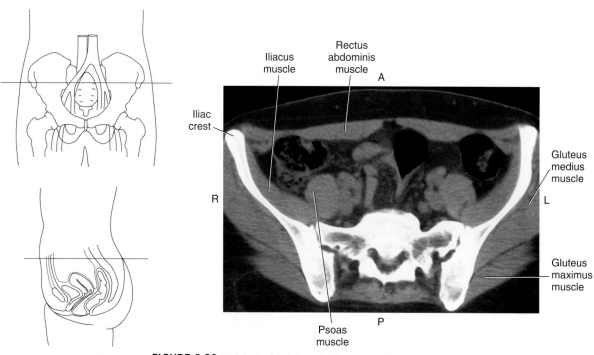

FIGURE 8.28 Axial CT of pelvis with iliacus muscle.

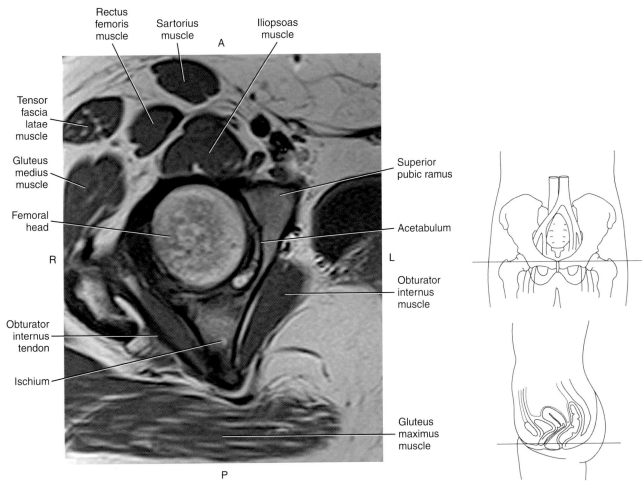

FIGURE 8.29 Axial, T1-weighted MRI of right hip with iliopsoas muscle.

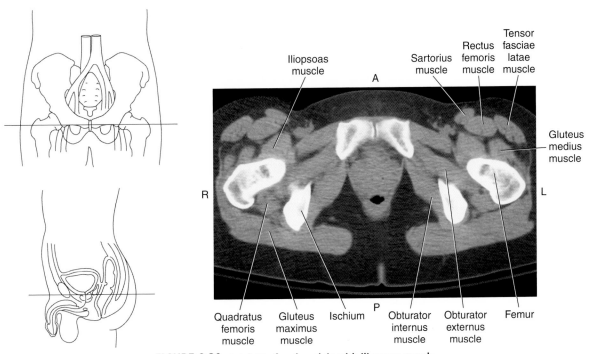

FIGURE 8.30 Axial CT of male pelvis with iliopsoas muscle.

TABLE 8.1	Muscles of the Pelvic Wall and Diaphragm		
Muscle	**Origin**	**Insertion**	**Function**
Piriformis	Ilium and sacrum	Greater trochanter of femur	Laterally rotates and adducts thigh
Obturator internus	Obturator foramen and pubic bone	Greater trochanter of femur (medial surface)	Laterally rotates thigh
Obturator externus	Obturator foramen	Greater trochanter of femur (trochanteric fossa)	Laterally rotates and adducts thigh
Iliacus	Iliac crest and sacrum	Lesser trochanter of femur (tendon fused with that of psoas muscle)	Flexes hip
Levator ani	Symphysis pubis and ischial spine	Coccyx	Supports pelvic viscera, flexes coccyx, elevates and retracts anus
Coccygeus	Ischial spine	Sacrum and coccyx	Assists in supporting the pelvic floor and flexes coccyx

Pelvic Diaphragm Muscles

The funnel-shaped pelvic diaphragm is a layer of muscles and fascia that forms the greatest majority of the pelvic floor. The primary muscles of the pelvic diaphragm are the levator ani and coccygeus muscles. The **levator ani** muscles are the largest and most important muscles of the pelvic floor, originating from the symphysis pubis and ischial spines to form winglike arches that attach to the coccyx. The levator ani muscle can be subdivided into the pubococcygeus, puborectalis, and iliococcygeus muscles. The two **coccygeus muscles** form the posterior portion of the pelvic floor, arising from the ischial spines and fanning out to attach to the lower sacrum and coccyx. Together, the levator ani and coccygeus muscles provide support for the pelvic contents (Figures 8.31 through 8.39 and Table 8.1).

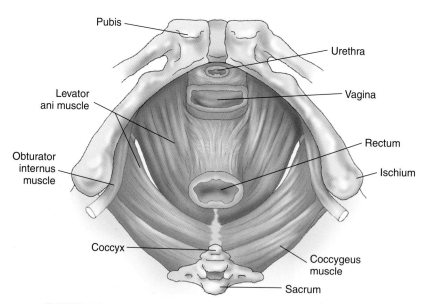

FIGURE 8.31 Inferior view of pelvic diaphragm muscles, female pelvis.

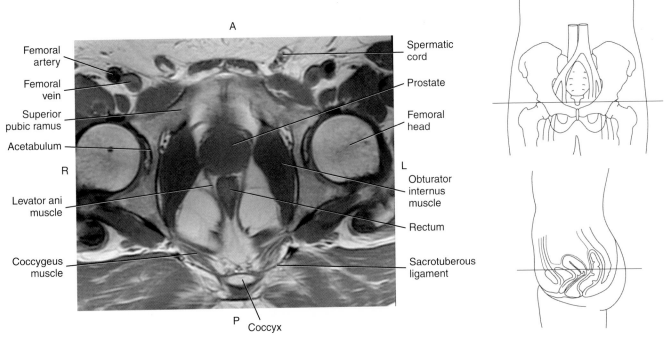

FIGURE 8.32 Axial, T1-weighted MRI of male pelvis with coccygeus muscles.

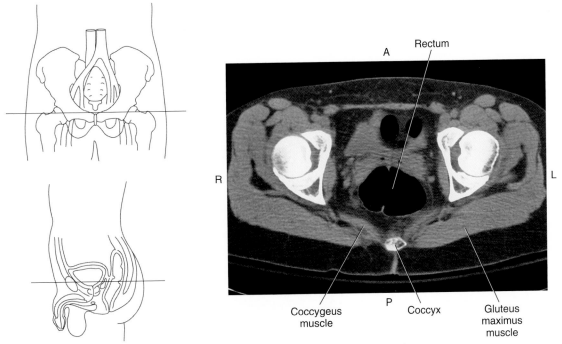

FIGURE 8.33 Axial CT of pelvis with coccygeus muscles.

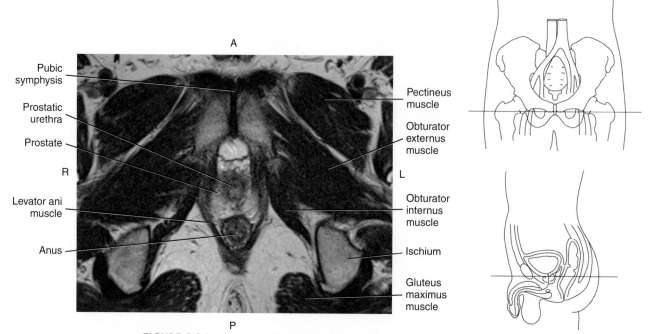

A

Pubic symphysis

Prostatic urethra

Prostate

R

Levator ani muscle

Anus

Pectineus muscle

Obturator externus muscle

L

Obturator internus muscle

Ischium

Gluteus maximus muscle

P

FIGURE 8.34 Axial, T2-weighted MRI of male pelvis with levator ani muscles.

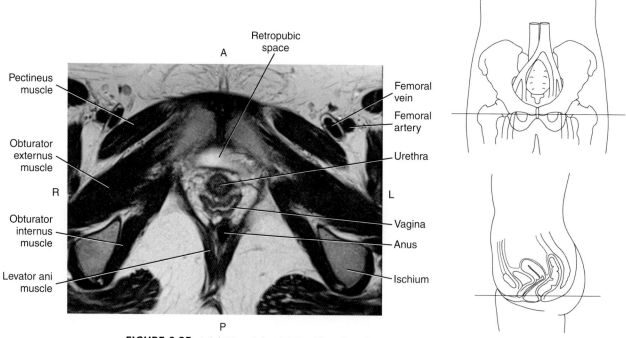

Retropubic space

A

Pectineus muscle

Obturator externus muscle

R

Obturator internus muscle

Levator ani muscle

Femoral vein

Femoral artery

L

Urethra

Vagina

Anus

Ischium

P

FIGURE 8.35 Axial, T2-weighted MRI of female pelvis with levator ani muscles.

S

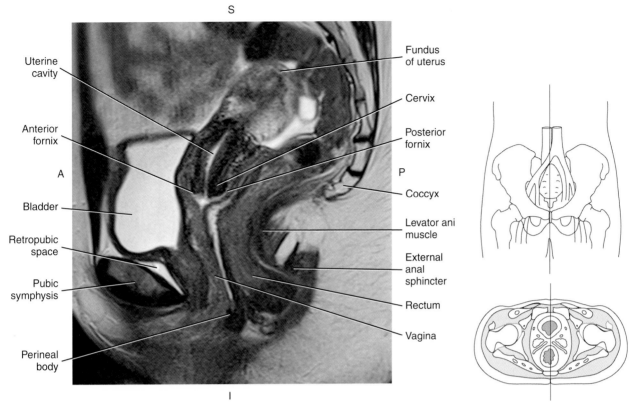

Uterine cavity

Anterior fornix

A

Bladder

Retropubic space

Pubic symphysis

Perineal body

Fundus of uterus

Cervix

Posterior fornix

P

Coccyx

Levator ani muscle

External anal sphincter

Rectum

Vagina

I

FIGURE 8.36 Sagittal, T2-weighted MRI of female pelvis with pelvic diaphragm muscles.

S

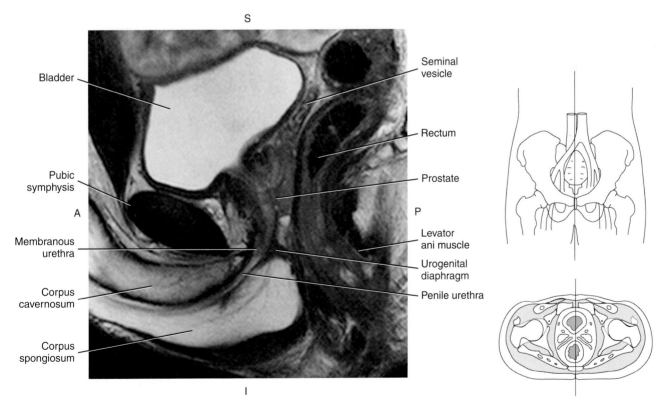

Bladder

Pubic symphysis

A

Membranous urethra

Corpus cavernosum

Corpus spongiosum

Seminal vesicle

Rectum

Prostate

P

Levator ani muscle

Urogenital diaphragm

Penile urethra

I

FIGURE 8.37 Sagittal, T2-weighted MRI of male pelvis with urogenital diaphragm.

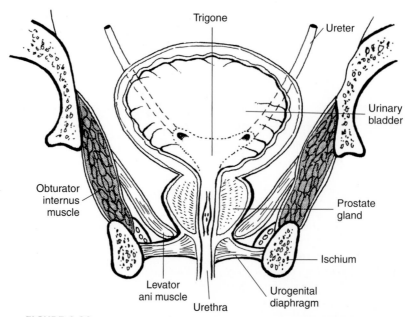

FIGURE 8.38 Coronal view of levator ani muscles and urogenital diaphragm.

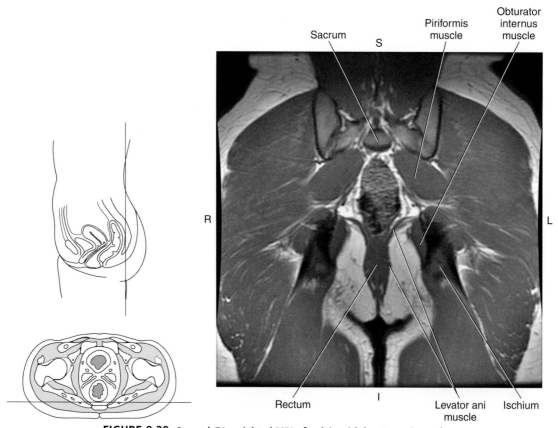

FIGURE 8.39 Coronal, T1-weighted MRI of pelvis with levator ani muscles.

Perineum

The **perineum** is the area located posterior to the pubic arches and anterior to the coccyx. The bony circumferential boundaries of the perineum are the inner edges of the pelvic outlet and consist of the following surface relationships: anteriorly by the pubic symphysis; laterally by the pubic rami, ischial rami, ischial tuberosities, and sacrotuberous ligaments; and posteriorly by the coccyx (Figure 8.40). The region is divided into two triangles, posterior and anterior, by an imaginary line joining the ischial tuberosities. The posterior triangle is the **anal triangle**, and the anterior triangle is the **urogenital triangle** commonly referred to as the **urogenital diaphragm**. The anal triangle contains the inferior one-third of the anal canal and its sphincter muscles, as well as ischioanal fossae. The urogenital diaphragm contains the openings of the urethra and vagina in the female and the urethra and root structures of the penis in the male (Figures 8.40 through 8.42). It is covered by a tough layer of fascia, called the perineal membrane, stretching between the pubic arches. Located at the center of the midpoint between the ischial tuberosities is the perineal body, which is a mass of muscle and fascia and is the site where the interlacing fibers of several muscles converge. In females, the perineal body is located between the vagina and rectum and in males it is located between the rectum and root of the penis (Figure 8.40).

The perineal body is an important structure in females due to its function as a support for the pelvic organs. When muscles connected to the perineal body stretch or tear (i.e., during childbirth), the muscular support of the pelvic floor can be compromised, resulting in prolapse of the pelvic organs. Injury to the perineal body due to trauma or infection can result in the formation of a fistula.

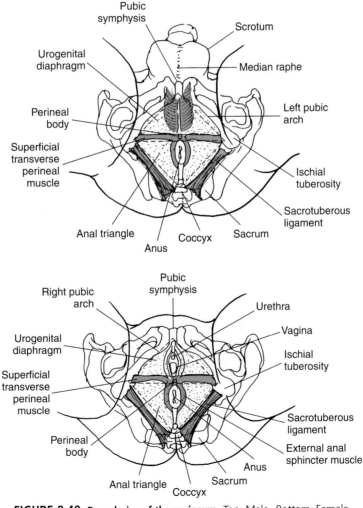

FIGURE 8.40 Boundaries of the perineum. *Top,* Male. *Bottom,* Female.

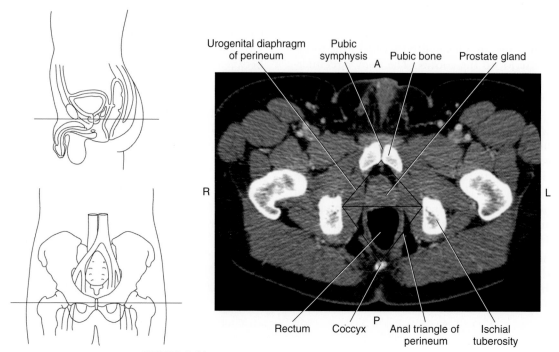

FIGURE 8.41 Axial CT with boundaries of male perineum.

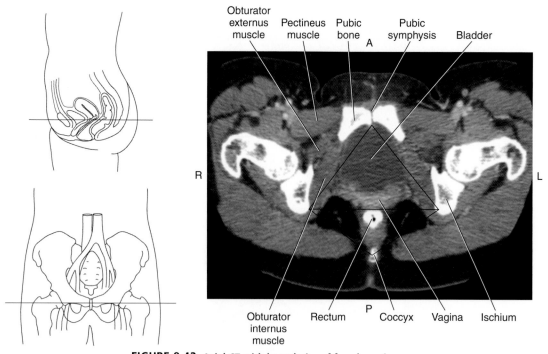

FIGURE 8.42 Axial CT with boundaries of female perineum.

VISCERA

The pelvic cavity contains the bladder, rectum, and internal reproductive organs.

Bladder

The **bladder** is a pyramid-shaped muscular organ that rests on the pelvic floor, immediately posterior to the symphysis pubis (Figures 8.43 through 8.47). It functions as a temporary reservoir for the storage of urine. In a normal adult, it takes approximately 200 to 250 mL of urine to accumulate before the urge to urinate is triggered. However, the bladder has the potential storage capacity of approximately 750 mL. When empty, the bladder has four surfaces (superior, posterior, and two inferolateral) and four angles (anterior, inferior, two posterolateral, and anterior). The **superior surface** (body) of the bladder is covered by peritoneum, allowing loops of ileum and sigmoid colon to rest on it. The **posterior surface** is referred to as the **fundus** or **base of the bladder**. This surface is closely related to the anterior wall of the vagina in the female and to the rectum in the male. The two **inferolateral surfaces** face inferior, lateral, and anterior and are in contact with the fascia covering the levator ani muscles (Figure 8.38). As urine is collected in the bladder, the superior and inferolateral surfaces distend accordingly while the posterior surface remains relatively fixed. The **inferior angle** is a funnel-shaped narrowing formed by the convergence of the inferolateral and posterior surfaces and is called the **neck of the bladder**, which is continuous with the urethra (Figure 8.43). The bladder neck contains the muscular **internal urethral sphincter**, which provides for involuntary control over the release of urine from the bladder. The two **posterolateral angles** mark the point where the ureters enter the bladder. The **anterior angle** is formed by the convergence of the superior and inferolateral surfaces and is referred to as the **apex** of the bladder.

The bladder is anchored to the pelvis by peritoneal ligaments. The apex is attached to the anterior abdominal wall by the **median umbilical ligament**, which is the remains of the fetal urachus (obliterated umbilical artery). Two **medial umbilical ligaments** from the body of the bladder ascend along with the median umbilical ligament to the umbilicus (Figure 8.48). The fibrous cords of these ligaments represent the obliterated remains of the two umbilical arteries, which provide blood to the placenta during fetal development. The bladder neck is held in place by the **puboprostatic ligament** in males and the **pubovesical ligament** in females. Three openings in the floor of the bladder form a triangular area called the **trigone** (Figure 8.38). Two of the openings are created by the ureters. The pelvic portions of the ureters run anterior to the internal iliac arteries and enter the posterolateral surface of the bladder at an oblique angle (Figures 8.49 and 8.51). The third opening is located in the apex of the trigone and is formed by the entrance to the urethra (Figures 8.38, 8.43 through 8.47, and 8.52).

The **urethra** is a muscular tube that drains urine from the bladder. In both genders, the urethra passes through the urogenital diaphragm, which contains the urethral sphincter muscle responsible for the voluntary closure of the bladder. The short (3-4 cm) female urethra is located in front of the anterior vaginal wall and descends inferiorly and anteriorly to terminate at the external urethral opening located between the clitoris and vagina (Figures 8.43, 8.44, and 8.52). The **male urethra** is much longer (18-20cm) and extends from the inferior portion of the bladder to the tip of the penis (Figures 8.45, 8.46, and 8.53). It can be subdivided into three regions: prostatic urethra, membranous urethra, and penile urethra. The prostatic **urethra** passes through the middle of the prostate gland. The **membranous urethra** is the shortest and narrowest portion of the urethra and is the portion that penetrates the urogenital diaphragm. The **penile urethra** is the longest portion, extending from the external urethral sphincter to the tip of the penis (Figures 8.45 and 8.46). The male urethra has the dual function to drain urine from the bladder and to receive secretions from the prostatic and ejaculatory ducts and the ducts of the bulbourethral glands.

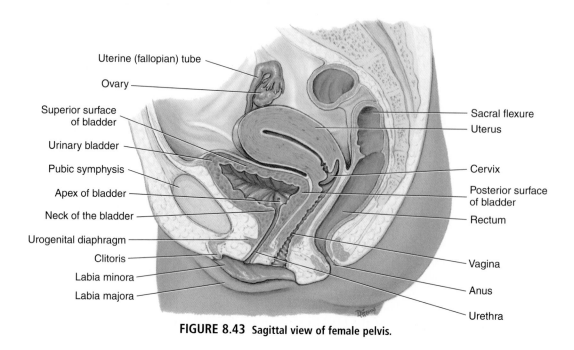

Uterine (fallopian) tube

Ovary

Superior surface
of bladder

Urinary bladder

Pubic symphysis

Apex of bladder

Neck of the bladder

Urogenital diaphragm

Clitoris

Labia minora

Labia majora

Sacral flexure

Uterus

Cervix

Posterior surface
of bladder

Rectum

Vagina

Anus

Urethra

FIGURE 8.43 Sagittal view of female pelvis.

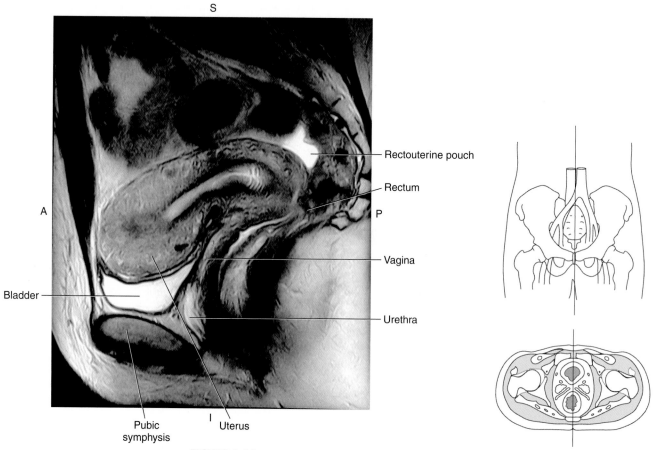

S

A

P

I

Rectouterine pouch

Rectum

Vagina

Urethra

Bladder

Pubic
symphysis

Uterus

FIGURE 8.44 Sagittal, T2-weighted MRI of female pelvis.

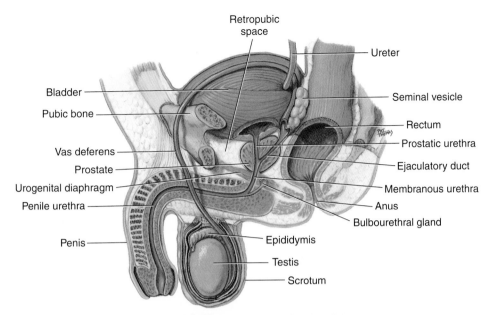

FIGURE 8.45 Sagittal view of male pelvis.

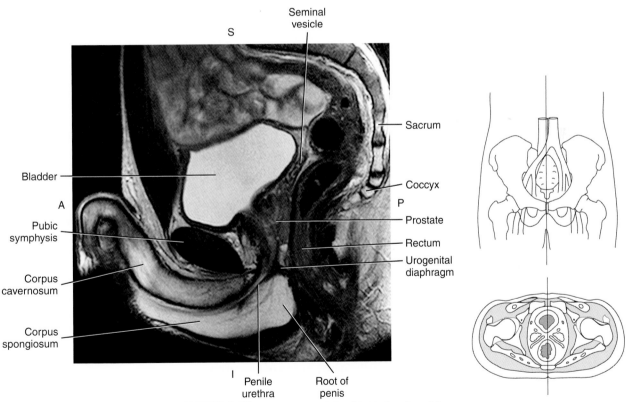

FIGURE 8.46 Sagittal, T2-weighted MRI of male pelvis.

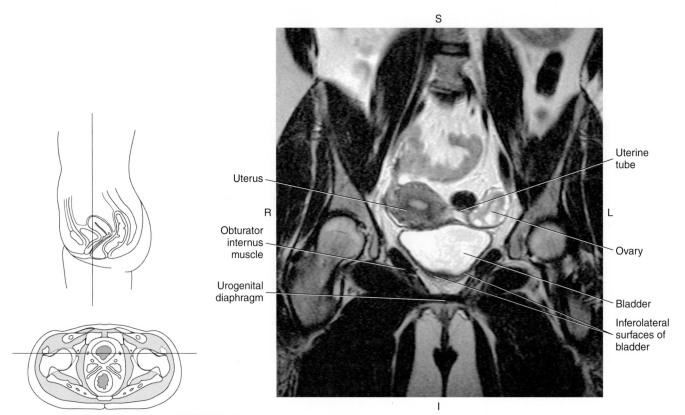

S

Uterine tube

Uterus

R

L

Obturator internus muscle

Ovary

Urogenital diaphragm

Bladder

Inferolateral surfaces of bladder

I

FIGURE 8.47 Coronal, T2-weighted MR of female pelvis with bladder.

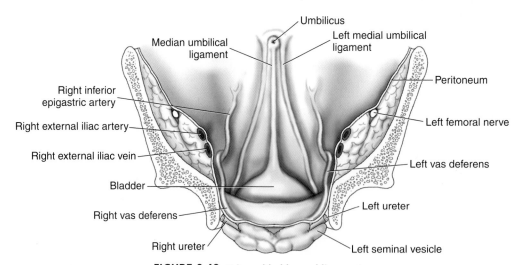

Umbilicus

Median umbilical ligament

Left medial umbilical ligament

Right inferior epigastric artery

Peritoneum

Right external iliac artery

Left femoral nerve

Right external iliac vein

Left vas deferens

Bladder

Right vas deferens

Left ureter

Right ureter

Left seminal vesicle

FIGURE 8.48 Urinary bladder and ligaments.

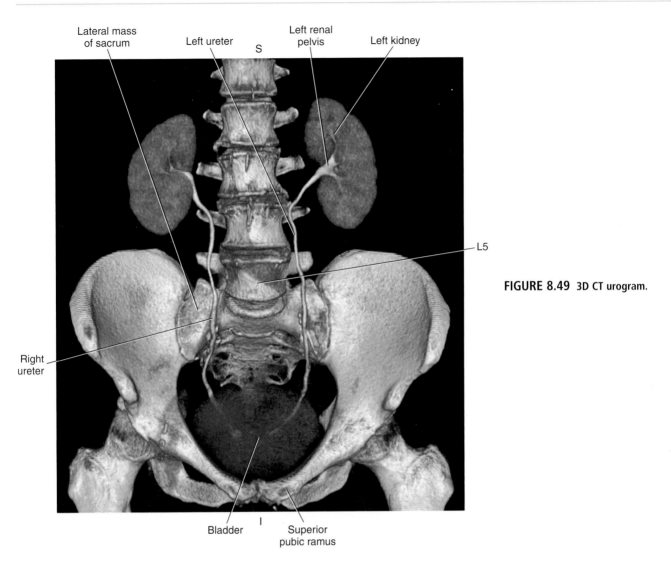

Lateral mass
of sacrum

Left ureter

Left renal
pelvis

Left kidney

S

L5

Right
ureter

Bladder

I

Superior
pubic ramus

FIGURE 8.49 3D CT urogram.

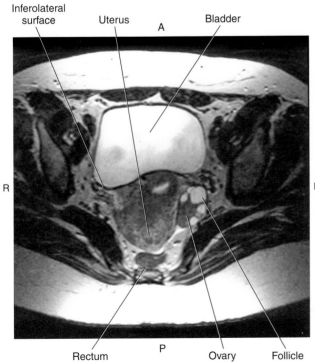

Inferolateral
surface

Uterus

A

Bladder

R

L

Rectum

P

Ovary

Follicle

FIGURE 8.50 Axial, T2-weighted MRI of female pelvis with bladder.

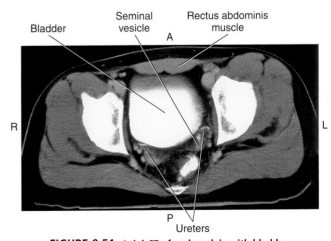

Bladder

Seminal
vesicle

Rectus abdominis
muscle

A

R

L

P

Ureters

FIGURE 8.51 Axial CT of male pelvis with bladder.

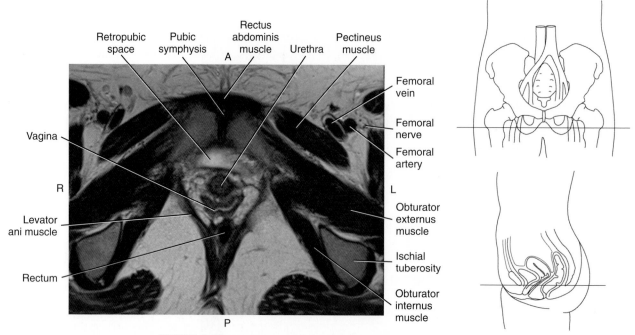

FIGURE 8.52 Axial, T1-weighted MRI of female pelvis with urethra.

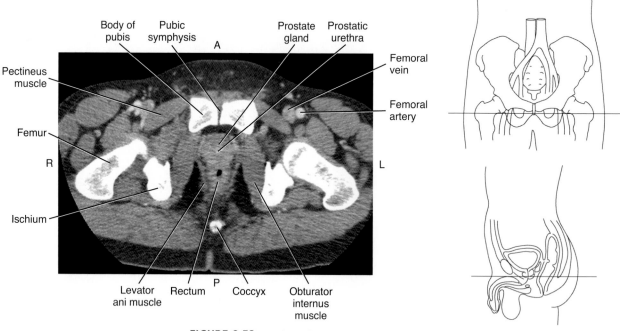

FIGURE 8.53 Axial CT of male pelvis with urethra.

Rectum

The rectum is the terminal part of the large intestine extending from S3 to the tip of the coccyx, approximately 15 cm long. It follows the anteroposterior curve of the sacrum and coccyx (**sacral flexure**) and ends by turning inferiorly and anteriorly (**perineal flexure**) to become the anal canal, which ends at the anus (Figures 8.43 through 8.46 and 8.54 through 8.57). Between the two flexures is a fold of tissue called the **transverse rectal fold** (**Kohlrausch's fold**) located 5 to 8 cm from the anus (Figure 8.54). It serves as a topographic landmark during a rectal examination marking the posterior side of the prostate in males and the vault of the vagina in females. The upper third of the rectum, the **rectal ampulla**, has considerable distensibility. As fecal material collects in this area, it triggers the urge to defecate. The **anal canal** is the distal portion of the rectum and contains small longitudinal folds called **rectal** or **anal columns**. The **anus** marks the exit of the anal canal and is under the involuntary control of the **internal anal sphincter**, a circular muscle layer within the rectal wall. The **external anal sphincter** consists of a ring of skeletal muscle fibers and is under voluntary control (Figures 8.40, 8.43, 8.45, and 8.54 through 8.57).

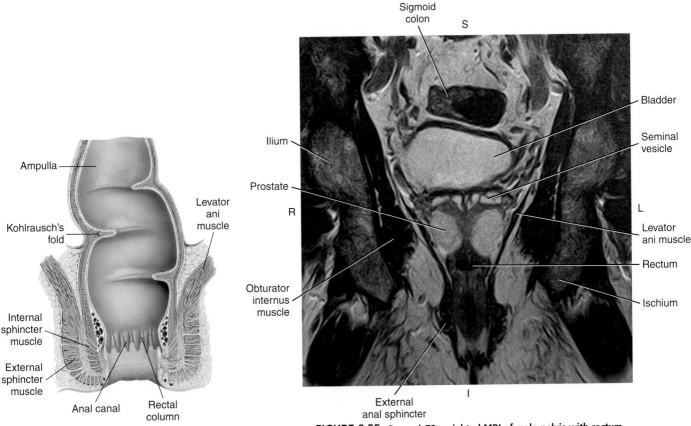

FIGURE 8.54 Coronal view of rectum.

FIGURE 8.55 Coronal, T2-weighted MRI of male pelvis with rectum.

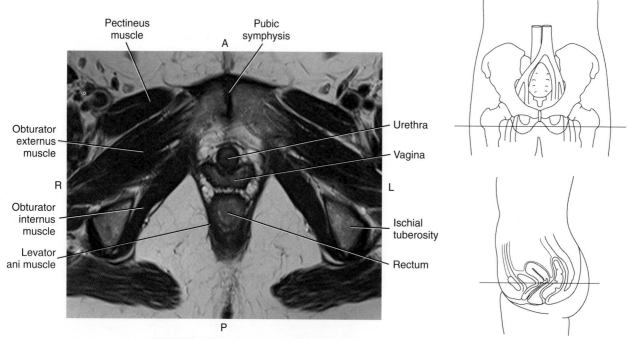

FIGURE 8.56 Axial, T2-weighted MRI of female pelvis with rectum.

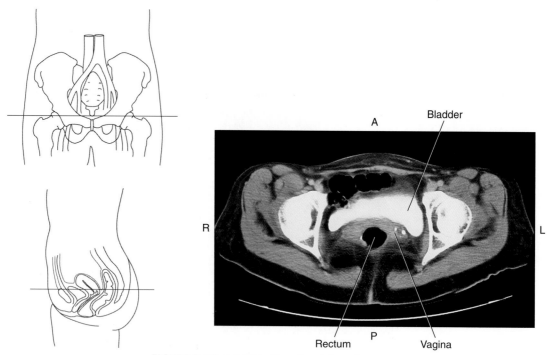

FIGURE 8.57 Axial CT of female pelvis with rectum.

Female Reproductive Organs

The female reproductive system is responsible for producing sex hormones and ova and functions to protect and support a developing embryo. The principal organs of the female reproductive system are located within the pelvic cavity and include the uterus, ovaries, uterine tubes, and vagina (Figures 8.58 through 8.60).

Uterus. The **uterus** is a pear-shaped muscular organ located in the anterior portion of the pelvic cavity between the bladder and the rectum (Figures 8.58 and 8.59). The uterus can be subdivided into two anatomic

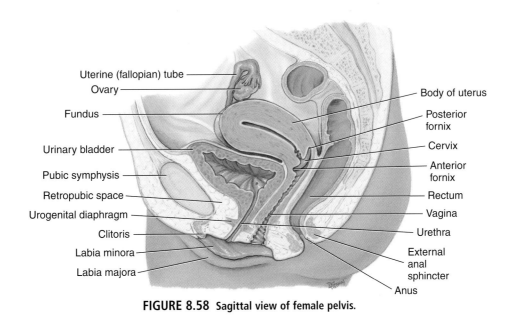

FIGURE 8.58 Sagittal view of female pelvis.

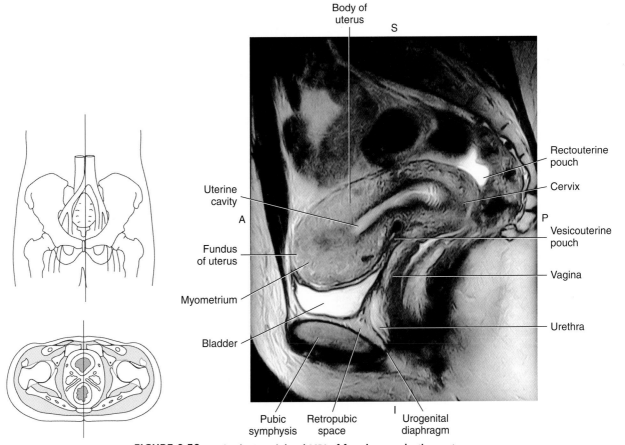

FIGURE 8.59 Sagittal, T2-weighted MRI of female reproductive system.

regions: body and cervix. The **body** is the largest division, comprising the upper two-thirds of the uterus. The rounded superior portion of the body is called the **fundus**, which is located just superior to the region where the uterine tubes enter the uterus. The lateral borders of the fundus contain the **cornua**, where the uterine tubes attach to the uterus. The narrow inferior third of the uterus is called the **cervix**, which communicates with the vagina. The narrow lumen within the cervix, called the **cervical canal**, is a conduit between the uterine cavity superiorly via the **internal os** and opens inferiorly into the vagina via the **external os** (Figure 8.60). The most common position of the uterus is with the body projecting superiorly and anteriorly over the bladder, with the fundus adjacent to the anterior abdominal wall and the cervix directed inferior and posteriorly into the vaginal vault. The wall of the uterus is composed of three layers: the **endometrium** is the inner glandular tissue lining the inner wall; the **myometrium** is the middle, muscular layer and the thickest component of the uterine wall; and the **perimetrium** is the outer layer consisting of a serous membrane that covers the fundus and posterior surface of the uterus. The endometrium is lined by a mucous membrane that is continuous with the inner lining of the vagina and uterine tubes. The thick myometrial layer is highly vascular and is responsible for the main contractive force during childbirth. The perimetrium is formed by peritoneum and is firmly attached to the myometrium. The uterus is the reproductive organ responsible for protecting the fetus during development (Figures 8.58 through 8.63).

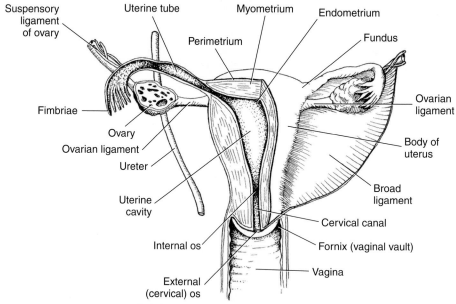

FIGURE 8.60 Anterior view of uterus.

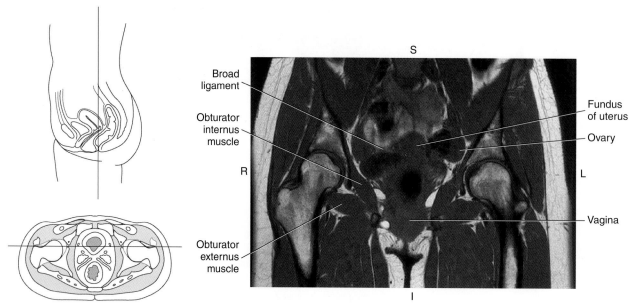

FIGURE 8.61 Coronal, T1-weighted MRI of female pelvis.

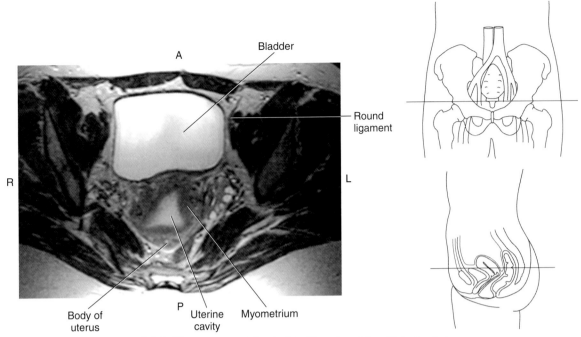

FIGURE 8.62 Axial, T2-weighted MRI of female pelvis with body of uterus.

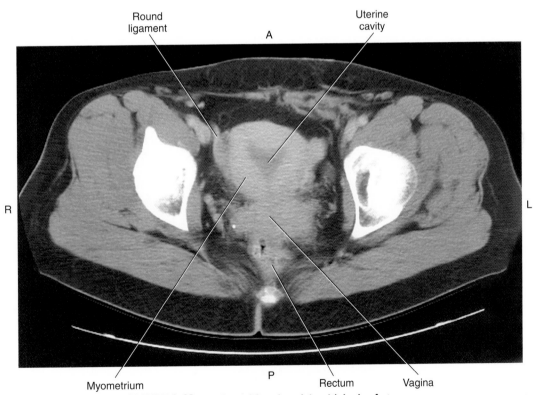

FIGURE 8.63 Axial CT of female pelvis with body of uterus.

Suspensory ligaments of the uterus. The uterus is stabilized by several pairs of suspensory ligaments formed by the peritoneum. The **round ligaments** extend laterally from the uterine cornu to the inner inguinal ring, through the inguinal canal, and anchor to the labia majora (Figures 8.62 through 8.65). They help keep the body flexed anteriorly (anteversion) and help prevent posterior movement of the uterus). The **uterosacral ligaments** extend from the lateral walls of the cervix to the anterior surface of the sacrum, preventing forward movement of the uterus (Figures 8.64 through 8.66). The **lateral cervical (cardinal) ligaments** extend like a fan from the lateral walls of the cervix and vagina and anchor into the fascia of the wall of the lesser pelvis. They help suspend the uterus above the bladder and help to prevent downward displacement of the uterus (Figures 8.65, and 8.67 through 8.69). Additional support is provided by the muscles and fascia of the pelvic floor.

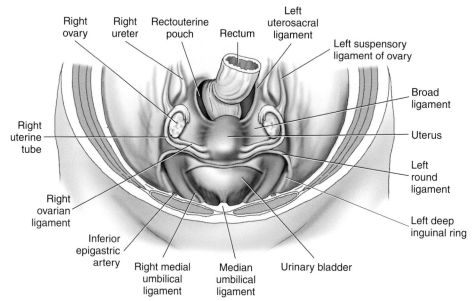

FIGURE 8.64 Anterior view of female pelvis with peritoneal ligaments.

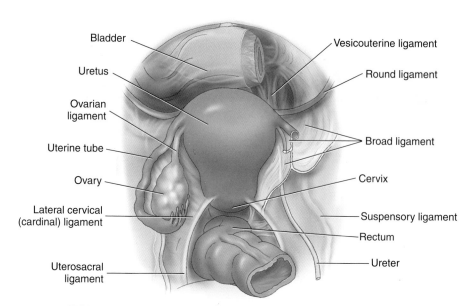

FIGURE 8.65 Superior view of female pelvis with peritoneal ligaments.

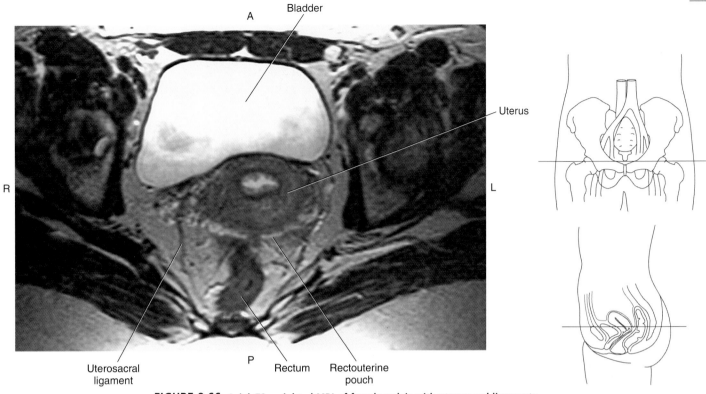

FIGURE 8.66 Axial, T2-weighted MRI of female pelvis with uterosacral ligaments.

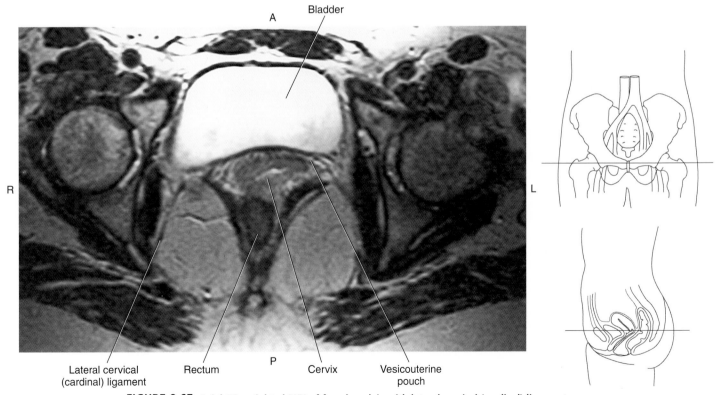

FIGURE 8.67 Axial, T2-weighted MRI of female pelvis with lateral cervical (cardinal) ligaments.

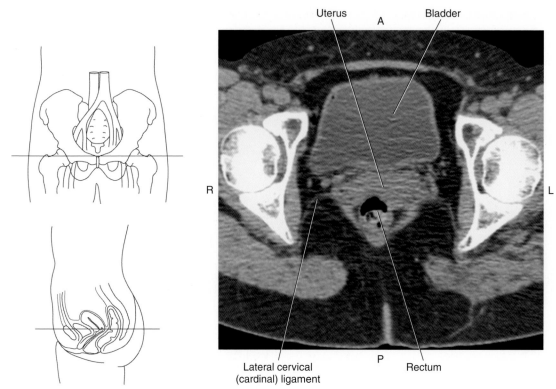

FIGURE 8.68 Axial CT of female pelvis with lateral cervical (cardinal) ligaments.

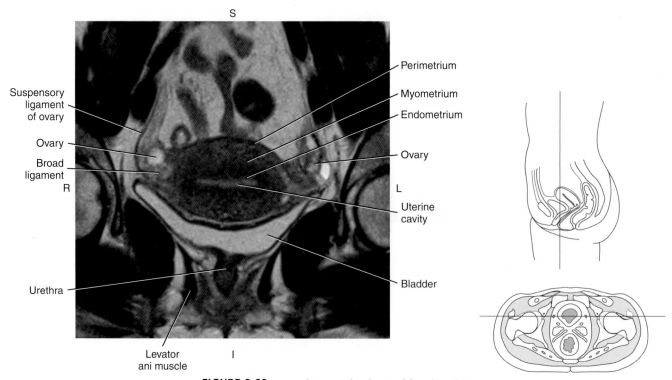

FIGURE 8.69 Coronal, T2-weighted MRI of female pelvis.

Ovaries. The paired **ovaries** are small almond-shaped organs located on either side of the uterus (Figures 8.60, and 8.70 through 8.73). They lie in a depression on the lateral walls of the pelvis and are held in place by the ovarian and suspensory ligaments (Figure 8.65). The cordlike **ovarian ligament** attaches the inferior aspect of the ovaries to the lateral surface of the uterus and uterine tubes (Figure 8.60). The **suspensory ligament** attaches the superior aspect of the ovaries to the lateral sides of the pelvic wall and contains the ovarian vessels (Figures 8.64 and 8.65). The ovaries are responsible for the production of **ova** and the production and secretion of

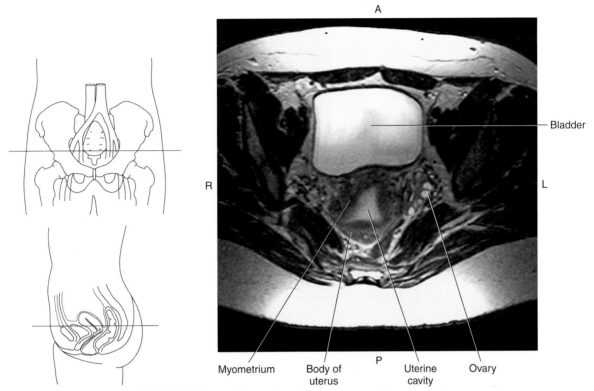

FIGURE 8.70 Axial, T2-weighted MRI of female pelvis with ovaries.

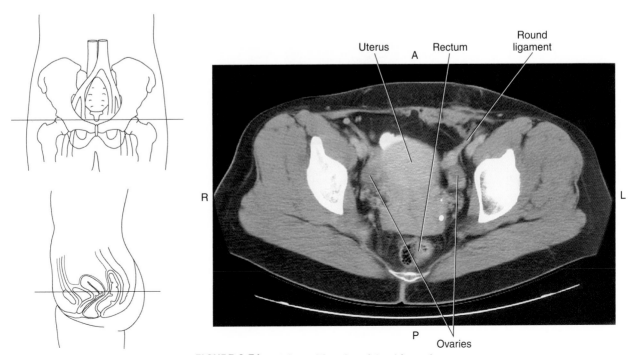

FIGURE 8.71 Axial CT of female pelvis with ovaries.

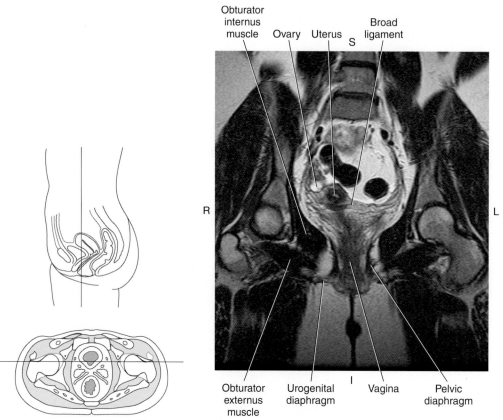

Obturator
internus   Ovary   Uterus   Broad
muscle   ligament
                        S

R   L

Obturator   Urogenital   Vagina   Pelvic
externus   diaphragm   diaphragm
muscle
                        I

FIGURE 8.72 Coronal, T2-weighted MRI of female pelvis with ovaries.

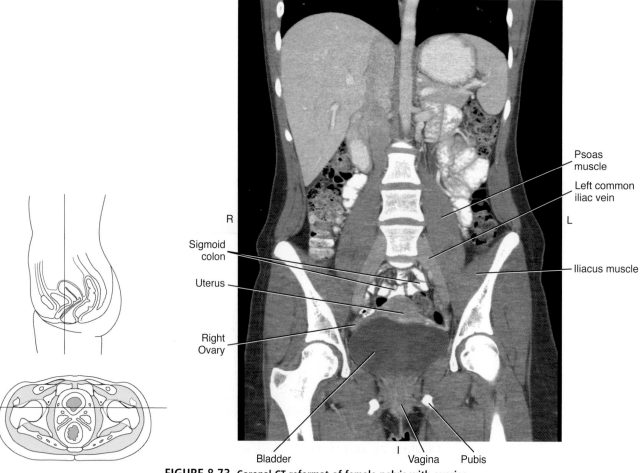

S

R   L

                                    Psoas
                                    muscle

                                    Left common
                                    iliac vein

Sigmoid
colon

Uterus   Iliacus muscle

Right
Ovary

Bladder   Vagina   Pubis
                I

FIGURE 8.73 Coronal CT reformat of female pelvis with ovaries.

estrogens and progesterone. Estrogens are responsible for the development and maintenance of female characteristics and reproductive organs. Progesterone is responsible for the uterine changes in preparation of pregnancy, such as the thickening of the uterine lining and decreasing the contractions of the uterine muscles.

 A follicular cyst represents the mature oocyte and its surrounding follicular cavity. Fluid increases within the cavity as the oocyte matures.

Uterine tubes. The **uterine (fallopian) tubes** are slender, muscular tubes (approximately 8-20 cm long) extending laterally from the body of the uterus to the peritoneum near the ovaries (Figures 8.60 and 8.65). They are supported by the broad ligament and at their distal end expand to form a funnel-shaped **infundibulum.** The infundibulum has numerous 1- to 2-cm fingerlike projections called **fimbriae,** which spread loosely over the surface of the ovaries (Figures 8.60 and 8.65). During ovulation, the fimbriae trap the ovum and sweep it into the uterine tubes. The proximal portion of the uterine tubes opens into the uterus, and the distal portion opens directly into the peritoneal cavity, immediately superior to the ovaries, thereby providing a direct route for pathogens to enter the pelvic cavity. The uterine tubes provide a method of transport for ova to reach the uterus from the ovaries.

Vagina. The **vagina** is an 8- to 10-cm muscular tube extending anteroinferiorly from the cervix of the uterus to the external vaginal orifice. The **vaginal vault** or **fornix** is the upper vaginal area that surrounds the cervical os like a ring and is commonly divided into **anterior** and **posterior fornices.** The vagina is located between the bladder and the rectum and functions as a receptacle for sperm and as the lower portion of the birth canal (Figures 8.58 through 8.60 and 8.72 through 8.75).

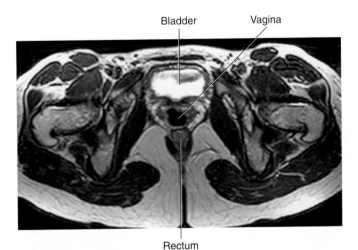
FIGURE 8.74 Axial, T2-weighted MRI of female pelvis with vagina.

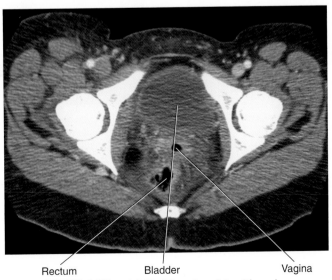
FIGURE 8.75 Axial CT of female pelvis with vagina.

Pelvic spaces. A peritoneal fold called the **broad ligament** encloses the ovaries, uterine tubes, and uterus (Figures 8.65, 8.69, 8.72 and 8.76). The broad ligament extends from the sides of the uterus to the walls and floor of the pelvis, preventing side-to-side movement of the uterus and dividing the pelvis into anterior and posterior pouches. The anterior **vesicouterine pouch** is located between the uterus and the posterior wall of the bladder, whereas the posterior **rectouterine pouch (pouch of Douglas)** lies between the uterus and rectum. In males, the posterior space is called the rectovesical pouch and is located between the rectum and seminal vesicles (Figures 8.66, 8.67, and 8.77). The pelvic spaces are common areas for the accumulation of fluid within the pelvis. Another space in the pelvis is the **retropubic space**, which is located between the pubic bones and the bladder and contains extraperitoneal fat and connective tissue for the expansion of the bladder (Figures 8.77 and 8.78).

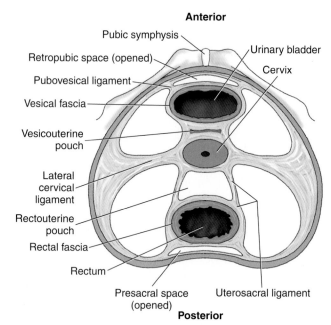

FIGURE 8.77 Superior view of pelvic spaces, Female.

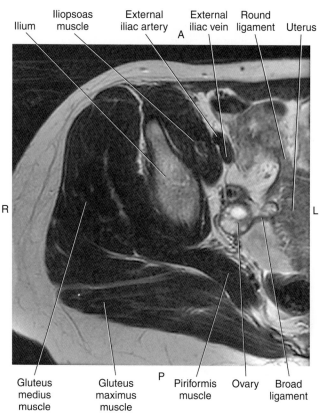

FIGURE 8.76 Axial, T2-weighted MRI of female pelvis with broad ligament.

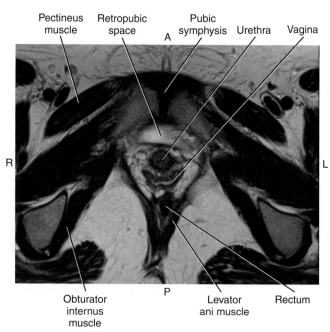

FIGURE 8.78 Axial, T2-weighted MRI of female pelvis with retropubic space.

Male Reproductive Organs

The principal structures of the male reproductive system are the testis, epididymis, vas deferens, ejaculatory duct, seminal vesicle, prostate gland, bulbourethral gland, and penis. All these structures, except the testes and penis, are located within the pelvic cavity (Figures 8.79 and 8.80).

Scrotum. The **scrotum** is a musculotendinous pouch that encloses the testis, epididymis, and lower portions of the spermatic cord (Figure 8.79 through 8.81). It is composed of three fascial layers and a connective tissue layer embedded with smooth muscle fibers called the **dartos tunica**. Internally, the dartos tunic forms a septum that divides the scrotum into right and left

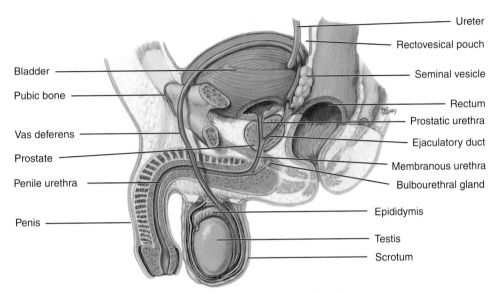

FIGURE 8.79 Sagittal view of male pelvis.

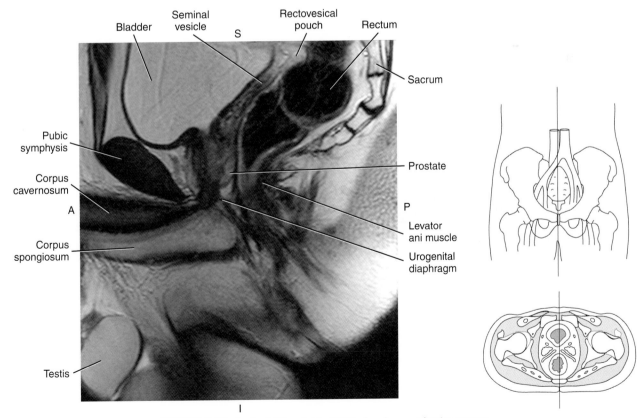

FIGURE 8.80 Sagittal, T2-weighted MRI of male reproductive system.

compartments (**median raphe**), each containing a testis (Figures 8.81, 8.82, and 8.84). The scrotum facilitates sperm formation by distending the testes outside the peritoneum in a cooler environment, in effect regulating the temperature of the testes. In cold temperatures, the dartos tunica responds by constricting and pulling the testis closer to the body. This gives the scrotum its wrinkled appearance.

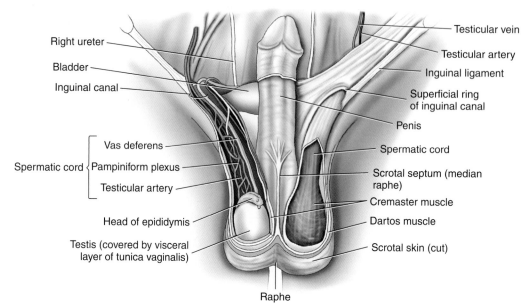

FIGURE 8.81 Coronal view of male reproductive system.

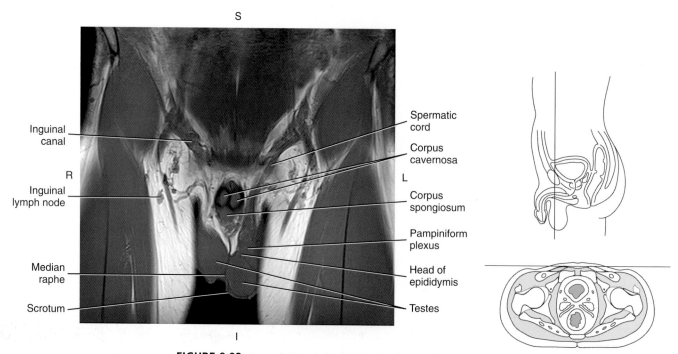

FIGURE 8.82 Coronal, T1-weighted MRI of male reproductive system.

Testes and epididymis. The paired **testes** are suspended in the fleshy, pouchlike scrotal sacs. Each testis is an ovoid organ that produces sperm and male sex hormones. The outer fibrous covering of the testes is the **tunica albuginea**, which also projects into each organ to create wedge-shaped lobules. Each testis is made up of several hundred lobules, with each lobule containing 1 to 4 seminiferous tubules, approximately 800 seminiferous tubules in total. The seminiferous tubules leave their respective lobule and converge in an area called the **rete testis**. From here, about 15 to 20 ductules leave the rete testis to enter the head of the epididymis. The **epididymis** is a tightly coiled tubular structure located on the supero-posterior surface of each testis. The **head** of the epididymis is located on the upper pole of each testis, whereas the **body** courses along the posterior surface to the **tail**, which is located under the lower pole of each testis. Sperm are transmitted from the testis to the **epididymis**, where they are stored as they undergo the final stages of maturation (Figures 8.79, and 8.81 through 8.87).

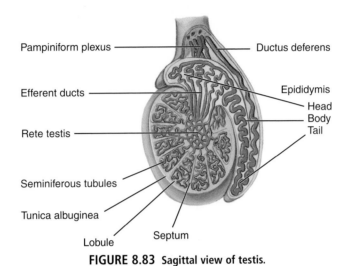

FIGURE 8.83 Sagittal view of testis.

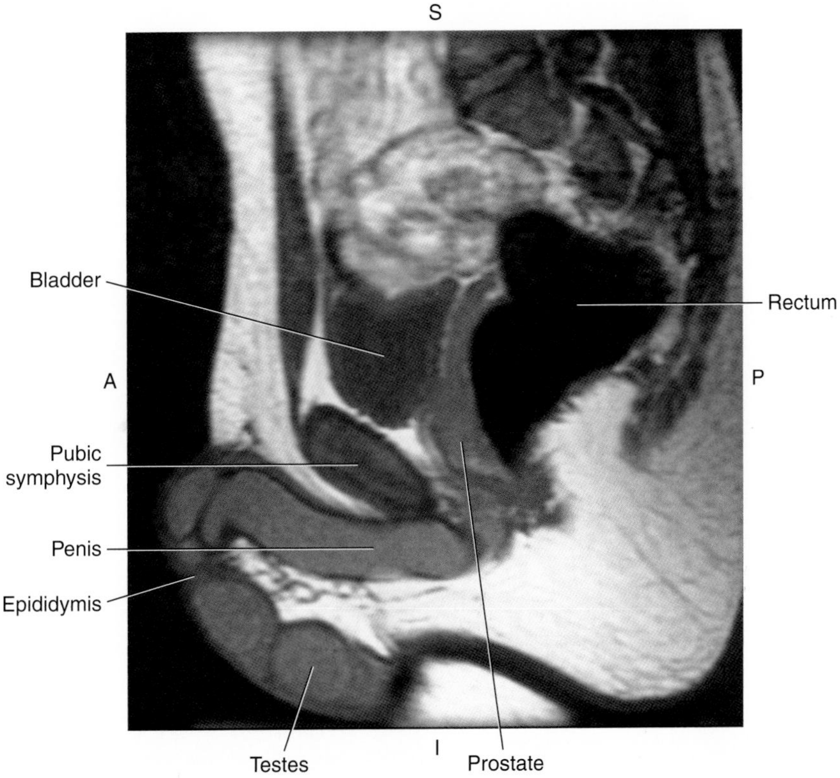

FIGURE 8.84 Sagittal, T1-weighted MRI of male pelvis with testes.

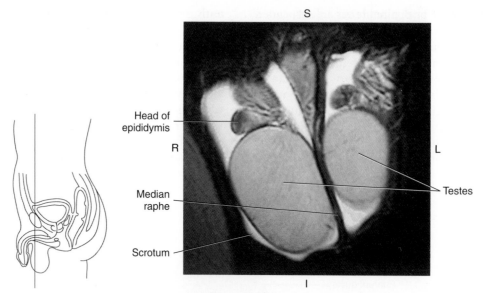

FIGURE 8.85 Coronal, T2-weighted MRI of male pelvis with testes.

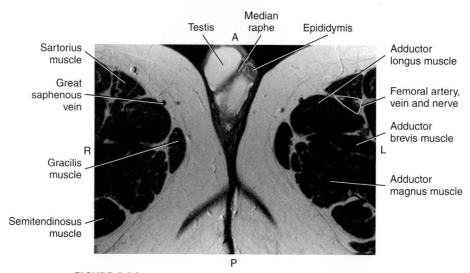

FIGURE 8.86 Axial, T2-weighted MRI of male pelvis with testes.

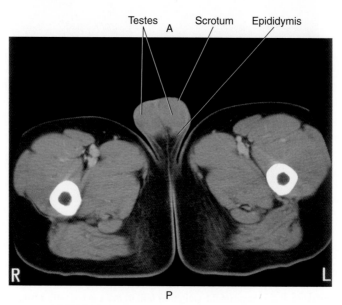

FIGURE 8.87 Axial CT of male pelvis with testes.

Vas deferens (ductus) and ejaculatory duct. As a continuation from the tail of the epididymis, the **vas deferens** is a long muscular tube that ascends in the posterior portion of the spermatic cord and traverses the inguinal canal, exiting at the deep inguinal ring (Figure 8.88). It then leaves the spermatic cord and passes along the lateral pelvic wall over the ureter to the posterior surface of the bladder, where it broadens and becomes the **ampulla** of the vas deferens. Near its proximal end, it joins with the duct of the seminal vesicle to form the **ejaculatory duct**, which empties into the prostatic urethra. Each vas deferens, along with a testicular artery and vein, is surrounded by the tough connective tissue and muscle of the paired **spermatic cords**. Within the spermatic cord is the **pampiniform plexus**, a group of interconnected veins that drain the blood from the testicles (Figures 8.81 and 8.83). The pampiniform plexus cools the blood in the testicular artery before it enters the testicles, helping to maintain a temperature that is conducive for optimal sperm production.

The spermatic cords begin at the inguinal ring and exit through the inguinal ligament to descend into the scrotum (Figures 8.81, 8.82, and 8.88 through 8.92).

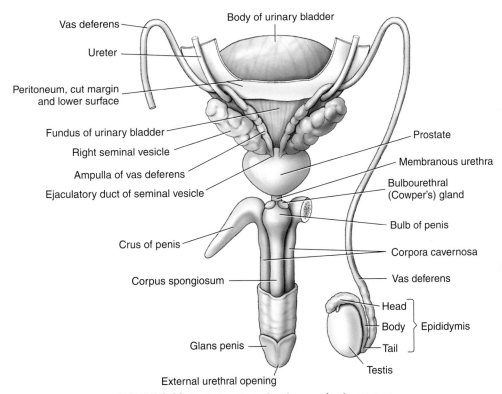

FIGURE 8.88 Posterior view of male reproductive system.

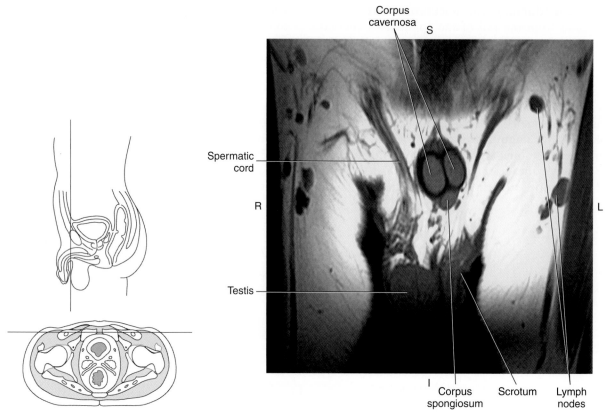

FIGURE 8.89 **Coronal, T1-weighted MRI of male pelvis with spermatic cords.**

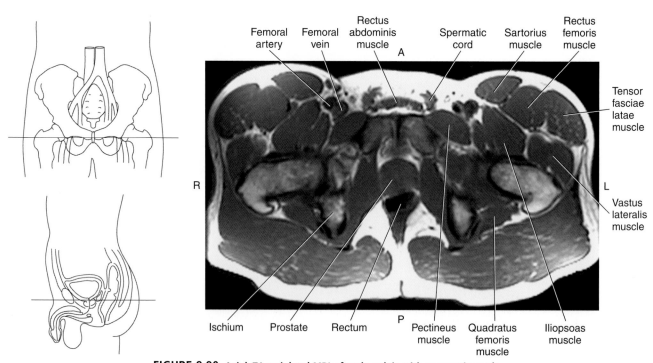

FIGURE 8.90 **Axial, T1-weighted MRI of male pelvis with spermatic cords.**

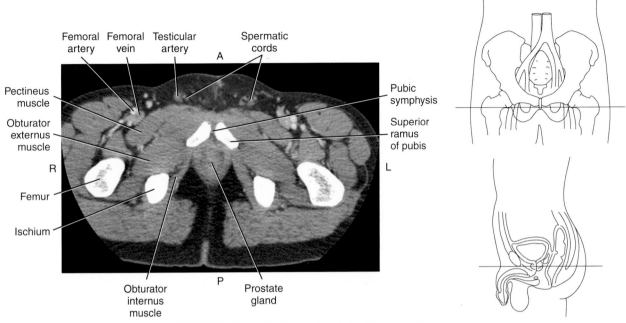

FIGURE 8.91 Axial CT of male pelvis with spermatic cords.

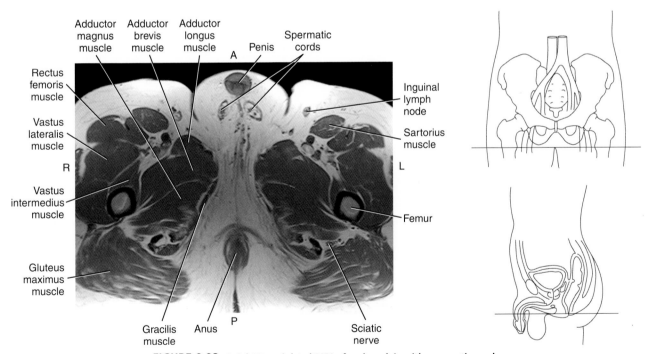

FIGURE 8.92 Axial, T2-weighted MRI of male pelvis with spermatic cords.

Seminal vesicles. The **seminal vesicles** are paired accessory glands consisting of coiled tubes that form two pouches, lateral to the vas deferens on the posterior inferior surface of the bladder. They lie superior to the prostate gland and produce fructose and a coagulating enzyme for the seminal fluid that mixes with sperm before ejaculation (Figures 8.79, 8.80, 8.88, and 8.93 through 8.96).

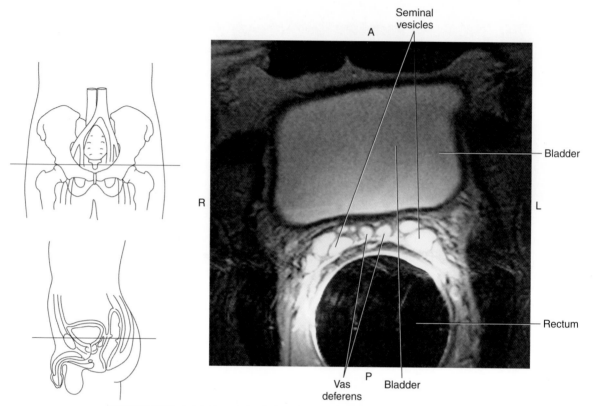

FIGURE 8.93 Axial, T2-weighted MRI of seminal vesicles, with endorectal coil.

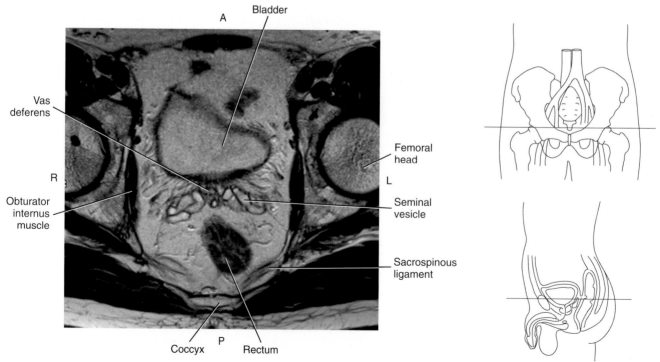

FIGURE 8.94 Axial, T2-weighted MRI of male pelvis with seminal vesicles.

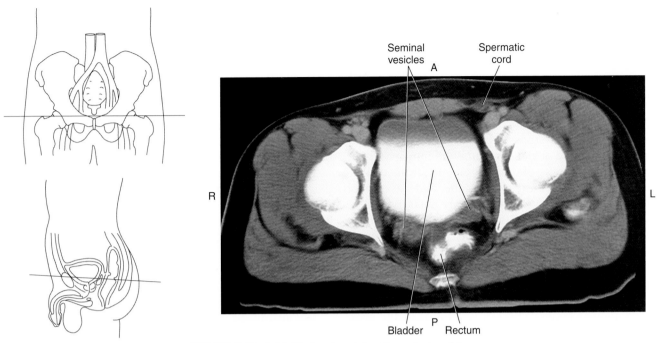

FIGURE 8.95   Axial CT of male pelvis with seminal vesicles.

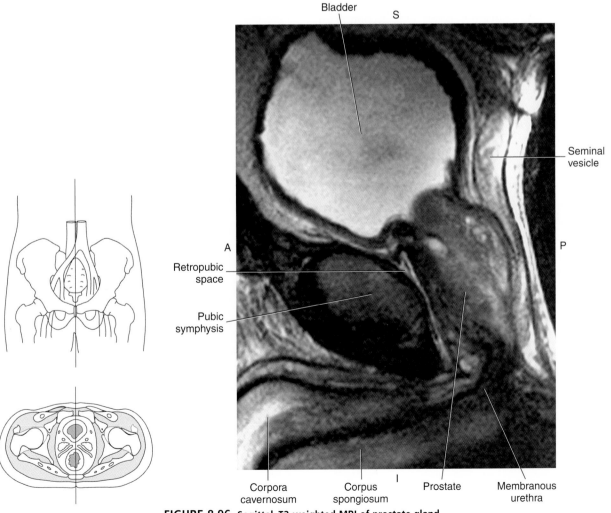

FIGURE 8.96   Sagittal, T2-weighted MRI of prostate gland.

Prostate gland. The **prostate gland** is the largest accessory gland of the male reproductive system. It secretes a thin, slightly alkaline fluid that forms a portion of the seminal fluid. The prostate gland is located inferior to the bladder and surrounds the prosthetic urethra, which courses through the anterior portion of the gland (Figures 8.79, 8.96, and 8.97). The prostate has a base adjacent to the neck of the bladder and an apex that is in contact with the urogenital diaphragm. The prostate gland is composed of glandular and fibromuscular tissue and surrounded by a fibrous capsule. It can be divided into two lateral lobes, a middle lobe, and an anterior fibromuscular portion. The ejaculatory ducts, which are extensions of the seminal vesicles, descend within the central zone of the gland and open into the prostatic urethra at the verumontanum. The **verumontanum** is a longitudinal mucosal fold that forms an elliptical segment of the prostatic urethra, marking the point where the ejaculatory ducts enter the urethra (Figure 8.98). The glandular tissue comprises two-thirds of the prostate's parenchymal tissue and can be divided into zonal anatomy in sectional imaging. The four main regions are the central, peripheral, transition, and anterior fibromuscular stroma (Figures 8.98 through 8.100). The **central zone** is located at the base of the prostate between the peripheral and transition zones and accounts for approximately 25% of the glandular tissue. It surrounds the ejaculatory ducts and narrows to an apex at the verumontanum. The **peripheral zone** is the larger of the zones, comprising approximately 70% of the glandular tissue. It extends from the base to the apex along the posterior or rectal surface of the gland and surrounds the distal urethra. The peripheral zone is separated from the central and transition zones by the surgical capsule. The **transition zone** forms only 5% of the glandular tissue. It consists of two small lobules that are located lateral to the proximal urethra between the verumontanum and the neck of the bladder. This is the portion of the glandular tissue that enlarges due to benign prostatic hypertrophy. The periurethral zone comprises less than 1% of the glandular tissue. It is found embedded along the smooth muscular wall of the urethra. The **anterior fibromuscular stroma** is devoid of glandular tissue and is composed of fibrous and muscular elements. As it extends laterally and posteriorly, it thins to form the fibrous capsule that surrounds the prostate gland.

> Cancer of the prostate gland is the second most common type of cancer in men, occurring with increasing frequency after the age of 55 years.

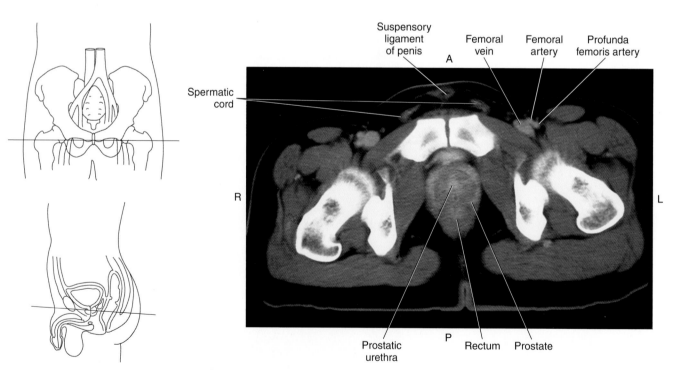

FIGURE 8.97 Axial CT of male pelvis with prostate gland.

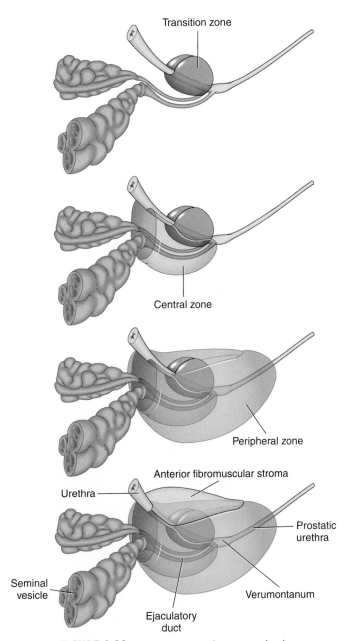

FIGURE 8.98 Zonal anatomy of prostate gland.

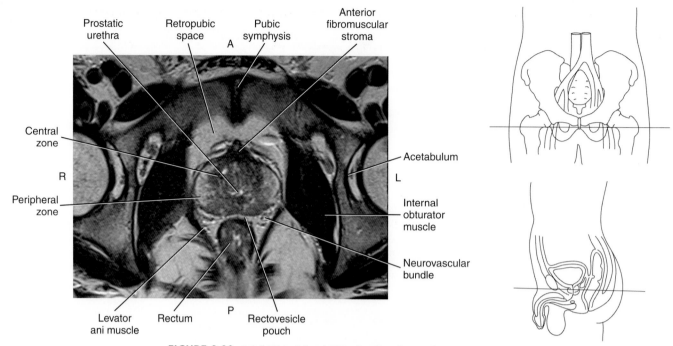

FIGURE 8.99 Axial, T2-weighted MRI of male pelvis with prostate gland.

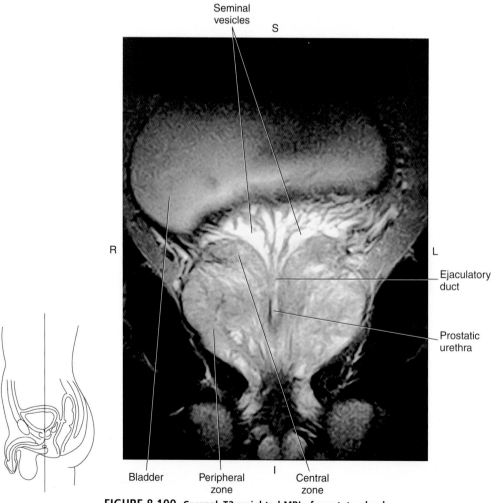

FIGURE 8.100 Coronal, T2-weighted MRI of prostate gland.

Bulbourethral glands. The two small, **bulbourethral glands** (Cowper's glands) lie posterolateral to the membranous urethra, embedded in the urogenital diaphragm. These glands secrete an alkaline fluid, which forms a portion of the seminal fluid, into the membranous urethra (Figure 8.101).

Penis. The **penis**, the external reproductive organ, is attached to the pubic arch via suspensory ligaments. It has two parts: the **root**, which is attached to the pubic arch, and the **body**, which remains free. Three cylindric masses of erectile tissue constitute the root of the penis: two corpus cavernosa and the corpus spongiosum. The **corpus cavernosa** consists of a network of collagen fibers and spaces that become enlarged when filled with blood, contributing to an erection. The **corpus spongiosum** consists mostly of a dense venous plexus and contributes to an erection. The two corpus cavernosa form the upper surface, whereas the corpus spongiosum forms the undersurface and contains the greater part of the urethra. At the root of the penis, the corpus cavernosa forms the **crura**, which attach along the ischiopubic ramus. The corpus spongiosum forms the **bulb** of the penis, which is located between the two crura and is firmly attached to the inferior aspect of the urogenital diaphragm. The distal end of the cylindric masses forms the **glans penis**, which surrounds the external urethral meatus (Figures 8.101 through 8.105).

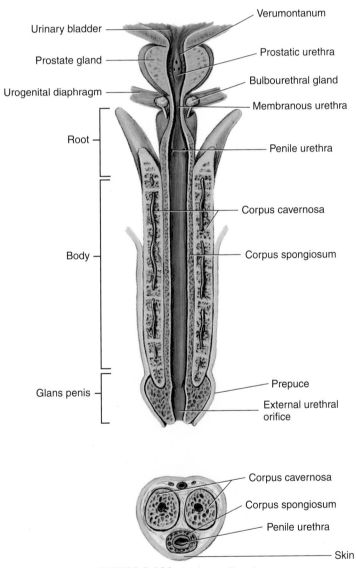

FIGURE 8.101 Anatomy of penis.

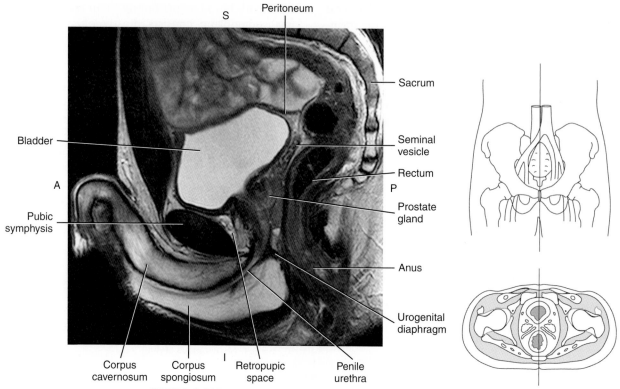

FIGURE 8.102 Sagittal, T2-weighted MRI of male pelvis with penis.

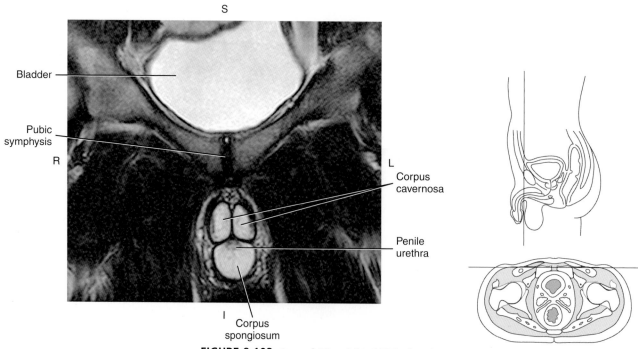

FIGURE 8.103 Coronal, T2-weighted MRI of penis.

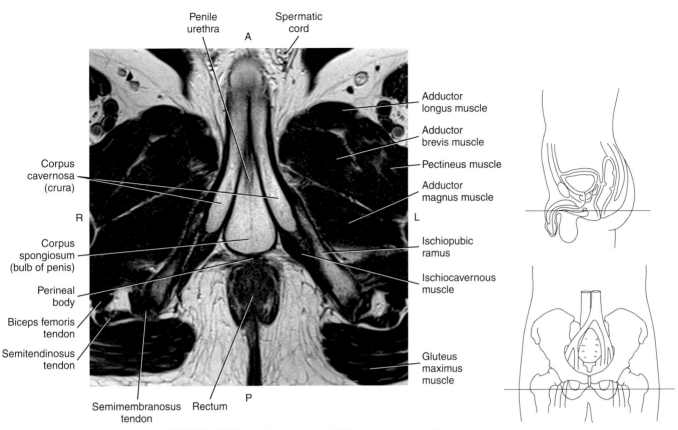

FIGURE 8.104   Axial, T2-weighted MRI of male pelvis with root of penis.

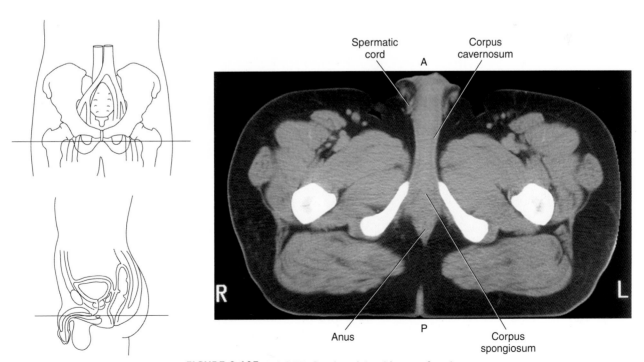

FIGURE 8.105   Axial CT of male pelvis with root of penis.

VASCULATURE

Arteries

The abdominal aorta descends into the pelvis anterior to the lumbar vertebra slightly to the left of midline. Extending from the dorsal wall of the aorta, just above the aortic bifurcation at the level of the fourth lumbar verterbae, is the **median (middle) sacral artery**, which continues caudally in front of the sacrum to the apex of the coccyx. The descending aorta bifurcates into the right and left **common iliac arteries** (Figures 8.106 through 8.108). Each common iliac artery bifurcates at the upper margin of the sacroiliac joint into the internal and external iliac arteries (Figure 8.109). The smaller **internal iliac artery** extends posteromedially into the pelvis just medial to the external iliac vein and branches into an anterior trunk and a posterior trunk. The **anterior trunk of the internal iliac artery** supplies blood to the perineum, gluteal region, and pelvic viscera. Branches of the anterior trunk of the internal iliac artery include the **obturator, umbilical, inferior vesical** in males, **uterine** and **vaginal** in females, **middle rectal, internal pudendal,** and **inferior gluteal arteries** (Figure 8.107). The **posterior trunk of the internal iliac artery** supplies blood to the posterior and lateral walls of the pelvis, iliac crest, and gluteal region. Branches of the posterior trunk include the **iliolumbar, lateral sacral,** and **superior gluteal arteries**. The large **external iliac artery** does not enter the true pelvis but extends along the pelvic brim to exit the iliac fossa and course under the inguinal ligament to supply the leg. The external iliac artery becomes the **femoral artery** at approximately the level of the anterior superior iliac spine. Branches of the external iliac artery include the **inferior epigastric artery**, which supplies blood to the muscles and skin of the anterior abdominal wall, and the **deep circumflex iliac artery**, which supplies blood to the lateral abdominal muscles (Figures 8.110 through 8.120 and Table 8.2).

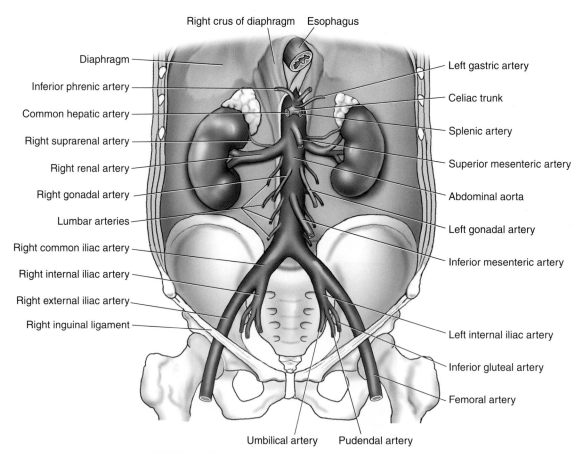

FIGURE 8.106 Anterior view of abdominal aorta and vessels.

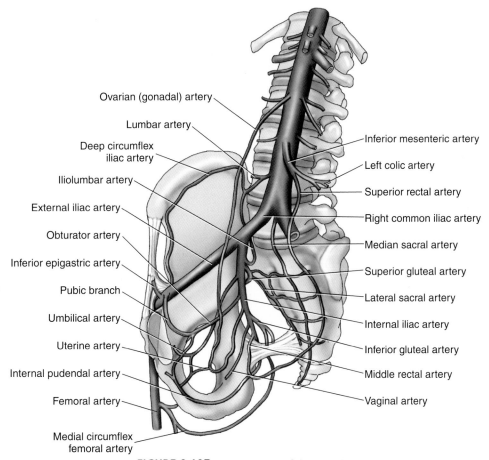

Ovarian (gonadal) artery

Lumbar artery

Deep circumflex
iliac artery

Iliolumbar artery

External iliac artery

Obturator artery

Inferior epigastric artery

Pubic branch

Umbilical artery

Uterine artery

Internal pudendal artery

Femoral artery

Medial circumflex
femoral artery

Inferior mesenteric artery

Left colic artery

Superior rectal artery

Right common iliac artery

Median sacral artery

Superior gluteal artery

Lateral sacral artery

Internal iliac artery

Inferior gluteal artery

Middle rectal artery

Vaginal artery

FIGURE 8.107 Anterior view of iliac arteries.

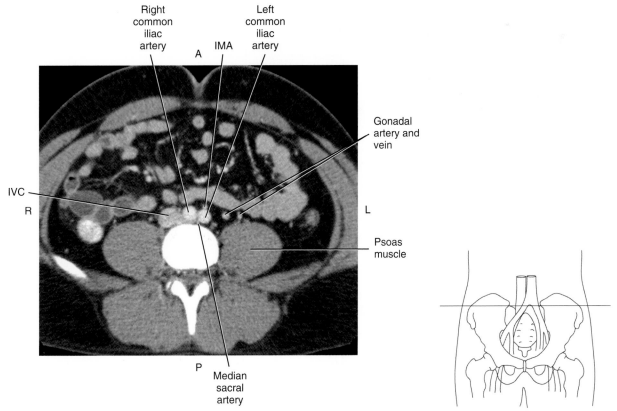

Right
common
iliac
artery

Left
common
iliac
artery

A

IMA

Gonadal
artery and
vein

IVC

R

L

Psoas
muscle

P

Median
sacral
artery

FIGURE 8.108 Axial CT of pelvis with common iliac vessels.

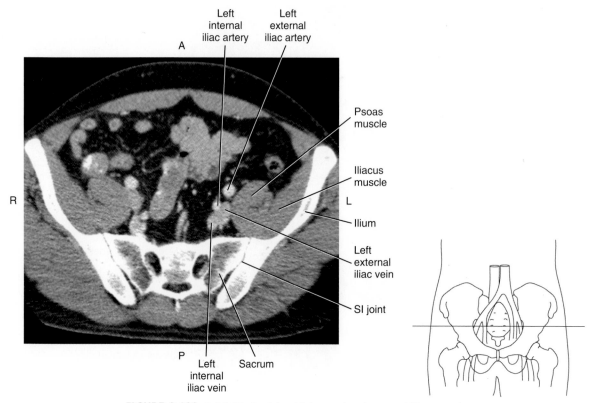

FIGURE 8.109 Axial CT of pelvis with internal and external iliac vessels.

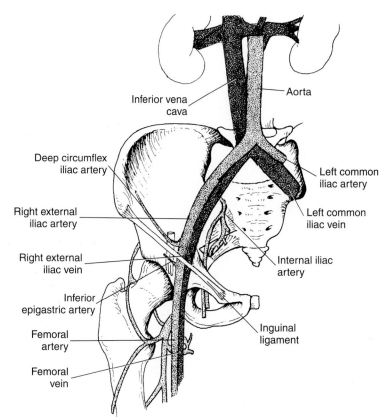

FIGURE 8.110 Anterior view of inferior vena cava and abdominal aorta.

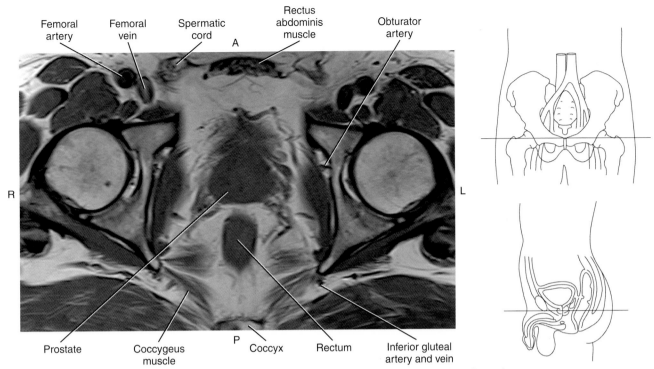

Femoral artery   Femoral vein   Spermatic cord   A   Rectus abdominis muscle   Obturator artery

R   L

Prostate   Coccygeus muscle   P   Coccyx   Rectum   Inferior gluteal artery and vein

FIGURE 8.111 Axial, T1-weighted MRI of pelvis with inferior gluteal vessels.

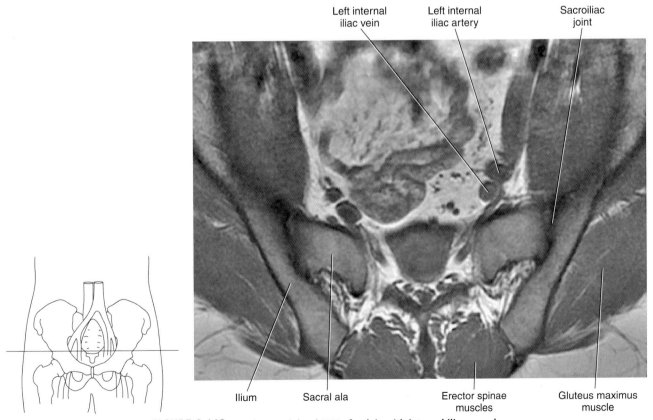

Left internal iliac vein   Left internal iliac artery   Sacroiliac joint

Ilium   Sacral ala   Erector spinae muscles   Gluteus maximus muscle

FIGURE 8.112 Axial, T1-weighted MRI of pelvis with internal iliac vessels.

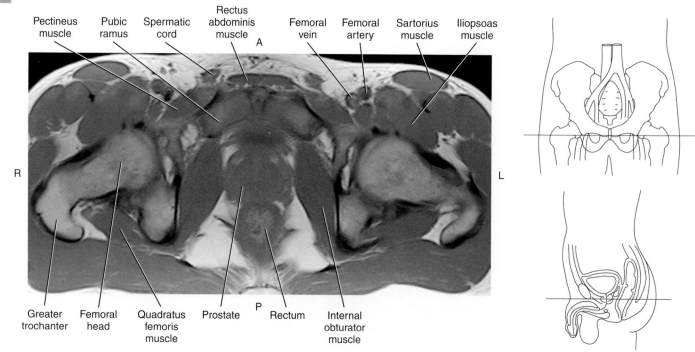

Pectineus muscle
Pubic ramus
Spermatic cord
Rectus abdominis muscle
A
Femoral vein
Femoral artery
Sartorius muscle
Iliopsoas muscle

R

L

Greater trochanter
Femoral head
Quadratus femoris muscle
Prostate
P
Rectum
Internal obturator muscle

FIGURE 8.113 Axial, T1-weighted MRI of pelvis with femoral artery and vein.

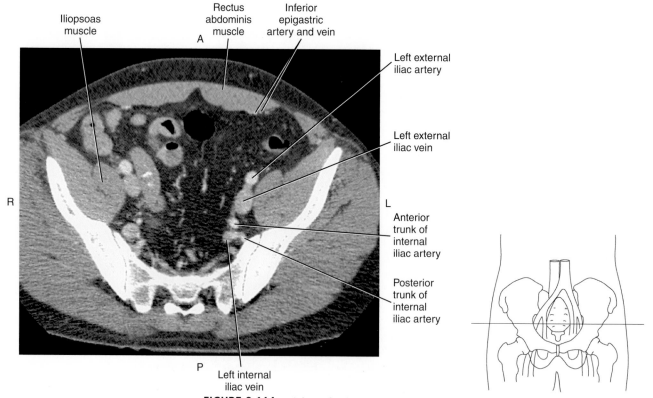

Iliopsoas muscle
Rectus abdominis muscle
A
Inferior epigastric artery and vein
Left external iliac artery
Left external iliac vein
L
Anterior trunk of internal iliac artery
Posterior trunk of internal iliac artery

R

P
Left internal iliac vein

FIGURE 8.114 Axial CT of pelvis with iliac vessels.

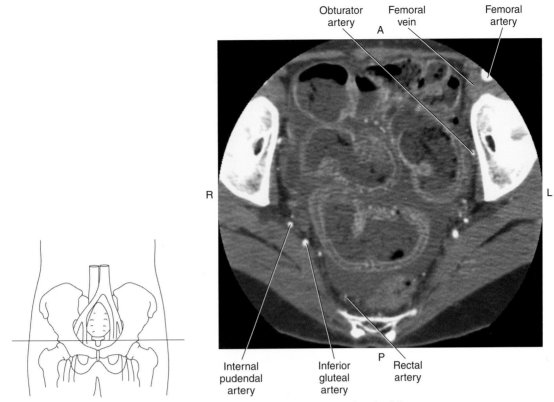

FIGURE 8.115 Axial CT of pelvis with internal pudendal artery.

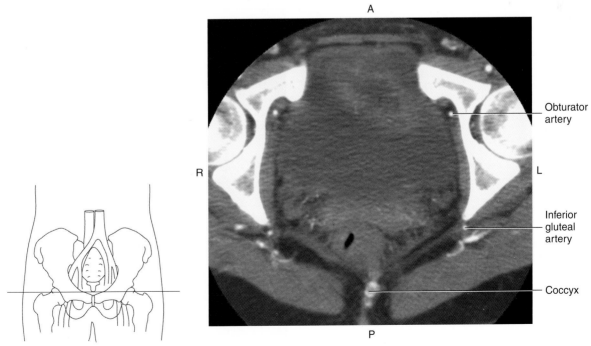

FIGURE 8.116 Axial CT of pelvis with obturator artery.

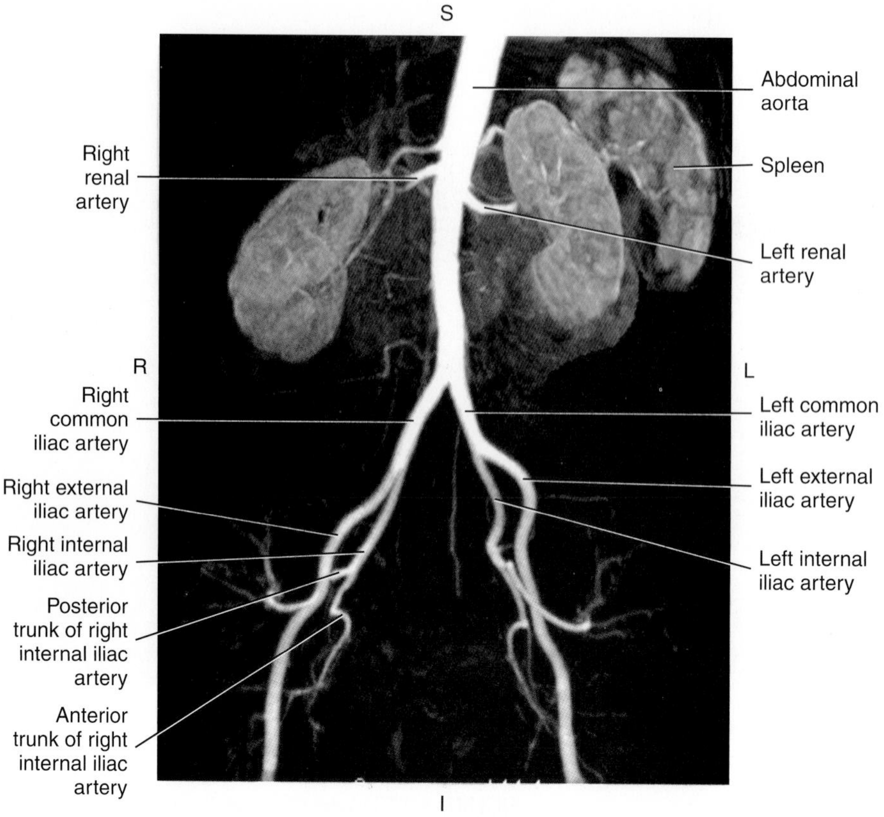

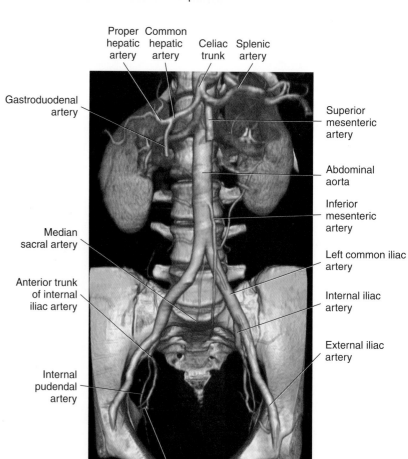

S

Right
renal
artery

Abdominal
aorta

Spleen

Left renal
artery

R

L

Right
common
iliac artery

Left common
iliac artery

Right external
iliac artery

Left external
iliac artery

Right internal
iliac artery

Left internal
iliac artery

Posterior
trunk of right
internal iliac
artery

Anterior
trunk of right
internal iliac
artery

I

FIGURE 8.117 MRA of descending aorta
and iliac vessels.

Proper   Common
hepatic   hepatic   Celiac   Splenic
artery   artery   trunk   artery

Gastroduodenal
artery

Superior
mesenteric
artery

Abdominal
aorta

Inferior
mesenteric
artery

Median
sacral artery

Left common iliac
artery

Anterior trunk
of internal
iliac artery

Internal iliac
artery

External iliac
artery

Internal
pudendal
artery

FIGURE 8.118 3D CTA of descending aorta and iliac
vessels.

Inferior gluteal artery

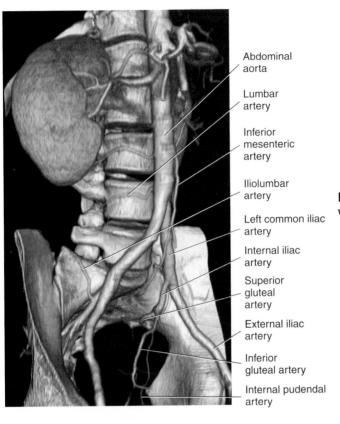

Abdominal aorta

Lumbar artery

Inferior mesenteric artery

Iliolumbar artery

Left common iliac artery

Internal iliac artery

Superior gluteal artery

External iliac artery

Inferior gluteal artery

Internal pudendal artery

FIGURE 8.119 Anterior oblique 3D CTA of descending aorta and iliac vessels.

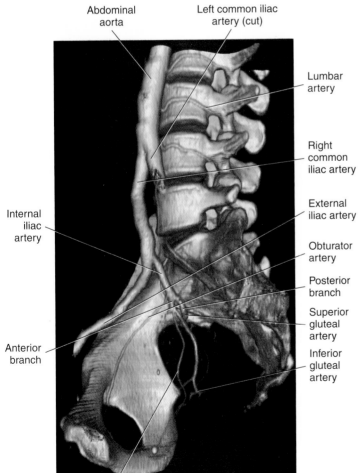

Abdominal aorta

Left common iliac artery (cut)

Lumbar artery

Right common iliac artery

External iliac artery

Obturator artery

Posterior branch

Superior gluteal artery

Inferior gluteal artery

Internal iliac artery

Anterior branch

Internal pudendal artery

FIGURE 8.120 3D CTA of iliac vessels.

TABLE 8.2	Branches of the Internal and External Iliac Arteries
Arterial Branch	**Structures Supplied**
Anterior Branch of Internal Iliac	
Obturator artery	Medial thigh
Umbilical artery	Superior bladder, vas deferens
Uterine artery	Uterus, cervix, and vagina
Vaginal artery	Vagina, posteroinferior bladder, pelvic part of urethra
Inferior vesicle artery	Prostate, seminal vesicles, and posteroinferior part of the bladder
Middle rectal artery	Distal end of rectum, prostate, and seminal vesicles or vagina
Internal pudendal artery	Anal canal and perineum
Inferior gluteal artery	Muscles and skin of the buttock and posterior surface of the thigh
Posterior Branch of Internal Iliac	
Iliolumbar artery	Psoas, iliacus, quadratus lumborum, gluteal muscles, and cauda equina
Lateral sacral artery	Spinal meninges, roots of the sacral nerves, and muscles and skin of dorsal sacrum
Superior gluteal artery	Obturator internus, piriformis, and gluteus muscles
Branches of External Iliac Artery	
Inferior epigastric artery	Ascends abdomen to anastomose with internal thoracic vessels to supply the anterior abdominal wall
Deep circumflex iliac artery	Ascends abdomen to anastomose with internal thoracic vessels to supply the lateral aspect of the anterior abdominal wall

Venous Drainage

Venous drainage of the pelvis follows a pattern similar to that of the arterial supply. Mainly the **internal iliac veins** and their tributaries drain the pelvis (Figures 8.121 and 8.122). However, there is some drainage through the **superior rectal, median (middle) sacral,** and **gonadal veins.** The internal iliac vein ascends the pelvis medial to the internal iliac artery as it returns blood from the pelvic viscera. Tributaries of the internal iliac vein are similar to that of the branches of the internal iliac artery with some differences, such as the iliolumbar vein, which usually drains into the common iliac vein. In addition,

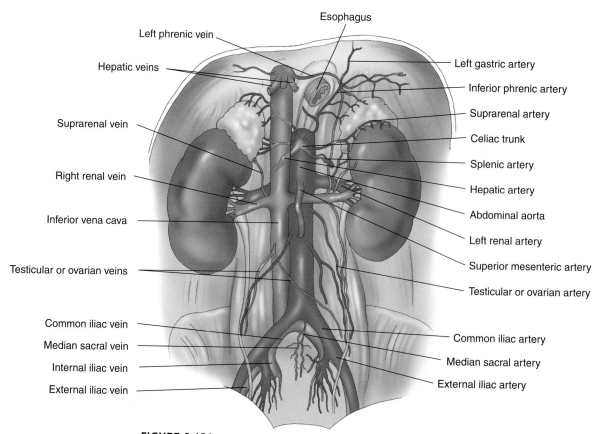

FIGURE 8.121 Anterior view of inferior vena cava and tributaries.

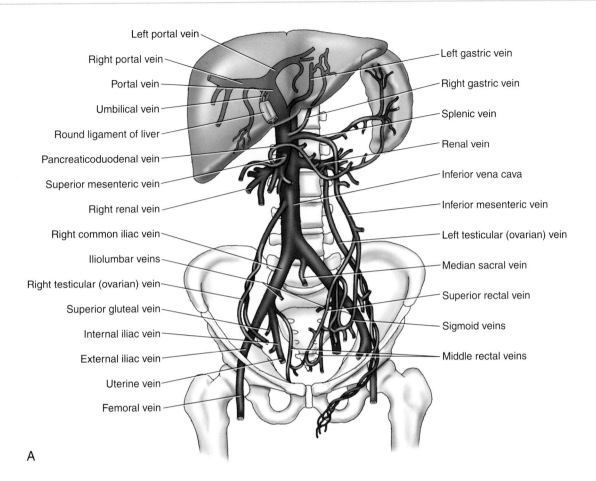

A

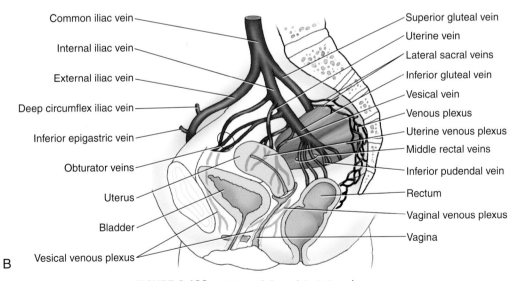

B

FIGURE 8.122 A, Veins of the pelvis. B, Female.

(Continued)

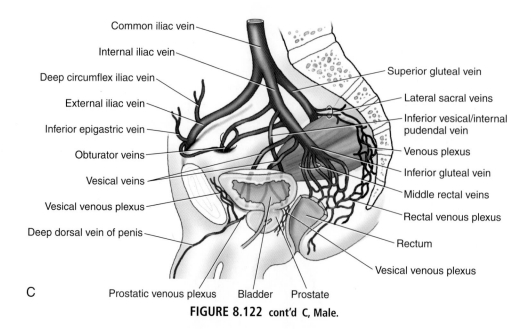

FIGURE 8.122 cont'd **C,** Male.

venous plexuses are formed by the veins in the pelvis and unite to drain mainly into the internal iliac vein (Figure 8.122). These plexuses include the uterine, vaginal, prostatic, vesical, and rectal. The **external iliac veins**, extensions of the femoral veins, return blood from the legs. Typically, both external iliac veins course medial to their respective external iliac artery and then change to a posterior position as they ascend to join the common iliac vein at approximately the level of the sacroiliac joint. The **common iliac vein** arises posterior to the common iliac artery from the junction of the internal and external iliac veins. The **inferior vena cava** is formed at the level of L5, just a little to the right of the midline, by the union of the common iliac veins. From this level it continues to ascend the abdomen to the right of the abdominal aorta (Figures 8.108 through 8.115).

LYMPH NODES

Pelvic lymph nodes include nodal chains or groups that accompany their corresponding vessels. Those nodal groups that correspond to pelvic vessels include the common iliac, internal iliac, external iliac, and sacral nodal groups (Figure 8.123). The **common iliac lymph nodes** form two groups along the surface of the common iliac artery: a lateral group and a median group. The **lateral common iliac group** receives lymph from the lower limb and pelvis via the external and internal iliac lymph nodes. The **median common iliac group** receives lymph directly from the pelvic viscera and indirectly through the internal iliac and sacral lymph nodes. The **obturator nodes,** which course along the midportion of the obturator internus muscle, are included in the medial common iliac group. The **external iliac lymph nodes** lie on the external iliac vessels and drain lymph from the lower limb, abdominal wall, bladder, and prostate in males or uterus and vagina in females. The **internal iliac lymph nodes** surround the internal iliac vessels and their branches. They receive lymph from all the pelvic viscera, deep parts of the perineum, and gluteal and thigh regions. **Sacral lymph nodes** lie along the median and lateral sacral arteries. They receive lymph from the posterior pelvic wall, rectum, neck of the bladder, and prostate

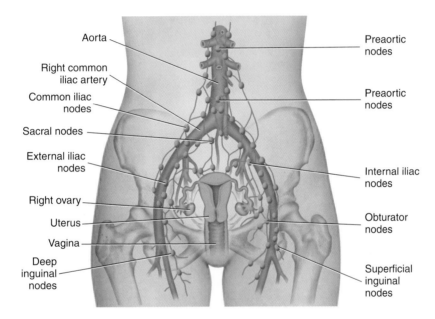

FIGURE 8.123 Anterior view of pelvic lymph nodes.

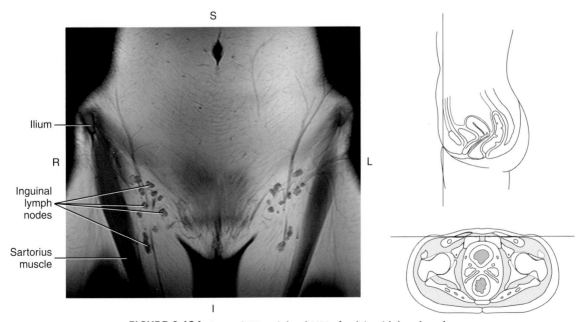

FIGURE 8.124 Coronal, T1-weighted MRI of pelvis with lymph nodes.

or cervix. The inguinal lymph nodes drain lymph from the lower limb, perineum, anterior abdominal wall as far superiorly as the umbilicus, gluteal region, and parts of the anal canal. They can be divided into the superficial inguinal lymph nodes that are situated distal to the inguinal ligament in the subcutaneous tissue anterior and medial to common femoral vessels. The deep inguinal lymph nodes are fewer in number and are situated medial to the femoral vessels at the approximate level of the ischial tuberosity. Pelvic lymph nodes are considered pathologically enlarged when they exceed 10 mm in the short axis (Figures 8.124 through 8.126).

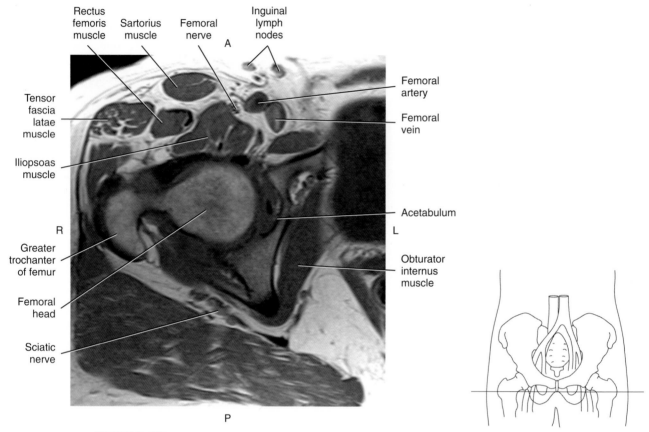

FIGURE 8.125 Axial, T1-weighted MRI of right hip with femoral vessels and inguinal lymph nodes.

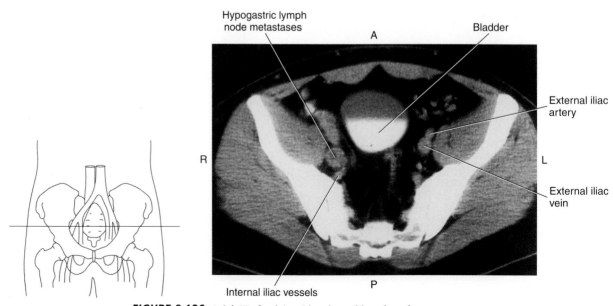

FIGURE 8.126 Axial CT of pelvis with enlarged lymph nodes.

9

Upper Extremity

It is sometimes on one's weakest limbs that one must lean in order to keep going.

Jean Rostand, Substance of Man

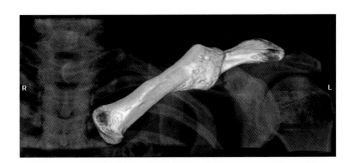

The intricate anatomy of the musculoskeletal system can make identification of the upper extremity anatomy challenging (Figure 9.1). A basic knowledge of the anatomy and kinesiology of these areas increases the ability to identify pathology or injury that may occur.

FIGURE 9.1 3D CT—healing fracture of the clavicle.

OBJECTIVES

- Identify the bony anatomy of the upper extremity.
- Identify the components that contribute to the glenoid labrum.
- Describe the joint capsules of the shoulder and elbow.
- List and describe the ligaments and tendons of each upper extremity joint.

- Identify and state the actions of the muscles, as well as their origin and insertion sites.
- Identify the major arteries and veins of the upper extremity.
- List and identify the nerves that innervate the upper extremity.

OUTLINE

SHOULDER

Bony Anatomy

The bony anatomy that comprises the shoulder girdle includes the clavicle, scapula, and humerus (Figures 9.2 and 9.3).

Clavicle. The clavicle connects the upper limb to the trunk of the body and provides attachments for several muscles and ligaments. The clavicle is a long, slender bone located anteriorly that extends transversely from the sternum to the acromion of the scapula. The widened **sternal end** of the clavicle articulates with the manubrium of the sternum to form the **sternoclavicular (SC)**

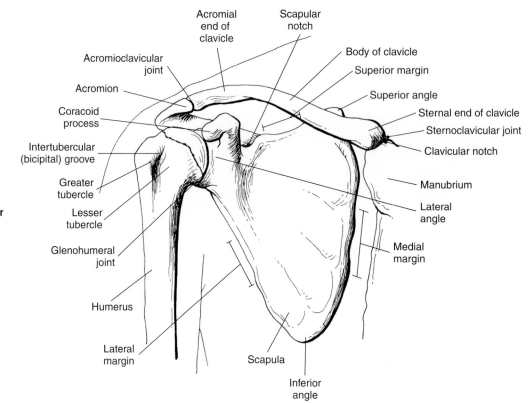

FIGURE 9.2 Anterior view of shoulder girdle.

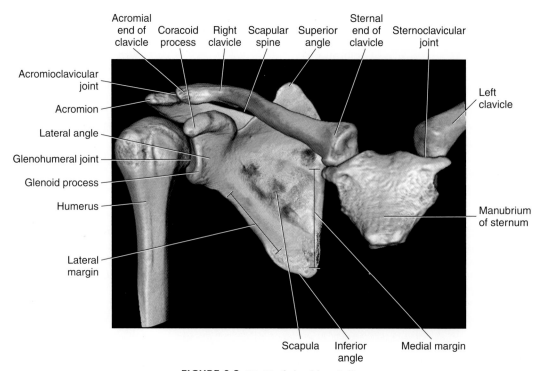

FIGURE 9.3 3D CT of shoulder girdle.

joint, and its flattened **acromial end** articulates with the acromion process of the scapula to form the **acromioclavicular (AC) joint.** The medial two thirds of the body of the clavicle are anteriorly convex, whereas the lateral one third is flattened and anteriorly concave (Figures 9.2 through 9.6).

Scapula. The scapula is a triangular-shaped flat bone that forms the posterior portion of the shoulder girdle. It has a medial margin (vertebral border), a lateral margin (axillary border), and a superior margin. The margins are separated by the superior, inferior, and lateral angles (Figures 9.2 and 9.3). The anterior surface

of the scapula, **subscapular fossa,** is flat and slightly concave. The posterior surface of the scapula is divided by the scapular spine into a smaller **supraspinous fossa** and a larger **infraspinous fossa** (Figure 9.7). Four projections of the scapula provide attachment sites for the muscles and ligaments contributing to the shoulder girdle. These include the **scapular spine, acromion, coracoid process,** and **glenoid process** (Figures 9.7 through 9.10). The scapular spine arises from the upper third of the posterior surface of the scapula and extends obliquely and laterally to give rise to the acromion process. Located on the anterolateral surface of the scapula

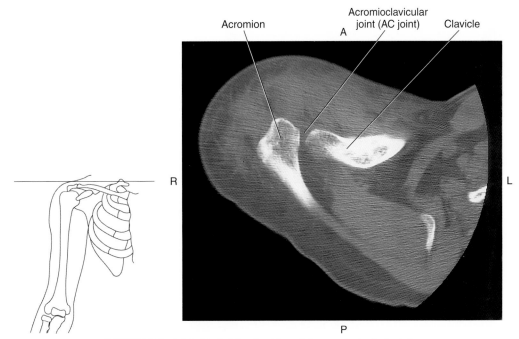

FIGURE 9.4 Axial CT of right shoulder with acromioclavicular joint.

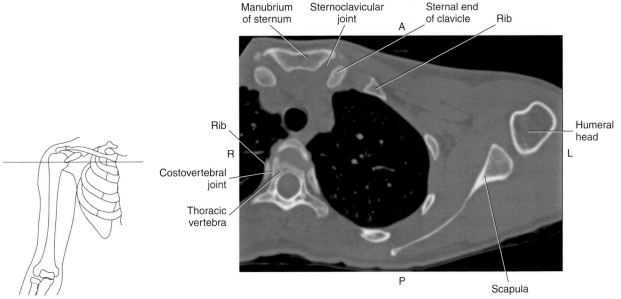

FIGURE 9.5 Axial CT of left shoulder with sternoclavicular joint.

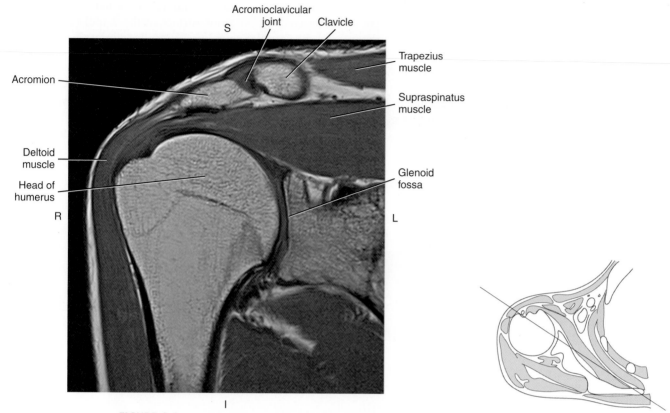

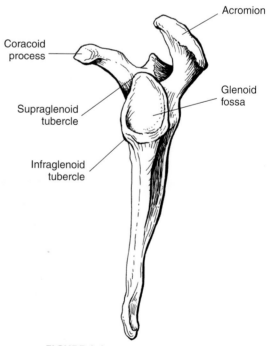

FIGURE 9.6 Coronal oblique, T1-weighted MRI of right shoulder with acromioclavicular joint.

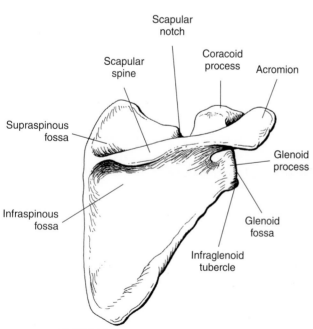

FIGURE 9.7 Posterior view of scapula.

FIGURE 9.8 Lateral view of scapula.

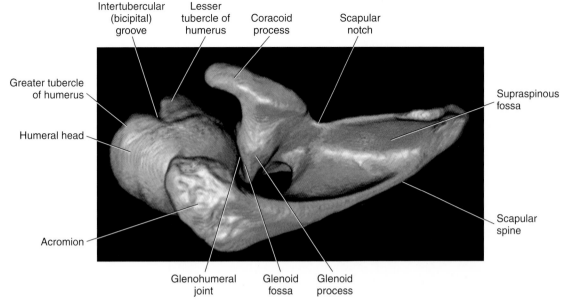

Intertubercular (bicipital) groove

Lesser tubercle of humerus

Coracoid process

Scapular notch

Greater tubercle of humerus

Humeral head

Supraspinous fossa

Acromion

Scapular spine

Glenohumeral joint

Glenoid fossa

Glenoid process

FIGURE 9.9 3D CT of superior aspect of scapula.

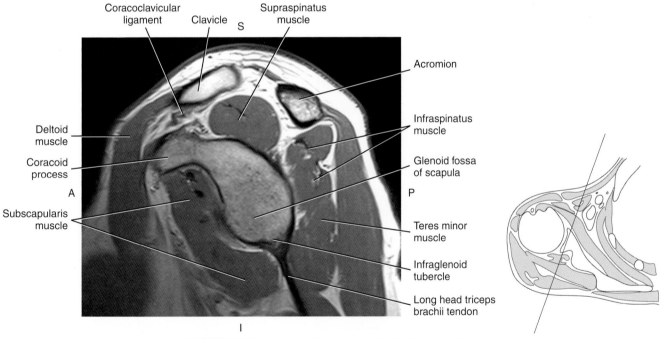

Coracoclavicular ligament

Clavicle

S

Supraspinatus muscle

Acromion

Deltoid muscle

Infraspinatus muscle

Coracoid process

Glenoid fossa of scapula

A

P

Subscapularis muscle

Teres minor muscle

Infraglenoid tubercle

Long head triceps brachii tendon

I

FIGURE 9.10 Sagittal oblique, T1-weighted MRI of shoulder.

is a beaklike process termed the **coracoid process**, which arises just medial to the glenoid process and functions to protect the shoulder joint, which lies beneath it. The coracoid process is an attachment site for the pectoralis minor, short head of the biceps brachii, and the coracobrachialis muscles. The **scapular notch** is located just medial to the coracoid process on the superior margin of the scapula and allows for the passage of the suprascapular nerve (Figure 9.2). The **glenoid process**, the largest of the projections, forms the lateral angle of the scapula and ends in

a depression called the **glenoid fossa (glenoid cavity)** (Figures 9.3 and 9.7 through 9.9). There are two tubercles associated with the glenoid fossa, an upper **supraglenoid tubercle** and a lower **infraglenoid tubercle**, which serve as attachment sites for the long heads of the biceps brachii and triceps brachii, respectively (Figures 9.8 and 9.10). The shallow articular surface of the glenoid fossa joins with the relatively large articular surface of the humeral head to create the freely moving **glenohumeral joint** (Figures 9.2, 9.3, 9.11, and 9.12).

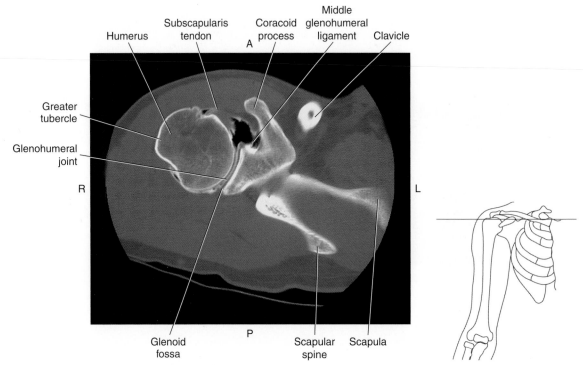

FIGURE 9.11 Axial CT of right shoulder, post-arthrogram.

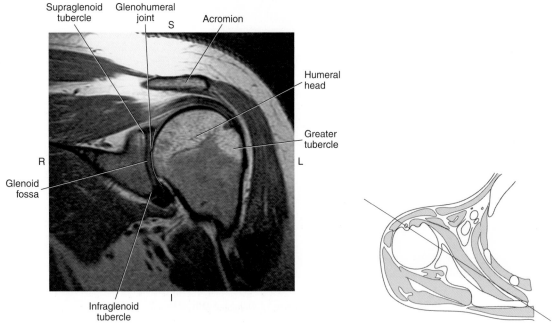

FIGURE 9.12 Coronal oblique, T1-weighted MRI of left shoulder.

Proximal humerus. The humerus is a long bone that articulates with the scapula superiorly and the radius and ulna inferiorly. It consists of a proximal end, a body (shaft), and a distal end (Figure 9.13). The proximal end is formed by the head of the humerus. Two tubercles project from the **humeral head** to provide attachment sites for tendons and ligaments. The **lesser tubercle** is located on the anterior surface of the humeral head, whereas the **greater tubercle** is located on the lateral surface of the

humeral head (Figures 9.12 through 9.15). The tubercles are separated by the **intertubercular (bicipital) groove** (Figures 9.9 and 9.13 through 9.15). The humerus has two necks, the more proximal **anatomic neck** and the **surgical neck,** located inferior to the tubercles just distal to the humeral head (Figures 9.13 and 9.16). In the middle of the body or shaft of the humerus, on the anterior surface, is the roughened area of the **deltoid tuberosity,** which provides attachment for the deltoid muscle (Figure 9.13).

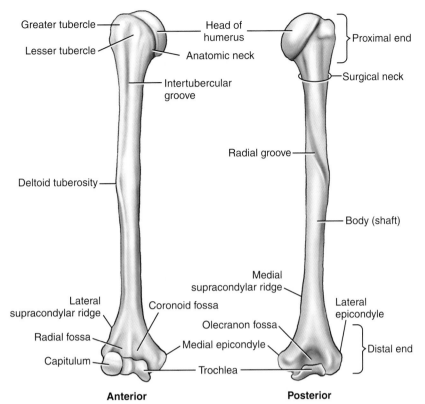

Greater tubercle
Lesser tubercle
Head of humerus
Anatomic neck
Proximal end
Intertubercular groove
Surgical neck
Radial groove
Deltoid tuberosity
Body (shaft)
Medial supracondylar ridge
Lateral supracondylar ridge
Coronoid fossa
Lateral epicondyle
Radial fossa
Olecranon fossa
Distal end
Capitulum
Medial epicondyle
Trochlea

Anterior   **Posterior**

FIGURE 9.13 **Humerus.** *Left,* Anterior view. *Right,* Posterior view.

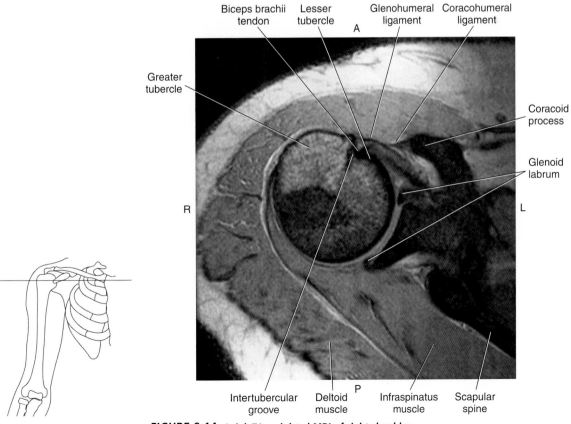

Biceps brachii tendon
Lesser tubercle
Glenohumeral ligament
Coracohumeral ligament
A
Greater tubercle
Coracoid process
Glenoid labrum
R
L
Intertubercular groove
Deltoid muscle
P
Infraspinatus muscle
Scapular spine

FIGURE 9.14 **Axial, T1-weighted MRI of right shoulder.**

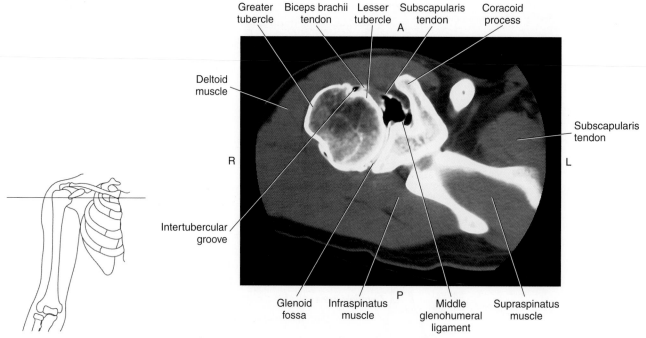

Greater tubercle   Biceps brachii tendon   Lesser tubercle   Subscapularis tendon   Coracoid process

Deltoid muscle

Subscapularis tendon

Intertubercular groove

Glenoid fossa   Infraspinatus muscle   Middle glenohumeral ligament   Supraspinatus muscle

FIGURE 9.15 Axial CT or right shoulder, post-arthrogram.

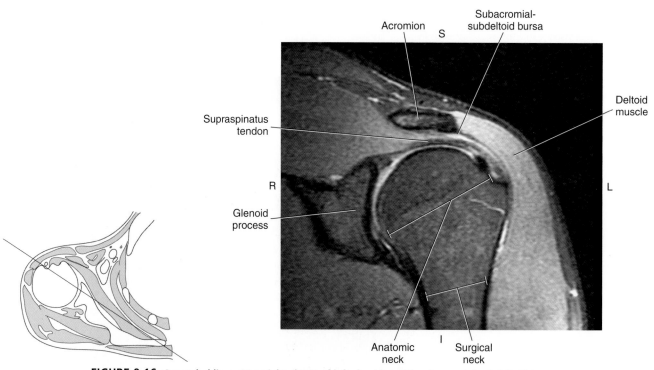

Acromion   Subacromial-subdeltoid bursa

Deltoid muscle

Supraspinatus tendon

Glenoid process

Anatomic neck   Surgical neck

FIGURE 9.16 Coronal oblique, T2-weighted MRI of left shoulder with subacromial-subdeltoid bursa.

Labrum and Ligaments

The outer rim of the glenoid fossa is surrounded by a fibrocartilaginous ring termed the **glenoid labrum**, which functions to deepen the articular surface of the glenoid fossa (Figure 9.17). Superiorly, the glenoid labrum blends with the long head of the biceps brachii muscle. In cross-section it appears triangular (Figures 9.14 and 9.18). The three **glenohumeral ligaments** (superior, middle, and inferior) thicken the fibrous capsule that surrounds the shoulder joint; they contribute to the formation of the glenoid labrum (Figures 9.17 and 9.19). They extend from the

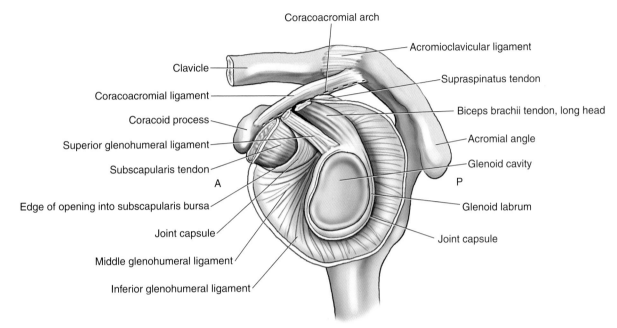

FIGURE 9.17 Lateral view of glenohumeral ligaments and glenoid labrum.

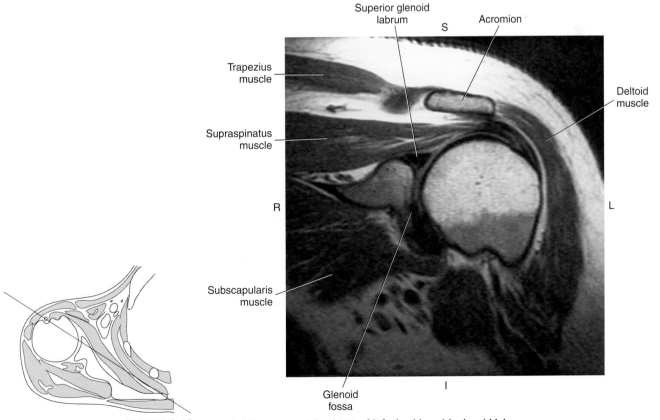

FIGURE 9.18 Coronal oblique, T1-weighted MRI of left shoulder with glenoid labrum.

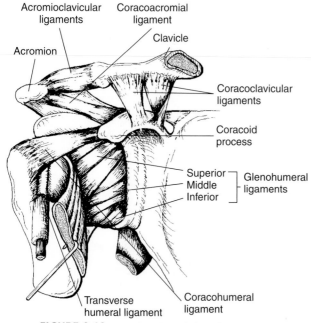

Acromioclavicular ligaments

Coracoacromial ligament

Acromion

Clavicle

Coracoclavicular ligaments

Coracoid process

Superior ⎤
Middle ⎬ Glenohumeral ligaments
Inferior ⎦

Transverse humeral ligament

Coracohumeral ligament

FIGURE 9.19 Anterior view of shoulder ligaments.

supraglenoid tubercle of the scapula to the lesser tubercle of the humerus. The **coracohumeral ligament** passes from the lateral side of the coracoid process of the scapula to the anatomic neck of the humerus (Figure 9.19). The **coracoacromial ligament** is another important ligament located on the anterior portion of the shoulder. As this ligament joins the coracoid process and acromion, it forms a strong bridge, termed the **coracoacromial arch**, which protects the humeral head and rotator cuff tendons from direct trauma and prevents displacement of the humeral head superiorly (Figures 9.17, 9.19 and 9.20). The **coracoclavicular ligaments** help to maintain the position of the clavicle, in relation to the acromion, by spanning the distance between the clavicle and coracoid process of the scapula (Figure 9.19). The **acromioclavicular ligament**, at the acromioclavicular joint, provides support for the superior surface of the shoulder (Figures 9.17 and 9.19). The **transverse humeral ligament** is a broad band of connective tissue passing from the greater tubercle to the lesser tubercle of the humerus, forming a bridge over the intertubercular groove for protection of the long head of the biceps tendon (Figure 9.19). The ligaments of the shoulder are demonstrated in Figures 9.20 through 9.35.

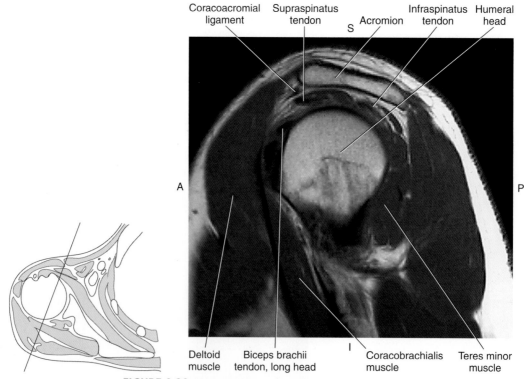

Coracoacromial ligament

Supraspinatus tendon

Acromion

Infraspinatus tendon

Humeral head

Deltoid muscle

Biceps brachii tendon, long head

Coracobrachialis muscle

Teres minor muscle

FIGURE 9.20 Sagittal oblique, T1-weighted MRI of shoulder.

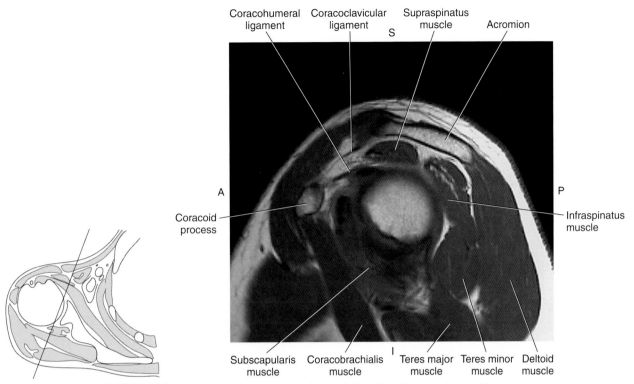

Coracohumeral ligament • Coracoclavicular ligament • Supraspinatus muscle • Acromion

S

A

P

Coracoid process

Infraspinatus muscle

I

Subscapularis muscle • Coracobrachialis muscle • Teres major muscle • Teres minor muscle • Deltoid muscle

FIGURE 9.21 Sagittal oblique, T1-weighted MRI of shoulder with coracohumeral ligament.

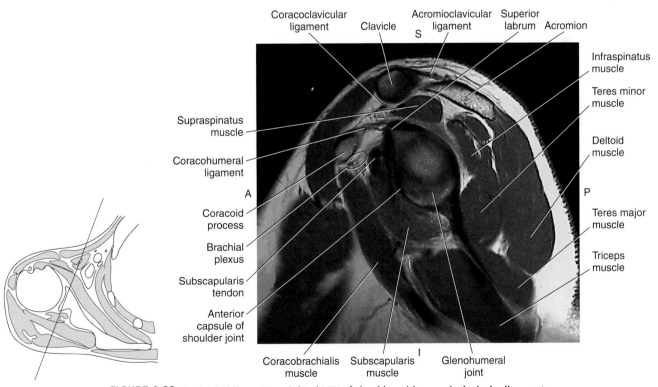

Coracoclavicular ligament • Clavicle • Acromioclavicular ligament • Superior labrum • Acromion

S

Infraspinatus muscle

Teres minor muscle

Supraspinatus muscle

Coracohumeral ligament

Deltoid muscle

A

P

Coracoid process

Teres major muscle

Brachial plexus

Subscapularis tendon

Triceps muscle

Anterior capsule of shoulder joint

I

Coracobrachialis muscle • Subscapularis muscle • Glenohumeral joint

FIGURE 9.22 Sagittal oblique, T1-weighted MRI of shoulder with acromioclavicular ligament.

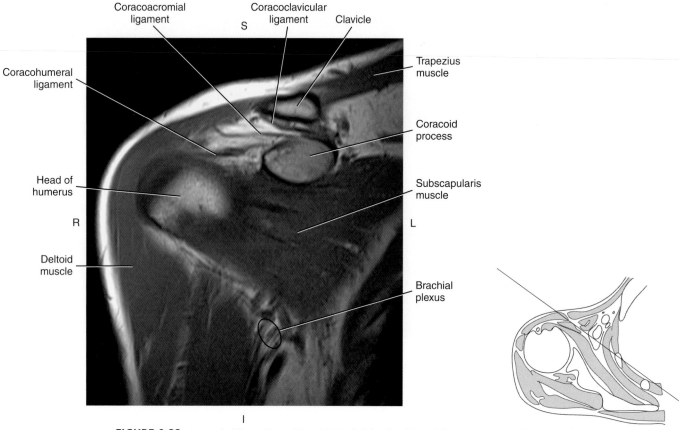

FIGURE 9.23 Coronal oblique, T1-weighted MRI of right shoulder with coracoacromial ligament.

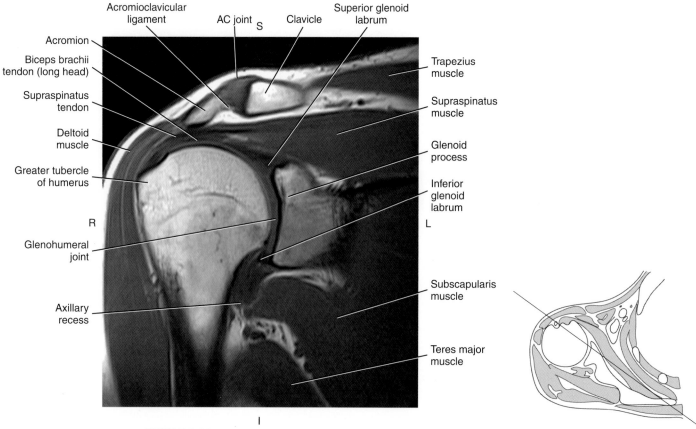

FIGURE 9.24 Coronal oblique, T1-weighted MRI of right shoulder with glenoid labrum.

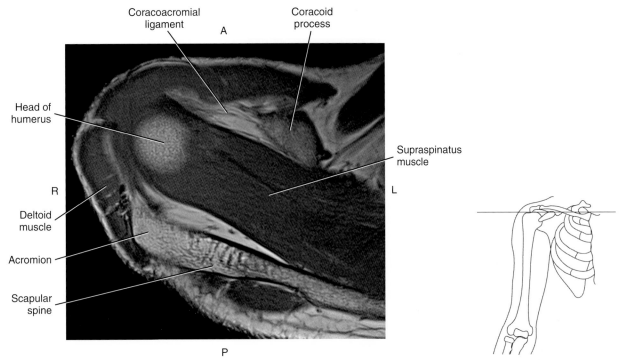

FIGURE 9.25 Axial, T1-weighted MRI of right shoulder with coracoacromial ligament.

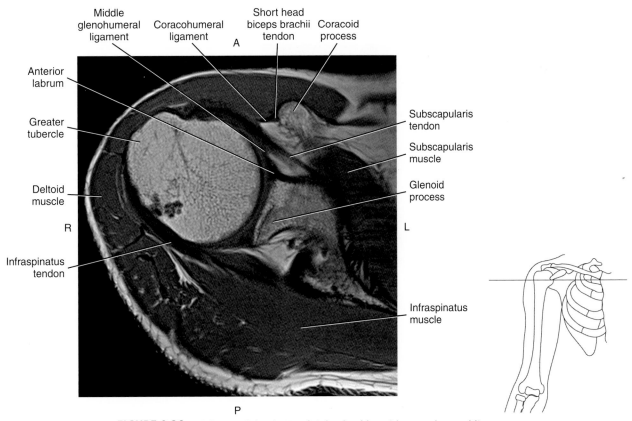

FIGURE 9.26 Axial, T1-weighted MRI of right shoulder with coracohumeral ligament.

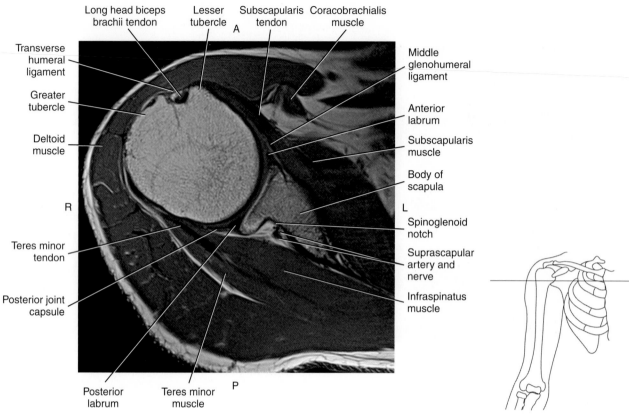

Long head biceps brachii tendon

Lesser tubercle

Subscapularis tendon

Coracobrachialis muscle

A

Transverse humeral ligament

Greater tubercle

Deltoid muscle

R

Teres minor tendon

Posterior joint capsule

Posterior labrum

Teres minor muscle

P

Middle glenohumeral ligament

Anterior labrum

Subscapularis muscle

Body of scapula

L

Spinoglenoid notch

Suprascapular artery and nerve

Infraspinatus muscle

FIGURE 9.27 Axial, T1-weighted MRI of right shoulder with glenoid labrum.

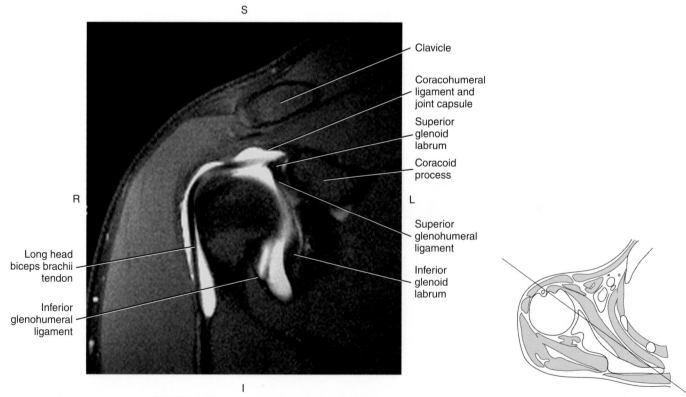

S

Clavicle

Coracohumeral ligament and joint capsule

Superior glenoid labrum

Coracoid process

R

L

Superior glenohumeral ligament

Inferior glenoid labrum

Long head biceps brachii tendon

Inferior glenohumeral ligament

I

FIGURE 9.28 Coronal oblique, T2-weighted MRI of right shoulder, post-arthrogram.

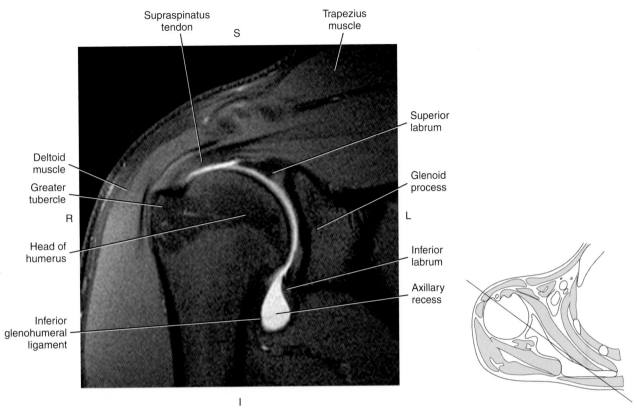

FIGURE 9. 29 Coronal oblique, T2-weighted MRI of right shoulder, post-arthrogram with axillary recess.

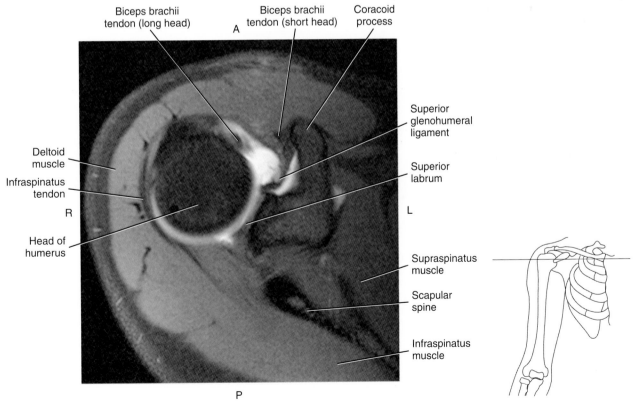

FIGURE 9.30 Axial, T2-weighted MRI of right shoulder, post-arthrogram.

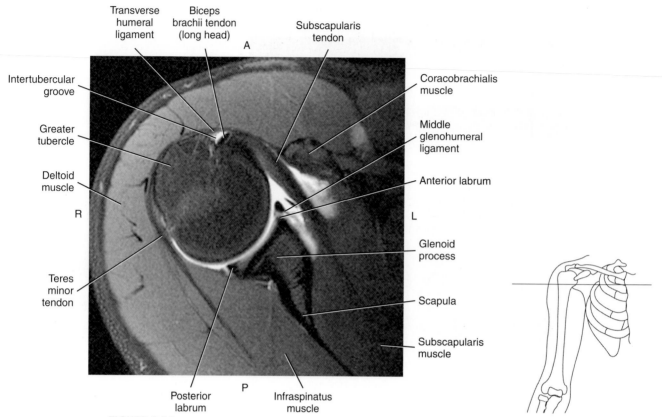

FIGURE 9.31 Axial, T2-weighted MRI of right shoulder, post-arthrogram with glenoid labrum.

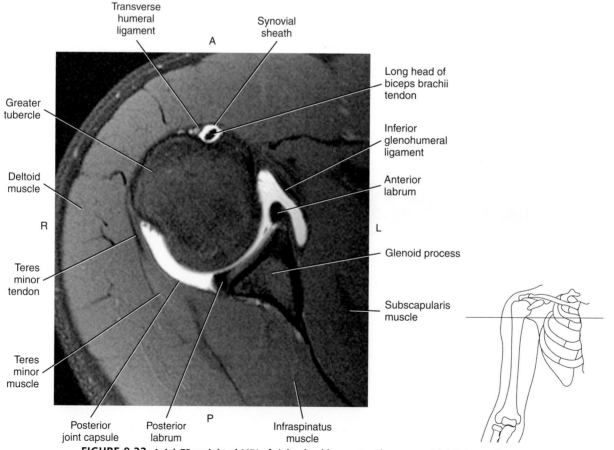

FIGURE 9.32 Axial, T2-weighted MRI of right shoulder, post-arthrogram with joint capsule.

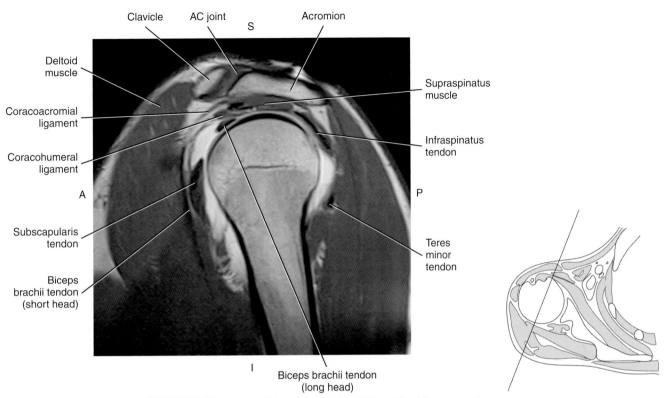

Clavicle AC joint S Acromion

Deltoid muscle

Coracoacromial ligament

Coracohumeral ligament

A

Subscapularis tendon

Biceps brachii tendon (short head)

Supraspinatus muscle

Infraspinatus tendon

P

Teres minor tendon

I Biceps brachii tendon (long head)

FIGURE 9.33 Sagittal oblique, T1-weighted MRI of shoulder, post-arthrogram.

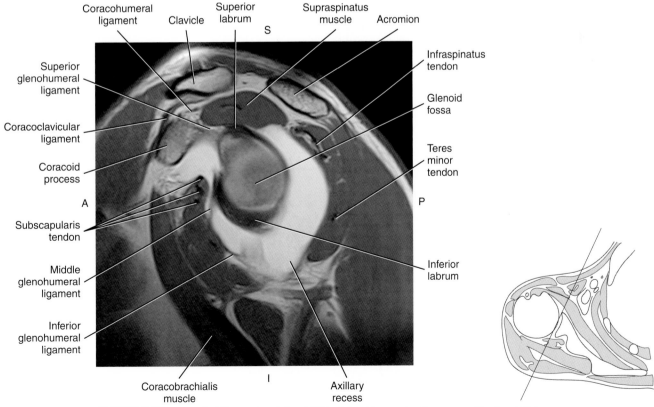

Coracohumeral ligament Clavicle Superior labrum S Supraspinatus muscle Acromion

Superior glenohumeral ligament

Coracoclavicular ligament

Coracoid process

A

Subscapularis tendon

Middle glenohumeral ligament

Inferior glenohumeral ligament

Infraspinatus tendon

Glenoid fossa

Teres minor tendon

P

Inferior labrum

Coracobrachialis muscle I Axillary recess

FIGURE 9.34 Sagittal oblique, T1-weighted MRI of shoulder, post-arthrogram with glenoid labrum.

P

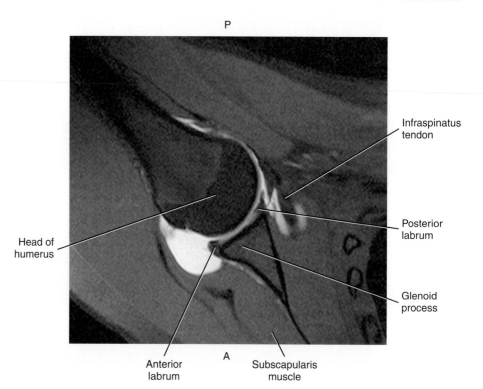

FIGURE 9.35 T2-weighted, MRI of right shoulder, post-arthrogram in abduction external rotation (ABER) position.

Infraspinatus tendon

Posterior labrum

Glenoid process

Head of humerus

Anterior labrum

A

Subscapularis muscle

Articular Joint Capsule

The **articular joint capsule** completely encloses the shoulder joint and is quite thin and loose to allow for extreme freedom of movement. When the arm is adducted, the capsule sags to form a pouchlike area termed the **axillary recess** (Figures 9.29 and 9.36). The capsule is attached medially to the glenoid fossa of the scapula and laterally to the anatomic neck of the

humerus. It is strengthened by several muscles and ligaments, including the rotator cuff muscles and the long head of the biceps brachii muscle, as well as the glenohumeral and coracohumeral ligaments. There are two openings of the joint capsule. The first is to allow for the passage of the long head of the biceps brachii, and the second establishes a communication between the joint and the subscapularis bursa. A synovial membrane lines

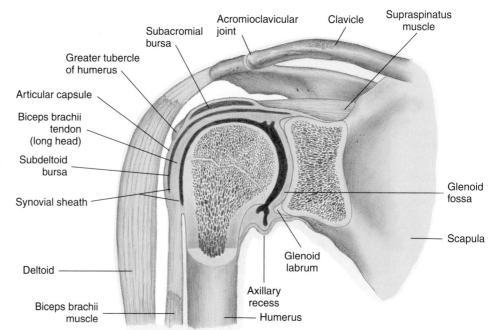

FIGURE 9.36 Anterior cross-section of shoulder joint.

Subacromial bursa

Acromioclavicular joint

Clavicle

Supraspinatus muscle

Greater tubercle of humerus

Articular capsule

Biceps brachii tendon (long head)

Subdeltoid bursa

Synovial sheath

Deltoid

Biceps brachii muscle

Humerus

Axillary recess

Glenoid labrum

Glenoid fossa

Scapula

the fibrous capsule and extends to the glenoid labrum and neck of the humerus. The synovial membrane provides a sheath for the tendon of the long head of the biceps brachii muscle, where it passes into the joint cavity through the intertubercular groove, extending as far as the surgical neck of the humerus (Figures 9.28 through 9.36).

Bursae

The tendons and ligaments of the shoulder joint are cushioned by several fluid-filled bursae. Bursae, within the shoulder, reduce friction where large muscles and tendons pass across the joint capsule. Two prominent shoulder bursae include the subacromial-subdeltoid and subscapular bursae (Figures 9.36 and 9.37). The **subacromial-subdeltoid bursa** is the main bursa of the shoulder and the largest bursa within the body. Beginning at the coracoid process, the bursa extends laterally over the superior surface of the supraspinatus and infraspinatus tendons, extends beyond the acromion, and continues beneath the deltoid muscle to the greater tubercle of the humerus. This bursa cushions the rotator cuff muscles and coracoacromial arch (Figure 9.16). The **subscapular bursa** is located between the subscapularis tendon and the scapula and communicates with the synovial cavity through an opening in the joint capsule. This bursa protects the subscapularis tendon, where it passes inferior to the coracoid process and over the neck of the scapula (Figure 9.37).

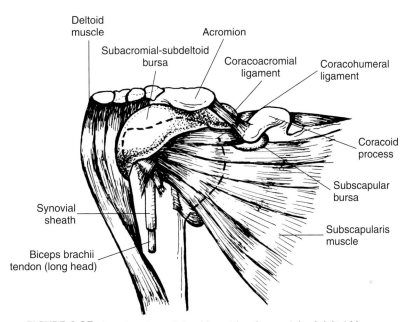

FIGURE 9.37 Anterior view of shoulder with subacromial-subdeltoid bursa.

Muscles and Tendons

Numerous muscles and their tendons provide stability for the shoulder joint and movement of the upper arm. These can be separated into four muscle groups: (1) muscles that connect the upper extremity to the vertebral column, (2) muscles of the scapula, (3) muscles that connect the upper extremity to the anterior thoracic wall, and (4) the muscles of the upper arm.

Muscles connecting the upper extremity to the vertebral column. Muscles connecting the upper extremity to the vertebral column include the following:

Trapezius
Levator scapulae
Latissimus dorsi
Rhomboid major
Rhomboid minor

Muscles connecting the upper extremity to the vertebral column are demonstrated in Figures 9.38 through 9.42 and are described in Table 9.1. The large triangular **trapezius muscle** covers the posterior aspect of the neck and superior half of the trunk (Figure 9.38). It connects the upper limb to the cranium via the external occipital protuberance and to the vertebral column via the spinous processes of C7-T12. The trapezius muscle functions to stabilize the scapula, as well as to elevate, retract, and depress the scapula. The **levator scapulae muscle** lies deep in the neck and functions to elevate and rotate the scapula. It extends from the transverse processes of C1-C4 to the superior angle and medial border of the scapula above its spine (Figure 9.38). The **latissimus dorsi** muscle covers the inferior portion of the back as it extends from the spinous processes of the inferior six thoracic vertebrae, iliac crest, and inferior three or four ribs to the distal end of the intertubercular groove of the humerus. The latissimus dorsi medially rotates, extends, and adducts the humerus. The **rhomboid muscles, major** and **minor,** lie deep to the trapezius muscle. The rhomboid major is wider than the rhomboid minor. They parallel each other as they span from the ligamentum nuchae and spinous processes of C7-T5 to the medial border of the scapula. They function to retract the scapula and fix the scapula to the thoracic wall (Figures 9.38 through 9.42).

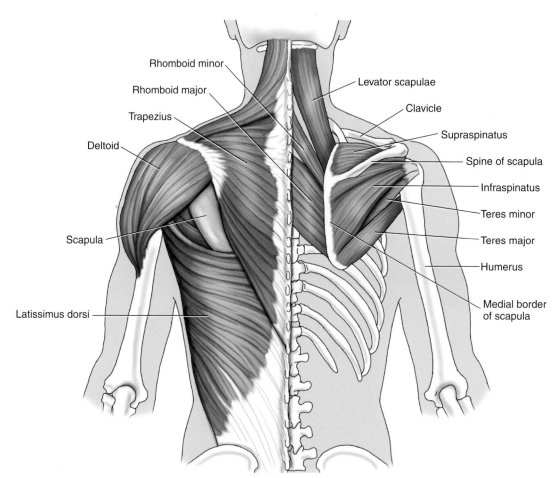

FIGURE 9.38 Posterior view of trapezius, rhomboid, levator scapula, and latissimus dorsi muscles.

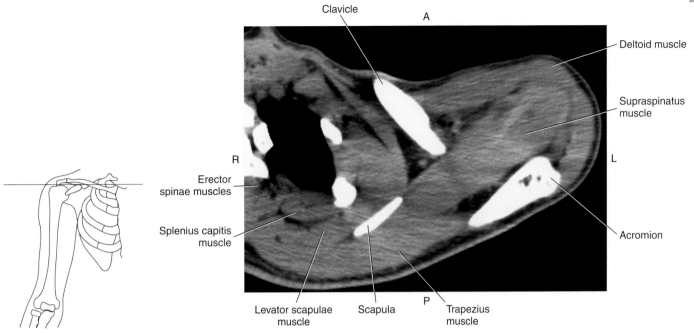

FIGURE 9.39 Axial CT of left shoulder.

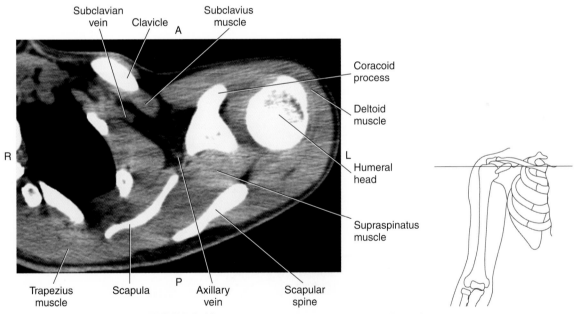

FIGURE 9.40 Axial CT of left shoulder with deltoid muscle.

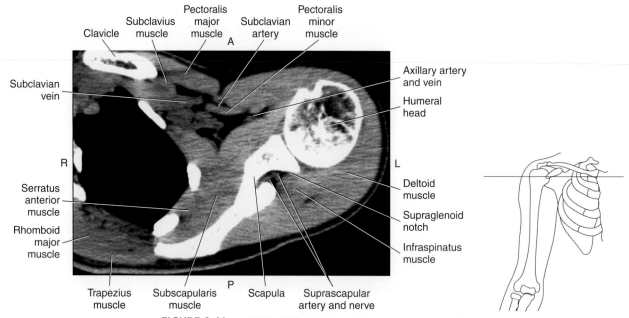

FIGURE 9.41 Axial CT of left shoulder with subscapularis muscle.

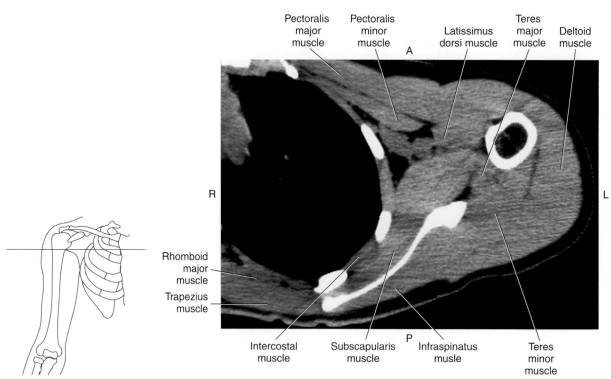

FIGURE 9.42 Axial CT of left shoulder with pectoralis muscles.

TABLE 9.1	Muscles Connecting the Upper Extremity to the Vertebral Column		
Muscle	Origin	Insertion	Primary Actions
Trapezius	External occipital protuberance, ligamentum nuchae, spinous processes of C7-T12	Clavicle acromion and spine of scapula	Stabilizes, elevates, retracts, and depresses scapula
Levator scapula	Transverse processes of C1-C4	Superior angle and medial border of scapula	Elevates scapula
Latissimus dorsi	Spinous process of T6-T12, iliac crest, and inferior three or four ribs	Intertubercular groove of the humerus	Extends, medially rotates, and adducts the humerus
Rhomboid major	Ligamentum nuchae and spinous processes of C7-T1	Medial border of scapula	Retracts scapula and fixes scapula to thoracic wall
Rhomboid minor	Spinous processes of T2-T5	Medial border of scapula	Retracts scapula and fixes scapula to thoracic wall

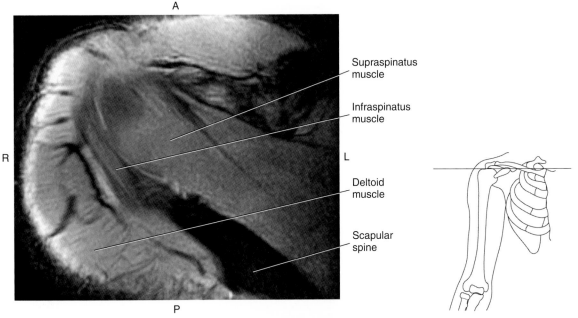

FIGURE 9.43 Axial, T1-weighted MRI of right shoulder.

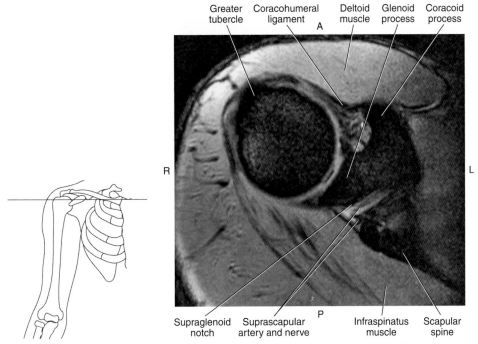

FIGURE 9.44 Axial, T1-weighted MRI of right shoulder with deltoid muscle.

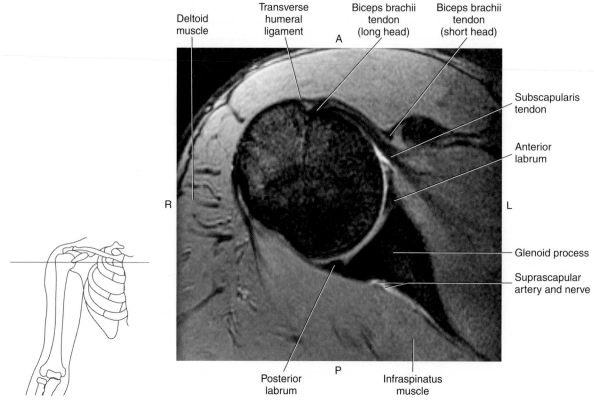

FIGURE 9.45 Axial, T1-weighted MRI of right shoulder with long head of biceps tendon.

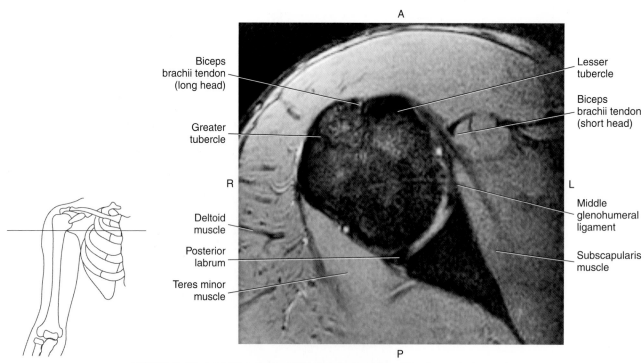

FIGURE 9.46 Axial, T1-weighted MRI of right shoulder with subscapularis muscle.

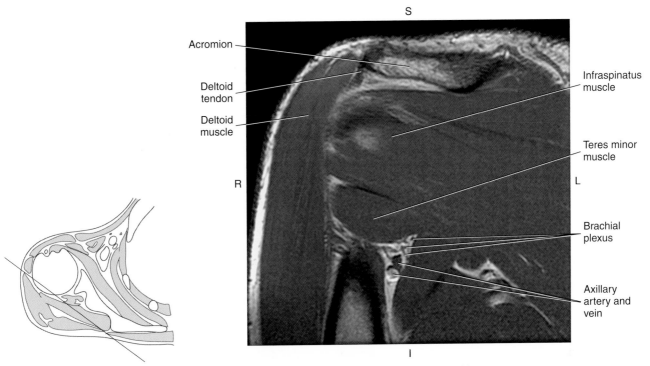

Acromion

Deltoid
tendon

Deltoid
muscle

R

Infraspinatus
muscle

Teres minor
muscle

L

Brachial
plexus

Axillary
artery and
vein

S

I

FIGURE 9.47 Coronal oblique, T1-weighted MRI of right shoulder.

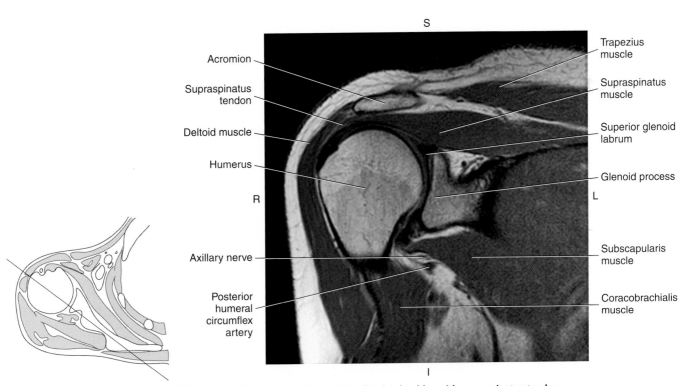

Acromion

Supraspinatus
tendon

Deltoid muscle

Humerus

R

Axillary nerve

Posterior
humeral
circumflex
artery

Trapezius
muscle

Supraspinatus
muscle

Superior glenoid
labrum

Glenoid process

L

Subscapularis
muscle

Coracobrachialis
muscle

S

I

FIGURE 9.48 Coronal oblique, T1-weighted MRI of right shoulder with supraspinatus tendon.

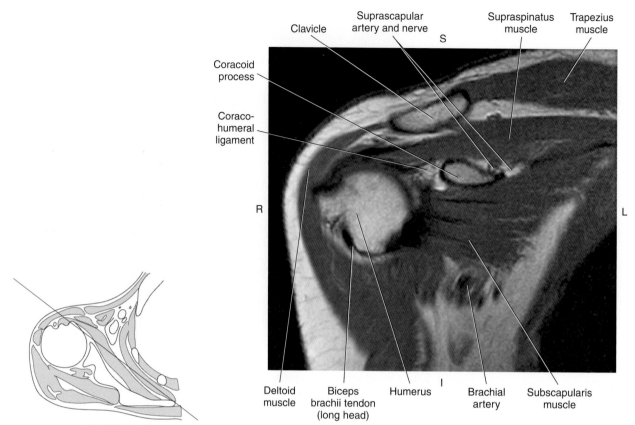

FIGURE 9.49 Coronal oblique, T1-weighted MRI of right shoulder with long head of biceps tendon.

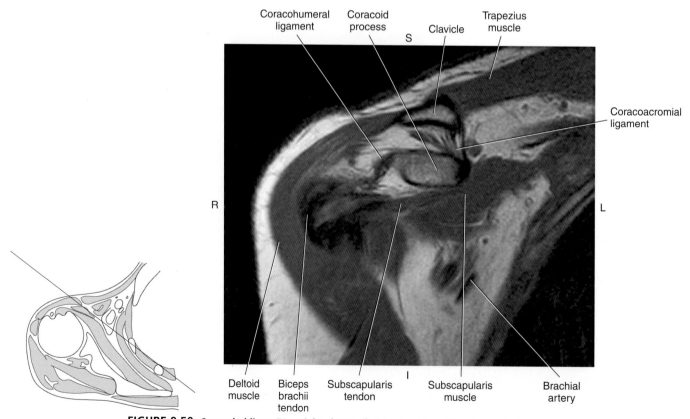

FIGURE 9.50 Coronal oblique, T1-weighted MRI of right shoulder with subscapularis tendon.

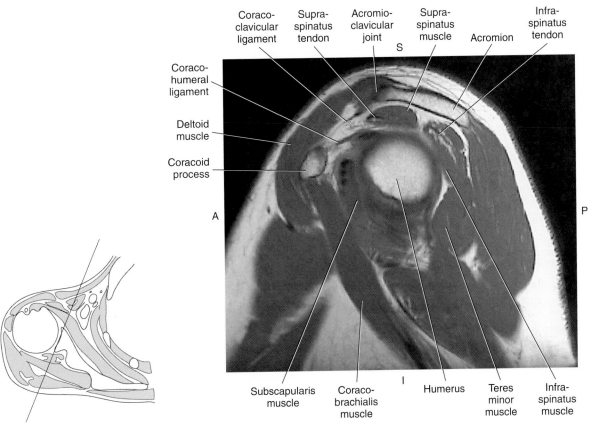

FIGURE 9.51 Sagittal oblique, T1-weighted MRI of shoulder.

Coraco-clavicular ligament
Supra-spinatus tendon
Acromio-clavicular joint
Supra-spinatus muscle
Acromion
Infra-spinatus tendon
Coraco-humeral ligament
Deltoid muscle
Coracoid process
S
A
P
Subscapularis muscle
Coraco-brachialis muscle
I
Humerus
Teres minor muscle
Infra-spinatus muscle

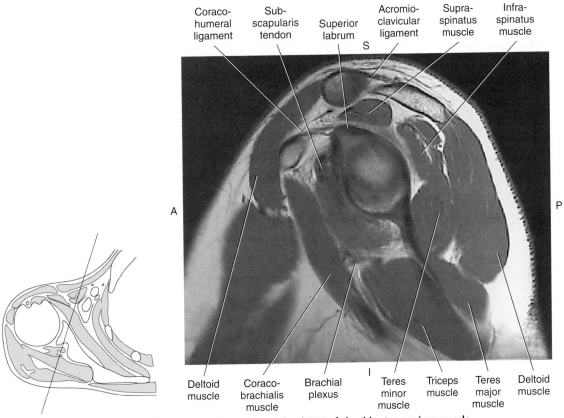

FIGURE 9.52 Sagittal oblique, T1-weighted MRI of shoulder teres minor muscle.

Coraco-humeral ligament
Sub-scapularis tendon
Superior labrum
Acromio-clavicular ligament
Supra-spinatus muscle
Infra-spinatus muscle
S
A
P
Deltoid muscle
Coraco-brachialis muscle
Brachial plexus
I
Teres minor muscle
Triceps muscle
Teres major muscle
Deltoid muscle

Muscles of the scapula. Muscles of the scapula include the following:

Deltoid
Teres major
Teres minor
Supraspinatus
Infraspinatus
Subscapularis

Muscles of the scapula are described in Table 9.2 and demonstrated in Figures 9.39 through 9.57. The large **deltoid muscle** originates on the clavicle, acromion, and scapular spine to blanket the shoulder joint as it extends to insert on the deltoid tuberosity of the humerus. This powerful muscle forms the rounded contour of the shoulder and functions primarily to abduct the arm (Figure 9.53). The **teres major muscle** is a flat rectangular muscle that adducts and medially rotates the arm. It extends from the inferior angle of the scapula to the medial aspect or lip of the intertubercular groove of the humerus (Figure 9.54, A). The four remaining muscles, **supraspinatus, infraspinatus, teres minor,** and **subscapularis,** closely surround the scapula and constitute the rotator cuff (Figures 9.54 through 9.57). The **rotator cuff** provides dynamic stability to the shoulder joint and allows for adduction, abduction, and rotation of the humerus. The supraspinatus, infraspinatus, and teres minor muscles are located on the posterior aspect of the scapula. The tendons of these muscles insert on the greater tubercle of the humerus. The **supraspinatus muscle** lies in the supraspinous fossa of the scapula and helps to abduct the arm. The tendon of the supraspinatus muscle is the most frequently injured tendon of the rotator cuff because of possible impingement as it extends under the acromioclavicular joint and continues over the humeral head (Figure 9.54, B). The **infraspinatus muscle** is a triangular muscle that lies below the scapular spine in the infraspinous fossa. It acts to laterally rotate the arm (Figure 9.54, A). Lying along the inferior border of the infraspinatus muscle is the elongated **teres minor muscle**, which also acts to laterally rotate the arm (Figure 9.54, B). The **subscapularis muscle** is the only muscle of the rotator cuff located on the anterior surface of the scapula; its tendon inserts on the lesser tubercle of the humerus (Figures 9.55 through 9.57). The subscapularis muscle acts to medially rotate the humerus. See sequential images through the shoulder (Figures 9.28 through 9.35 and 9.39 through 9.52).

> The majority of rotator cuff lesions are a result of chronic impingement of the supraspinatus tendon against the acromial arch. The most susceptible area is approximately 1 cm from the insertion site of the supraspinatus tendon. This location is commonly referred to as the **critical zone.**

TABLE 9.2	Scapular Muscles		
Muscle	**Proximal/Medial Attachment**	**Distal/Lateral Attachment**	**Primary Action**
Deltoid	Clavicle, acromion, and spine of scapula	Deltoid tuberosity of humerus	Flexes, medially rotates abductor, extensor and lateral rotator of humerus
Teres major	Inferior angle of scapula	Intertubercular groove of humerus	Adducts and medially rotates humerus
Teres minor	Axillary border of scapula	Greater tubercle of humerus	Laterally rotates humerus, stabilizes glenohumeral joint
Supraspinatus	Supraspinous fossa of scapula	Greater tubercle of humerus	Abducts humerus and stabilizes glenohumeral joint
Infraspinatus	Infraspinous fossa of scapula	Greater tubercle of humerus	Laterally rotates humerus and stabilizes glenohumeral joint
Subscapularis	Subscapular fossa of scapula	Lesser tubercle of humerus	Medially rotates humerus and stabilizes glenohumeral joint

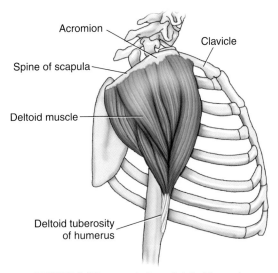

FIGURE 9.53 Lateral view of deltoid muscle.

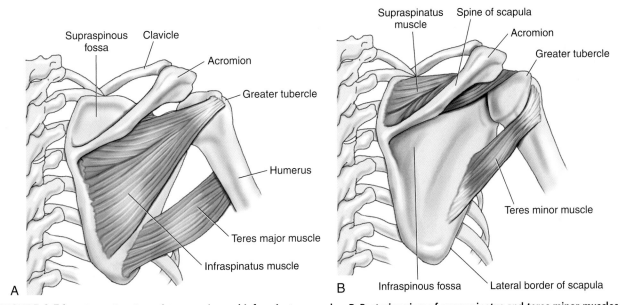

A

B

FIGURE 9.54 A, Posterior view of teres major and infraspinatus muscles. B, Posterior view of supraspinatus and teres minor muscles.

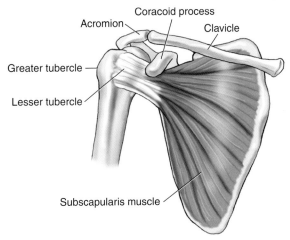

FIGURE 9.55 Anterior view of subscapularis muscle.

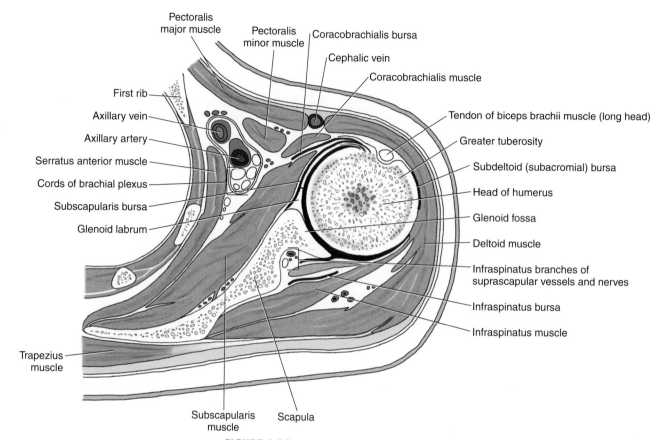

Pectoralis major muscle

Pectoralis minor muscle

Coracobrachialis bursa

Cephalic vein

Coracobrachialis muscle

First rib

Axillary vein

Axillary artery

Serratus anterior muscle

Cords of brachial plexus

Subscapularis bursa

Glenoid labrum

Tendon of biceps brachii muscle (long head)

Greater tuberosity

Subdeltoid (subacromial) bursa

Head of humerus

Glenoid fossa

Deltoid muscle

Infraspinatus branches of suprascapular vessels and nerves

Infraspinatus bursa

Infraspinatus muscle

Trapezius muscle

Subscapularis muscle

Scapula

FIGURE 9.56 Axial view of shoulder muscles.

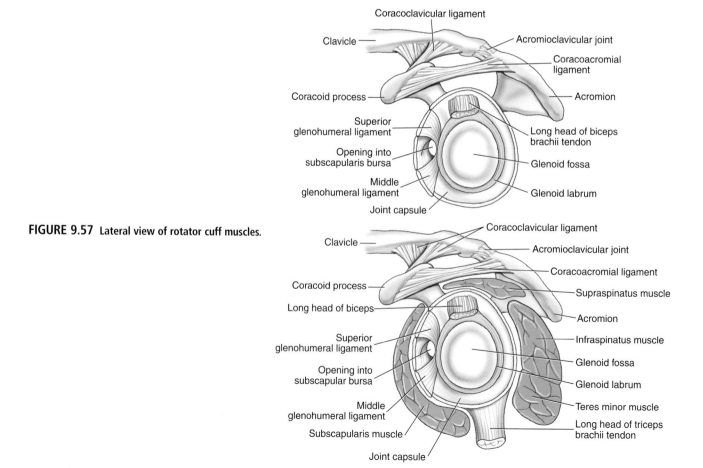

Coracoclavicular ligament

Clavicle

Acromioclavicular joint

Coracoacromial ligament

Coracoid process

Acromion

Superior glenohumeral ligament

Long head of biceps brachii tendon

Opening into subscapularis bursa

Glenoid fossa

Middle glenohumeral ligament

Glenoid labrum

Joint capsule

FIGURE 9.57 Lateral view of rotator cuff muscles.

Coracoclavicular ligament

Clavicle

Acromioclavicular joint

Coracoacromial ligament

Coracoid process

Supraspinatus muscle

Long head of biceps

Acromion

Superior glenohumeral ligament

Infraspinatus muscle

Opening into subscapular bursa

Glenoid fossa

Glenoid labrum

Middle glenohumeral ligament

Teres minor muscle

Subscapularis muscle

Long head of triceps brachii tendon

Joint capsule

Muscles connecting the upper extremity to the anterior and lateral thoracic walls. Muscles connecting the upper extremity to the anterior and lateral thoracic walls include the following:

Pectoralis major
Pectoralis minor
Serratus anterior
Subclavius

Muscles connecting the upper extremity to the anterior and lateral thoracic walls are demonstrated in Figures 9.39 through 9.52, 9.58, and 9.59 and described in Table 9.3. The **pectoralis muscles (major and minor)**, located on the anterior surface of the chest, primarily aid in the movement of the upper limb (Figure 9.58). The large fan-shaped **pectoralis major** muscle covers the superior part of the thorax as it spans from the sternum, clavicle, and cartilaginous attachments of the upper six ribs to the lateral aspect or lip of the intertubercular groove of the humerus. Its primary functions are to adduct, medially rotate, flex, and extend the humerus and to assist in forced inspiration. The smaller triangular-shaped **pectoralis minor** lies beneath the pectoralis major muscle and acts to depress the scapula and assist the serratus anterior muscle in pulling the scapula forward (Figure 9.58). The **serratus (sawlike) anterior**

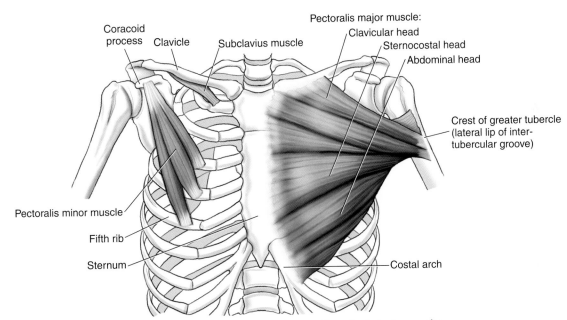

FIGURE 9.58 Anterior view of pectoralis and subclavius muscles.

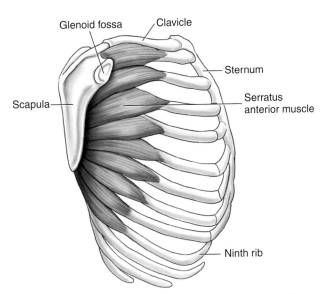

FIGURE 9.59 Anterior view of serratus anterior muscle.

TABLE 9.3	Muscles Connecting the Upper Extremity to the Anterior and Lateral Thoracic Wall		
Muscle	**Proximal/Medial Attachment**	**Distal/Lateral Attachment**	**Primary Action**
Pectoralis major	Medial half of clavicle, manubrium and body of sternum, and six upper costal cartilages	Lateral lip intertubercular groove of humerus	Adducts, medially rotates, and flexes humerus.
Pectoralis minor	Anterior surface of third to fifth ribs	Coracoid process of the scapula	Depresses and downwardly rotates scapula. Assists in scapular protraction and stabilizes scapula
Serratus anterior	Angles of first to eighth or ninth ribs	Medial border of scapula	Rotates, stabilizes and protracts scapula
Subclavius	First rib and cartilage	Inferior surface of the clavicle	Stabilizes the clavicle and depresses the shoulder

muscle is visualized on the lateral border of the thorax. It extends from the first through eighth ribs to the medial border of the scapula. The primary action of the serratus anterior muscle is to protract and stabilize the scapula (Figure 9.59). The **subclavius**, a small triangular-shaped muscle that spans between the first rib and clavicle, acts to stabilize the clavicle and depress the shoulder (Figure 9.58).

Muscles of the upper arm. The muscles of the upper arm can be divided into ventral and dorsal groups according to their position. The ventral group contains the biceps brachii, brachialis, and coracobrachialis muscle, and the dorsal group consists of the triceps brachii and anconeus muscles. These muscles are demonstrated in Figures 9.60 through 9.74 and described in Table 9.4.

Ventral group. The **biceps brachii muscle** is located on the anterior surface of the humerus and acts as a strong flexor of the forearm. The biceps brachii muscle is named "biceps" because of its two expanded heads of proximal attachment (long and short). The **tendon of the long head** arises from the supraglenoid tubercle and courses through the intertubercular (bicipital) groove to merge with the tendon from the short head. The **short head** of the biceps brachii muscle originates from the coracoid process and joins with the long head to create the biceps brachii muscle, which terminates in two tendons. The stronger tendon inserts on the radial tuberosity, and the other tendon creates the **bicipital aponeurosis**, which radiates into the fascia of the forearm (Figure 9.60).

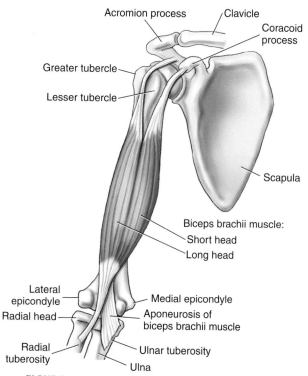

FIGURE 9.60 Anterior view of biceps brachii muscle.

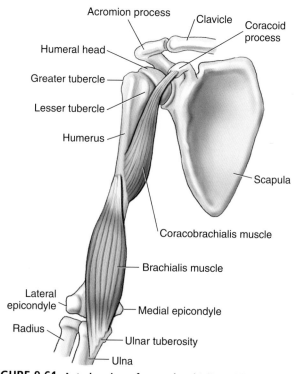

FIGURE 9.61 Anterior view of coracobrachialis and brachialis muscles.

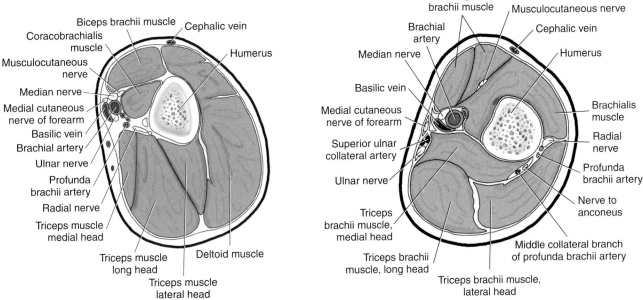

FIGURE 9.62 Axial view of humerus, proximal one-third, left arm.

FIGURE 9.63 Axial view of humerus, midhumerus, left arm.

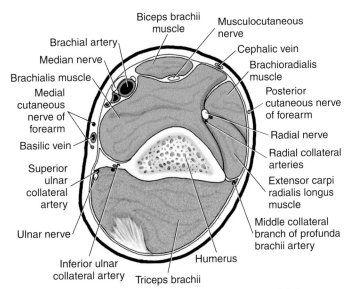

FIGURE 9.64 Axial view of humerus, distal one-third, left arm.

The **brachialis muscle** originates from the anterior surface of the distal humerus and covers the anterior surface of the elbow joint before inserting on the ulnar tuberosity and the coronoid process. The brachialis muscle is considered to be the most important flexor muscle of the elbow joint (Figure 9.61). The **coracobrachialis** is a long, narrow muscle located in the superomedial aspect of the arm. It arises from the coracoid process along with the short head of the biceps brachii and extends to insert on the medial surface of the humerus. The primary action of the coracobrachialis muscle is to assist with flexion and adduction of the arm, but it also helps hold the head of the humerus within the joint capsule (Figures 9.61 through 9.72).

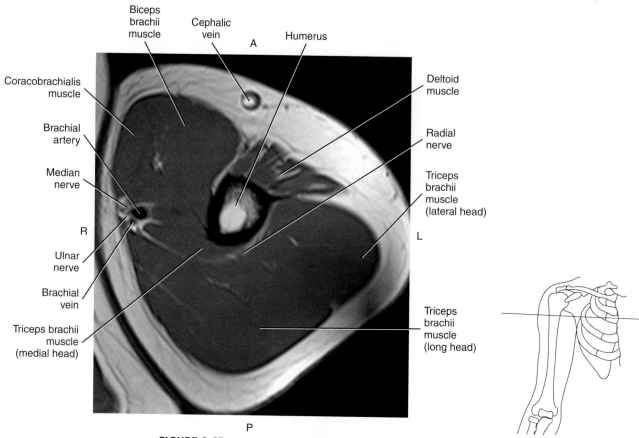

FIGURE 9.65 Axial, T1-weighted MRI of proximal humerus, left arm.

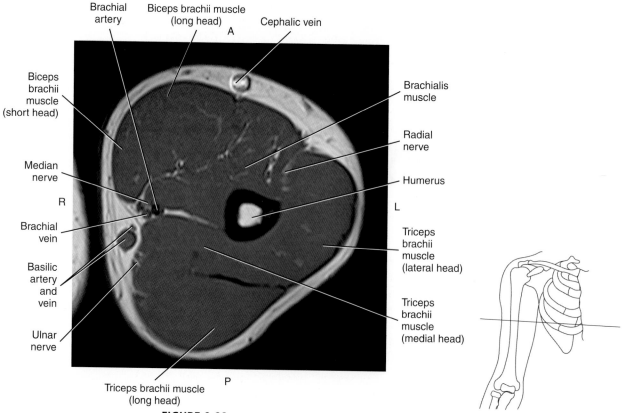

FIGURE 9.66 Axial, T1-weighted MRI of midhumerus, left arm.

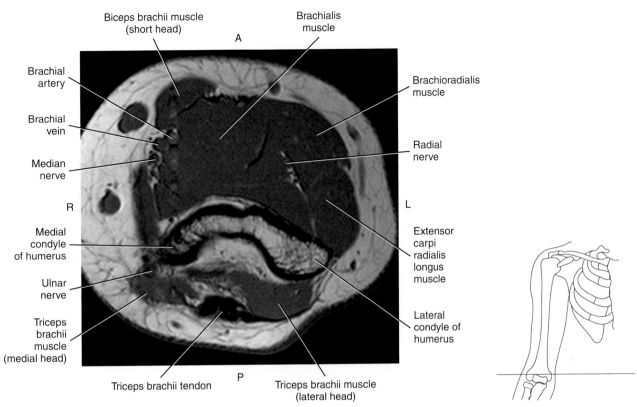

FIGURE 9.67 Axial, T1-weighted MRI of distal humerus, left arm.

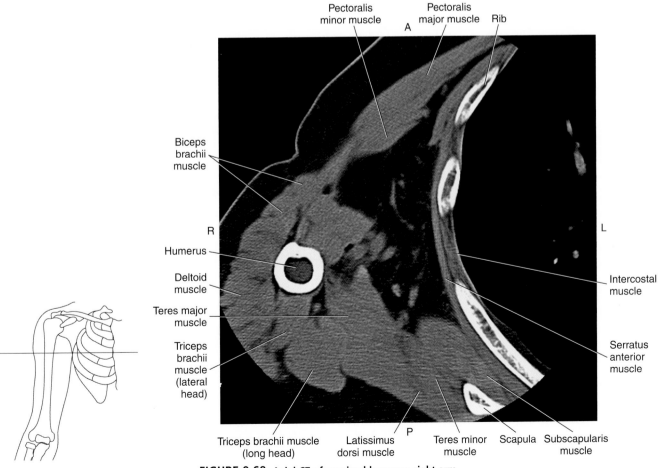

FIGURE 9.68 Axial CT of proximal humerus, right arm.

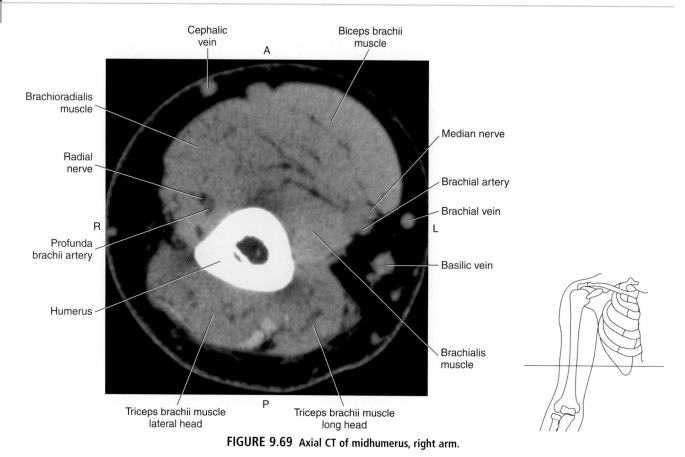

FIGURE 9.69 Axial CT of midhumerus, right arm.

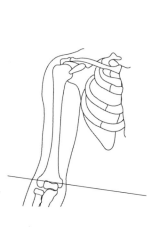

FIGURE 9.70 Axial CT of distal humerus, right arm.

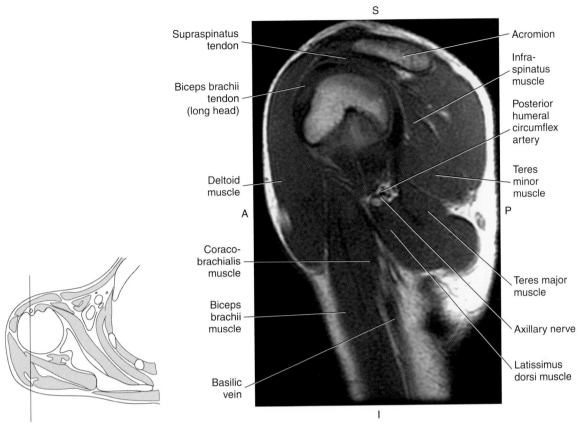

S

Supraspinatus tendon

Acromion

Infra-spinatus muscle

Biceps brachii tendon (long head)

Posterior humeral circumflex artery

Deltoid muscle

Teres minor muscle

A

P

Coraco-brachialis muscle

Teres major muscle

Biceps brachii muscle

Axillary nerve

Basilic vein

Latissimus dorsi muscle

I

FIGURE 9.71 Sagittal, T1-weighted MRI of humerus.

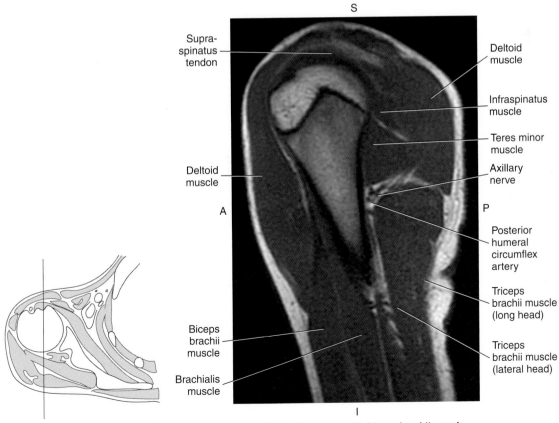

S

Supra-spinatus tendon

Deltoid muscle

Infraspinatus muscle

Teres minor muscle

Deltoid muscle

Axillary nerve

A

P

Posterior humeral circumflex artery

Triceps brachii muscle (long head)

Biceps brachii muscle

Triceps brachii muscle (lateral head)

Brachialis muscle

I

FIGURE 9.72 Sagittal, T1-weighted MRI of humerus with biceps brachii muscle.

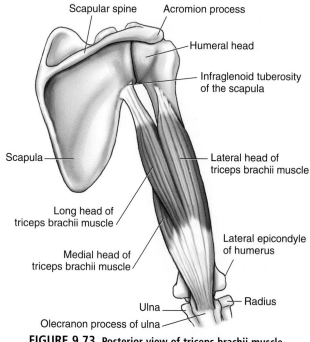

FIGURE 9.73 Posterior view of triceps brachii muscle.

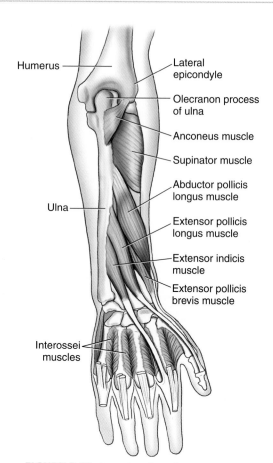

FIGURE 9.74 Posterior view of anconeus muscle.

TABLE 9.4	Muscles of the Upper Arm		
Muscle	**Proximal Attachment**	**Distal Attachment**	**Primary Action**
Biceps brachii	Long head—supraglenoid tubercle of scapula Short head—coracoid process of scapula	Bicipital aponeurosis and radial tuberosity	Supinates and flexes forearm
Brachialis	Distal humerus	Ulner tuberosity and coronoid process	Flexion of elbow joint
Coracobrachialis	Coracoid process of scapula	Middle third medial surface of humerus	Assists to flex and adduct the arm
Triceps brachii	Long head—infraglenoid tubercle of scapula Medial head—posterior surface of humerus below radial groove Lateral head—posterior surface of humerus below greater tubercle	Proximal end of olecranon process of the ulna	Chief extensor of forearm, long head steadies head of humerus if abducted
Anconeus	Lateral epicondyle of humerus	Olecranon process of the ulna	Assists triceps brachii in extension of elbow

Dorsal group. The **triceps brachii muscle** is located on the posterior surface of the humerus and is the main extensor of the forearm. It is named triceps because of its three heads of proximal attachment (**long, medial,** and **lateral**). The **long head** of the triceps originates from the infraglenoid tubercle of the scapula, the **medial head** originates from the entire dorsal surface of the humerus distal to the radial groove, and the **lateral head** arises from the dorsal surface and lateral intermuscular septum of the humerus.

All three heads join in a common tendon that inserts on the olecranon process of the ulna and the posterior joint capsule (Figure 9.73). The small, triangular **anconeus muscle** originates on the lateral epicondyle and crosses obliquely to insert on the dorsal surface of the olecranon process, close to the tendon of the triceps brachii (Figure 9.74). It assists the triceps brachii in extension and also provides dynamic joint stability to the lateral joint capsule. For images of the upper arm, see Figures 9.62 through 9.74.

ELBOW

The elbow is a complex hinge-pivot joint created by the articulations of the humerus, radius, and ulna. All three articulations communicate with each other within a single joint capsule. The radius and ulna are the bones of the forearm, with the radius located on the lateral side. The **radioulnar** and **radiohumeral** articulations create the pivot joint that aids in supination and pronation of the elbow. The radiohumeral and **ulnohumeral** articulations form the hinge joint that allows for flexion and extension (Figures 9.75 through 9.78).

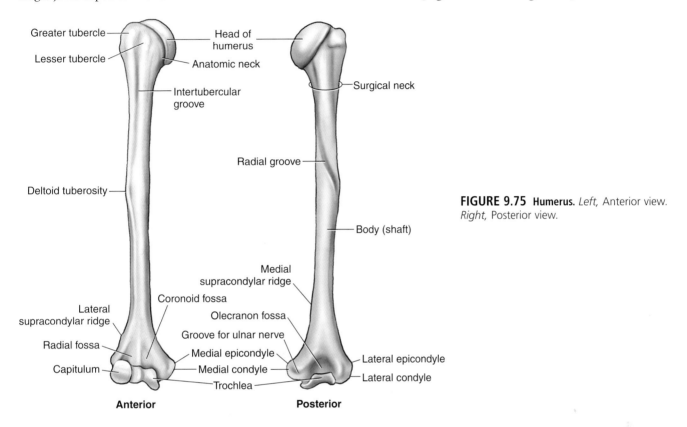

FIGURE 9.75 Humerus. *Left,* Anterior view. *Right,* Posterior view.

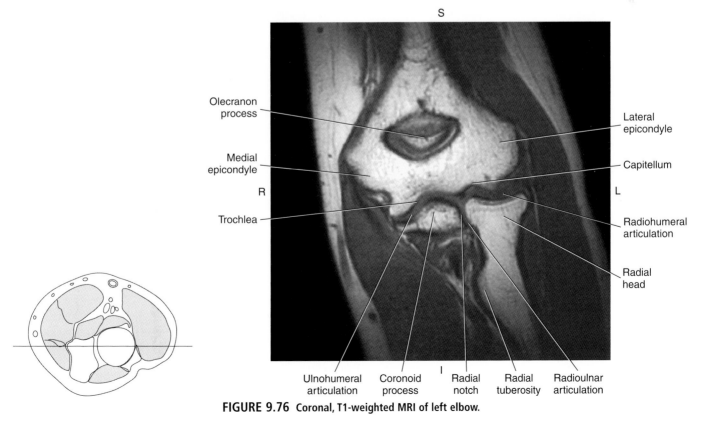

FIGURE 9.76 Coronal, T1-weighted MRI of left elbow.

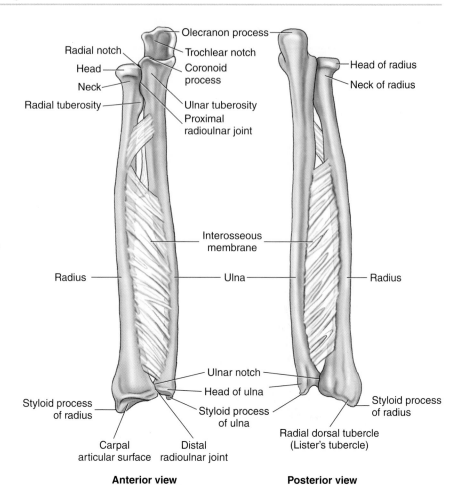

FIGURE 9.77 Radius and ulna. *Left,* Anterior view. *Right,* Posterior view.

Olecranon process
Trochlear notch
Radial notch
Head
Coronoid process
Neck
Ulnar tuberosity
Radial tuberosity
Proximal radioulnar joint

Head of radius
Neck of radius

Interosseous membrane

Radius   Ulna   Radius

Ulnar notch
Head of ulna
Styloid process of radius
Styloid process of ulna
Styloid process of radius

Radial dorsal tubercle (Lister's tubercle)

Carpal articular surface   Distal radioulnar joint

Anterior view   **Posterior view**

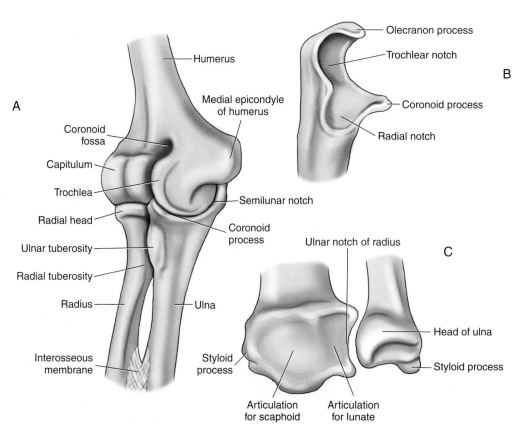

Humerus

Medial epicondyle of humerus

A

Coronoid fossa
Capitulum
Trochlea
Radial head
Ulnar tuberosity
Radial tuberosity
Radius   Ulna

Semilunar notch
Coronoid process

Interosseous membrane

Olecranon process
Trochlear notch

B

Coronoid process
Radial notch

Ulnar notch of radius

C

Styloid process

Head of ulna

Styloid process

Articulation for scaphoid   Articulation for lunate

FIGURE 9.78 Anatomy of the elbow and distal forearm. A, Elbow in medial view. **B,** Proximal ulna in lateral view. **C,** Distal radius and ulna.

Bony Anatomy

Distal humerus. The distal portion of the humerus has two distinct prominences termed the **medial** and **lateral condyles**, with associated **epicondyles**, which provide attachment sites for tendons and ligaments (Figure 9.75). The medial epicondyle serves as the site of origin for the common flexor tendon, pronator teres muscle, and medial collateral ligament, whereas the lateral epicondyle serves as the attachment site for the common extensor tendon, supinator muscle, and lateral collateral ligament. Just lateral to the medial epicondyle along its posterior surface is a shallow groove containing the ulnar nerve. Two depressions located on the distal humerus are the anterior **coronoid fossa** and the deep posterior **olecranon fossa**. These depressions accommodate the coronoid and olecranon processes of the proximal ulna (Figures 9.75, 9.76, and 9.78). The distal humerus has two cartilage-covered articular surfaces—the capitellum and the trochlea for articulation with the radius and ulna (Figure 9.76). The lateral of the two surfaces is the **capitellum**, a rounded projection that articulates with the concave surface of the radial head. The **trochlea** is more medial and has the appearance of an hourglass if viewed in the horizontal plane. The shape of the trochlea helps keep the ulna in position during flexion between the distal humerus and proximal radius (Figures 9.76 and 9.78).

Radius: proximal radius. The radius is a long, slender bone with a proximal portion that consists of the radial head, neck, and tuberosity. The **radial head** has a flat cartilage-covered depression or **fossa** (fovea of the radius) that articulates with the capitellum of the humerus. In addition, the articular circumference of the radial head articulates against the radial notch of the ulna during supination and pronation. The radial head is attached to the body of the radius by the narrow **radial neck**. Located at the distal portion of the neck on the medial side of the radius is a roughened projection termed the **radial tuberosity**. The radial tuberosity serves as the attachment point for the biceps brachii muscle (Figures 9.77 through 9.79).

> Because of its superficial location, the ulnar nerve is the most frequently injured nerve of the body.

Distal radius. The broadened distal end of the radius includes the cartilage-covered carpal articular surface, the ulnar notch, and the radial styloid process. The

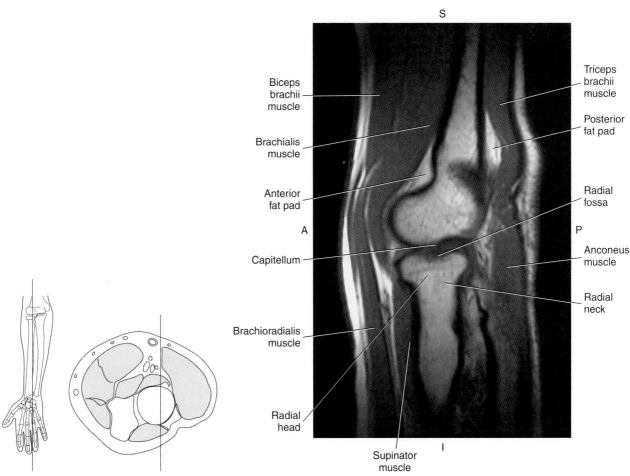

FIGURE 9.79 Sagittal, T1-weighted MRI of elbow with proximal radius.

carpal articular surface articulates with the scaphoid and lunate bones of the wrist. The **ulnar notch** articulates with the ulna, and the **styloid process** serves as an attachment site for the extensor pollicis longus and extensor carpi radialis tendons. The dorsal surface of the radius contains several grooves that serve as passages for the extensor tendons. Along with the grooves, a prominent ridge is located on the dorsal surface termed the **radial dorsal tubercle,** or **Lister's tubercle,** a common site for the formation of bony spurs (Figure 9.77).

Ulna: proximal ulna. The ulna is located medial within the forearm. The proximal ulna consists of the olecranon and coronoid processes and the trochlear and radial notches. The superficial dorsal surface is formed by the hook-shaped **olecranon process,** which is the attachment site for the triceps brachii muscle. The **trochlear notch** is a half-moon–shaped concave articular surface that curves around the trochlea of the humerus. This articulation allows for flexion and extension of the elbow. Located on the anterior portion of the distal end of the trochlear notch is a small beaklike process called the **coronoid process.** Just distal and lateral to the coronoid process is a flattened depression called the **radial notch** which is covered by articular cartilage for articulation with the radial head. Immediately distal to the coronoid process is a roughened bony surface termed the **ulnar tuberosity.** The tendon of the brachialis muscle inserts on both the coronoid process and the ulnar tuberosity (Figures 9.77, 9.78, 9.80, and 9.81).

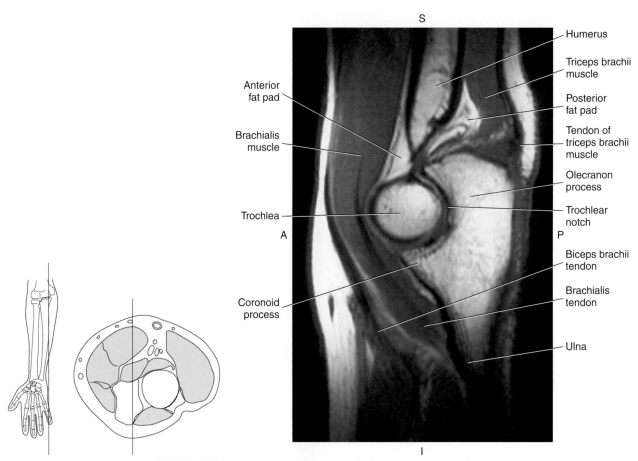

FIGURE 9.80 Sagittal, T1-weighted MRI of elbow with proximal ulna.

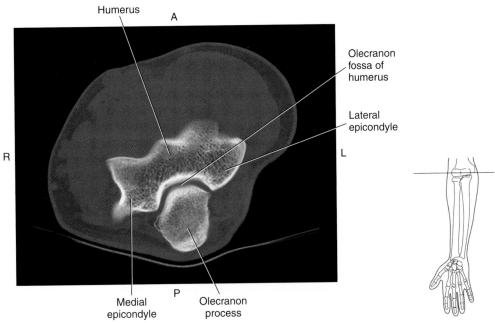

FIGURE 9.81 Axial CT of left elbow.

Ulna: distal ulna. The smaller, distal end of the ulna has two prominent projections. The larger, rounded projection is an articular eminence termed the **head of the ulna.** It articulates with the ulnar notch of the radius and the triangular fibrocartilage complex. The small conical projection on the medial surface is called the **ulnar styloid process,** which serves as the attachment site for the ulnar collateral ligament of the wrist. Another structure that is important in stabilizing and strengthening the connection between the radius and ulna is the **interosseous membrane,** a strong fibrous sheath stretching between the interosseous borders of both bones (Figure 9.77).

Joint capsule and fat pads. The entire elbow joint is surrounded by a relatively loose joint capsule that allows for the movements of flexion and extension. The joint capsule is weaker anteriorly and posteriorly but is reinforced medially and laterally by the strong radial and ulnar collateral ligaments (discussed in the next section). Located within the olecranon and coronoid fossas are fat pads that fill the space between the synovial membrane and joint capsule (Figures 9.79, 9.80, and 9.82 through 9.85). The fat pads help cushion the area where the olecranon and coronoid processes move during flexion and extension of the elbow. There are two clinically important bursae located in the elbow: the olecranon bursa and the distal bicipitoradial bursa. The **olecranon bursa** is located within the subcutaneous tissue overlying the olecranon process (Figure 9.82). The distal **bicipitoradial bursa** lies between the insertion of the biceps tendon and the humerus.

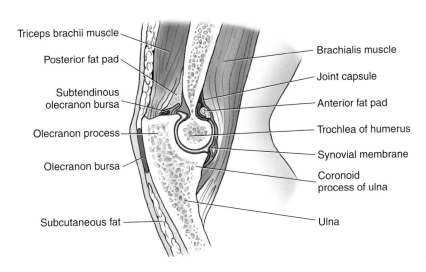

FIGURE 9.82 Sagittal view of elbow at midjoint.

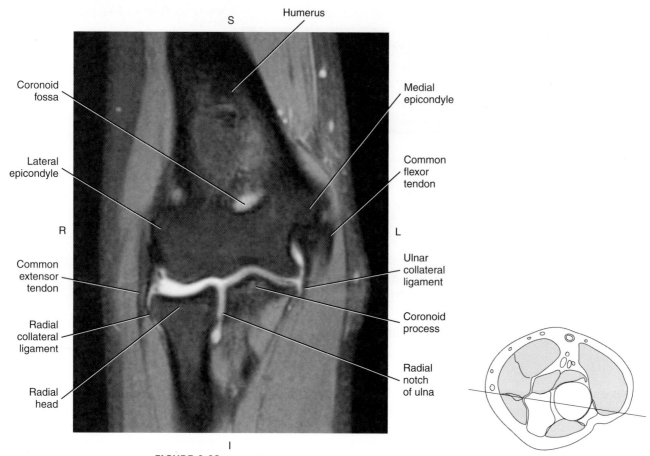

FIGURE 9.83 Coronal, T2-weighted MRI of right elbow, post-arthrogram.

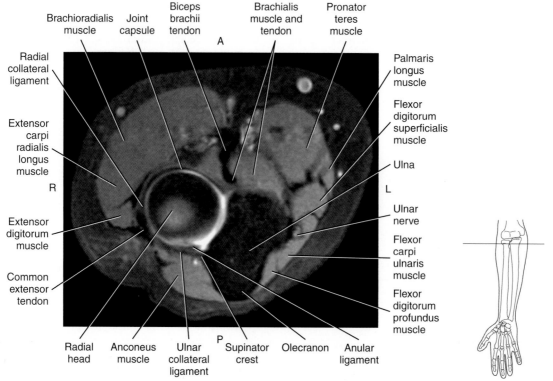

FIGURE 9.84 Axial, T2-weighted MRI of right elbow, post-arthrogram.

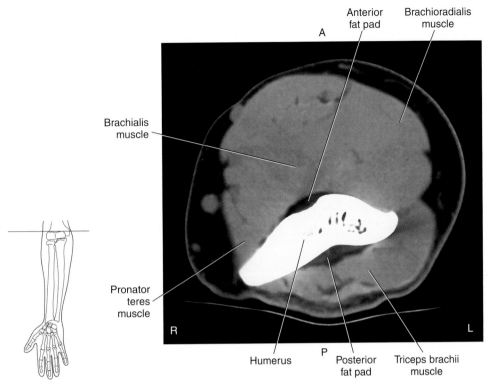

FIGURE 9.85 **Axial CT of right elbow with fat pads.**

Ligaments

The stability of the elbow joint primarily depends on the collateral ligaments, which are woven into the lateral portions of the joint capsule. The **ulnar (medial) collateral ligament** consists of three components: an anterior band, a posterior band, and a transverse band (ligament of Cooper) (Figures 9.86 through 9.89). The anterior band, which is the strongest, extends from the medial epicondyle of the humerus to the medial aspect of the coronoid process. The posterior band originates along with the anterior band from the medial epicondyle of the humerus and inserts on the medial aspect of the olecranon process, forming a triangular plate. The weaker transverse band stretches between the medial surfaces of the coronoid and olecranon processes to unite the anterior and posterior bands. The ulnar collateral ligament forms the floor of the **cubital tunnel** for passage of the ulnar nerve (Figures 9.86 through 9.89).

Reinforcing the lateral side is the triangular radial (lateral) collateral ligament. The radial collateral ligament originates from the lateral epicondyle of the humerus, adjacent to and beneath the common extensor tendons, and spreads distally to insert on the anular ligament and the anterior and posterior margins of the radial notch of the ulna (Figures 9.88 and 9.90). The **anular ligament** forms a fibrous ring that encircles the radial head, with a narrow portion that tightens around the radial neck to prevent inferior displacement of the radius (Figures 9.86 and 9.90 through 9.92). The anular ligament is considered a key structure in the proximal radioulnar joint, allowing the head of the radius to rotate freely. Just distal to the anular ligament is the **quadrate ligament**, a small band of tissue that passes from the radial notch of the ulna to the neck of the radius to provide stability to the joint during supination and pronation.

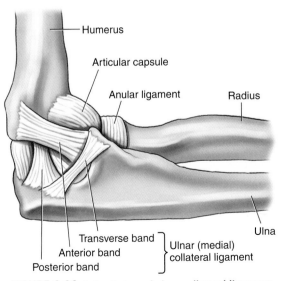

FIGURE 9.86 **Lateral view of ulnar collateral ligament.**

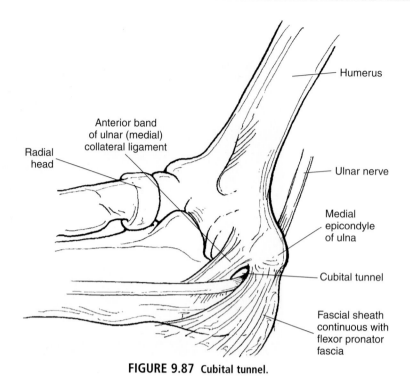

FIGURE 9.87 Cubital tunnel.

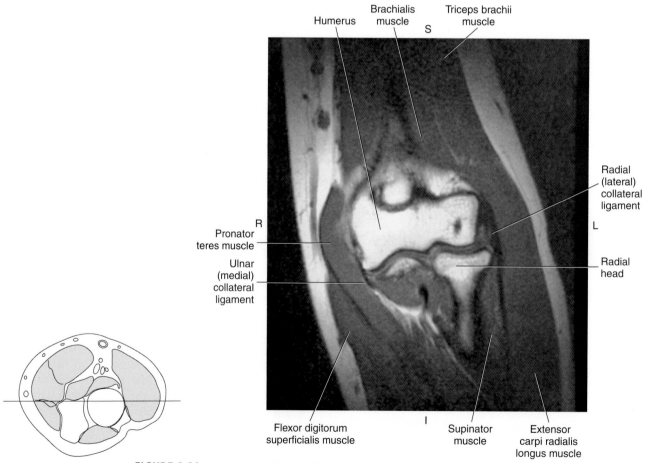

FIGURE 9.88 Coronal, T1-weighted MRI of left elbow with collateral ligaments.

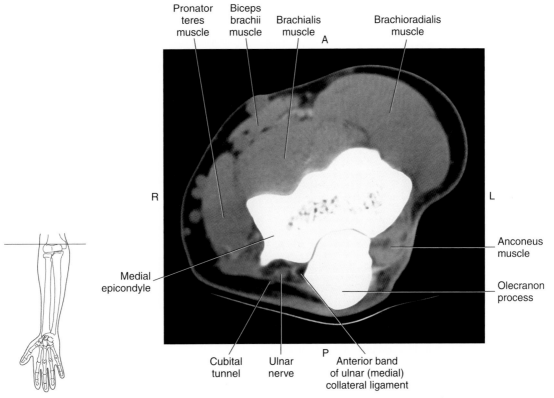

FIGURE 9.89 Axial CT of left elbow with ulnar nerve and cubital tunnel.

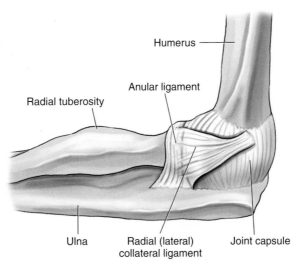

FIGURE 9.90 Lateral view of radial (lateral) collateral ligament.

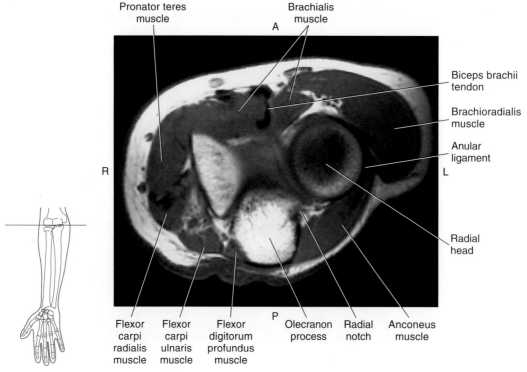

Pronator teres muscle
Brachialis muscle
Biceps brachii tendon
Brachioradialis muscle
Anular ligament
Radial head
A
R
L
P
Flexor carpi radialis muscle
Flexor carpi ulnaris muscle
Flexor digitorum profundus muscle
Olecranon process
Radial notch
Anconeus muscle

FIGURE 9.91 Axial, T1-weighted MRI of left elbow with anular ligament.

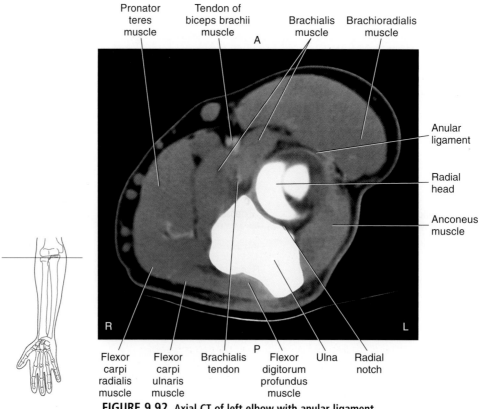

Pronator teres muscle
Tendon of biceps brachii muscle
Brachialis muscle
Brachioradialis muscle
Anular ligament
Radial head
Anconeus muscle
A
R
L
P
Flexor carpi radialis muscle
Flexor carpi ulnaris muscle
Brachialis tendon
Flexor digitorum profundus muscle
Ulna
Radial notch

FIGURE 9.92 Axial CT of left elbow with anular ligament.

Muscles of the Forearm

One method to classify the muscles of the forearm is to use the radius, ulna, and interosseous membrane to divide them into a ventral group (the flexors) and a dorsal group (the extensors). The two groups can be further divided into superficial and deep muscles. The muscles of the forearm are described in Table 9.5.

Ventral Group—superficial muscles

Pronator teres
Flexor carpi radialis
Palmaris longus
Flexor carpi ulnaris
Flexor digitorum superficialis

TABLE 9.5	Muscles of the Forearm		
Muscle	**Origin**	**Insertion**	**Primary Actions**
Ventral-Superficial Group			
Pronator teres	Humeral head—common flexor tendon Ulnar head—near coronoid process of ulna	Lateral surface of radius, midshaft	Pronates and flexes forearm
Flexor carpi radialis	Common flexor tendon	Base of second metacarpal	Flexes and abducts hand
Palmaris longus	Common flexor tendon	Distal half of flexor retinaculum	Flexes wrist
Flexor carpi ulnaris	Humeral head—common flexor tendon Ulnar head—olecranon process	Humeral head—distal half of flexor retinaculum Ulnar head—pisiform, hook of hamate, fifth metacarpal	Flexes wrist and adducts hand
Flexor digitorum superficialis	Humeral head—common flexor tendon Ulnar head—coronoid process Radial head—anterior surface of proximal half of radius	Lateral sides of middle phalanges of second to fifth fingers	Flexes middle and proximal phalanges of second to fifth fingers
Ventral-Deep Group			
Flexor digitorum profundus	Anterior surface of proximal ulna	Bases of distal phalanges of fourth or fifth figner	Flexes distal phalanges of fourth or fifth finger at distal interphalangeal joint
Flexor pollicis longus	Anterior surface of radius and interosseous membrane	Base of distal phalanx of thumb	Flexes phalanges of thumb
Pronator quadratus	Anterior and radial aspects of distal ulna	Anterior surface of distal radius	Pronates forearm
Dorsal-Superficial Group			
Brachioradialis	Proximal two-thirds of supracondylar ridge of humerus	Distal radius, base of styloid process on lateral surface	Weak forearm flexion
Extensor carpi radialis longus	Lateral supracondylar ridge of humerus	Dorsal aspect base of second metacarpal	Extend and abduct hand at wrist joint
Extensor carpi radialis brevis	Common extensor tendon	Dorsal aspect base of third metacarpal	Extend and abduct hand at wrist joint
Extensor digitorum	Common extensor tendon	Extensor expansions of second to fifth fingers	Extends second to fifth fingers at metacarpophalangeal joints
Extensor digiti minimi	Common extensor tendon	Extensor expansion of fifth finger	Extends fifth finger at metacarpophalangeal joint
Extensor carpi ulnaris	Common extensor tendon	Dorsal aspect of base of fifth metacarpal	Extends and adducts hand at wrist joint
Dorsal-Deep Group			
Abductor pollicis longus	Posterior surface of proximal ulna, radius, and interosseous membrane	Base of first metacarpal	Abducts thumb and extends thumb at carpometacarpal joint
Extensor pollicis brevis	Posterior surface of distal third of radius and interosseous membrane	Dorsal aspect of base of proximal phalanx of thumb	Extends proximal phalanx of thumb at metacarpophalangeal joint
Extensor pollicis longus	Posterior surface of middle third of ulna and interosseous membrane	Dorsal aspect of base of distal phalanx of thumb	Extends distal phalanx of thumb at interphalangeal joint
Extensor indicis	Posterior surface distal third of ulna and interosseous membrane	Extensor expansion of second finger	Supinate forearm
Supinator	Lateral epicondyle of humerus; radial and collateral ligaments; supinator fossa; crest of ulna	Lateral, posterior, and anterior surface of proximal third and radius	Supinate forearm

All five of the superficial muscles in the ventral group have an origin from the **common flexor tendon** off the medial epicondyle of the humerus. These muscles are demonstrated in Figures 9.93 through 9.106.

The **pronator teres muscle** has two heads of origin. Its humeral head originates from the common flexor tendon, whereas the ulnar head originates near the coronoid process of the ulna. The pronator teres muscle courses obliquely before inserting on the lateral surface of the radius at midshaft. It works in conjunction with the pronator quadratus muscle to pronate the forearm (Figure 9.93).

The **flexor carpi radialis muscle** originates from the common flexor tendon and is located medial to the pronator teres. Its tendon passes through the carpal tunnel before inserting on the palmar surface of the base of the second metacarpal. Its actions include flexion and radial deviation of the hand at the wrist joint (Figure 9.93).

The **palmaris longus muscle** originates from the common flexor tendon and passes superficial to the flexor retinaculum to merge with the palmar aponeurosis. It acts to flex the hand and tighten the palmar aponeurosis (Figure 9.93).

The **flexor carpi ulnaris muscle** is the most medial of the superficial muscles located in the anterior portion of the forearm. It has two heads: The humeral head originates from the common flexor tendon, and the ulnar head originates from the olecranon process. It inserts onto the pisiform, hook of the hamate, and fifth metacarpal and acts to flex and adduct (ulnar deviation) the hand at the wrist joint (Figure 9.93).

The **flexor digitorum superficialis muscle** is the largest muscle of the superficial muscles in the forearm. It arises from three heads: the humeral head from the common flexor tendon, the ulnar head from the coronoid process, and the radial head from the anterior surface of the proximal half of the radius. Just before reaching the flexor retinaculum, the muscle divides into four tendons that share a common synovial sheath through the carpal tunnel. After passing under the flexor retinaculum, the tendons insert on the lateral sides of the middle phalanges of the second to fifth digits. The flexor digitorum superficialis is a strong flexor of the middle and proximal phalanges of the second through fifth digits (Figure 9.93).

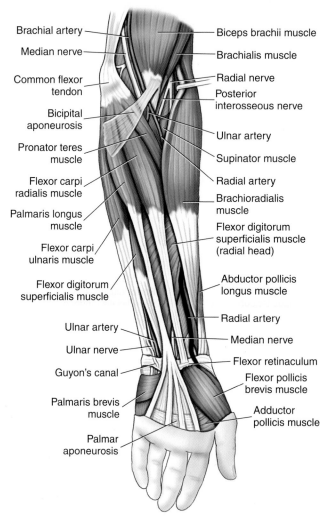

FIGURE 9.93 Anterior view of superficial flexor muscles of forearm.

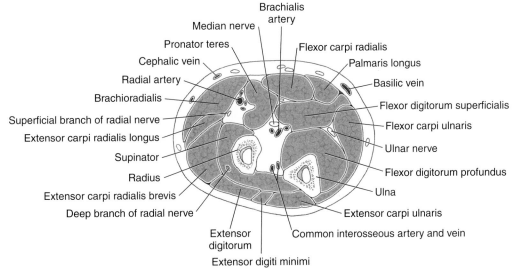

Median nerve
Brachialis artery
Pronator teres
Cephalic vein
Radial artery
Brachioradialis
Superficial branch of radial nerve
Extensor carpi radialis longus
Supinator
Radius
Extensor carpi radialis brevis
Deep branch of radial nerve
Extensor digitorum
Extensor digiti minimi
Flexor carpi radialis
Palmaris longus
Basilic vein
Flexor digitorum superficialis
Flexor carpi ulnaris
Ulnar nerve
Flexor digitorum profundus
Ulna
Extensor carpi ulnaris
Common interosseous artery and vein

FIGURE 9.94 Axial view of forearm, proximal one-third, right arm.

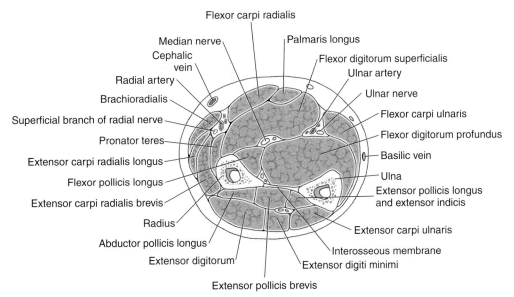

Flexor carpi radialis
Median nerve
Cephalic vein
Radial artery
Brachioradialis
Superficial branch of radial nerve
Pronator teres
Extensor carpi radialis longus
Flexor pollicis longus
Extensor carpi radialis brevis
Radius
Abductor pollicis longus
Extensor digitorum
Extensor pollicis brevis
Palmaris longus
Flexor digitorum superficialis
Ulnar artery
Ulnar nerve
Flexor carpi ulnaris
Flexor digitorum profundus
Basilic vein
Ulna
Extensor pollicis longus and extensor indicis
Extensor carpi ulnaris
Interosseous membrane
Extensor digiti minimi

FIGURE 9.95 Axial view of forearm, mid-forearm, right arm.

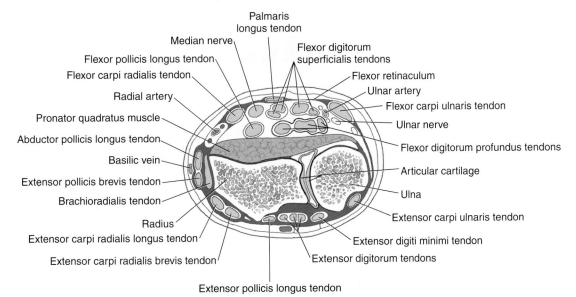

Palmaris longus tendon
Median nerve
Flexor pollicis longus tendon
Flexor carpi radialis tendon
Radial artery
Pronator quadratus muscle
Abductor pollicis longus tendon
Basilic vein
Extensor pollicis brevis tendon
Brachioradialis tendon
Radius
Extensor carpi radialis longus tendon
Extensor carpi radialis brevis tendon
Extensor pollicis longus tendon
Flexor digitorum superficialis tendons
Flexor retinaculum
Ulnar artery
Flexor carpi ulnaris tendon
Ulnar nerve
Flexor digitorum profundus tendons
Articular cartilage
Ulna
Extensor carpi ulnaris tendon
Extensor digiti minimi tendon
Extensor digitorum tendons

FIGURE 9.96 Axial view of forearm, distal one-third, right arm.

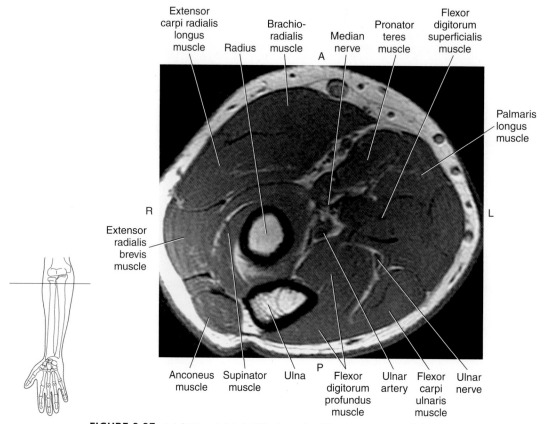

FIGURE 9.97 Axial, T1-weighted MRI of proximal forearm muscles, right arm.

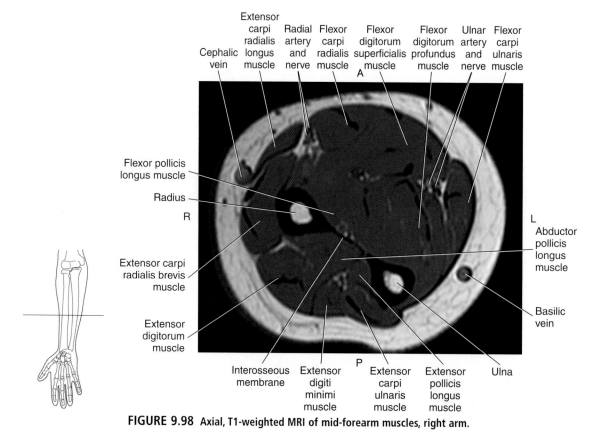

FIGURE 9.98 Axial, T1-weighted MRI of mid-forearm muscles, right arm.

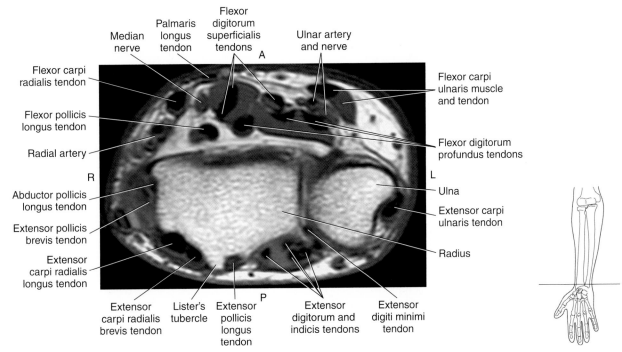

FIGURE 9.99 Axial, T1-weighted MRI of distal forearm, right arm.

Median nerve
Palmaris longus tendon
Flexor digitorum superficialis tendons
Ulnar artery and nerve
A
Flexor carpi radialis tendon
Flexor pollicis longus tendon
Radial artery
R
Abductor pollicis longus tendon
Extensor pollicis brevis tendon
Extensor carpi radialis longus tendon
Flexor carpi ulnaris muscle and tendon
Flexor digitorum profundus tendons
L
Ulna
Extensor carpi ulnaris tendon
Radius
Extensor carpi radialis brevis tendon
Lister's tubercle
Extensor pollicis longus tendon
P
Extensor digitorum and indicis tendons
Extensor digiti minimi tendon

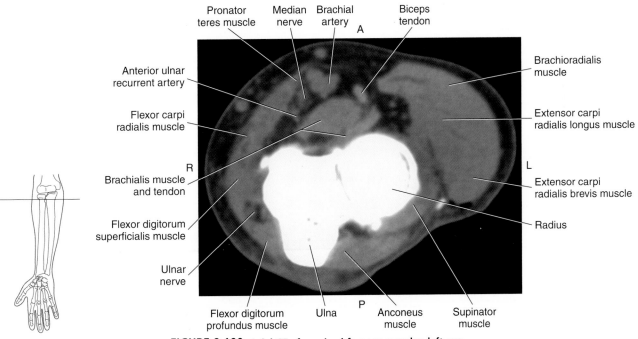

FIGURE 9.100 Axial CT of proximal forearm muscles, left arm.

Pronator teres muscle
Median nerve
Brachial artery
A
Biceps tendon
Anterior ulnar recurrent artery
Flexor carpi radialis muscle
R
Brachialis muscle and tendon
Flexor digitorum superficialis muscle
Ulnar nerve
Flexor digitorum profundus muscle
Ulna
P
Anconeus muscle
Supinator muscle
Brachioradialis muscle
Extensor carpi radialis longus muscle
L
Extensor carpi radialis brevis muscle
Radius

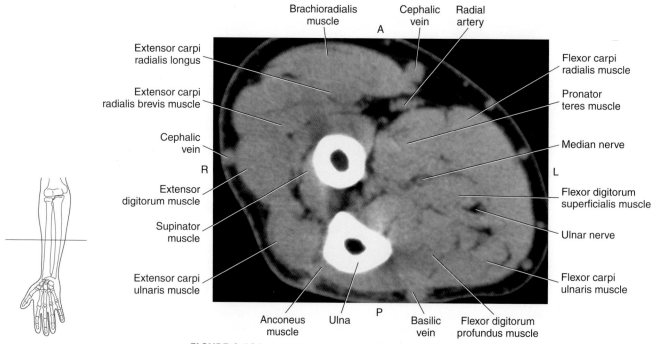

FIGURE 9.101 Axial CT of mid-forearm muscles, left arm.

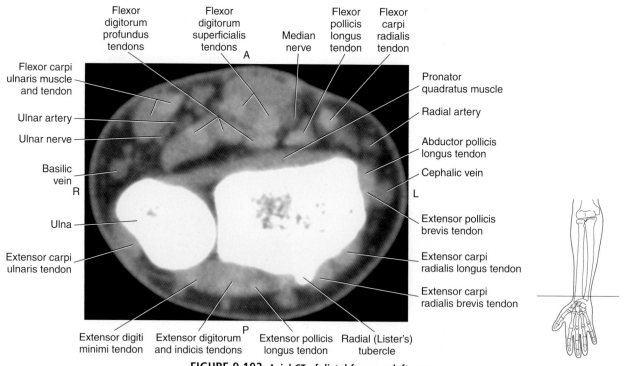

FIGURE 9.102 Axial CT of distal forearm, left arm.

S

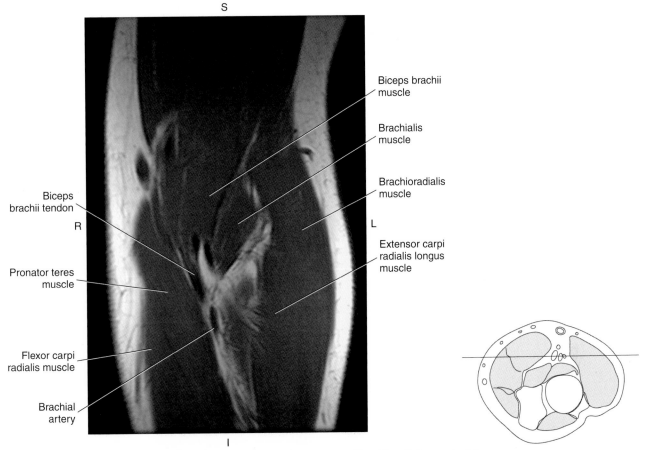

Biceps brachii
muscle

Brachialis
muscle

Brachioradialis
muscle

Biceps
brachii tendon

R

L

Extensor carpi
radialis longus
muscle

Pronator teres
muscle

Flexor carpi
radialis muscle

Brachial
artery

I

FIGURE 9.103 Coronal, T1-weighted MRI of brachioradialis muscle, left arm.

S

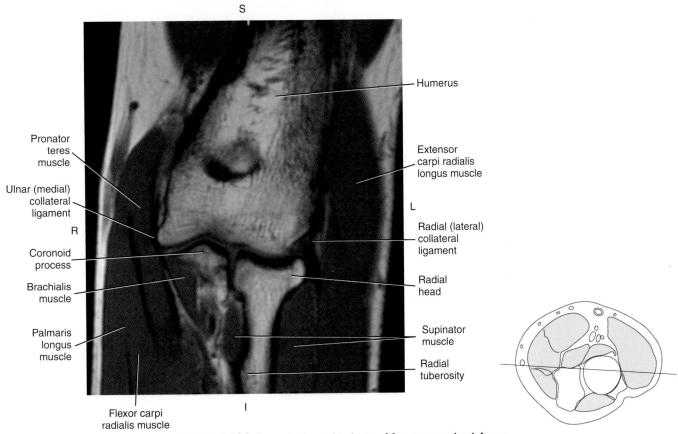

Humerus

Pronator
teres
muscle

Extensor
carpi radialis
longus muscle

Ulnar (medial)
collateral
ligament

L

R

Radial (lateral)
collateral
ligament

Coronoid
process

Radial
head

Brachialis
muscle

Palmaris
longus
muscle

Supinator
muscle

Radial
tuberosity

Flexor carpi
radialis muscle

I

FIGURE 9.104 Coronal, T1-weighted MRI of forearm muscles, left arm.

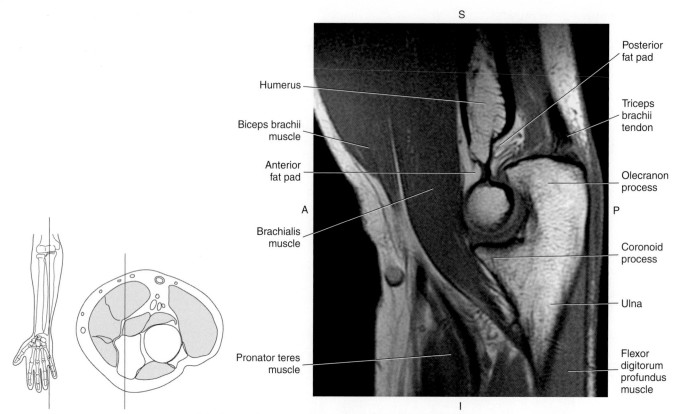

FIGURE 9.105 Sagittal, T1-weighted MRI of forearm muscles.

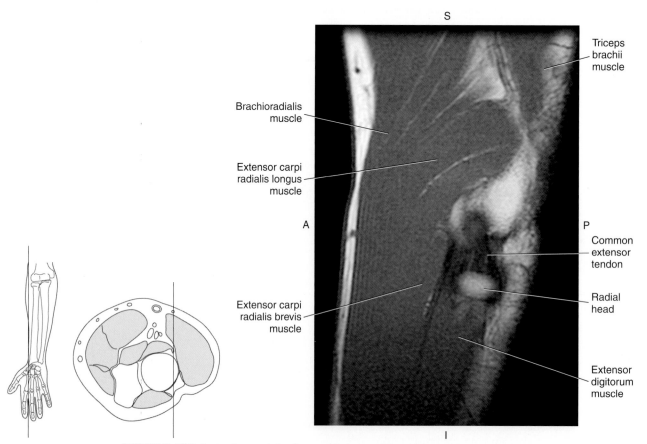

FIGURE 9.106 Sagittal, T1-weighted MRI of forearm with common extensor tendon.

Ventral group—deep muscles

Flexor digitorum profundus
Flexor pollicis longus
Pronator quadratus

The muscles of the ventral group are demonstrated on Figures 9.94 through 9.107. The **flexor digitorum profundus muscle** is a long, thick muscle responsible for flexing the distal interphalangeal joints of the fingers. It originates from the anterior surface of the proximal ulna and extends medially to the interosseous membrane. Similar to the flexor digitorum superficialis, the flexor digitorum profundus divides into four tendons before reaching the flexor retinaculum. The four tendons pass deep in the carpal tunnel and continue distally to insert on the distal phalanges, where they pair up with the flexor digitorum superficialis to provide flexion of the middle and proximal phalanges of the second through fifth digits (Figure 9.107, B).

The **flexor pollicis longus muscle** arises from the anterior surface of the radius and adjacent interosseous membrane and runs lateral to the flexor digitorum profundus to cover the anterior aspect of the radius. After passing through the carpal tunnel, the flexor pollicis longus tendon runs between the flexor pollicis brevis and adductor pollicis brevis muscles to insert at the base of the first distal phalanx (Figure 9.107, A and B).

The **pronator quadratus**, a quadrangular muscle, is the deepest muscle in the anterior aspect of the forearm. It arises from the anterior and radial aspect of the distal ulna and passes transversely to insert on the anterior surface of the distal radius. The deep fibers of this muscle help bind the radius and ulna together along with the interosseous membrane. The pronator quadratus is the prime mover in pronation of the forearm (Figure 9.107).

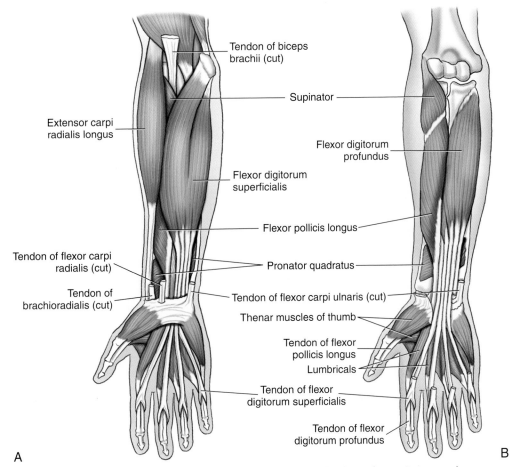

FIGURE 9.107 Anterior view of forearm muscles. A, Superficial muscles. **B,** Deep muscles.

Dorsal group—superficial muscles

Brachioradialis
Extensor carpi radialis longus
Extensor carpi radialis brevis
Extensor digitorum
Extensor digiti minimi
Extensor carpi ulnaris

The muscles of the superficial dorsal group are demonstrated in Figures 9.94 through 9.106 and 9.108. The **brachioradialis** is an extensor muscle lying along the lateral border of the forearm. This large muscle arises from the upper two thirds of the supracondylar ridge of the humerus and attaches distally to the radial styloid process. The brachioradialis flexes the forearm at the elbow and assists with pronation and supination (Figure 9.108).

The **extensor carpi radialis longus muscle** arises just distal to the brachioradialis on the lower third of the supracondylar ridge of the humerus. It runs posterior and deep to the brachioradialis to insert on the base of the second metacarpal. It acts as an extensor and abductor of the hand at the wrist joint (Figure 9.108).

The other superficial muscles (extensor carpi radialis brevis, extensor digitorum, extensor digiti minimi, extensor carpi ulnaris) arise from a **common extensor** tendon attached to the lateral epicondyle of the humerus. At the level of the elbow they appear as one structure but become more distinct distally as they insert on various structures about the wrist and hand.

The **extensor carpi radialis brevis muscle** has components that arise from the radial collateral and anular ligaments, as well as the common extensor tendon. It runs along the dorsal surface of the wrist to insert at the base of the third metacarpal and acts to extend and abduct the hand at the wrist joint (Figure 9.108).

The **extensor digitorum muscle** is the main extensor of the second to fifth digits and occupies much of the posterior surface of the forearm. It arises from the common extensor tendon and divides into four individual tendinous slips just proximal to the wrist. The four tendons run in a single synovial sheath as they pass under the extensor retinaculum. The tendons insert into the extensor expansions of the second through fifth digits, helping to form the extensor hoods (see the section on ligaments of the finger). In addition, small slips of the tendon spread out and run to the bases of the proximal phalanges and to the capsules of the metacarpophalangeal joints (Figure 9.108). The extensor digitorum muscle extends and spreads the fingers and extends the hand at the wrist joint. The **extensor digiti minimi muscle** arises from the common extensor tendon and passes

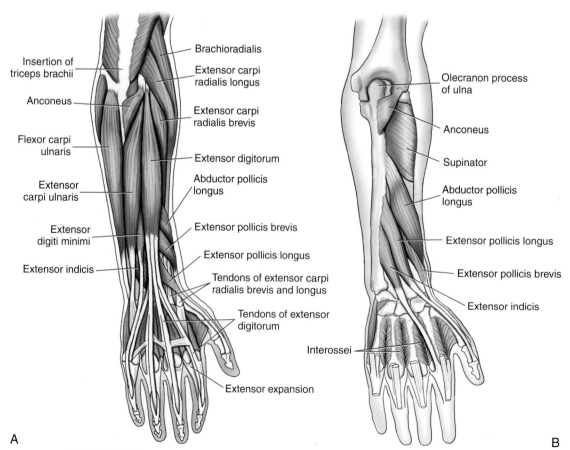

FIGURE 9.108 Posterior view of forearm muscles. A, Superficial muscles. **B,** Deep muscles.

under the extensor retinaculum in its own synovial compartment. It then divides into two tendinous slips that insert on the proximal phalanx of the fifth digit to help with extension of the little finger (Figure 9.108).

The **extensor carpi ulnaris** is a long, slender muscle that arises from the common extensor tendon and runs along the medial and dorsal side of the ulna to insert on the base of the fifth metacarpal. Its main actions include extension of the hand at the wrist joint and adduction of the hand, resulting in ulnar deviation (Figure 9.108).

Dorsal group—deep muscles

Abductor pollicis longus
Extensor pollicis brevis
Extensor pollicis longus
Extensor indicis
Supinator

The deep muscles of the dorsal group consist of four extensors that act on either the first or second digit and include the supinator muscle. These muscles are demonstrated in Figures 9.94 through 9.106 and 9.108.

The three deep extensors that act on the first digit are the abductor pollicis longus, extensor pollicis brevis, and the extensor pollicis longus muscles. The long, slender **abductor pollicis longus muscle** arises from the dorsal surfaces of the ulna and radius and from the interosseous membrane. It inserts at the base of the first metacarpal to abduct and extend the thumb (Figure 9.108).

The short **extensor pollicis brevis muscle** arises from the dorsal surfaces of the ulna and radius and from the interosseous membrane just distal to the abductor pollicis longus muscle. It inserts at the base of the proximal phalanx of the first digit and works together with the abductor pollicis longus to extend and abduct the thumb (Figure 9.108).

The **extensor pollicis longus muscle** arises from the dorsal surface of the ulna and interosseous membrane just distal to the abductor pollicis longus muscle. After passing through the extensor retinaculum, it crosses over the extensor carpi radialis longus and brevis to insert at the base of the distal phalanx of the first digit. Its main action is to extend the distal phalanx of the first digit, but it can also abduct the hand (Figure 9.108).

The **extensor indicis muscle** arises from the distal third of the dorsal ulna and the interosseous membrane and runs with the extensor digitorum muscle through the extensor retinaculum to insert on the dorsal aponeurosis of the second digit. It functions with the extensor digitorum muscle to extend the index finger, as if pointing (Figure 9.108).

The **supinator muscle** originates from two heads: oblique and transverse. The oblique head originates from the lateral epicondyle and collateral ligament, whereas the transverse head originates from the supinator crest of the ulna. Both heads wrap laterally around the proximal radius to insert on the posterolateral and anterior surfaces of the proximal radius to supinate the forearm (Figure 9.108).

WRIST AND HAND

The complex anatomy of the wrist and hand provides for a multitude of movements unmatched by any other joint of the body.

Bony Anatomy

The bony anatomy of the wrist and hand consists of the distal radius and ulna, 8 carpal bones, 5 metacarpals, and 14 phalanges (Figure 9.109). Both the distal radius and ulna have a conical styloid process that acts as an attachment site for ligaments. The radial styloid process is located on the lateral surface of the radius, whereas the ulnar styloid process is located on the posteromedial side of the ulna. The carpal bones are arranged in proximal and distal rows. Located in the proximal row of carpal bones are the **scaphoid (navicular)**, **lunate (semilunar)**, **triquetral (triquetrum)**, and **pisiform bones**. The pisiform is considered a sesamoid bone that is embedded in the tendon of the flexor carpi ulnaris. The distal row consists of the **trapezium (greater multangular)**, **trapezoid (lesser multangular)**, **capitate (os magnum)**, and **hamate (unciform)** bones (Figures 9.109 through 9.123). The five **metacarpals** are small tubular bones with a proximal end (base), distal end (head), and middle (body) portion. The 14 **phalanges** that make up the fingers, like the metacarpals, consist of a proximal (base), distal (head), and middle (body) portion. Each digit consists of three phalanges (proximal, middle, and distal), except for the thumb (first digit), which has only two phalanges (proximal and distal).

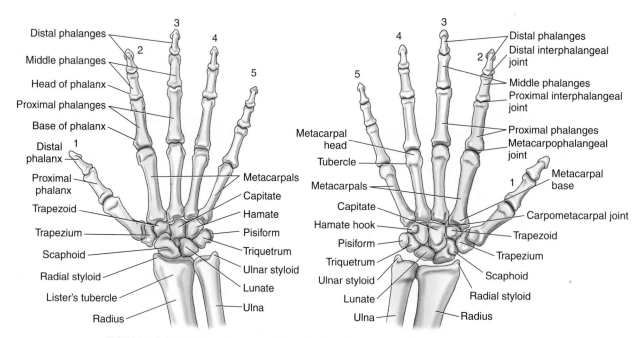

FIGURE 9.109 Osseous structures of hand and wrist. *Left,* Dorsal view. *Right,* Palmar view.

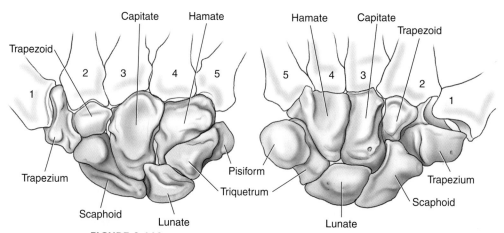

FIGURE 9.110 Carpal bones. *Left,* Dorsal view. *Right,* Palmar view.

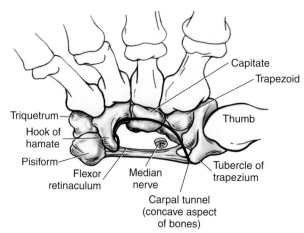

FIGURE 9.111 Carpal tunnel.

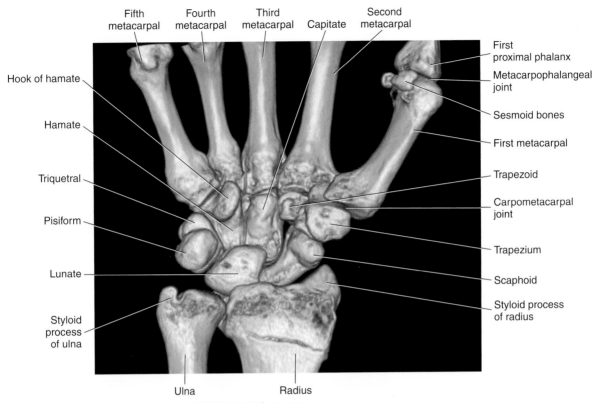

Fifth metacarpal • Fourth metacarpal • Third metacarpal • Capitate • Second metacarpal

Hook of hamate

Hamate

Triquetral

Pisiform

Lunate

Styloid process of ulna

First proximal phalanx

Metacarpophalangeal joint

Sesmoid bones

First metacarpal

Trapezoid

Carpometacarpal joint

Trapezium

Scaphoid

Styloid process of radius

Ulna • Radius

FIGURE 9.112 3D CT of wrist, palmar aspect.

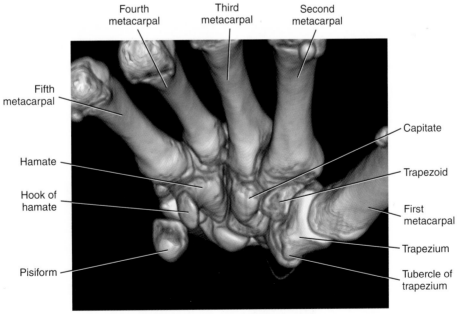

Fourth metacarpal • Third metacarpal • Second metacarpal

Fifth metacarpal

Hamate

Hook of hamate

Pisiform

Capitate

Trapezoid

First metacarpal

Trapezium

Tubercle of trapezium

FIGURE 9.113 3D CT of carpal tunnel.

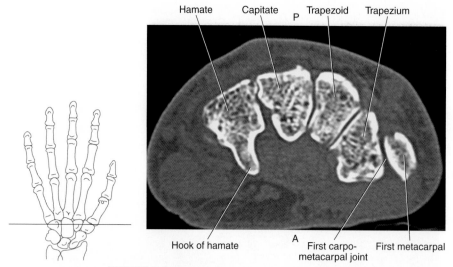

FIGURE 9.114 Axial CT of wrist with distal carpals.

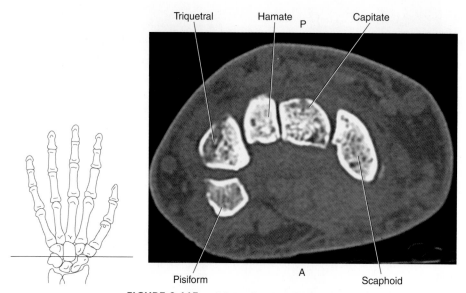

FIGURE 9.115 Axial CT of wrist, midcarpals.

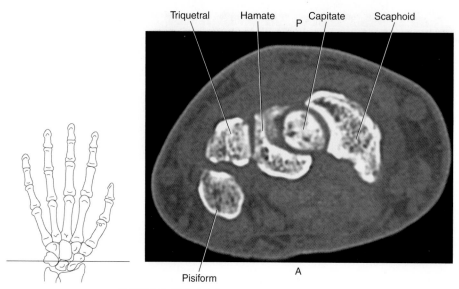

FIGURE 9.116 Axial CT of wrist with pisiform.

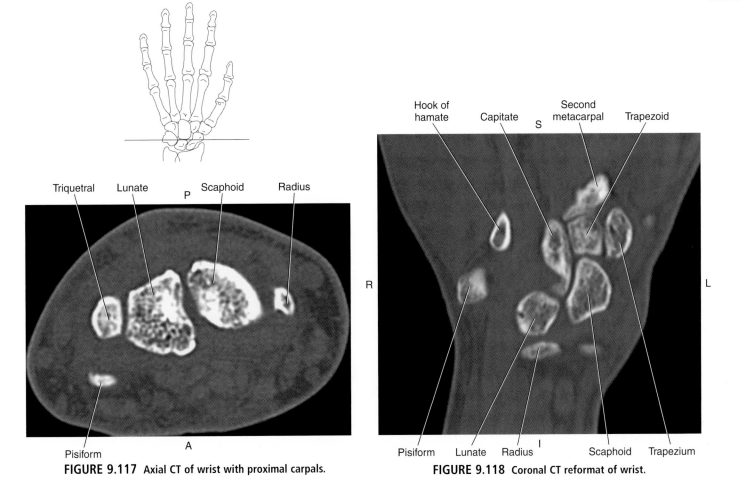

Triquetral Lunate P Scaphoid Radius

Pisiform

A

FIGURE 9.117 Axial CT of wrist with proximal carpals.

Hook of hamate Capitate S Second metacarpal Trapezoid

R L

Pisiform Lunate Radius I Scaphoid Trapezium

FIGURE 9.118 Coronal CT reformat of wrist.

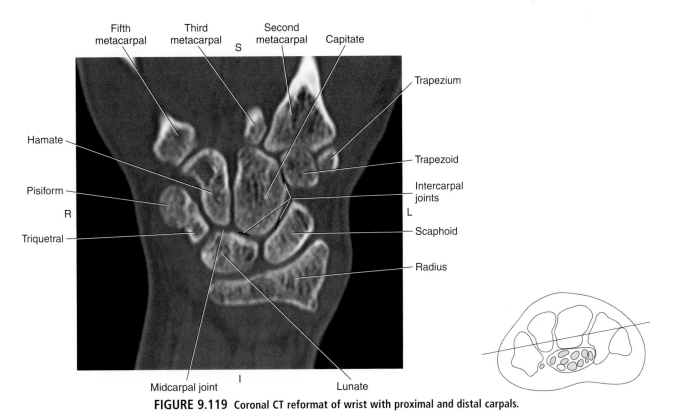

Fifth metacarpal Third metacarpal S Second metacarpal Capitate

Trapezium

Hamate

Trapezoid

Pisiform

Intercarpal joints

R L

Triquetral

Scaphoid

Radius

Midcarpal joint I Lunate

FIGURE 9.119 Coronal CT reformat of wrist with proximal and distal carpals.

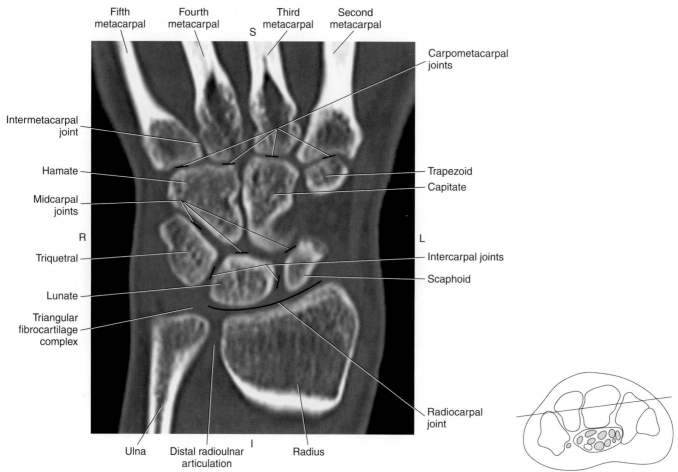

FIGURE 9.120 Coronal CT reformat of wrist with intercarpal joints.

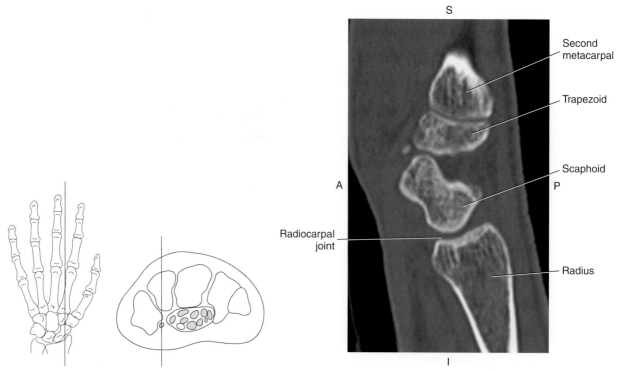

FIGURE 9.121 Sagittal CT reformat of wrist with scaphoid.

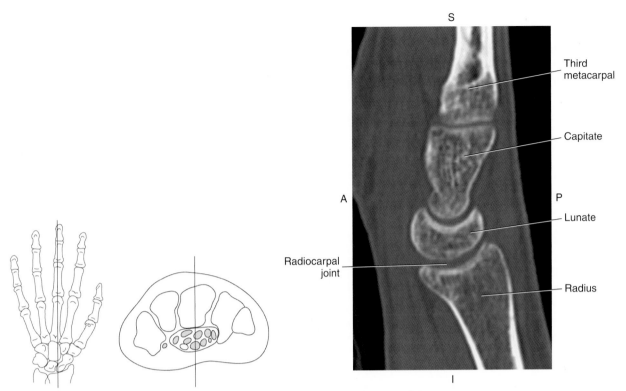

FIGURE 9.122 Sagittal CT reformat of wrist with lunate.

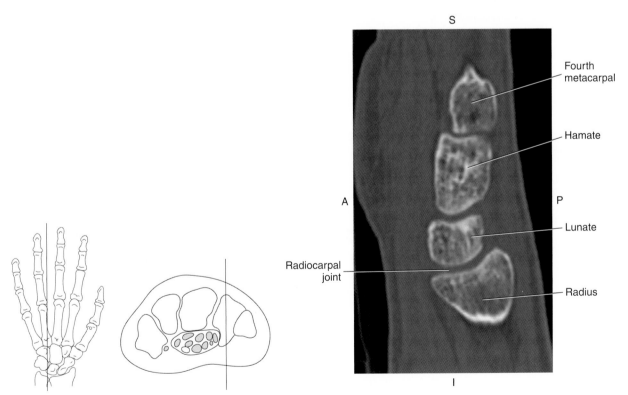

FIGURE 9.123 Sagittal CT reformat of wrist with hamate.

Joints

The joints of the wrist and hand are quite complex and consist of the following: distal radioulnar articulation, radiocarpal articulation (proximal joint of hand), mid-carpal articulation (distal joint of hand), intercarpal articulations (articulations between proximal and distal carpals), carpometacarpal articulations (between carpals and metacarpals), the intermetacarpal articulations (between bases of metacarpals two through five) and the interphalangeal joints (between phalanges of each digit) (Figures 9.120 and 9.124).

Joints of the wrist. The **distal radioulnar articulation**, also called the **distal radioulnar joint (DRUJ)**, is created when the ulnar notch of the radius moves around the articular circumference of the ulna, providing the movements of supination and pronation. The main stabilizing element of the DRUJ is an articular disk called the **triangular fibrocartilage complex (TFCC)**. The TFCC is a fan-shaped band of fibrous tissue that originates on the medial surface of the distal radius and traverses horizontally to insert on the ulnar styloid process (Figures 9.124 through 9.126). It rotates against the distal surface of the ulnar head during pronation and supination and separates the ulna from the carpal bones. The proximal surface of the **radiocarpal articulation** is formed by the articular carpal surface of the radius and the TFCC, whereas the distal surface is formed by the articular surfaces of the scaphoid, lunate, and triquetrum and the interosseous ligaments connecting them (Figures 9.120 through 9.124). The **mid-carpal joint** is formed by the articulations between the proximal and distal carpal rows (Figures 9.119 and 9.124). The articulation between the carpals within each row creates the **intercarpal joints** (Figures 9.119, 9.120, and 9.124). The **carpometacarpal** joints are formed by the articulations between the carpus and the five metacarpals (Figure 9.120 and 9.124). The carpometacarpal joint of the thumb is an independent joint formed by the articular surfaces of the trapezium and first metacarpal, creating a pure saddle joint. The carpometacarpal articulations of the two to five digits are amphiarthrotic joints with little mobility (Figures 9.114 and 9.124). The **intermetacarpal articulation** exists between the bases of the metacarpals and is joined by the palmar and dorsal **metacarpal ligaments** (Figure 9.124).

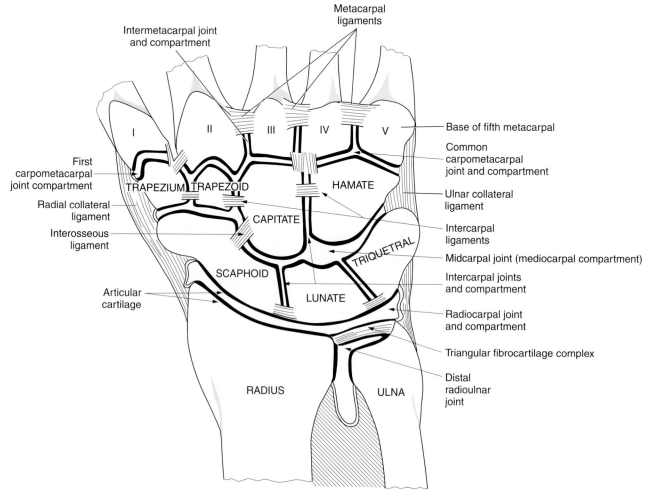

FIGURE 9.124 Anterior cross-section view of wrist joint.

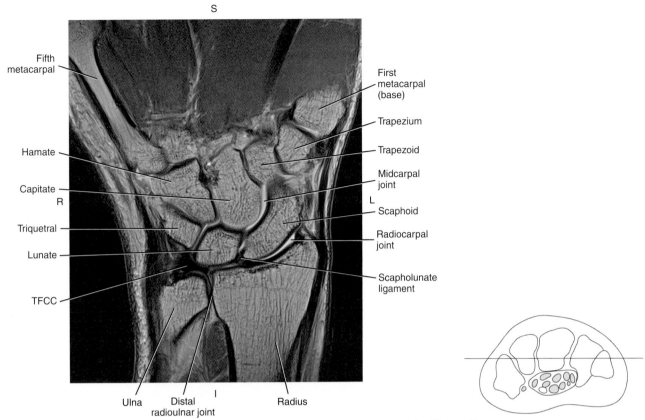

S

Fifth
metacarpal

First
metacarpal
(base)

Trapezium

Hamate

Trapezoid

Capitate

Midcarpal
joint

R   L

Scaphoid

Triquetral

Radiocarpal
joint

Lunate

Scapholunate
ligament

TFCC

Ulna   Distal   I   Radius
          radioulnar joint

FIGURE 9.125 Coronal, T2-weighted MRI of wrist with triangular fibrocartilage complex.

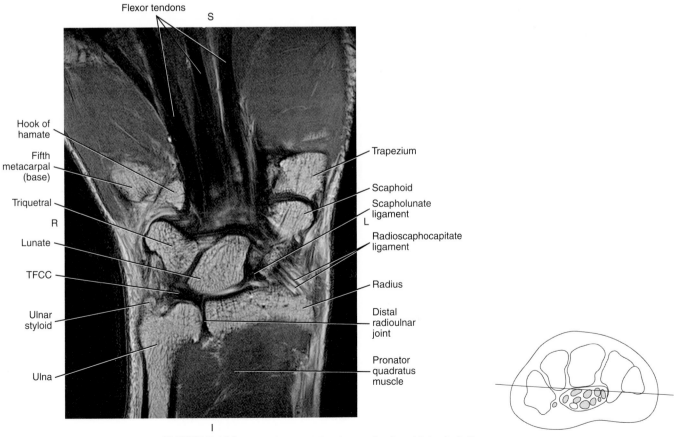

Flexor tendons
S

Hook of
hamate

Trapezium

Fifth
metacarpal
(base)

Scaphoid

Scapholunate
ligament

Triquetral

R   L

Radioscaphocapitate
ligament

Lunate

TFCC

Radius

Ulnar
styloid

Distal
radioulnar
joint

Ulna

Pronator
quadratus
muscle

I

FIGURE 9.126 Coronal, T2-weighted MRI of wrist with intrinsic ligaments.

Joints of the hand. The articulation of the phalanges of the second through fifth digits creates three interphalangeal joints: the **metacarpophalangeal (MCP) joints** classified as condyloid joints, **proximal interphalangeal (PIP),** and **distal interphalangeal (DIP).** The proximal and distal interphalangeal joints are classified as hinge joints (Figure 9.109). The first digit, which consists of 2 phalanges, has just two joints: the MCP joint, classified as a saddle joint, and an interphalangeal joint, classified as a hinge joint (Figures 9.109 and 9.112).

Ligaments and Fascia

Numerous ligaments provide additional stability to the wrist. The **extrinsic ligaments** reinforce the joint cavity surrounding the carpal region and include **palmar** and **dorsal radial carpal ligaments,** the radial and **ulnar collateral ligaments,** and the **TFCC** (Figures 9.124 through 9.127). The many articulations between the carpal bones are supported by the **intercarpal ligaments** or **intrinsic ligaments,** which connect the carpal bones to each other (Figures 9.124 through 9.126). The configuration of the intrinsic ligaments, metacarpal ligaments, and

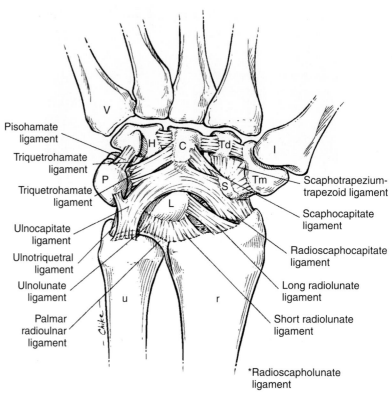

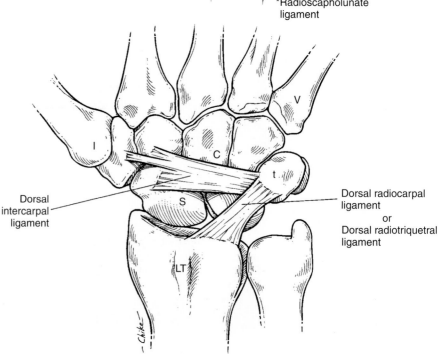

FIGURE 9.127 Extrinsic ligaments of wrist.
Top, Palmar view. *Bottom,* Dorsal view.

triangular fibrocartilage complex creates five different joint compartments that can be demonstrated by arthrography: (1) compartment of the first carpometacarpal articulation, (2) common carpometacarpal compartment, (3) mediocarpal compartment, (4) intermetacarpal compartment, and (5) radiocarpal compartment (Figure 9.124). The **carpal tunnel** is created by the concave arrangement of the carpal bones (Figures 9.111, 9.113, and 9.128). A thick ligamentous band called the **flexor retinaculum (transverse carpal ligament)** stretches across the carpal tunnel to create an enclosure for the passage of

tendons and the median nerve (Figures 9.128, 9.129, and 9.131 through 9.137). The flexor retinaculum inserts medially on the pisiform and hook of the hamate and spans the wrist to insert laterally on the scaphoid and trapezium. In addition to the carpal tunnel, another tunnel called **Guyon's canal** is formed where the ulnar extension of the flexor retinaculum continues over the pisiform and hamate. This creates a potential site for compression of the ulnar nerve (Figures 9.128, *top*, and 9.132). The **extensor retinaculum (dorsal carpal ligament)**, located dorsally, is much thinner. It attaches medially to the ulnar styloid process, triquetrum, and pisiform, and laterally to the lateral margin of the radius (Figure 9.129, *right*). Along its course it forms six fibro-osseous tunnels for the passage of the synovial sheaths containing the extensor tendons (Figures 9.128, *bottom* and 9.130 through 9.133).

> Compression of the median nerve as it passes through the carpal tunnel is called **carpal tunnel syndrome**. Symptoms include pain and numbness of the fingers supplied by the median nerve.

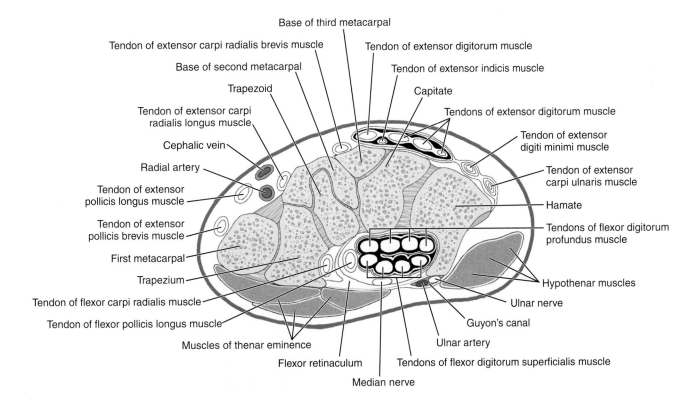

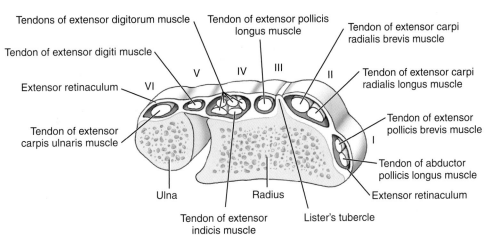

FIGURE 9.128 Axial view of carpal tunnel and flexor tendons. *Top,* Extensor tendons. *Bottom,* Compartments.

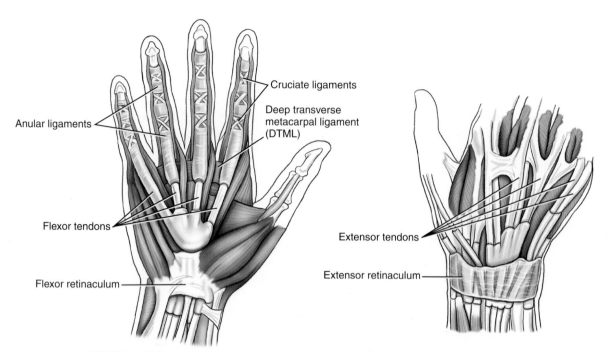

FIGURE 9.129 Left, Palmar view of flexor tendons. Right, Dorsal view of extensor tendons.

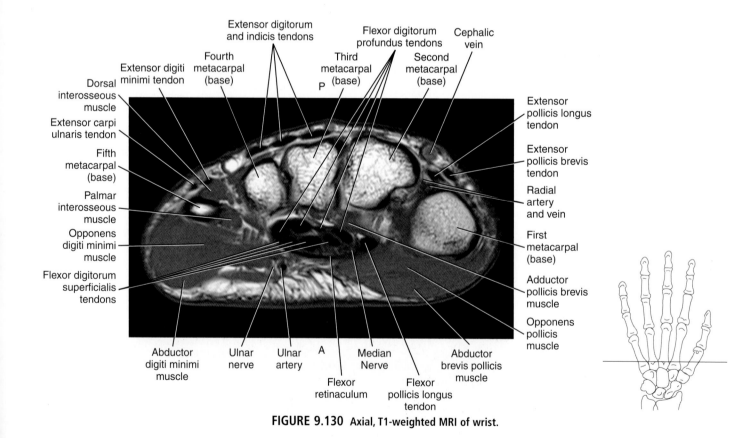

FIGURE 9.130 Axial, T1-weighted MRI of wrist.

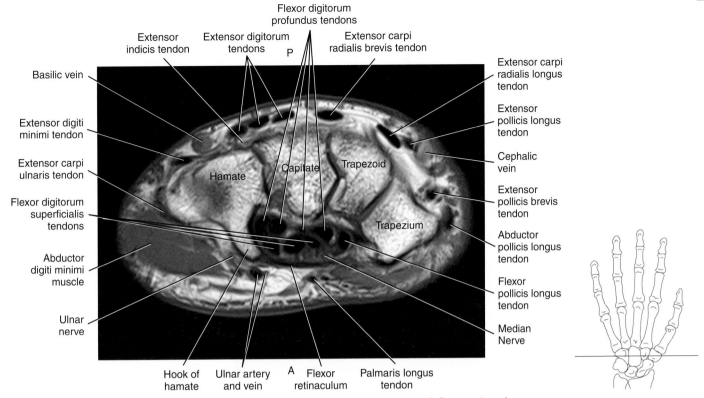

FIGURE 9.131 Axial, T1-weighted MRI of wrist with flexor retinaculum.

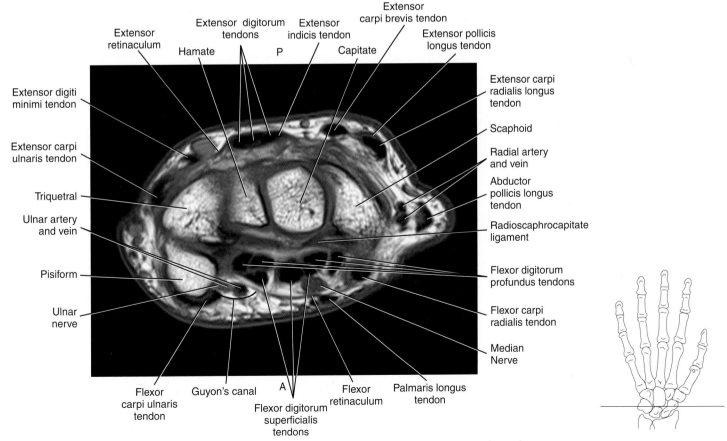

FIGURE 9.132 Axial, T1-weighted MRI of wrist with Guyon's canal.

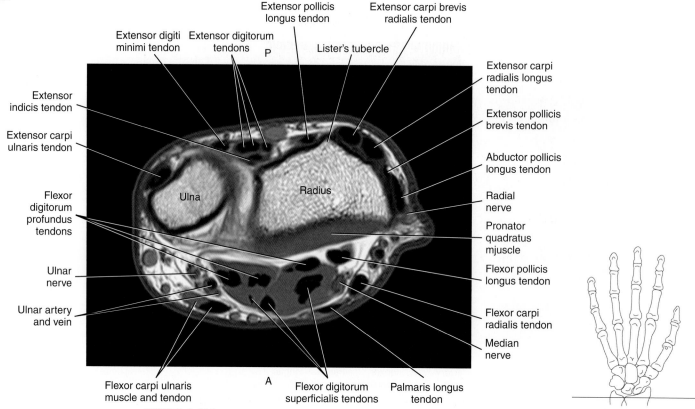

FIGURE 9.133 Axial, T1-weighted MRI of wrist with compartments of extensor tendons.

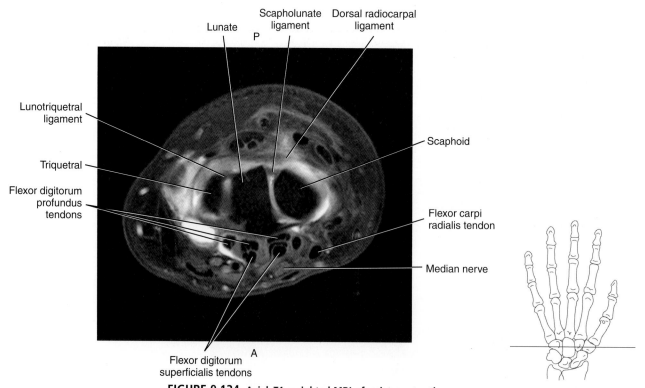

FIGURE 9.134 Axial, T1-weighted MRI of wrist, post arthrogram.

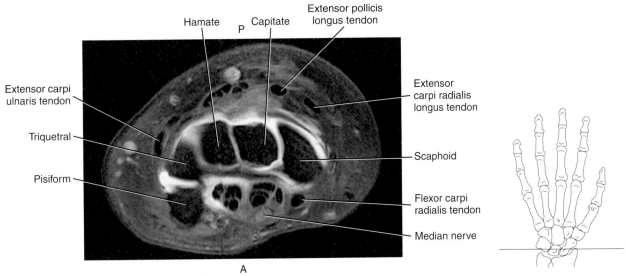

FIGURE 9.135 Axial, T1-weighted MRI of proximal wrist, post-arthrogram.

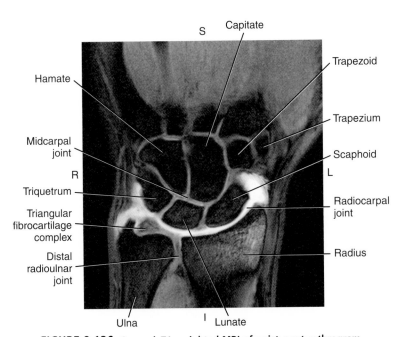

FIGURE 9.136 Coronal, T1-weighted MRI of wrist, post-arthrogram.

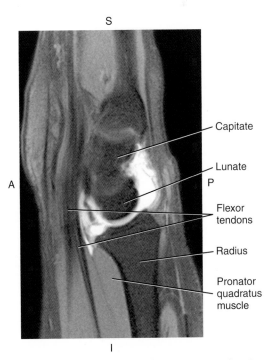

FIGURE 9.137 Sagittal, T1-weighted MRI of wrist, post-arthrogram.

Ligaments of the fingers. The MCP and interphalangeal joints each have a palmar plate (ligament) and two collateral ligaments. The **palmar plate** (**ligament**) is a thick, dense fibrocartilaginous tissue that covers the palmar surface of the joints. The palmar plate runs between and is connected to the collateral ligaments, creating the floor of the interphalangeal and MCP joints (Figure 9.138). The **deep transverse metacarpal ligament** (**DTML**) consists of a series of short ligaments

that connect the palmar plate of the metacarpal heads (Figure 9.129). The DTML prevents separation of the metacarpals. Along the palmar surface of the fingers, the ligamentous structures of the radial and ulnar **collateral ligaments**, radial and ulnar **accessory collateral ligaments**, and palmar plates provide stability for the MCP and interphalangeal joints (Figure 9.138). There is a fibro-osseous tunnel along the palmar aspect of each finger for the passage of the flexor tendons. The tunnel is created by well-defined areas of thickening of the tendon sheath and is called the **anular pulley system**. It is composed of five **anular pulleys** and three **cruciate pulleys**, which are important structures that prevent the displacement of the tendons during flexion of the fingers (Figure 9.139). The dorsal surface of the hand and fingers contains the **extensor mechanism** or **extensor hood** (Figures 9.140 through 9.144). The extensor hood consists of the digital extensor tendon, extensor hood proper, and insertions of the lumbricals and interossei muscles and serves to maintain the integrity of the extensor tendons along the path of the MCP and interphalangeal joints.

FIGURE 9.138 Palmar plate. *Top,* Lateral view. *Bottom,* Anatomy.

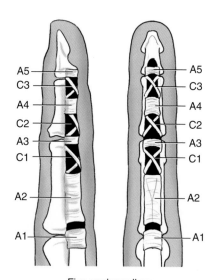

Five anular pulleys
Three cruciate pulleys

FIGURE 9.139 Anular pulley system. *Left,* Sagittal view. *Right,* Palmar view.

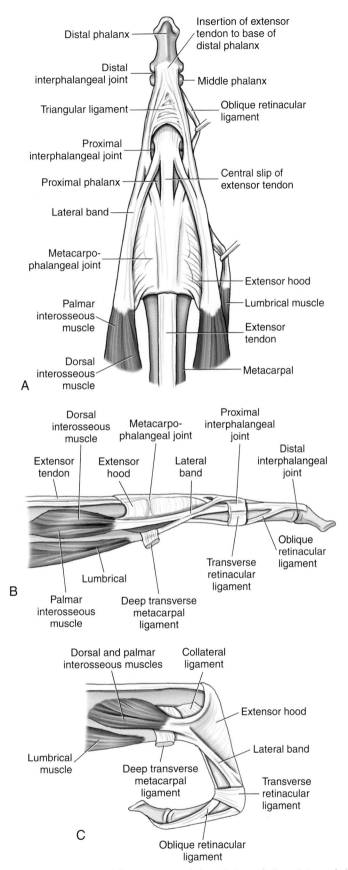

FIGURE 9.140 Extensor mechanism of finger. A, Dorsal view. **B,** Lateral view. **C,** Lateral view in flexion.

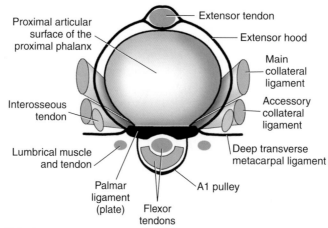

FIGURE 9.141 Axial view of metacarpophalangeal joint structures.

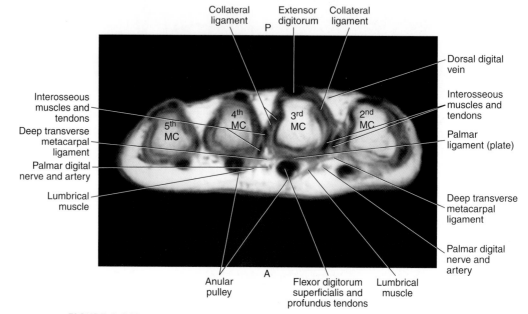

FIGURE 9.142 Axial, T1-weighted MRI of metacarpals.

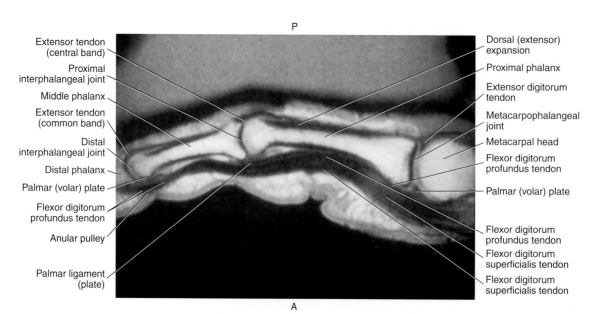

FIGURE 9.143 Sagittal, T1-weighted MRI of finger.

Muscles and Tendons

The numerous muscles of the forearm become tendinous just before the wrist joint. The many tendons located in the wrist can be divided into **flexor (palmar)** and **extensor (dorsal) tendon groups** (Figures 9.129, 9.145, and 9.146). The flexor tendon group collectively flexes the fingers and wrist. As this group courses through the carpal tunnel, the tendons appear to be arranged in two discrete rows (Figures 9.128, *top*, and 9.131). The tendons of the extensor group span the superficial surface of the wrist to extend the fingers and wrist (Figures 9.128 through 9.137).

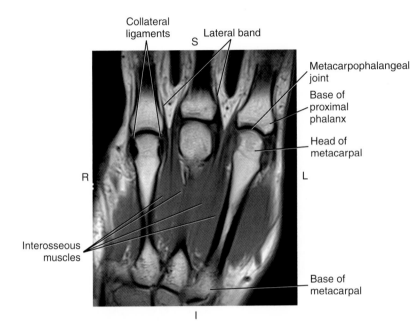

FIGURE 9.144 Coronal, T1-weighted MRI of finger.

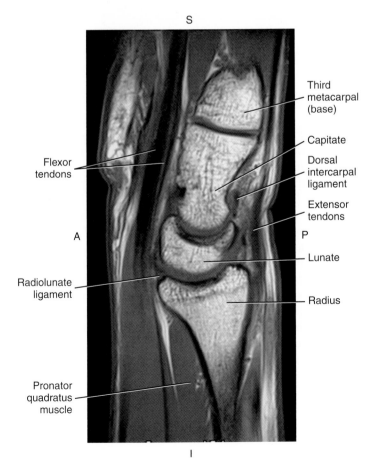

FIGURE 9.145 Sagittal, T1-weighted MRI of wrist with flexor and extensor tendons.

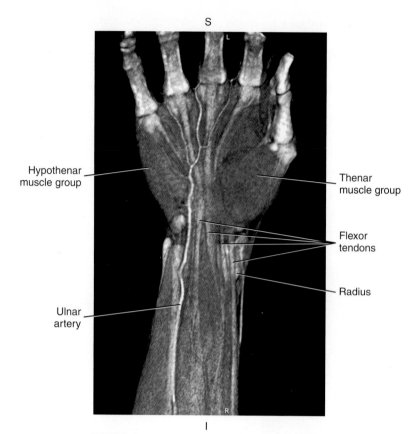

Hypothenar
muscle group

Thenar
muscle group

Flexor
tendons

Radius

Ulnar
artery

FIGURE 9.146 3D CT of wrist with flexor tendons.

Muscles of the hand. The muscles of the hand can be divided into three groups: (1) metacarpal group (muscles of the metacarpals are considered to be the central muscles of the hand), (2) thenar group (muscles involving the thumb and creating the thenar eminence on the radial side), and (3) hypothenar group (muscles involving the fifth digit and creating the hypothenar eminence on the ulnar side). These muscles are demonstrated in Figures 9.147 through 9.154.

Metacarpal group. The **metacarpal muscle group** includes the interossei and lumbrical muscles. There are seven short **interossei muscles** in the metacarpal muscle group: three single-headed muscles located on the palmar surface and four double-headed muscles located on the dorsal surface (Figure 9.147, A and B). The four **palmar interossei** muscles arise from the first, second, fourth, and fifth metacarpals and insert on the corresponding proximal phalanges, frequently radiating into the corresponding tendons of the dorsal aponeurosis. These muscles are responsible for flexion at the MCP joints and extension at the interphalangeal joints. The **dorsal interossei** arise from two heads on the sides of

the five metacarpal bones to insert on the proximal phalanges and radiate onto the dorsal aponeurosis. Like their palmar counterparts, the dorsal interossei flex at the MCP joints and extend at the interphalangeal joints. The four small **lumbrical** muscles arise from the tendons of the flexor digitorum profundus and pass to the radial side of the corresponding finger to insert on the extensor expansion covering the dorsal surface of the finger (Figure 9.148). The lumbricals flex the first phalanges at the MCP joints and extend the second and third phalanges at the interphalangeal joints. These muscles are demonstrated in Figures 9.147 through 9.154.

Thenar group. The four muscles of the **thenar group** are the abductor pollicis brevis, flexor pollicis brevis, adductor pollicis, and opponens pollicis. The **abductor pollicis brevis** is a thin, flat superficial muscle arising from the transverse carpal ligament, navicular, and trapezium (Figure 9.149). It runs inferiorly and laterally to insert on the base of the first phalanx of the thumb to abduct the thumb. The **flexor pollicis brevis** has two heads: The superficial or lateral head arises from the flexor retinaculum, and the deep or medial head arises from the trapezium, trapezoid, and capitate. This muscle inserts on the radial and ulnar base of the first phalanx to flex, adduct, and abduct the thumb (Figure 9.149). Frequently, a sesamoid bone can be found in the insertion tendon on the radial side. The **adductor pollicis** also has two heads: The transverse head arises from the dorsal aspect of the third metacarpal, and the oblique head arises from numerous slips off the capitate, bases of the second and third metacarpals, and the sheath of the flexor carpi radialis tendon. The adductor pollicis inserts onto the base of the first phalanx of the thumb to provide adduction and assist in the opposition and flexion of the thumb (Figures 9.148 and 9.149). The **opponens pollicis** provides the main opposition for the thumb but also assists with adduction. It arises from the trapezium and flexor retinaculum and inserts onto the radial aspect of the first metacarpal (Figures 9.148 and 9.149). These muscles are also demonstrated in Figures 9.148 through 9.154.

Hypothenar group. The hypothenar group consists of three muscles: abductor digiti minimi, flexor digiti minimi brevis, and opponens digiti minimi. The **abductor digiti minimi** muscle arises from the pisiform and the flexor retinaculum to end in a flat tendon that inserts onto the ulnar base of the first phalanx of the little finger (Figures 9.148 and 9.149). The abductor digiti minimi muscle is the main abductor of the little finger. The **flexor digiti minimi brevis** muscle arises from the flexor retinaculum and the hook of the hamate. It fuses with the tendon of the abductor digiti minimi to insert on the base of the first phalanx of the fifth digit (Figures 9.148 and 9.149). The flexor digiti minimi brevis flexes at the MCP joint. Like the flexor digiti minimi brevis muscle, the **opponens digiti minimi** arises from the hook of the hamate and the flexor retinaculum (Figure 9.148). It inserts on the ulnar surface of the fifth metacarpal to bring the little finger into the position for opposition. For the hand muscles, see Figures 9.148 through 9.154.

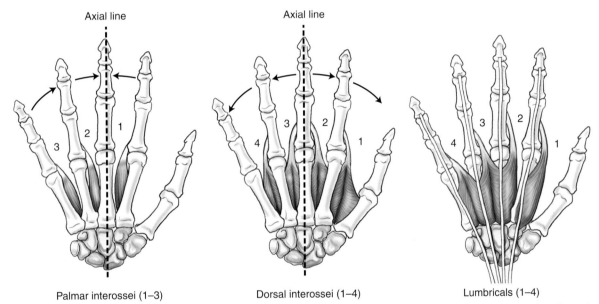

FIGURE 9.147 Left, Palmar view of interosseous muscles. Center, Dorsal view of interosseous muscles. Right, Lumbrical muscles.

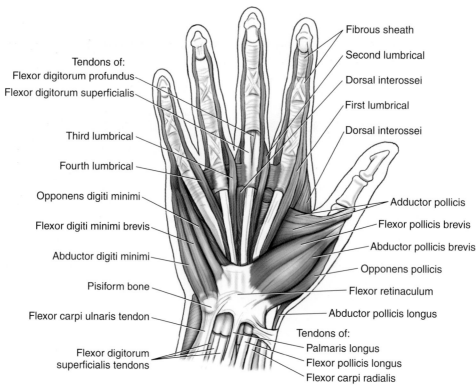

Tendons of:
Flexor digitorum profundus
Flexor digitorum superficialis

Third lumbrical

Fourth lumbrical

Opponens digiti minimi

Flexor digiti minimi brevis

Abductor digiti minimi

Pisiform bone

Flexor carpi ulnaris tendon

Flexor digitorum
superficialis tendons

Fibrous sheath

Second lumbrical

Dorsal interossei

First lumbrical

Dorsal interossei

Adductor pollicis

Flexor pollicis brevis

Abductor pollicis brevis

Opponens pollicis

Flexor retinaculum

Abductor pollicis longus

Tendons of:
Palmaris longus
Flexor pollicis longus
Flexor carpi radialis

FIGURE 9.148 Palmar view of flexor pollicis brevis, flexor digiti minimi, abductor pollicis brevis, opponens pollicis, and abductor digiti minimi muscles.

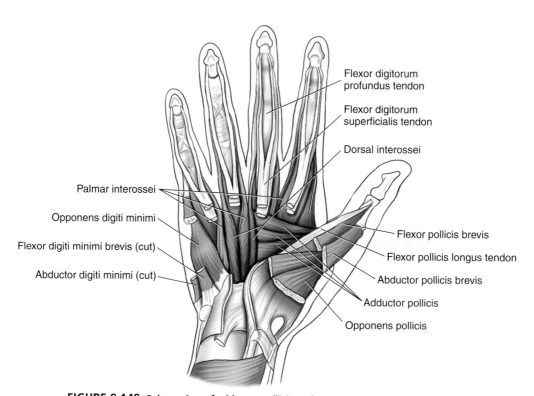

Palmar interossei

Opponens digiti minimi

Flexor digiti minimi brevis (cut)

Abductor digiti minimi (cut)

Flexor digitorum
profundus tendon

Flexor digitorum
superficialis tendon

Dorsal interossei

Flexor pollicis brevis

Flexor pollicis longus tendon

Abductor pollicis brevis

Adductor pollicis

Opponens pollicis

FIGURE 9.149 Palmar view of adductor pollicis and opponens digiti minimi muscles.

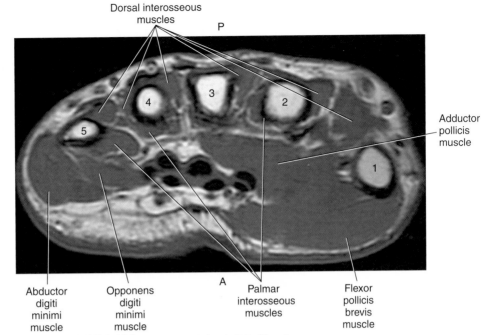

Dorsal interosseous muscles

P

Adductor pollicis muscle

Abductor digiti minimi muscle

Opponens digiti minimi muscle

A

Palmar interosseous muscles

Flexor pollicis brevis muscle

FIGURE 9.150 Axial, T1-weighted MRI of hand.

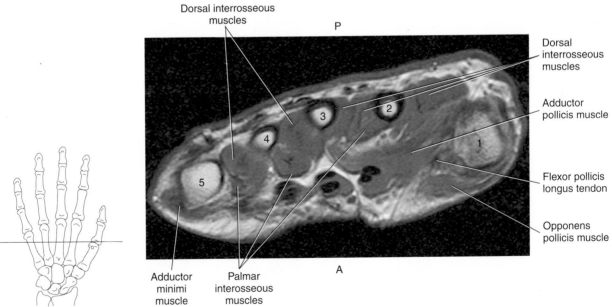

Dorsal interrosseous muscles

P

Dorsal interrosseous muscles

Adductor pollicis muscle

Flexor pollicis longus tendon

Opponens pollicis muscle

Adductor minimi muscle

Palmar interosseous muscles

A

FIGURE 9.151 Axial, T1-weighted MRI of hand with dorsal interosseous muscles.

S

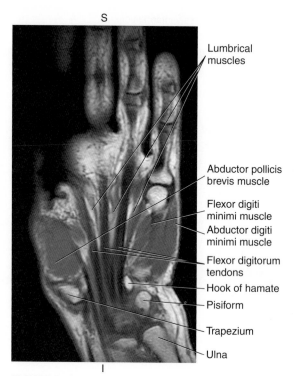

Lumbrical
muscles

Abductor pollicis
brevis muscle

Flexor digiti
minimi muscle

Abductor digiti
minimi muscle

Flexor digitorum
tendons

Hook of hamate

Pisiform

Trapezium

Ulna

I

FIGURE 9.152 Coronal, T1-weighted MRI of wrist and hand.

S

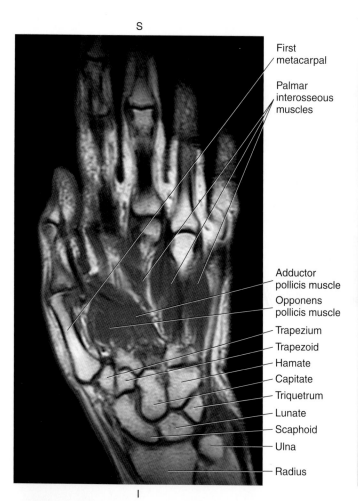

First
metacarpal

Palmar
interosseous
muscles

Adductor
pollicis muscle

Opponens
pollicis muscle

Trapezium

Trapezoid

Hamate

Capitate

Triquetrum

Lunate

Scaphoid

Ulna

Radius

I

FIGURE 9.153 Coronal, T1-weighted MRI of wrist and hand with palmar interosseous muscles.

S

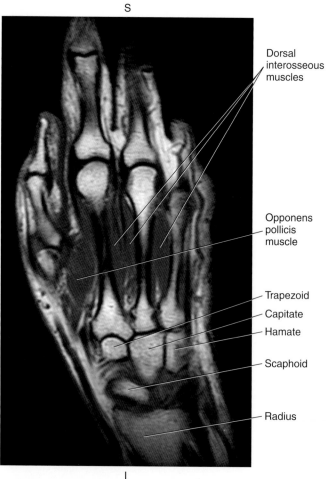

Dorsal
interosseous
muscles

Opponens
pollicis
muscle

Trapezoid

Capitate

Hamate

Scaphoid

Radius

I

FIGURE 9.154 Coronal, T1-weighted MRI of wrist and hand with opponens pollicis muscle.

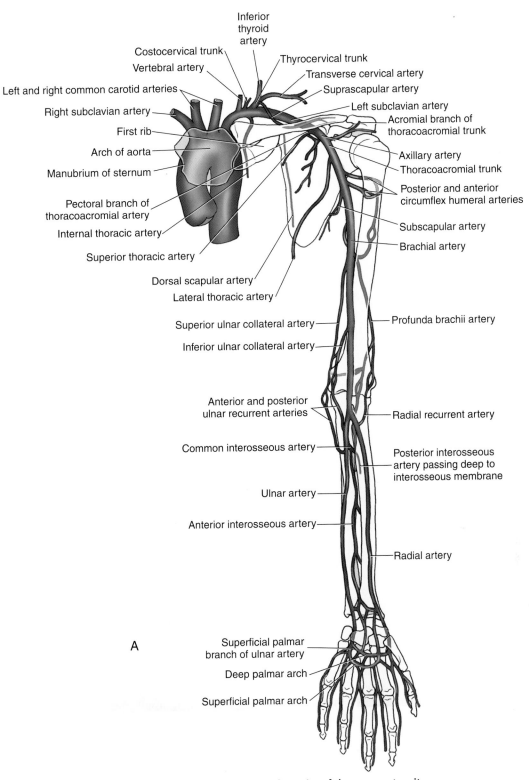

Inferior
thyroid
artery

Costocervical trunk

Vertebral artery

Thyrocervical trunk

Transverse cervical artery

Left and right common carotid arteries

Suprascapular artery

Right subclavian artery

Left subclavian artery

Acromial branch of
thoracoacromial trunk

First rib

Arch of aorta

Axillary artery

Thoracoacromial trunk

Manubrium of sternum

Posterior and anterior
circumflex humeral arteries

Pectoral branch of
thoracoacromial artery

Subscapular artery

Internal thoracic artery

Brachial artery

Superior thoracic artery

Dorsal scapular artery

Lateral thoracic artery

Superior ulnar collateral artery

Profunda brachii artery

Inferior ulnar collateral artery

Anterior and posterior
ulnar recurrent arteries

Radial recurrent artery

Common interosseous artery

Posterior interosseous
artery passing deep to
interosseous membrane

Ulnar artery

Anterior interosseous artery

Radial artery

A

Superficial palmar
branch of ulnar artery

Deep palmar arch

Superficial palmar arch

FIGURE 9.155 A, Anterior view of arteries of the upper extremity.

(Continued)

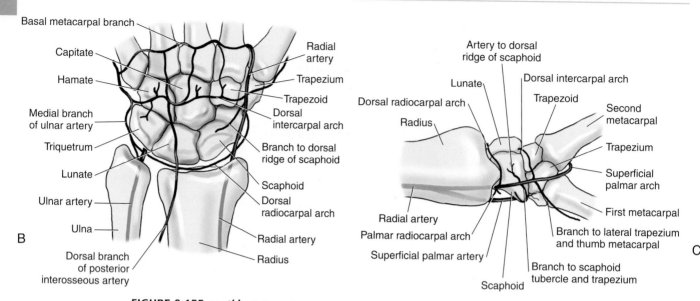

FIGURE 9.155 cont'd   B, Posterior view of arteries in wrist. **C,** Lateral view of arteries of wrist.

NEUROVASCULATURE

The neurovasculature of the upper extremity is composed primarily of the branches of the axillary and brachial arteries, their accompanying deep veins, a system of superficial veins, and the brachial plexus that innervates the upper extremity.

Arterial Supply

Shoulder. The primary arteries supplying the shoulder region include the axillary and brachial arteries (Figure 9.155). The **axillary artery** begins at the lateral border of the first rib as a continuation of the subclavian artery. It ends at the inferior border of the teres major muscle, where it passes into the arm and becomes the brachial artery. The axillary artery and its branches supply blood to numerous thoracic and shoulder structures, including the first and second intercostal spaces, axillary lymph nodes, mammary gland in women, and scapular, serratus anterior, pectoral, latissimus dorsi, deltoid, and triceps brachii muscles. The branches of the axillary artery typically include the superior thoracic, thoracoacromial, lateral thoracic, subscapular artery, and anterior and posterior humeral circumflex arteries. The **brachial artery** is the principal arterial supply to the arm. It courses inferiorly on the medial side of the humerus and then continues anterior to the cubital fossa of the elbow. The brachial artery is relatively superficial and palpable throughout its course. It accompanies the median nerve, which crosses anterior to the artery in the middle of the arm. During its course, the brachial artery gives rise to numerous muscular branches, which include the profunda brachii, superior ulnar collateral, and inferior ulnar collateral arteries (Figures 9.155 through 9.160).

Elbow. The brachial artery divides at the cubital fossa into the radial and ulnar arteries (Figure 9.155, A).

The **radial artery** begins at the level of the head of the radius within the anterior compartment of the forearm. It courses beneath the brachioradialis muscle and then continues its course just deep to the skin, along the lateral side of the anterior forearm to the wrist. It passes anterior to the radial styloid process to enter the hand. The most proximal branch of the radial artery is the **radial recurrent artery,** which supplies the brachioradialis, supinator, and brachialis muscles and the elbow joint. Within the forearm, the radial artery gives off several direct muscular branches. The **ulnar artery** also gives rise to several branches that supply the elbow and forearm. The first branch of the ulnar artery is the **anterior ulnar recurrent artery,** which supplies the brachialis and pronator teres muscles. It courses just anterior to the medial condyle of the humerus to anastomose with the inferior ulnar collateral branch of the brachial artery. The **posterior ulnar recurrent artery** courses behind the medial epicondyle of the humerus to anastomose with the superior ulnar collateral branch of the brachial artery. It supplies the flexor carpi ulnaris, pronator teres, and anconeus muscles. The **common interosseous artery** branches from the ulnar artery and almost immediately bifurcates into the **anterior** and **posterior interosseous arteries.** These arteries and their branches supply the median nerve, deep flexor and extensor muscles of the forearm, superficial extensor muscles of the forearm, and radius and ulna (Figures 9.155, A, 9.156, B, C, 9.157, 9.159, and 9.160).

Wrist and hand. The terminal branches of the radial and ulnar arteries form the palmar arches of the wrist and hand. These arches emit branches that serve the wrist, palm, and digits (Figures 9.155 and 9.157). The **palmar**

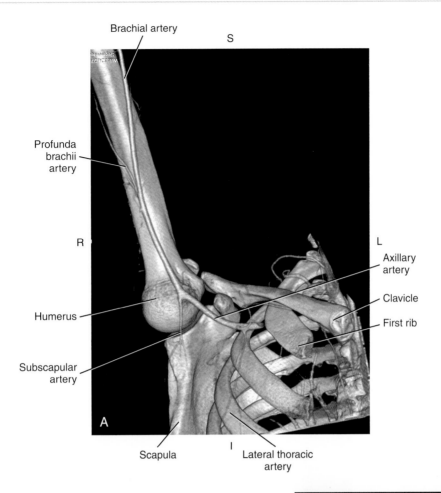

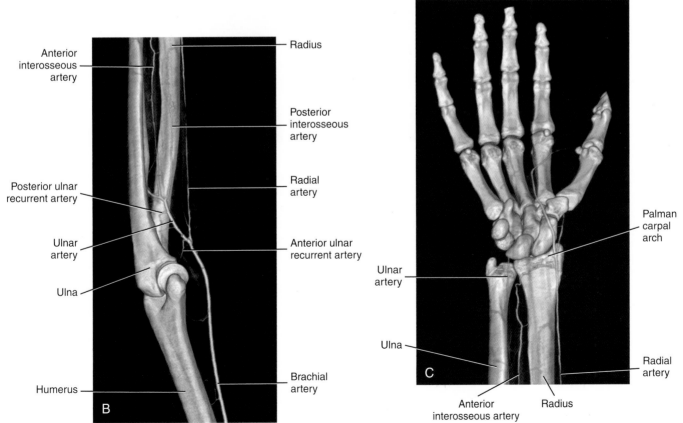

FIGURE 9.156 A, 3D CT of axillary artery. B, 3D CT of brachial artery. C, 3D CT of radial and ulnar arteries.

Palmar metacarpal artery   Common palmar digital artery   Proper palmar digital artery

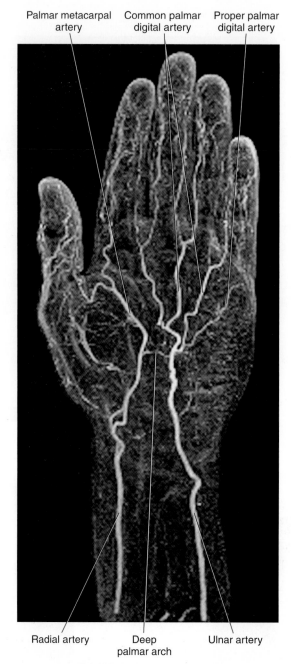

Radial artery   Deep palmar arch   Ulnar artery

FIGURE 9.157 MRA of hand.

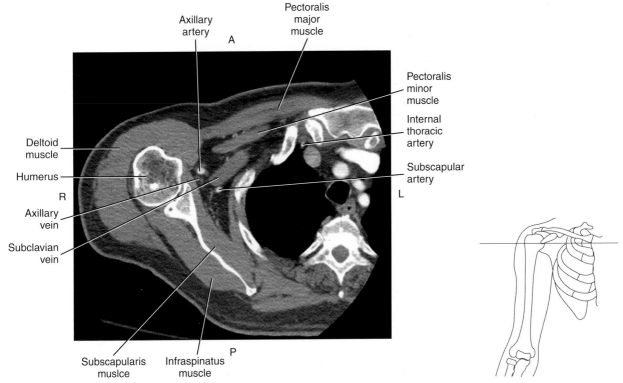

FIGURE 9.158 Axial CT of right shoulder with axillary artery.

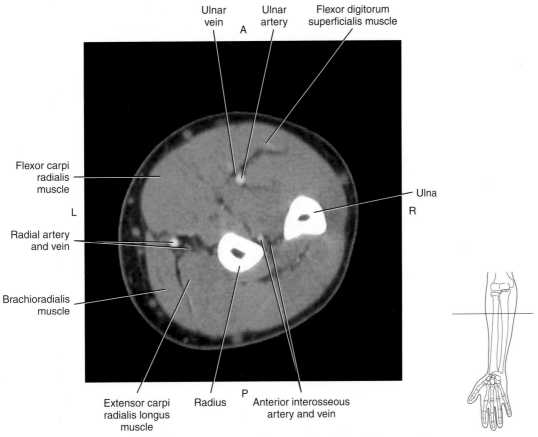

FIGURE 9.159 Axial CT of right forearm with radial and ulnar arteries.

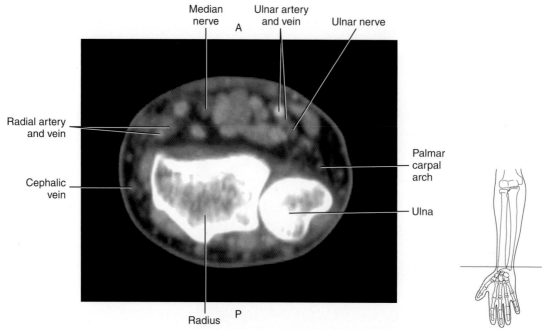

FIGURE 9.160 Axial CT of right wrist with radial and ulnar arteries.

radiocarpal arch or network is formed by the palmar carpal branches from the radial and ulnar arteries, the anterior interosseous artery, also a branch of the ulnar artery, and a recurrent branch from the deep palmar arch. These vessels supply the carpal bones and joints (Figure 9.155, A and C). The **dorsal radiocarpal arch** or network is formed by dorsal carpal branches of the radial and ulnar arteries. The dorsal carpal arch also receives contributions from the anterior and posterior interosseous arteries. The arch lies close to the dorsal surface of the carpals and gives rise to three dorsal metacarpal arteries and branches that supply the distal regions of the ulna and radius, carpal bones, and intercarpal joints (Figure 9.155). The superficial palmar branch of the radial artery anastomoses with the superficial palmar branch of the ulnar artery to form the **superficial palmar arch**. This arch gives rise to three common palmar digital arteries that anastomose with the palmar metacarpal arteries from the deep palmar arch (Figure 9.155, A and C). The **deep palmar arch** is formed by deep palmar branches of the radial and ulnar arteries and is located approximately 1 cm proximal to the superficial palmar arch. The deep palmar arch also gives rise to a recurrent branch that anastomoses with the palmar carpal branches of the radial and ulnar arteries (Figure 9.155, A).

Venous Drainage

The veins of the upper extremity are divided into deep and superficial groups (Figure 9.161). Numerous anastomoses occur between the groups. The superficial venous system consists of extensive venous networks that are especially well developed within the upper extremity

along with their accompanying arteries of the same name. The deep veins are often double and repeatedly anastomose with one another.

Shoulder. The veins of the upper arm include the brachial, cephalic, and basilic (Figure 9.161). The two deep **brachial veins** ascend the arm, one on either side of the brachial artery. The brachial veins begin in the elbow from the union of the ulnar and radial veins and end in the **axillary vein** near the lower margin of the subscapularis muscle. The two deep brachial veins may join to form one brachial vein during part of their course. The superficial veins of the upper arm include the cephalic and basilic. The **cephalic vein** courses from the radial side of the dorsal venous arch of the hand and then ascends to the midpoint of the forearm, where it curves around to the ventral surface of the forearm and ascends the lateral aspect of the upper arm, along the anterolateral border of the biceps brachii muscle, to open into the axillary vein, just below the clavicle. It drains the superficial parts of the lateral hand and lateral forearm. The **basilic vein** originates from the medial end of the dorsal venous arch of the hand. It then ascends the ulnar side of the forearm, along the medial surface of the biceps brachii muscle in the upper arm, to form the axillary vein. The basilic vein drains the superficial parts of the medial side of the hand and medial side of the forearm. The large **axillary vein** lies on the medial side of the axillary artery. It extends from the lower border of the teres major muscle to the lateral surface of the first rib to continue as the **subclavian vein**. The axillary vein receives tributaries that correspond to the branches of the axillary artery (Figures 9.158 and 9.161).

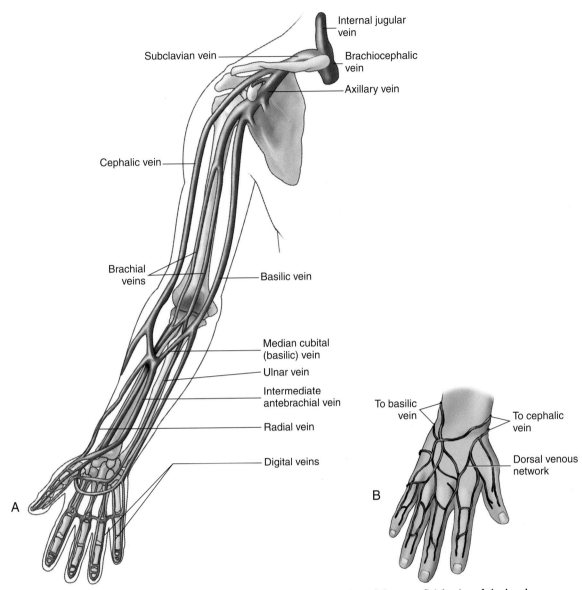

FIGURE 9.161 A, Anterior view of upper extremity veins. B, Posterior view of the superficial veins of the hand.

Elbow. The large deep vein of the elbow is the **brachial vein**, which is formed by the union of the **radial** and **ulnar veins**. The superficial veins of the elbow include the cephalic, median cubital, basilic, and intermediate (median) antebrachial veins. The **cephalic vein** courses along the radial side of the elbow and may give rise to the **median cubital vein**, which ascends in an oblique and medial course to create an anastomosis between the basilic and cephalic veins (Figure 9.161). The median cubital vein is a common site for venipuncture. The **basilic vein** courses along the posteromedial aspect of the forearm, crosses the elbow, then takes a deep course in the axilla to join the brachial vein. The **intermediate (median) antebrachial vein** transports blood from the superficial palmar venous arch and anterior forearm. It ascends the ventral side of the forearm on the ulnar side and typically ends in the basilic vein (Figures 9.94 through 9.102).

Wrist and hand. The superficial venous system forms a network at the dorsum of the hand termed the **dorsal venous network (arch)**. It is fed by the subcutaneous dorsal metacarpal veins of the fingers and continues to the distal forearm, where it drains into three major superficial veins: the **cephalic, basilic,** and **intermediate (median) antebrachial veins** of the forearm. These large superficial veins anastomose frequently as they course superiorly. The **deep** and **superficial palmer venous arches** of the hand empty into the **radial** and **ulnar veins** that then unite to form the **brachial vein** of the arm (Figures 9.128, 9.130 through 9.133, and 9.161).

Innervation

The **brachial plexus**, also described in Chapter 4, is a large network of nerves that innervate the upper limb (Figures 9.22, 9.23, 9.47, and 9.162). It extends from

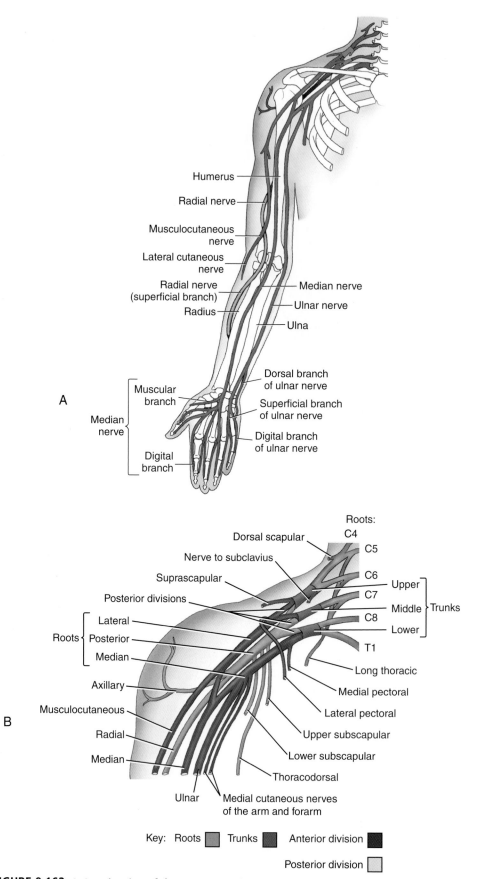

A

Humerus
Radial nerve
Musculocutaneous nerve
Lateral cutaneous nerve
Radial nerve (superficial branch)
Radius
Median nerve
Ulnar nerve
Ulna
Dorsal branch of ulnar nerve
Muscular branch
Superficial branch of ulnar nerve
Median nerve
Digital branch
Digital branch of ulnar nerve

B

Roots:
C4
Dorsal scapular
C5
Nerve to subclavius
C6
Upper
Suprascapular
C7
Middle   Trunks
Posterior divisions
C8
Lower
Lateral
Roots   Posterior
T1
Median
Long thoracic
Axillary
Medial pectoral
Musculocutaneous
Lateral pectoral
Radial
Upper subscapular
Median
Lower subscapular
Thoracodorsal
Ulnar   Medial cutaneous nerves of the arm and forearm

Key: Roots ▧   Trunks ▧   Anterior division ■
Posterior division ▢

FIGURE 9.162 A, Anterior view of the upper extremity nerves. B, Anterior view of the brachial plexus.

the neck into the axilla. The brachial plexus is formed by the union of the ventral rami of nerves C5-C8 and the greater part of the T1 ventral ramus. The ventral rami from C5 and C6 unite to form a **superior trunk**, the ventral ramus of C7 continues as the **middle trunk**, and the ventral rami of C8 and T1 unite to form an **inferior trunk**. Each of these trunks divides into an anterior and posterior division. The anterior divisions supply the anterior (flexor) parts of the upper limb, and the **posterior divisions** supply the posterior (extensor) parts of the upper limb. These divisions form three cords (**posterior, lateral, and medial**), which continue to divide to form the **median, ulnar, musculocutaneous,** and **radial nerves** (sequential Figures 9.62 through 9.67). These nerves supply the muscles of the forearm and hand. The **median nerve** descends the cubital fossa deep to the median cubital vein. It supplies the pronator teres muscle of the arm and all the superficial and deep flexor muscles of the forearm, except the flexor carpi ulnaris muscle. It gives off an anterior interosseous branch that descends within the forearm to supply the flexor digitorum profundus muscle. The median nerve courses through the carpal tunnel of the wrist, typically superficial to the flexor tendons (Figure 9.163). It supplies flexors of the hand, skin of the wrist, thenar eminence, palm of the hand, and sides of the first three digits and lateral half of the fourth. At the elbow, the **ulnar nerve** passes between the medial epicondyle of the humerus and the olecranon process within the cubital tunnel to enter the medial side of the flexor compartment of the forearm (Figures 9.87 and 9.162). Posterior to the medial epicondyle, the ulnar nerve is superficial and easily palpable. It supplies the flexor carpi ulnaris muscle and the medial side of the flexor digitorum profundus muscle in the forearm before entering the hand. The ulnar nerve passes under the flexor retinaculum, along with the ulnar artery, to enter the palmar compartment of the hand (Figure 9.163). At this point, the ulnar nerve divides into superficial and deep terminal branches that supply the ulnar flexors of the hand, as well as the skin on the medial side of the palm, medial half of the dorsum of the hand, fifth digit, and medial half of the fourth digit. The **musculocutaneous nerve** descends to the lateral side of the arm and elbow to innervate the flexors in the arm and the skin of the forearm, wrist, and thenar region of the hand (Figure 9.162). It emits branches that supply both heads of the biceps brachii muscle, the brachialis muscle, and the elbow joint. It innervates the skin of the dorsal surface of the arm. A continuation of the musculocutaneous nerve is the **lateral cutaneous nerve**, which terminates

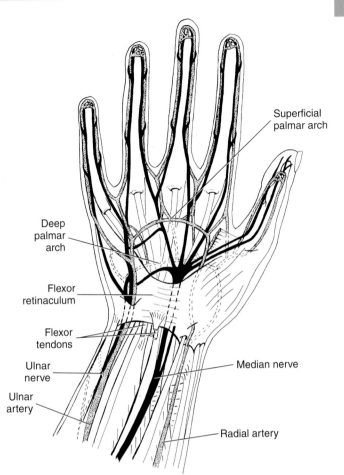

FIGURE 9.163 Coronal view of neurovasculature of hand and wrist.

into cutaneous branches that supply the skin covering the radial side of the wrist and the thenar eminence. The **radial nerve** is the largest branch of the brachial plexus. It passes inferolaterally around the body of the humerus in the radial groove (Figure 9.162). It continues inferiorly between the brachialis and brachioradialis muscles to the level of the lateral epicondyle of the humerus, where it divides into deep and superficial branches. The deep branches supply all the extensors in the arm and forearm, and the cutaneous branches innervate the skin on the dorsal side of the arm and hand. The superficial branch, the direct continuation of the radial nerve, is entirely sensory. It supplies skin and fascia over the lateral two thirds of the dorsum of the hand, the dorsum of the thumb, and proximal parts of the lateral three and one half digits on their dorsal surfaces (Figures 9.93 through 9.102).

10

Lower Extremity

And well observe Hippocrates' old rule,
the only medicine for the foote is rest.

Thomas Nash (1567-1601)
Summers' Last Will and Testament

The complex anatomy of the lower extremity is responsible for bearing the entire upper body weight and for accommodating the demands of movement placed on this system (Figure 10.1).

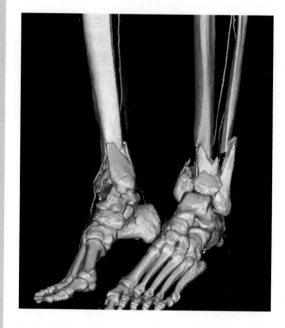

FIGURE 10.1 Multiple fractures of the distal tibia and fibula.

OBJECTIVES

- Identify the bony anatomy of the lower extremity.
- Identify and state the actions of the lower extremity muscles, as well as their origins and insertions.
- Describe the labrum and articular capsule of the hip.
- List and describe the ligaments, retinacula, and tendons of the lower extremity joints.

- Define and identify the meniscus and articular capsule of the knee.
- Identify the bursae of the hip and knee.
- List and identify the major arteries and veins of the lower extremity.
- Describe the nerves that innervate the lower extremity.

OUTLINE

HIP

The hip provides strength to carry the weight of the body in an erect position. This synovial ball-and-socket joint, created by the articulation of the femoral head with the acetabulum of the pelvis, allows for a wide range of motion.

Bony Anatomy

Acetabulum. A cuplike cavity termed the **acetabulum** is created by the three bones of the pelvis: **ilium, ischium,** and **pubis** (Figure 10.2). (See also chapter 8, Bony Anatomy of the Pelvis.) In axial cross-section, this area can be divided into sections known as the **anterior** and **posterior columns** (Figure 10.3). Within the acetabulum is a centrally located, nonarticulating depression called the **acetabular fossa**. It is formed mainly by the ischium and is filled with fat (Figure 10.4). A continuation of the acetabular fossa is the **acetabular notch**, which interrupts the smooth circumference of the acetabular rim below and functions as an attachment site for the transverse acetabular ligament (Figure 10.2).

Femur. The **femur** is the longest, heaviest, and strongest bone in the body. The proximal end of the femur consists of a head, a neck, and two large processes: the greater and

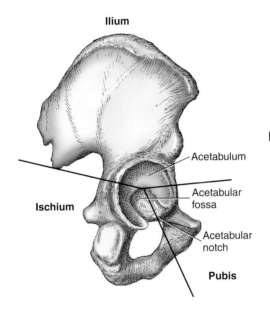

FIGURE 10.2 Lateral aspect of right hip.

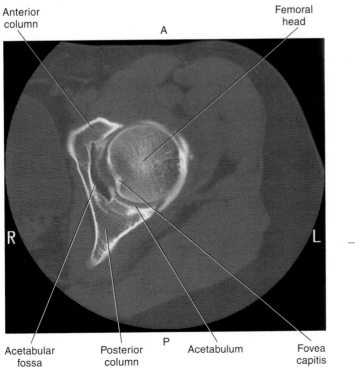
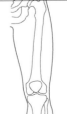

FIGURE 10.3 Axial CT of left hip joint, post arthrogram.

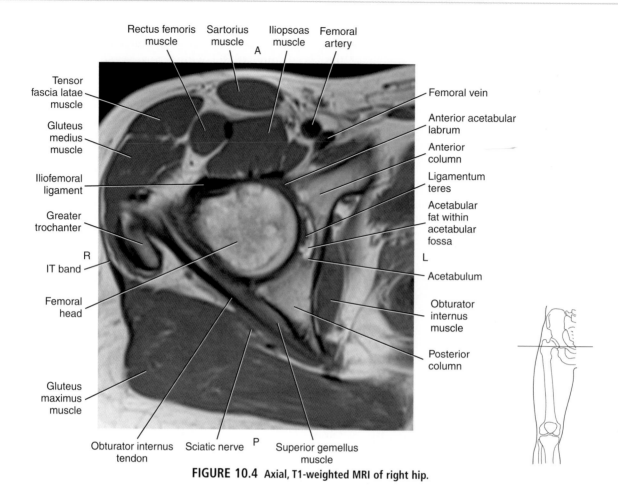

Rectus femoris muscle   Sartorius muscle   Iliopsoas muscle   Femoral artery   A

Tensor fascia latae muscle
Gluteus medius muscle
Iliofemoral ligament
Greater trochanter
R
IT band
Femoral head
Gluteus maximus muscle

Femoral vein
Anterior acetabular labrum
Anterior column
Ligamentum teres
Acetabular fat within acetabular fossa
L
Acetabulum
Obturator internus muscle
Posterior column

Obturator internus tendon   Sciatic nerve   P   Superior gemellus muscle

FIGURE 10.4 Axial, T1-weighted MRI of right hip.

lesser trochanters (Figures 10.5 and 10.6). On the proximal portion of the femur is the smooth, rounded femoral head. The **femoral head** is covered entirely by articular cartilage, with the exception of a small centrally located pit termed the **fovea capitis**. The fovea capitis is an attachment site for the **ligamentum teres**, which transmits blood vessels to the femoral head (Figures 10.3 through 10.6). Connecting the head of the femur to the femoral shaft is the **femoral neck**. The neck extends obliquely from the head at an angle of approximately 120 degrees in an inferolateral direction to meet the shaft (Figure 10.5). The result of this angle is increased freedom of movement within the hip joint. At the distal end of the neck are two large bony prominences termed **trochanters** (Figures 10.5 through 10.8). The **greater trochanter** is situated at the junction of the neck with the shaft. The superior portion of the greater trochanter projects above the neck and curves slightly posteriorly and medially (Figures 10.4, 10.7, 10.9, and 10.10). The greater trochanter provides attachment for several muscles of the gluteal region. The **lesser trochanter** is at the posteromedial portion of the proximal shaft and gives insertion to the tendon of the iliopsoas (Figures 10.6, 10.9, and 10.10). The prominent ridge extending posteriorly between the trochanters at the base of the neck is the **intertrochanteric crest** (Figures 10.9 and 10.11). It provides an attachment site for the

ischiofemoral ligament and part of the quadratus femoris tendon. Connecting the trochanters anteriorly is the less prominent ridge termed the **intertrochanteric line**, which provides attachment for the iliofemoral ligament and part of the vastus lateralis tendon (Figures 10.9 and 10.10). On the proximal and posterior end of the femoral shaft is a raised ridge termed the **linea aspera**. Its medial and lateral lips provide attachment sites for muscles of the posterior and medial compartments of the thigh. The **pectineal line** runs from the medial lip of the linea aspera to the lesser trochanter of the femur (Figures 10.9 and 10.11). It is the insertion site for the tendon of the pectineus muscle. The lateral lip is very rough and runs almost vertically upward to the base of the greater trochanter. The widened portion of the lateral lip, the **gluteal tuberosity**, is an attachment site for the gluteus maximus and adductor magnus muscles (Figures 10.9 and 10.11). The linea aspera extends down to the popliteal surface of the femur.

Avascular necrosis (AVN) is a major concern following subcapital fractures of the femoral head. Disruption of the arterial supply to the femoral head is the most significant factor leading to AVN.

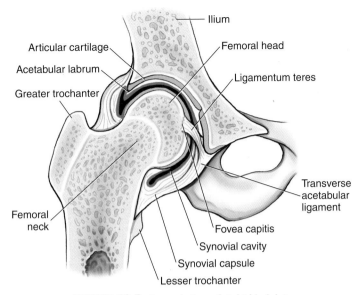

Ilium

Articular cartilage

Acetabular labrum

Greater trochanter

Femoral head

Ligamentum teres

Femoral
neck

Transverse
acetabular
ligament

Fovea capitis

Synovial cavity

Synovial capsule

Lesser trochanter

FIGURE 10.5 Coronal view of right hip joint.

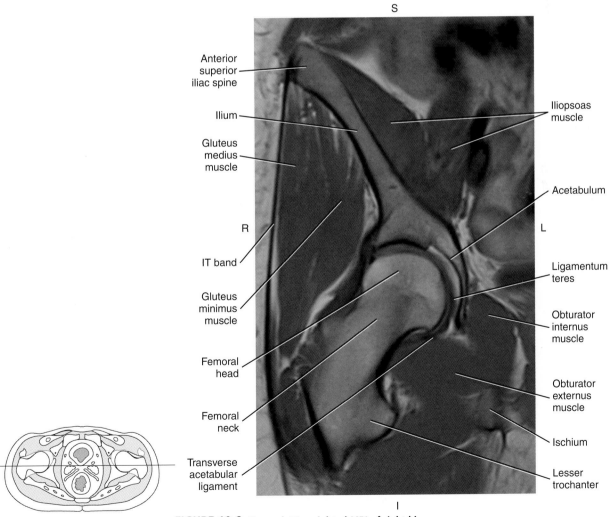

S

Anterior
superior
iliac spine

Ilium

Gluteus
medius
muscle

Iliopsoas
muscle

Acetabulum

R

L

IT band

Ligamentum
teres

Gluteus
minimus
muscle

Obturator
internus
muscle

Femoral
head

Obturator
externus
muscle

Femoral
neck

Ischium

Transverse
acetabular
ligament

Lesser
trochanter

I

FIGURE 10.6 Coronal, T1-weighted MRI of right hip.

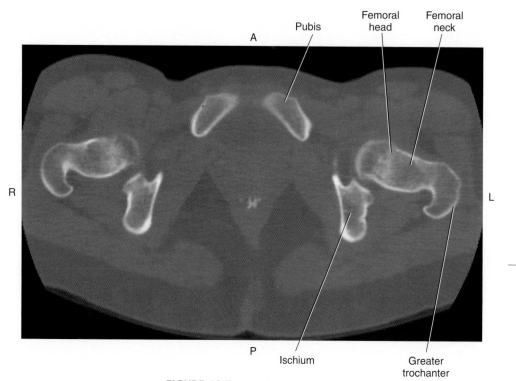

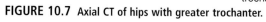

FIGURE 10.7 Axial CT of hips with greater trochanter.

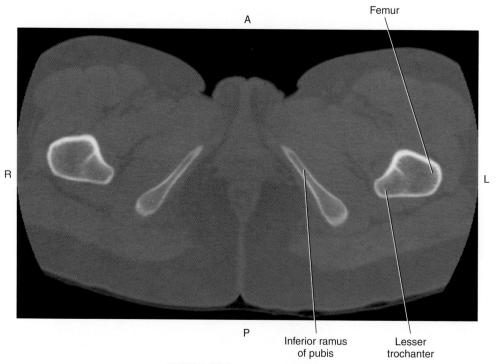

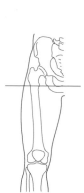

FIGURE 10.8 Axial CT of hips with lesser trochanter.

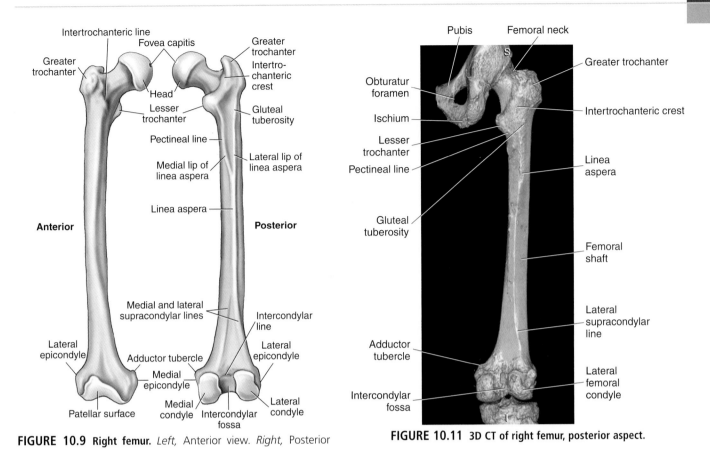

FIGURE 10.9 Right femur. *Left,* Anterior view. *Right,* Posterior view.

FIGURE 10.11 3D CT of right femur, posterior aspect.

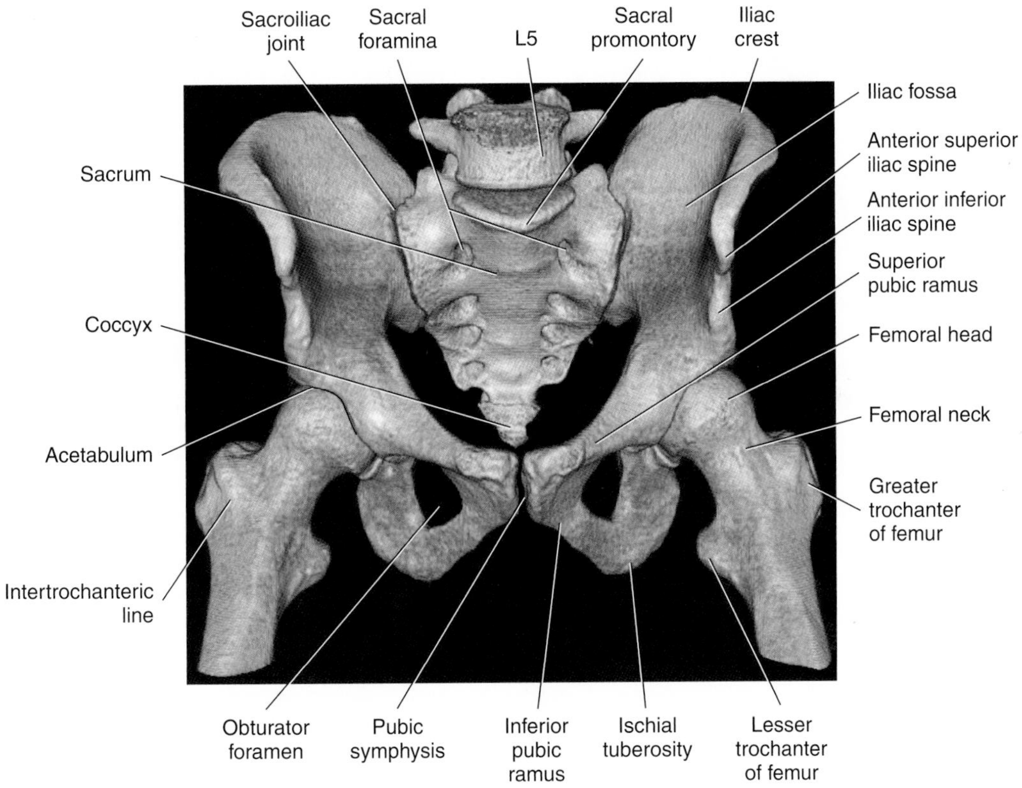

FIGURE 10.10 3D CT of pelvis and hips.

Labrum and Ligaments

The femoral head is held to the acetabulum by the acetabular labrum and several major ligaments. The acetabular labrum, transverse acetabular ligament, iliofemoral ligament, ischiofemoral ligament, pubofemoral ligament, and ligamentum teres are demonstrated in Figures 10.12 through 10.26.

Labrum. The **acetabular labrum** creates a fibrocartilaginous rim attached to the margin of the acetabulum. This labrum closely surrounds the femoral head, helping to hold it in place by deepening the acetabular fossa, which adds increased stability to the joint (Figure 10.12).

Ligaments. The inferior margin of the acetabulum is incomplete and is reinforced by the **transverse acetabular ligament**, a portion of the acetabular labrum that spans

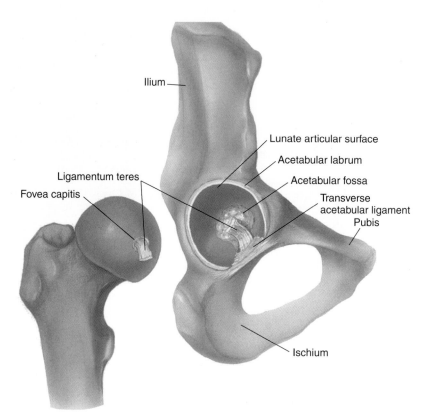

FIGURE 10.12 Femoral acetabulum and labrum.

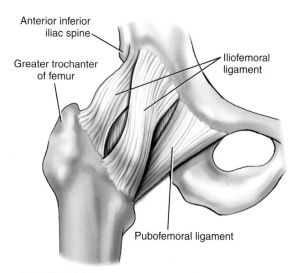

FIGURE 10.13 Anterior view of right hip joint capsule.

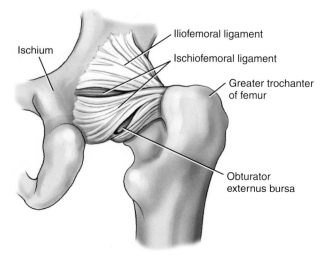

FIGURE 10.14 Posterior view of right hip joint capsule.

Sartorius Iliopsoas   Femoral Femoral Femoral
muscle   muscle   A   head   artery   vein

Tensor fasciae
latae muscle

Rectus
femoris muscle

Iliofemoral
ligament

Gluteus
medius
muscle

R

Iliotibial
band

Greater
trochanter

Obturator
internus tendon

Obturator artery
and vein

Obturator
internus muscle

L

Ischiofemoral
ligament

Superior gemellus
muscle

Sciatic
nerve

Gluteus
maximus
muscle

P

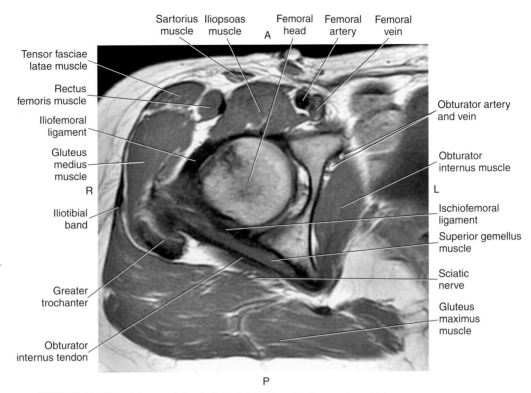
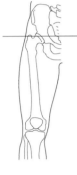

FIGURE 10.15 Axial, T1-weighted MRI of right hip with ligaments and labrum.

Iliopsoas   Femoral   Femoral Femoral Femoral
muscle   head   A   nerve   artery   vein

Tensor fasciae
latae muscle

Rectus
femoris muscle

Iliofemoral
ligament

Gluteus
medius
muscle

Iliotibial
band

R

Greater
trochanter

Transverse
acetabular
ligament

Superior pubic
ramus

Ligamentum
teres

Obturator
internus muscle

Ischiofemoral
ligament

L

Ischium

Inferior gemellus
muscle

Sciatic nerve

Gluteus
maximus
muscle

P

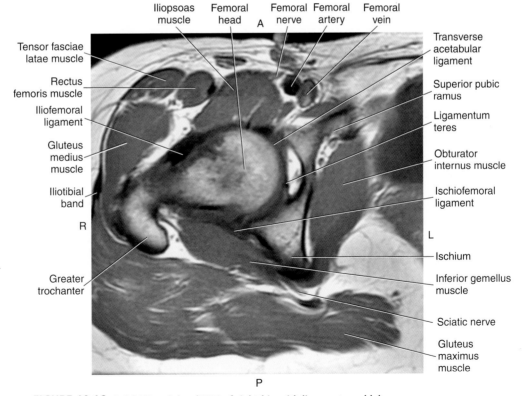
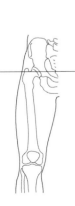

FIGURE 10.16 Axial, T1-weighted MRI of right hip with ligaments and labrum.

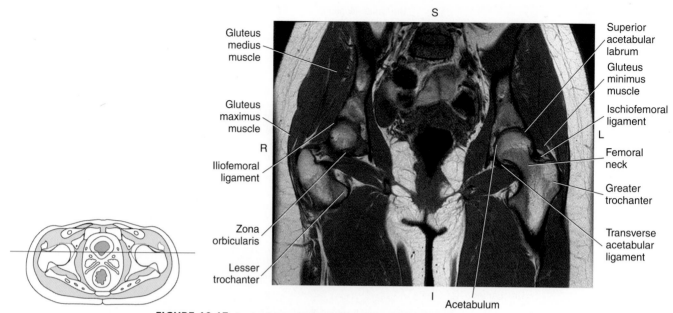

FIGURE 10.17 Coronal, T1-weighted MRI of hips with ligaments and labrum.

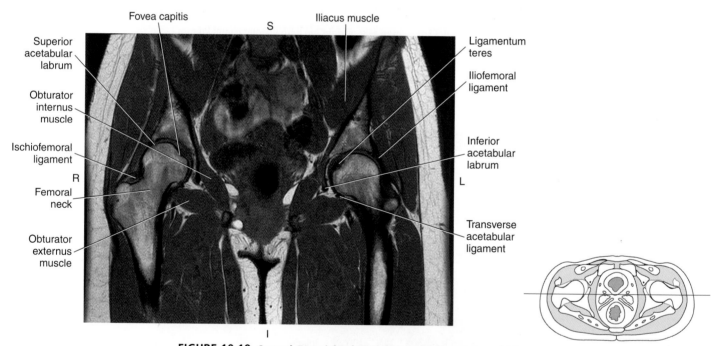

FIGURE 10.18 Coronal, T1-weighted MRI of hips with ligaments and labrum.

the acetabular notch at the inferior edge of the acetabulum (Figures 10.2, 10.12, 10.20, and 10.24). As the transverse acetabular ligament abridges the acetabular notch, it transforms it into the acetabular foramen, which allows nerves and blood vessels to pass to and from the hip joint. The **iliofemoral ligament** is among the strongest of the body, with many stabilizing functions as it spans from the anterior inferior iliac spine and rim of the acetabulum to insert on the intertrochanteric line of the femur (Figures 10.13 and 10.14). A primary function of this ligament is

to provide a thick reinforcement to the anterior part of the hip joint. The **ischiofemoral** and **pubofemoral ligaments**, though difficult to distinguish, present a spiral configuration of femoral attachment (Figures 10.13 and 10.14). The ischiofemoral ligament arises from the ischium and courses in a spiral above the femoral neck to insert on the posterior femoral neck, whereas the pubofemoral ligament arises from the superior pubic ramus to radiate and insert onto the iliofemoral ligament and intertrochanteric line. The spiral configuration of these two

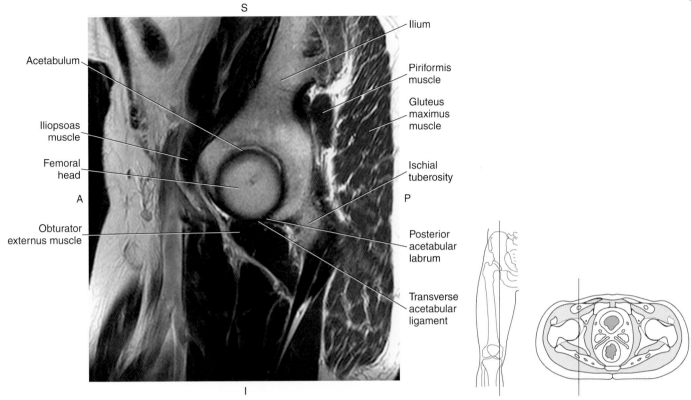

FIGURE 10.19 Sagittal, T1-weighted MRI of hip with ligaments and labrum.

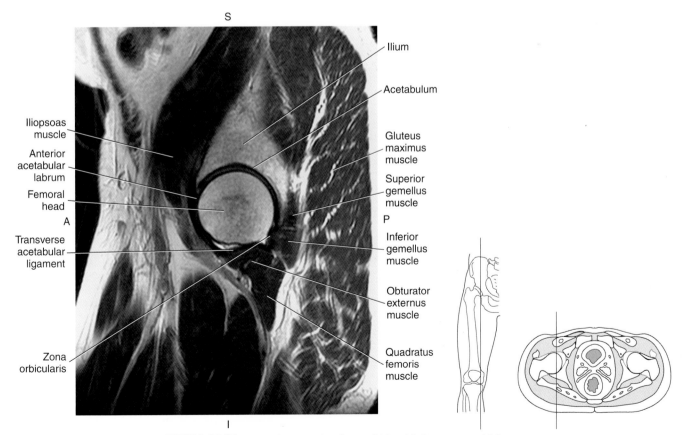

FIGURE 10.20 Sagittal, T1-weighted MRI of hip with ligaments and labrum.

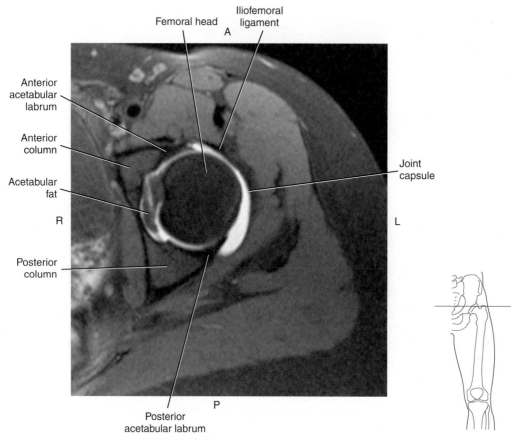

Femoral head

Iliofemoral ligament

A

Anterior acetabular labrum

Anterior column

Acetabular fat

R

L

Joint capsule

Posterior column

P

Posterior acetabular labrum

FIGURE 10.21 Axial, MR arthrogram of left hip.

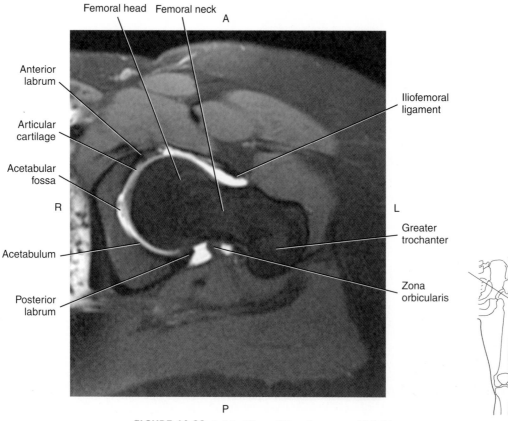

Femoral head   Femoral neck

A

Anterior labrum

Articular cartilage

Acetabular fossa

R

L

Iliofemoral ligament

Greater trochanter

Acetabulum

Posterior labrum

Zona orbicularis

P

FIGURE 10.22 Axial oblique, MR arthrogram of left hip.

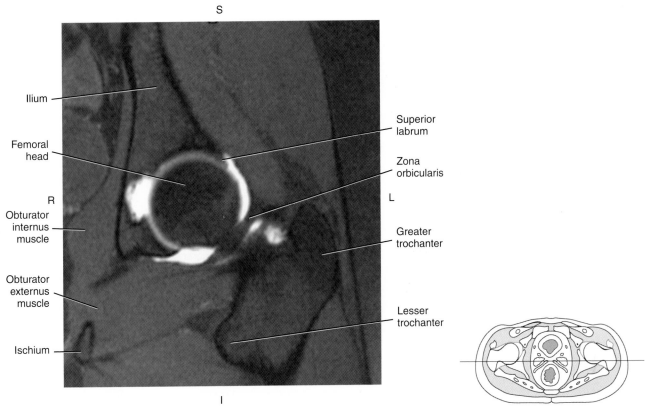

Ilium

Femoral
head

R

Obturator
internus
muscle

Obturator
externus
muscle

Ischium

Superior
labrum

Zona
orbicularis

L

Greater
trochanter

Lesser
trochanter

FIGURE 10.23 Coronal, MR arthrogram of left hip.

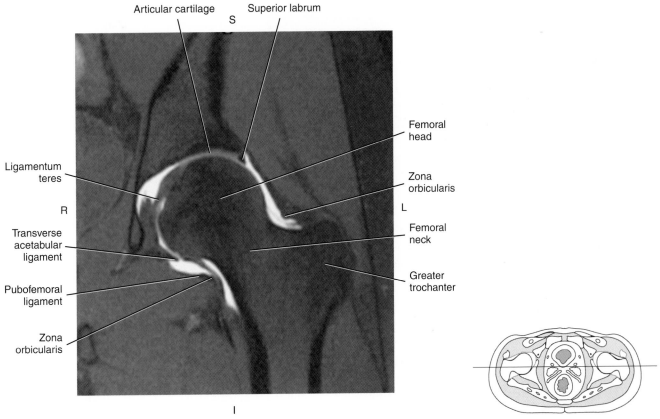

Articular cartilage   Superior labrum

Ligamentum
teres

R

Transverse
acetabular
ligament

Pubofemoral
ligament

Zona
orbicularis

Femoral
head

Zona
orbicularis

L

Femoral
neck

Greater
trochanter

FIGURE 10.24 Coronal, MR arthrogram of left hip.

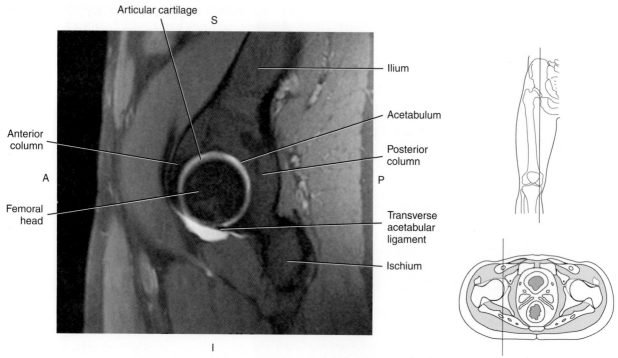

FIGURE 10.25 Sagittal, MR arthrogram of hip with transverse acetabular ligament.

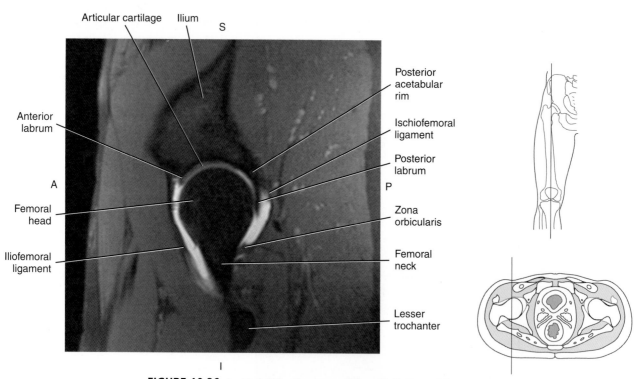

FIGURE 10.26 Sagittal, MR arthrogram of hip with ilofemoral ligament.

ligaments is unique to humans and ensures the stability and function while controlling the overall position of the lower limb. The **ligamentum teres** is a somewhat flattened band that extends from the fovea capitis of the femoral head to attach to the rim of the acetabular notch, as well as blend with the transverse acetabular ligament (Figure 10.12 and 10.24). This ligament contains the artery to the head of the femur. The ligamentum teres has little influence as a ligament but can assist to prevent dislocation of the hip. Ligaments of the hip are identified in Figures 10.15 through 10.26.

Joint Capsule

The **fibrous capsule** of the hip is strong and dense. It forms a sleeve that encloses the hip joint and most of the neck of the femur. Proximally, it is attached to the edge of the acetabulum, just distal to the acetabular labrum, and to the transverse acetabular ligament. Distally, the fibrous capsule is attached to the femoral neck, intertrochanteric line, and the greater trochanter, anteriorly. Posteriorly it attaches to the neck, just proximal to the intertrochanteric crest. The capsule consists of two sets of fibers: circular and longitudinal. The circular fibers are deep and form the **zona orbicularis**, a sling or collar around the femoral neck that constricts the capsule and helps to hold the femoral head in the acetabulum (Figures 10.20, 10.23, 10.24, and 10.26). Extending upward from the femoral neck are the longitudinal fibers, termed **retinacula**, that are most abundant at the superoanterior portion of the capsule. The retinacula contain blood vessels that supply the head and neck of the femur. They are reinforced by distinct bands or accessory ligaments, including the iliofemoral, pubofemoral, and ischiofemoral ligaments (Figures 10.13 through 10.26).

The **synovial capsule** of the hip joint lines the internal surface of the fibrous capsule. The synovial capsule forms a sleeve for the ligamentum teres, lines the acetabular fossa, and covers the fatty pad in the acetabular notch (Figure 10.5). It is attached to the edges of the acetabular fossa and to the transverse acetabular ligament. The synovial capsule protrudes inferior to the fibrous capsule on the posterior aspect and forms the obturator externus bursa, which protects the tendon of the obturator externus muscle (Figure 10.14).

Bursae

There are many bursae located around the hip owing to the number of muscles associated with this joint. The hip bursae vary in number and position and act to reduce friction at locations where tendons and muscle pass over bone. Major bursae of the hip include the trochanteric, iliopsoas, and ischial. The bursae that make up the **trochanteric (subgluteus maximus) bursae** are located between the insertion site of the gluteus muscles, as well as the vastus lateralis muscle to the greater trochanter of the femur. The **iliopsoas (iliopectineal) bursa** is situated between the iliopsoas tendon and the lesser trochanter of the femur. Located between the ischial tuberosity and the gluteus maximus muscle is the **ischial bursa** (Figure 10.27).

> Snapping hip syndrome is a condition characterized by a snapping or popping sensation when the hip is flexed and extended and may cause discomfort or pain. The most common cause of the snapping sound is due to tendons catching on bony prominences with movement of the hip. The hip bursae, greater trochanteric and iliopsoas, may become inflamed with this syndrome and result in pain due to bursitis.

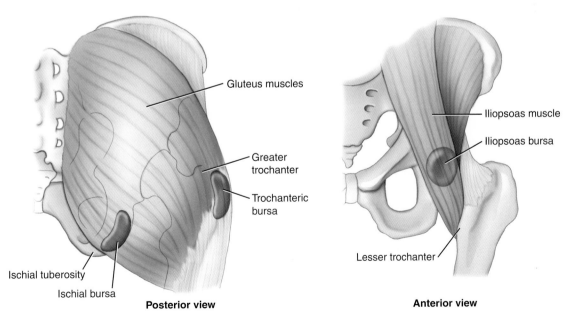

Posterior view   Anterior view

FIGURE 10.27 Hip Bursa.

Muscles of the Hip and Thigh

A complex arrangement of muscles around the hip joint and thigh produces the movements of the hip. They are described in this section as gluteal muscles and muscles of the thigh and are illustrated in Figures 10.28 through 10.54 and Table 10.1. The muscles of the gluteal region

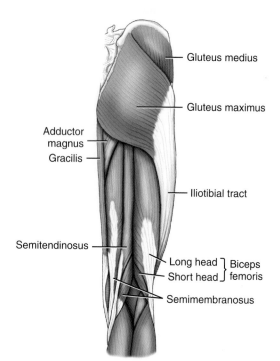

FIGURE 10.28 Posterior view of superficial muscles, right hip, and thigh.

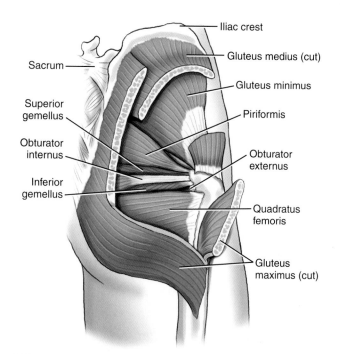

FIGURE 10.29 Posterior view of deep muscles, right hip, and thigh.

and thigh muscles may be separated into compartments by thickened sheets of deep fascia, thus allowing muscles of the lower extremity to be classified according to specific compartments in which they are located, such as gluteal, medial, and posterior compartments of the thigh.

Muscles of the gluteal compartment. The superficial gluteal muscles include the gluteus maximus, gluteus medius, and gluteus minimus. The **gluteus maximus muscle** is the largest and most superficial of the gluteal muscle group. It is situated on the posterior aspect of the hip joint, acts primarily as a powerful extensor of the hip, and is responsible for maintaining the erect position. The gluteus maximus originates from the ilium, sacrum, and coccyx to insert just distal to the gluteal tuberosity of the greater trochanter (Figures 10.28 through 10.36). The **gluteus medius muscle** is located on the lateral and upper part of the buttock. It originates from the iliac crest, just lateral to the gluteus maximus muscle, and is partially covered by the gluteus maximus along its medial one-third. The gluteus medius is fan-shaped as it spans from the iliac crest to insert on the superolateral aspect of the greater trochanter of the femur (Figures 10.29 through 10.36). The **gluteus minimus muscle** is the smallest of the gluteal muscles. It is triangular and completely covered by the gluteus medius. The upper attachment of the gluteus minimus is from the gluteal surface of the ilium, just inferior to that of the gluteus medius. Its tendon attaches to the anterosuperior aspect of the greater trochanter of the femur (Figures 10.29 through 10.36). The gluteus medius and minimus muscles act to abduct and medially rotate the thigh.

The deep group of muscles include the piriformis, obturator internus, obturator externus, gemellus, and quadratus femoris, which are mainly lateral rotators of the thigh at the hip joint and act to stabilize the hip joint. The **piriformis muscle** originates from the inner surface of the sacrum between the sacral foramina. It passes laterally and anteriorly through the greater sciatic foramen to attach to the superior boundary of the greater trochanter of the femur (Figures 10.29, 10.32, and 10.35). The actions of the piriformis muscle include lateral rotation and abduction of the thigh. The **obturator internus muscle** is a thick fan-shaped muscle that originates from the inner border of the obturator foramen and travels through the lesser sciatic foramen. At this point it changes shape as it becomes tendinous and courses laterally to attach to the greater trochanter of the femur (Figures 10.6, 10.29, 10.33, and 10.36). Its primary actions are the same as those of the piriformis muscle: lateral rotation and abduction of the thigh. The **obturator externus muscle** arises from the outer border of the obturator foramen in the pelvis to essentially mirror the obturator internus muscle. It courses laterally around the posterior side of the neck of the femur to insert into the medial side of the greater trochanter and

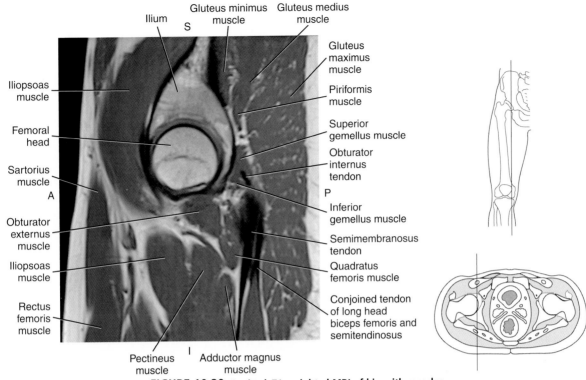

FIGURE 10.30 Sagittal, T1-weighted MRI of hip with muscles.

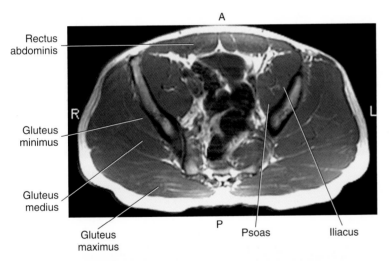

FIGURE 10.31 Axial, T1-weighted MRI of gluteal region with psoas muscle.

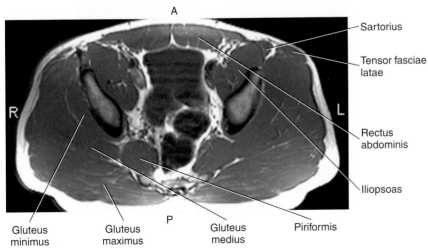

FIGURE 10.32 Axial, T1-weighted MRI of gluteal region with piriformis muscle.

FIGURE 10.33 Axial, T1-weighted MRI of gluteal region with obturator muscles.

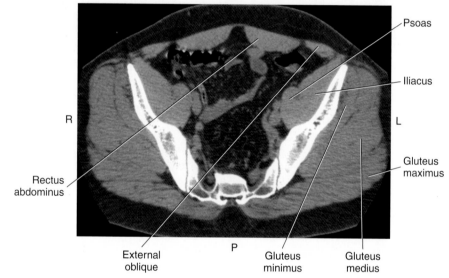

FIGURE 10.34 Axial CT of gluteal region with psoas muscle.

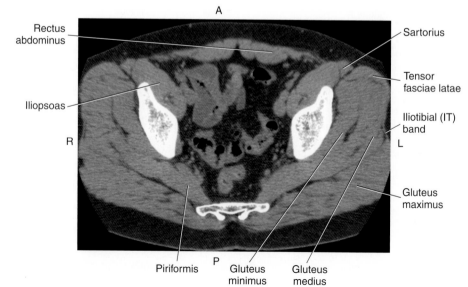

FIGURE 10.35 Axial CT of gluteal region with piriformis muscle.

acts to laterally rotate the thigh (Figures 10.6, 10.29, 10.33, and 10.36). The two **gemellus muscles** (superior and inferior) are located along the superior and inferior boundaries of the obturator internus muscle and tendon (Figure 10.29). The **superior gemellus muscle** arises from the ischial spine, whereas the **inferior gemellus muscle** arises from the ischial tuberosity. Both muscles join with the tendon of the obturator internus muscle to insert into the medial surface of the greater trochanter (Figures 10.15, 10.16, 10.20, 10.29, and 10.30). The gemellus muscles also act to laterally

rotate and abduct the thigh. The rectangular **quadratus femoris muscle** is located inferior to the obturator internus and gemellus muscles. It arises from the lateral border of the ischial tuberosity and then courses laterally to insert on the intertrochanteric crest of the femur. The primary action of the quadratus femoris muscle is lateral rotation of the thigh (Figures 10.29, 10.30, 10.33, and 10.36). The muscles of the gluteal compartment are identified in Figures 10.28 through 10.36, and their functions are presented in Table 10.1.

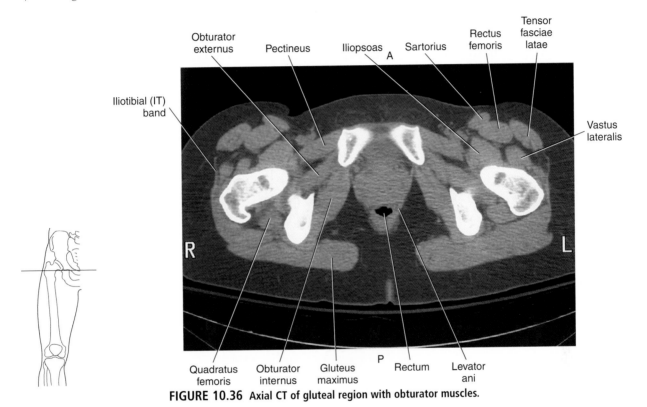

FIGURE 10.36 Axial CT of gluteal region with obturator muscles.

TABLE 10.1	Muscles of the Gluteal Region		
Muscle	**Proximal Insertion**	**Distal Insertion**	**Action**
Gluteus maximus	Ilium, sacrum, coccyx	Gluteal tuberosity of greater trochanter	Extensor of the hip, maintains erect position of the body
Gluteus medius	Iliac crest	Greater trochanter	Abducts and medially rotates the thigh
Gluteus minimus	Gluteal surface of ilium	Greater trochanter	Abducts and medially rotates the thigh
Piriformis	Sacrum	Greater trochanter	Lateral rotation and abduction of the thigh
Obturator internus	Obturator foramen	Greater trochanter	Lateral rotation and abduction of the thigh
Obturator externus	Obturator foramen	Greater trochanter	Lateral rotation of the thigh
Superior gemellus	Ischial spine	Greater trochanter	Lateral rotation and abduction of the thigh
Inferior gemellus	Ischial tuberosity	Greater trochanter	Lateral rotation and abduction of the thigh
Quadratus femoris	Ischial tuberosity	Intertrochanteric crest	Lateral rotation of the thigh

Muscles of the anterior thigh compartment. The muscles in the anterior compartment of the thigh act both to flex the hip joint and extend the knee joint. They include the iliopsoas muscle of the pelvis and the sartorius, quadriceps femoris, and tensor fasciae latae of the leg. These muscles are demonstrated in Figures 10.37 through 10.54 and described in Table 10.2. The powerful **iliopsoas muscle** is composed of the psoas major and iliacus muscles (Figures 10.34, 10.35, and 10.37). The **psoas major muscle** arises from the transverse processes of the lumbar vertebrae and courses inferiorly within the pelvis. It exits the pelvis as it courses under the inguinal ligament to enter the anterior compartment of the thigh. The tendon of the psoas major joins with the tendon of the iliacus muscle to pass anterior to the hip joint capsule and attach to the lesser trochanter of the femur. The **iliacus muscle** arises from the iliac fossa and courses along the lateral side of the psoas major muscle in the pelvis. These muscles act conjointly in flexing the thigh at the hip and stabilizing the hip joint. The **sartorius muscle** is known as the longest muscle in the body; it extends from the anterior superior iliac spine to the medial surface of the tibia near the tuberosity (Figures 10.37 and 10.40 through 10.54). It acts to flex, abduct, and laterally rotate the thigh. The biggest muscle in the body is the **quadriceps femoris muscle**, which covers almost all of the anterior surface and sides of the femur. It originates as four heads (**rectus femoris, vastus lateralis, vastus medialis,** and **vastus intermedius**) to create a powerful extensor of the knee (Figures 10.37 through 10.54). The superior ends of the four heads of the quadriceps femoris muscle arise from different locations, but their inferior tendons merge to form the **quadriceps tendon** that courses over the patella and continues as the

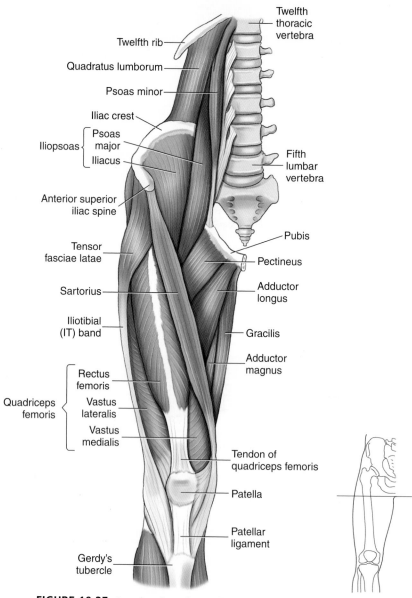

FIGURE 10.37 Anterior view of superficial muscles, right hip, and thigh.

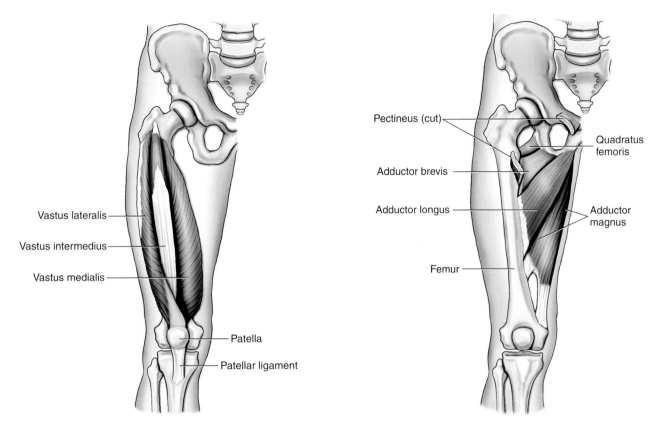

FIGURE 10.38 Anterior view of quadriceps muscle group.

FIGURE 10.39 Anterior view of adductor muscle group.

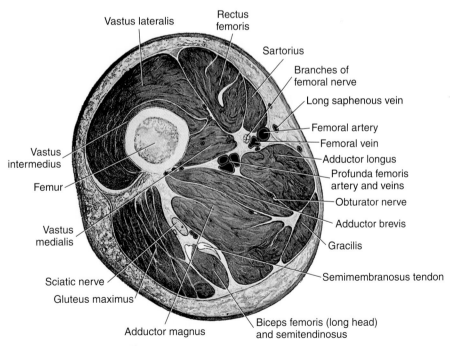

FIGURE 10.40 Axial view of right femur, proximal one-third.

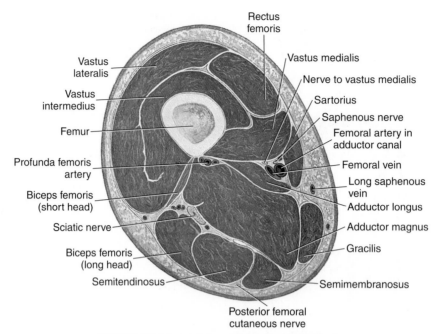

FIGURE 10.41 Axial view of right femur, midthigh.

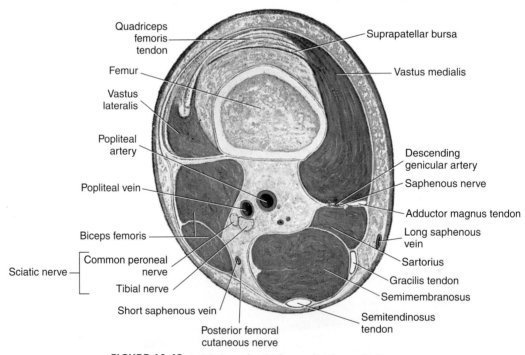

FIGURE 10.42 Axial view of right femur, distal one-third.

patellar ligament in the knee (Figure 10.37). The rectus femoris originates from the anterior inferior iliac spine, the vastus lateralis from the greater trochanter and lateral lip of the linea aspera of the femur, the vastus medialis from the intertrochanteric line and medial lip of the linea aspera of the femur, and the vastus intermedius from the anterior and lateral surfaces of the body of the femur. All the parts of the quadriceps femoris act to

extend the leg at the knee joint and, through the actions of the rectus femoris, flex the hip joint. The **tensor fascia latae muscle** is a short, thick, teardrop-shaped muscle located on the anterolateral aspect of the thigh, enclosed between two layers of the fascia. As its name implies, it tightens the lateral fascia, thereby enabling the thigh muscles to act with increased power. It abducts, medially rotates, flexes the thigh, and helps to keep the knee

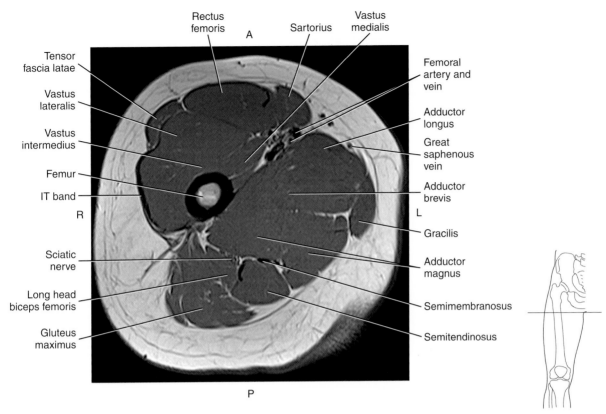

FIGURE 10.43 Axial, T1-weighted MRI of right proximal femur.

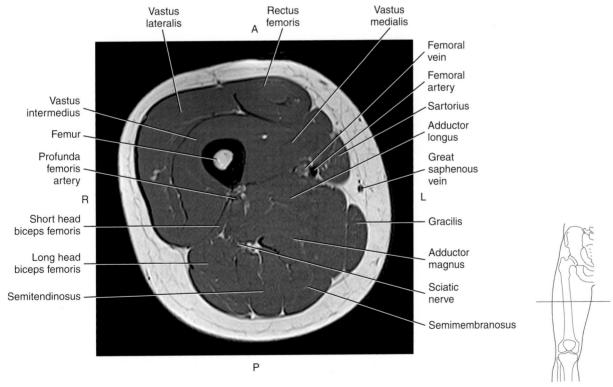

FIGURE 10.44 Axial, T1-weighted MRI of right midfemur.

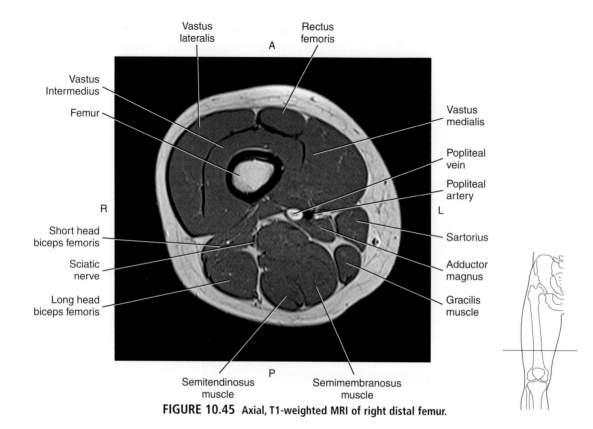

FIGURE 10.45   Axial, T1-weighted MRI of right distal femur.

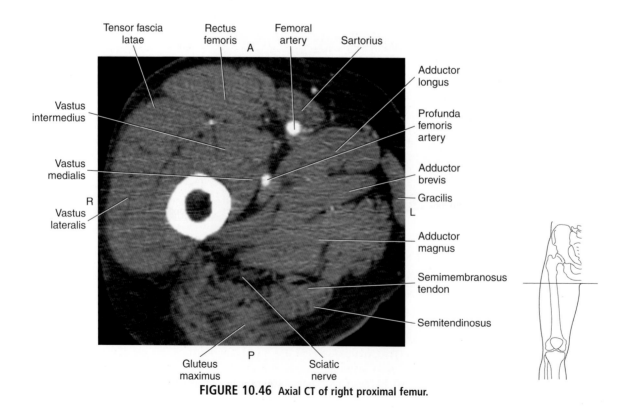

FIGURE 10.46   Axial CT of right proximal femur.

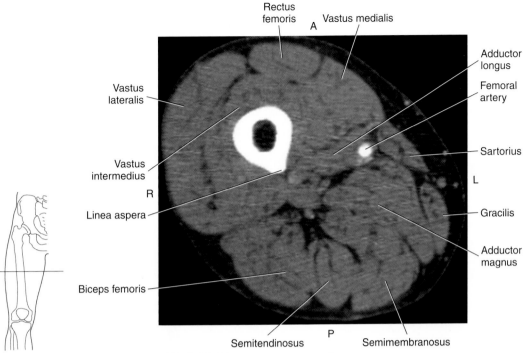

FIGURE 10.47 Axial CT of right midfemur.

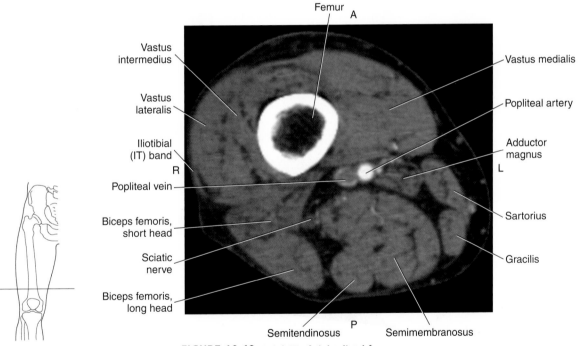

FIGURE 10.48 Axial CT of right distal femur.

extended. It originates from the anterior superior iliac spine and anterior part of the iliac crest and ends where the muscle inserts in the iliotibial band (Figures 10.32, 10.33, 10.35 through 10.37 and 10.43). The **iliotibial band**, also called the **IT band**, is a long, wide band of fascia that lies over the muscles on the outer surface of the thigh. This band is a thickening of the normal fascia that surrounds the entire leg. It arises from tendinous fibers of the tensor fascia latae and the gluteus maximus muscles. Acting almost like a ligament, this tendon helps mainly to stabilize the knee joint but also acts in flexing and extending the knee. It extends downward to insert on the lateral condyle of the tibia at Gerdy's tubercle (Figures 10.37, 10.43, and 10.49).

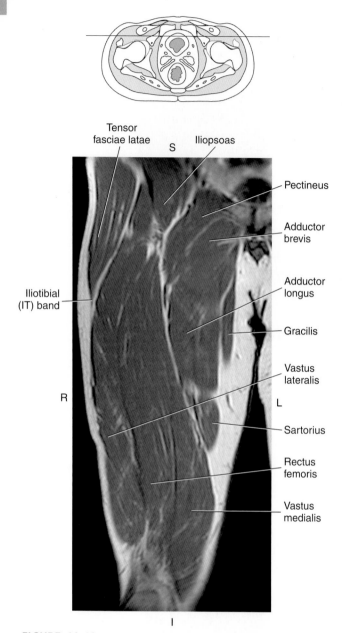

FIGURE 10.49 Coronal, T1-weighted MRI of right hip and thigh muscles.

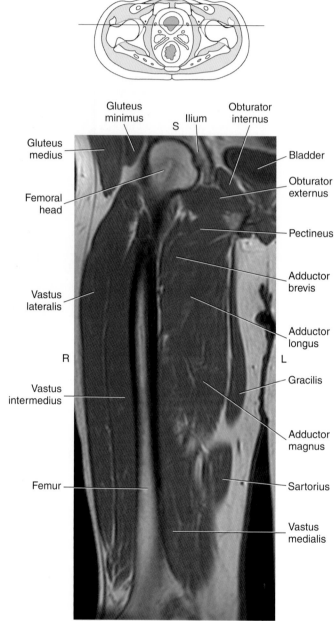

FIGURE 10.50 Coronal, T1-weighted MRI of right hip and thigh muscles.

Muscles of the medial thigh compartment. Adduction is the primary action of the medial thigh muscles. These muscles include the gracilis, pectineus, adductor longus, adductor brevis, and adductor magnus muscles, which are demonstrated in Figures 10.37 through 10.54 and described in Table 10.2. The long straplike **gracilis muscle** lies along the medial side of the thigh and knee. The gracilis muscle extends from the inferior ramus of the pubis and is the only medial thigh muscle to cross the knee joint as it inserts onto the anterior surface of the tibia just inferior to the medial condyle. In addition

to adducting the thigh, the gracilis muscle acts to flex the leg and helps to medially rotate the thigh (Figures 10.37 and 10.40 through 10.51). Arising from the pectineal line of the pubis is the short, flat **pectineus muscle**. It lies medial to the psoas major muscle in the superior thigh, then narrows as it courses inferiorly to insert on the medial lip of the linea aspera, at the pectineal line, distal to the lesser trochanter of the femur. It acts to adduct and flex the thigh (Figures 10.33, 10.36, 10.37, 10.49, and 10.50). The adductor muscle group, as named, acts to adduct the thigh and is composed of three

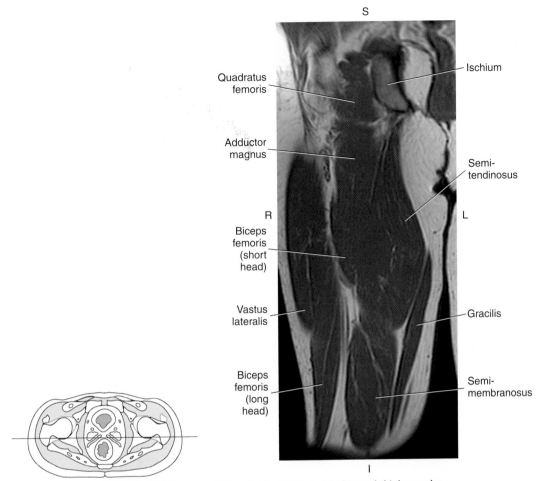

FIGURE 10.51 Coronal, T1-weighted MRI of right hip and thigh muscles.

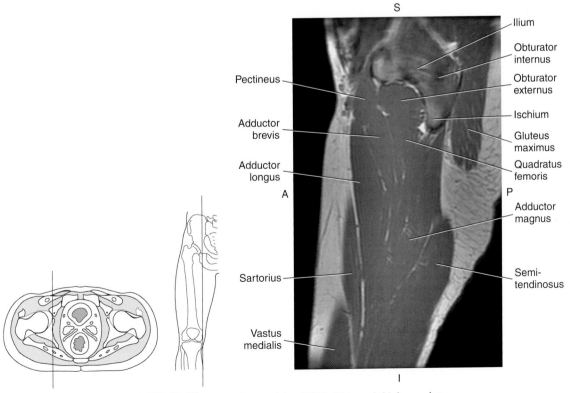

FIGURE 10.52 Sagittal, T1-weighted MRI of hip and thigh muscles.

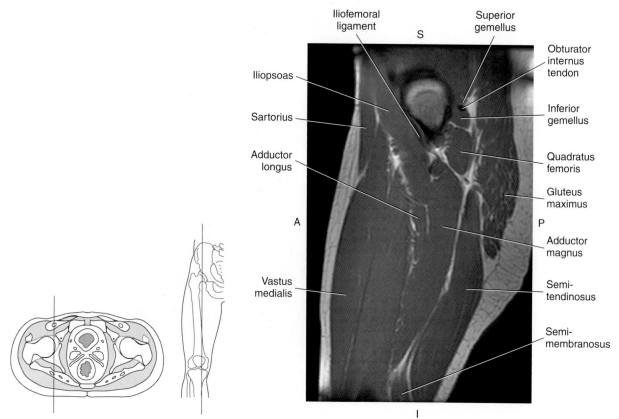

FIGURE 10.53 Sagittal, T1-weighted MRI of hip and thigh muscles.

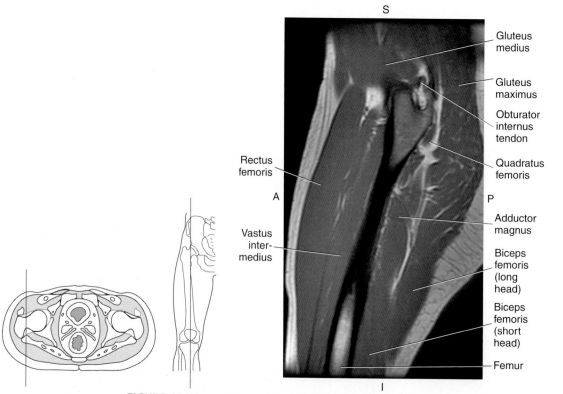

FIGURE 10.54 Sagittal, T1-weighted MRI of hip and thigh muscles.

TABLE 10.2	Muscles of the Thigh		
Muscle	**Proximal Insertion**	**Distal Insertion**	**Action**
Anterior Thigh			
Psoas major	Transverse processes of lumbar vertebrae	Lesser trochanter	Flexes the thigh at hip and stabilizes the hip joint
Iliacus	Iliac fossa	Lesser trochanter	Flexes the thigh at hip and stabilizes the hip joint
Sartorius	Anterior superior iliac spine and iliac crest	Medial surface of tibia	Flexes, abducts, and laterally rotates the thigh
Tensor fascia latae	Anterior superior iliac spine	Iliotibial tract	Abducts, medially rotates, and flexes the thigh; helps to maintain extension of the knee
Quadriceps Femoris			
Rectus femoris	Anterior inferior iliac spine	Patellar ligament	Extends the leg at knee joint and flexes the hip joint
Vastus lateralis	Greater trochanter and lateral lip of linea aspera	Patellar ligament	Extends leg at knee joint
Vastus medialis	Intertrochanteric line and medial lip of linea aspera	Patellar ligament	Extends leg at knee joint
Vastus intermedius	Anterior and lateral surfaces femoral body	Patellar ligament	Extends leg at knee joint
Medial Thigh			
Gracilis	Inferior pubic ramus	Anterior surface of tibia	Adducts thigh, flexes leg, and medially rotates thigh
Pectineus	Pectineal line of pubis	Medial lip of linea aspera	Adducts and flexes the thigh
Adductor longus	Pubic bone	Middle third of linea aspera	Adducts the thigh
Adductor brevis	Pubic bone	Superior linea aspera	Adducts the thigh
Adductor magnus	Pubic bone	Linea aspera and adductor tubercle of medial condyle of knee	Adducts the thigh
Posterior Thigh ***Hamstrings***			
Semitendinosus	Ischial tuberosity	Anterior tibia, medial side	Extend the thigh, flex and medially rotate the leg, and extend the trunk when hip and knee are flexed
Semimembranosus	Ischial tuberosity	Medial condyle of tibia, posterior aspect	Extend the thigh, flex and medially rotate the leg, and extend the trunk when hip and knee are flexed
Biceps femoris		Lateral surface of fibular head	Flex the leg at the knee and laterally rotate the leg when hip is flexed
Long head	Ischial tuberosity		
Short head	Lateral lip of linea aspera		

muscles: the **adductor longus, adductor brevis,** and **adductor magnus** (Figures 10.39 and 10.40 through 10.50). These muscles originate at the pubic bone and fan out to insert along the length of the medial aspect of the femur. The adductor longus muscle is the most anterior muscle in the adductor group and attaches to the middle third of the linea aspera of the femur. The shorter adductor brevis muscle lies deep to the pectineus and adductor longus muscles. Its distal attachment is between the lesser trochanter and superior end of the linea aspera of the femur. The largest and most medial of the adductor group is the adductor magnus. It is situated posterior to the adductor brevis and adductor longus and anterior to the semitendinosus and semimembranosus muscles. It forms a large triangular sheet of muscle in the thigh and is composed of two parts, an adductor part and a hamstring part. The adductor portion of the adductor magnus has an extensive distal attachment on the linea aspera of the femur, whereas the hamstring part attaches to adductor tubercle on top of the medial condyle of the femur.

Muscles of the posterior thigh compartment. The semitendinosus, semimembranosus, and biceps femoris muscles are collectively known as the **hamstrings** (Figures 10.28 and 10.40 through 10.54). They make up the large mass of muscles that can be palpated on the posterior aspect of the thigh and are involved with extension of the hip, flexion of the knee, and rotation of the flexed knee. The **semitendinosus muscle** extends from the ischial tuberosity, courses on the medial aspect of the femur, then continues inferiorly around the medial tibial condyle and attaches to the medial side of the anterior tibial surface (Figures 10.28, 10.40 through 10.48, and 10.52 through 10.54). It, along with the **semimembranosus muscle,** acts to extend the thigh, flex and medially rotate the leg, and extend the trunk when the thigh and leg are flexed. The semimembranosus also originates from the ischial tuberosity but attaches to the posterior part of the medial condyle of the tibia (Figures 10.28, 10.40 through 10.48, and 10.52 through 10.54). The **biceps femoris muscle,** as named, has two heads (long and short). The long head extends from the ischial tuberosity, whereas the short head extends from the lateral lip of the linea aspera of the femur. The biceps femoris extends inferiorly over the lateral part of the posterior surface of the knee to insert on the lateral surface of the fibular head (Figures 10.48, 10.51, and 10.54). It acts to flex the leg at the knee joint and laterally rotates the leg when the leg is flexed.

KNEE AND LOWER LEG

Bony Anatomy

The bones that contribute to the knee joint and lower leg are the femur, tibia, patella, and fibula (Figures 10.55 and 10.56). Cartilage covers the articular surfaces of the femur, tibia, and patella and helps to provide smooth movement within the knee joint.

Distal femur. The distal portion of the femur broadens into two articular cartilage-covered projections called the medial and lateral condyles (Figures 10.57 through 10.61). The **lateral femoral condyle** is wider in front than in the back, whereas the **medial femoral condyle**

remains more consistent in width. The femoral condyles are anteriorly connected by the smooth **patellar surface** and posteriorly separated by the **intercondylar fossa** (Figures 10.57 and 10.58). On the side of each condyle is a raised edge called the **medial** and **lateral epicondyle** for the attachment of ligaments and muscles (Figures 10.59 and 10.60). A small projection located above the medial epicondyle is the **adductor tubercle,** which serves as an attachment for a portion of the adductor magnus muscle (Figures 10.9 and 10.11). On the posterior surface of the distal femur is a triangular area called the **popliteal surface.** The base of the triangle is located at the **intercondylar line,** which marks the beginning of the intercondylar fossa. The sides of the triangle are formed by the **medial** and **lateral supracondylar lines,** which are continuations of the linea aspera (Figures 10.9 and 10.11).

Tibia. The **tibia** has a widened proximal end that has two cartilaginous projections: the **medial** and **lateral condyles** (Figure 10.62). The superior articular surface of both condyles has flattened surfaces called **tibial plateaus** for articulation with the femoral condyles (Figures 10.62 and 10.63). The tibial condyles are separated by the **intercondylar eminence (tibial spine),** which ends in two peaks called the **medial** and **lateral intercondylar tubercles.** The intercondylar tubercles and the

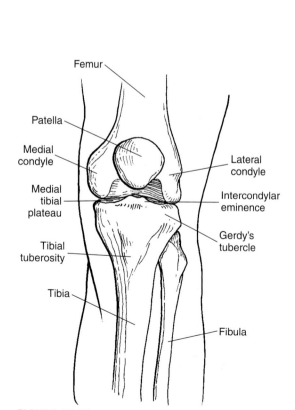

FIGURE 10.55 Anterior view of left knee joint.

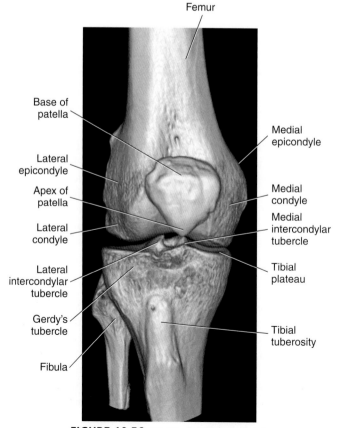

FIGURE 10.56 3D CT of right knee joint.

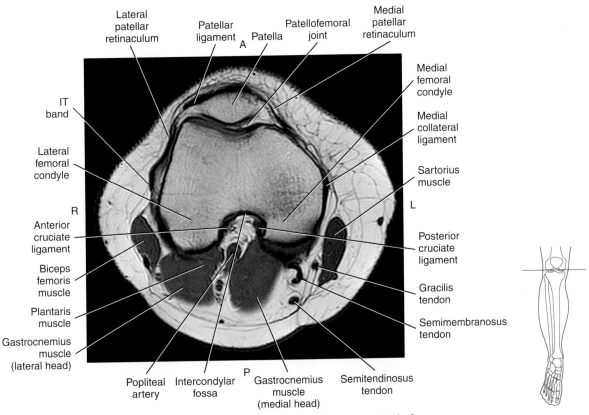

FIGURE 10.57 Axial, T1-weighted MRI of distal right femur.

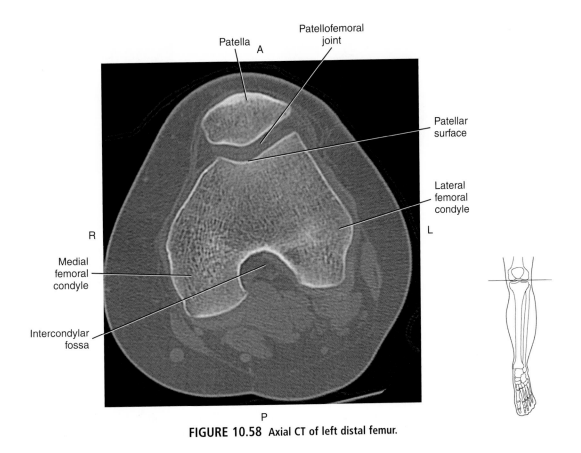

FIGURE 10.58 Axial CT of left distal femur.

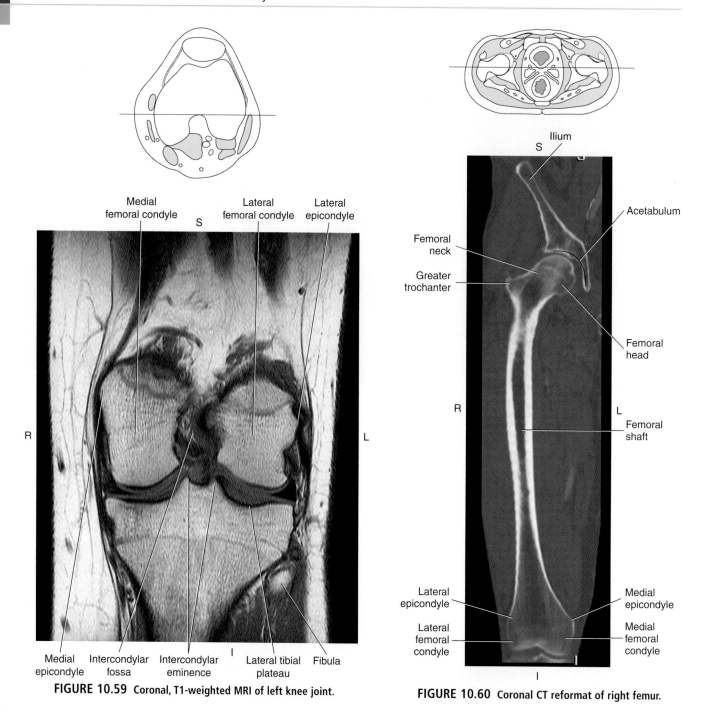

Medial femoral condyle   **Lateral femoral condyle**   **Lateral epicondyle**

S

R   L

Medial epicondyle   **Intercondylar fossa**   **Intercondylar eminence**   I   **Lateral tibial plateau**   **Fibula**

FIGURE 10.59 Coronal, T1-weighted MRI of left knee joint.

Ilium

S

Femoral neck   Acetabulum

Greater trochanter   Femoral head

R   L

Femoral shaft

Lateral epicondyle   Medial epicondyle

Lateral femoral condyle   Medial femoral condyle

I

FIGURE 10.60 Coronal CT reformat of right femur.

roughened areas around them serve as attachment sites for the cruciate ligaments and meniscus (Figures 10.55, 10.56, 10.59, and 10.62). The lateral tibial condyle has a small articular surface called the **articular fibular surface**, which articulates with the head of the fibula (Figure 10.64). The shaft of the tibia is triangular with a sharp anterior edge or crest that contains a bony projection called the **tibial tuberosity** for the attachment of the patellar ligament (Figures 10.65 and 10.66). Lateral and superior to the tibial tuberosity is the attachment site for the iliotibial (IT) band on a roughened area of the

lateral tibial condyle commonly called **Gerdy's tubercle** (Figures 10.37 and 10.56). The **medial margin** of the shaft lies directly beneath the skin and is devoid of muscle, and the **lateral surface** serves as the attachment site for the interosseous membrane. The **posterior surface** has an obliquely oriented bony ridge called the **soleal (popliteal) line**, which gives rise to tendon fibers of the soleus muscle (Figure 10.62). The distal tibia has a flattened articular end with a medial extension that forms the **medial malleolus** (Figures 10.62, 10.67, and 10.68). The posterior surface of the medial malleolus has a small

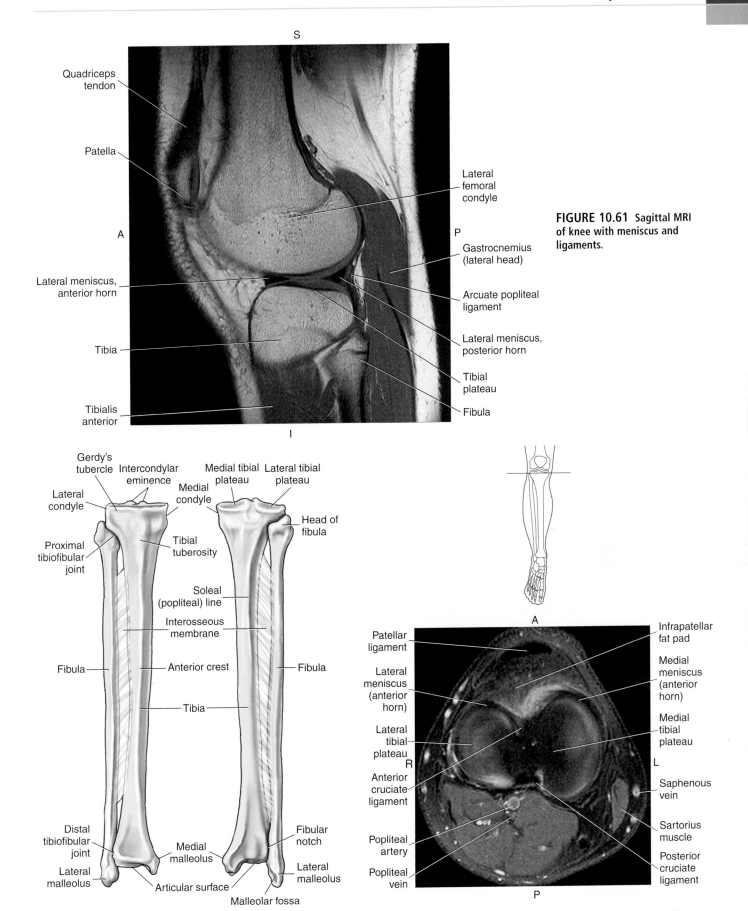

S

Quadriceps tendon

Patella

A

Lateral meniscus, anterior horn

Tibia

Tibialis anterior

I

Lateral femoral condyle

P

Gastrocnemius (lateral head)

Arcuate popliteal ligament

Lateral meniscus, posterior horn

Tibial plateau

Fibula

FIGURE 10.61 Sagittal MRI of knee with meniscus and ligaments.

Gerdy's tubercle   Intercondylar eminence

Medial tibial plateau   Lateral tibial plateau

Lateral condyle

Medial condyle

Proximal tibiofibular joint

Tibial tuberosity

Head of fibula

Soleal (popliteal) line

Interosseous membrane

Fibula

Anterior crest

Fibula

Tibia

Distal tibiofibular joint

Medial malleolus

Fibular notch

Lateral malleolus

Articular surface

Lateral malleolus

Malleolar fossa

FIGURE 10.62 Tibia and fibula. *Left,* Anterior view. *Right,* Posterior view.

A

Patellar ligament

Lateral meniscus (anterior horn)

Lateral tibial plateau

R

Anterior cruciate ligament

Popliteal artery

Popliteal vein

P

Infrapatellar fat pad

Medial meniscus (anterior horn)

Medial tibial plateau

L

Saphenous vein

Sartorius muscle

Posterior cruciate ligament

FIGURE 10.63 Axial, T1-weighted MRI of right knee with tibial plateau.

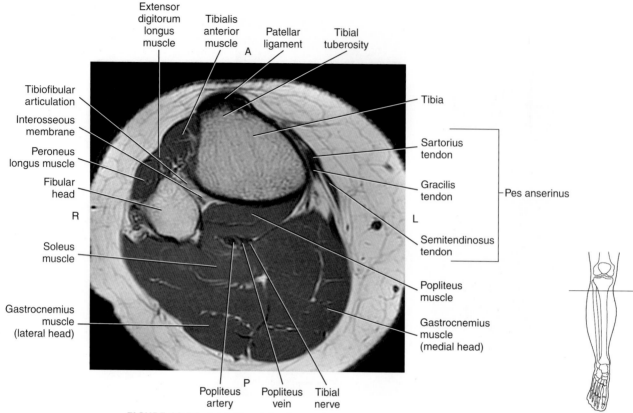

FIGURE 10.64 Axial, T1-weighted MRI of right knee with tibiofibular articulation.

Extensor digitorum longus muscle
Tibialis anterior muscle
A
Patellar ligament
Tibial tuberosity

Tibiofibular articulation
Interosseous membrane
Peroneus longus muscle
Fibular head
R
Soleus muscle
Gastrocnemius muscle (lateral head)

Tibia
Sartorius tendon
Gracilis tendon
L
Semitendinosus tendon
Pes anserinus
Popliteus muscle
Gastrocnemius muscle (medial head)

P
Popliteus artery
Popliteus vein
Tibial nerve

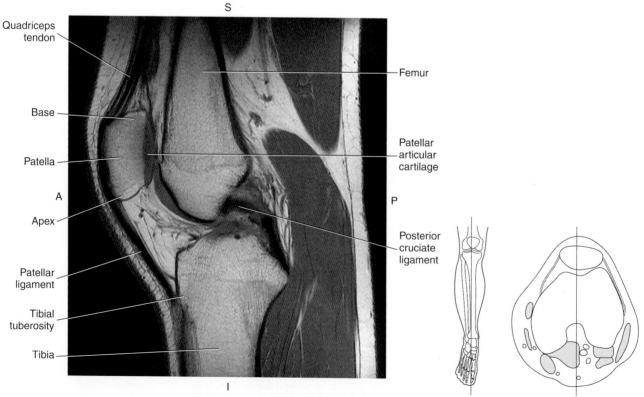

FIGURE 10.65 Midsagittal, T1-weighted MRI of tibia.

S

Quadriceps tendon
Base
Patella
A
Apex
Patellar ligament
Tibial tuberosity
Tibia

Femur
Patellar articular cartilage
P
Posterior cruciate ligament

I

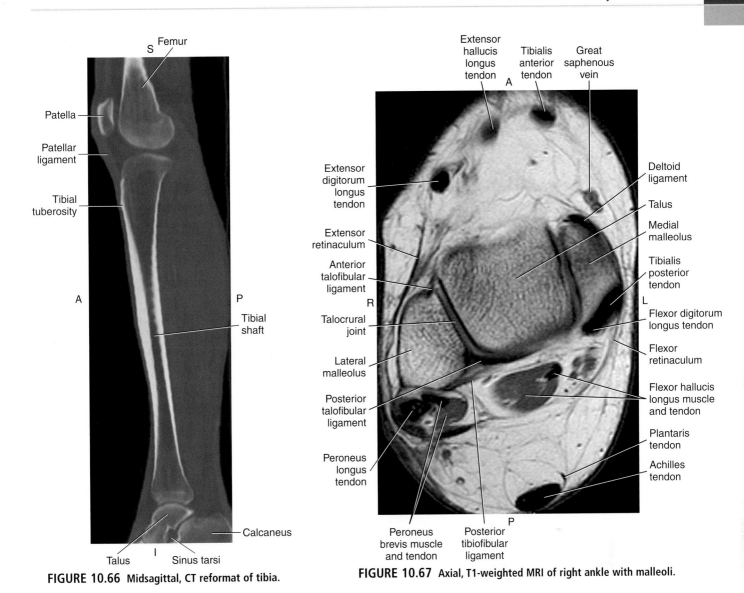

Femur
S
Patella
Patellar ligament
Tibial tuberosity
A
P
Tibial shaft
Calcaneus
Talus
I
Sinus tarsi

FIGURE 10.66 Midsagittal, CT reformat of tibia.

Extensor hallucis longus tendon
Tibialis anterior tendon
Great saphenous vein
A
Extensor digitorum longus tendon
Deltoid ligament
Talus
Medial malleolus
Extensor retinaculum
Anterior talofibular ligament
Tibialis posterior tendon
R
L
Talocrural joint
Flexor digitorum longus tendon
Lateral malleolus
Flexor retinaculum
Posterior talofibular ligament
Flexor hallucis longus muscle and tendon
Plantaris tendon
Peroneus longus tendon
Achilles tendon
P
Peroneus brevis muscle and tendon
Posterior tibiofibular ligament

FIGURE 10.67 Axial, T1-weighted MRI of right ankle with malleoli.

A
Talus
Medial malleolus
R
L
Lateral malleolus
P

FIGURE 10.68 Axial CT of left ankle with malleoli.

indentation, the **malleolar groove**, for the passage of the tibialis posterior and flexor digitorum longus tendons (Figure 10.67). On the lateral side of the distal tibia is a shallow indentation called the **fibular notch**, which provides a fibrous attachment with the distal fibula (Figure 10.62).

Fibula. The fibula is a long, relatively thin bone that has expanded proximal and distal ends. It is covered by muscles of the lower leg almost along its entire length. The proximal end is the **head of the fibula**, which ends in a sharp superior apex. Medially it has an articular surface for articulation with the lateral condyle of the tibia (Figures 10.62, and 10.64). The distal end forms the **lateral malleolus**, which extends farther distally than the medial malleolus of the tibia (Figures 10.67 and 10.68). The medial surface of the lateral malleolus has an **articular facet** that articulates with the talus. Posterior to the malleolar articular surface is a small cavity called the **malleolar fossa**, which is where the posterior talofibular ligament is anchored (Figures 10.62 and 10.67).

Patella and patellofemoral joint. The **patella** is the largest sesamoid bone in the body and is embedded within the quadriceps tendon. It is a subcutaneous, flat, triangular bone with the broad **base** facing proximally and the pointed **apex** facing distally (Figure 10.69). The patella has an **anterior** and **posterior surface** and three borders: **superior, medial,** and **lateral.** The base of the patella has roughened areas for the attachment of the rectus femoris and vastus intermedius muscles, whereas the roughened medial and lateral borders receive attachment for the vastus medialis and lateralis muscles. The posterior surface is covered with the thickest articular cartilage found in the body and is centrally divided by a broad **vertical ridge** into **medial** and **lateral facets.** The larger lateral facet articulates with the lateral femoral condyle, and the smaller medial facet articulates with the medial femoral condyle (Figure 10.70). The patella protects the anterior joint surface of the knee and functions to increase the leverage of the quadriceps extensor system (Figures 10.57, 10.58, 10.65, and 10.66).

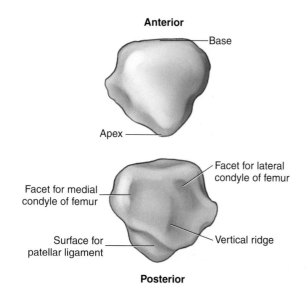

FIGURE 10.69 Patella. *Top,* Anterior view. *Bottom,* Posterior view.

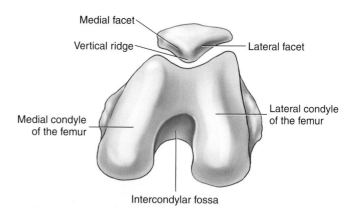

FIGURE 10.70 Patellofemoral joint with intercondylar fossa of femur.

Knee Joint

The **knee** is the largest and one of the most complex joints of the body. The bones that contribute to the knee joint are the femur, tibia, and patella (Figures 10.55 and 10.56). The knee has three separate articulations: two **femorotibial** and a **patellofemoral articulation** within the same synovial membrane. A supporting network of menisci, ligaments, tendons, and muscles functions together in order to meet the demands made on the knee.

Joint capsule. The joint capsule of the knee consists of a strong, fibrous membrane that is medially, laterally, and posteriorly reinforced by extracapsular ligaments.

These include the patellar, fibular collateral, tibial collateral, oblique popliteal, and arcuate ligaments. Anteriorly, the capsule blends with the quadriceps tendon and the medial and lateral retinacula. The synovial membrane of the knee is the largest and most extensive synovial cavity in the body. It lines the inner surface of the fibrous membrane attaching to the articular margins of the femur, tibia and patella. It is reflected across the anterior surface of the cruciate ligaments, so they are located intracapsular but extrasynovial (Figure 10.71). Synovial recesses can be found close to the patella, popliteus tendon, and behind each femoral condyle.

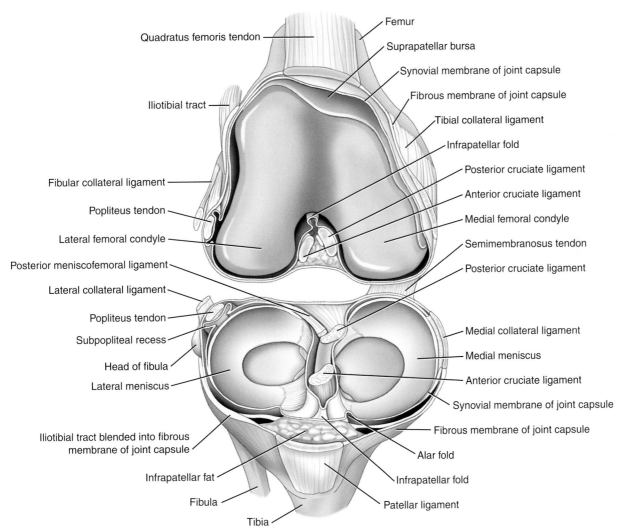

FIGURE 10.71 Knee joint (anterosuperior view).

Menisci. Located between the femoral condyles and tibial plateaus are the paired **menisci** (Figures 10.72 through 10.79). These C-shaped menisci, composed of fibrous connective tissue, cushion the articulation between the femoral condyles and tibial plateaus and are commonly divided into **anterior** and **posterior horns.** In cross-section they appear wedge-shaped, with a thickened outer margin that flattens medially (Figures 10.73 and 10.74). Their outer margins fuse with the joint capsule, and their anterior and posterior horns attach to the intercondylar eminence of the tibia. The menisci differ in size and shape. The **medial meniscus** is crescent-shaped, with the posterior horn being wider than the anterior horn. The medial meniscus is attached to the medial collateral ligament, making it far less mobile than the lateral meniscus. The **lateral meniscus** almost forms a closed ring with anterior and posterior horns of approximately the same width. Two ligaments arise from the posterior horn of the lateral meniscus. The **posterior meniscofemoral ligament (ligament of Wrisberg)** passes behind the posterior cruciate ligament to attach to the medial femoral condyle. The **anterior meniscofemoral ligament (ligament of Humphry)** connects the posterior horn to the medial condyle, passing in front of the posterior cruciate ligament. The two menisci are connected anteriorly by the **transverse ligament** (Figures 10.72, 10.73, and 10.79).

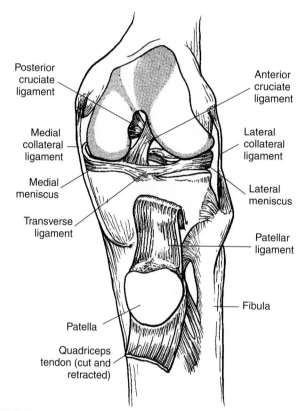

FIGURE 10.72 Anterior view of meniscus and ligaments of knee.

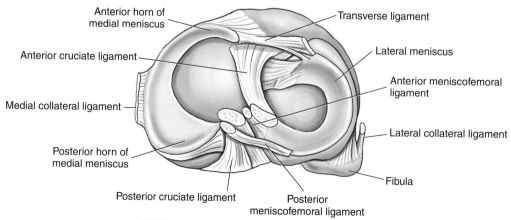

FIGURE 10.73 Superior view of right knee joint.

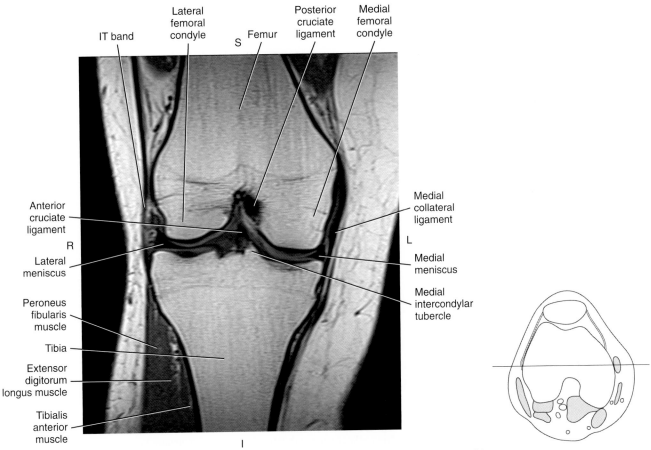

FIGURE 10.74 Coronal, T1-weighted MRI of right knee with meniscus and ligaments.

Labels (figure 10.74): IT band; Lateral femoral condyle; S; Femur; Posterior cruciate ligament; Medial femoral condyle; Anterior cruciate ligament; R; Lateral meniscus; Peroneus fibularis muscle; Tibia; Extensor digitorum longus muscle; Tibialis anterior muscle; I; Medial collateral ligament; L; Medial meniscus; Medial intercondylar tubercle

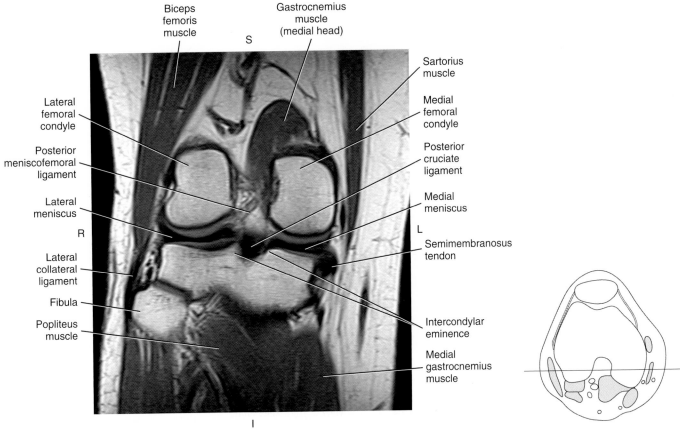

FIGURE 10.75 Coronal, T1-weighted MRI of right knee with posterior meniscofemoral ligament.

Labels (figure 10.75): Biceps femoris muscle; S; Gastrocnemius muscle (medial head); Sartorius muscle; Lateral femoral condyle; Medial femoral condyle; Posterior meniscofemoral ligament; Posterior cruciate ligament; Lateral meniscus; Medial meniscus; R; L; Lateral collateral ligament; Semimembranosus tendon; Fibula; Popliteus muscle; Intercondylar eminence; Medial gastrocnemius muscle; I

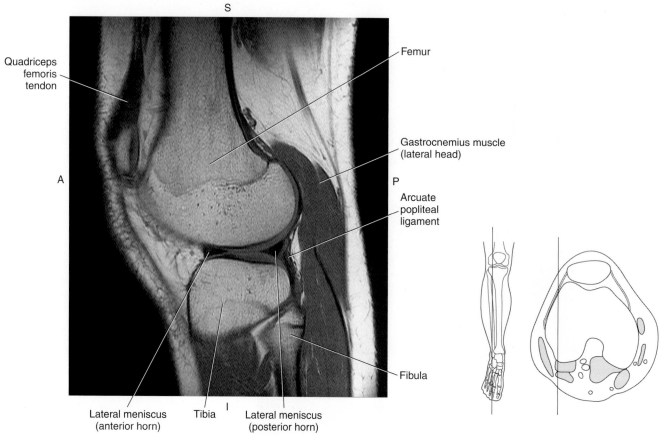

S

Quadriceps
femoris
tendon

Femur

A

Gastrocnemius muscle
(lateral head)

P

Arcuate
popliteal
ligament

Fibula

Lateral meniscus
(anterior horn)

Tibia

I

Lateral meniscus
(posterior horn)

FIGURE 10.76 Sagittal, T1-weighted MRI of knee with lateral meniscus and arcuate ligament.

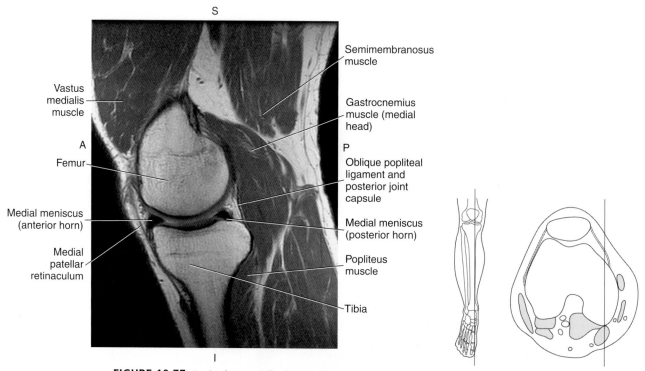

S

Vastus
medialis
muscle

Semimembranosus
muscle

A

Gastrocnemius
muscle (medial
head)

Femur

P

Oblique popliteal
ligament and
posterior joint
capsule

Medial meniscus
(anterior horn)

Medial meniscus
(posterior horn)

Medial
patellar
retinaculum

Popliteus
muscle

Tibia

I

FIGURE 10.77 Sagittal, T1-weighted MRI of knee with medial meniscus and retinaculum.

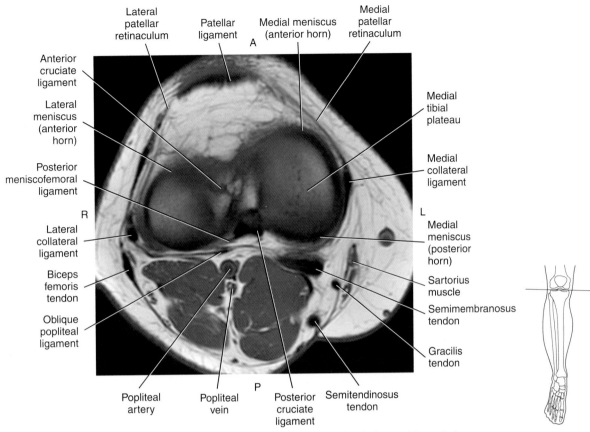

FIGURE 10.78 Axial, T1-weighted MRI of right knee with menisci.

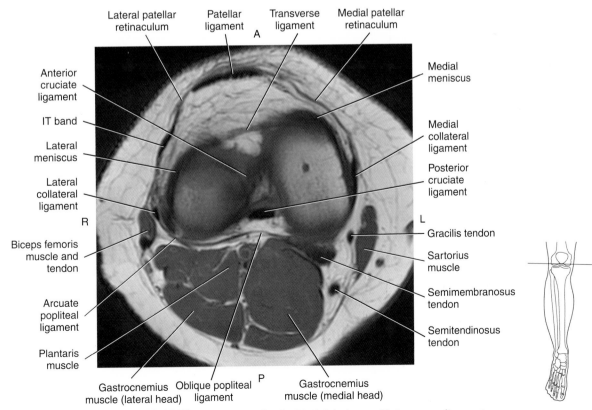

FIGURE 10.79 Axial, T1-weighted MRI of right knee with transverse ligament.

Ligaments. The ligaments of the knee are divided into external (extracapsular) and internal (intracapsular) ligaments. The external ligaments are arranged around the knee and serve to strengthen and support the joint capsule. The internal ligaments are found within the joint capsule and serve to provide stability to the tibia and femur. Ligaments of the knee are identified in Figures 10.80 through 10.98.

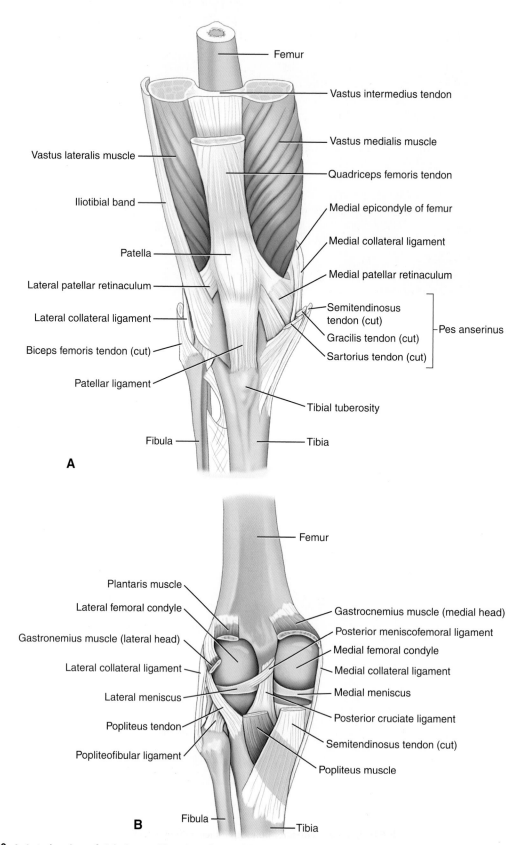

FIGURE 10.80 A, Anterior view of right knee with retinaculum and ligaments. B, Posterior view of right knee with joint capsule and ligaments.

External ligaments. The **external ligaments** of the knee include the collateral, patellar, and patellar retinaculum, oblique popliteal, and arcuate popliteal ligaments (Figures 10.80 and 10.81). The collateral ligaments provide support for the knee by reinforcing the joint capsule on the medial and lateral sides (Figures 10.72 through 10.75). The **medial collateral (tibial collateral) ligament** is a flattened triangular ligament that originates from the medial femoral epicondyle and extends to the medial tibial condyle, continuing to the medial shaft of the tibia. Along its path it fuses with the medial meniscus. The shorter, **lateral collateral (fibular collateral) ligament** is more of a rounded cord arising from the lateral femoral epicondyle and attaching to the head of the fibula. The anterior joint capsule is strengthened by the patellar ligament and patellar retinaculum. The **patellar ligament** is the strong thick band representing the continuation of the quadriceps tendon and extends from the patella to the tibial tuberosity (Figures 10.80 A, 10.87, 10.88, and 10.92 through 10.96). The **patellar retinaculum** is formed mainly by fibrous extensions and fascia of various muscles about the knee (Figures 10.79 and 10.80 A). The **medial patellar retinaculum** is formed mainly by fibers from the vastus medialis muscle and runs distally to attach to the tibia anterior to the medial collateral ligament. The **lateral patellar retinaculum** consists of fibers from the vastus lateralis and rectus femoris muscles, as well as the iliotibial band and attaches distally to the lateral margin of the tibial tuberosity to increase stability of the lateral joint capsule (Figures 10.80 A and 10.93 through 10.95). The oblique and arcuate popliteal ligaments help reinforce the dorsal surface of the joint capsule. The **oblique popliteal ligament** is an expansion of the semimembranosus tendon that reinforces the central region of the posterior joint capsule. It extends laterally to attach to the intercondylar line of the femur (Figures 10.77, 10.79, 10.81, 10.90, and 10.98). The inferolateral portion of the posterior capsule is strengthened by the **arcuate popliteal ligament** as it passes superiorly from the apex of the fibular head to spread out over the posterior capsule with fibers continuing to the posterior intercondylar area and to the posterior surface of the lateral femoral condyle (Figures 10.76, 10.81, 10.82, and 10.87).

Internal ligaments. Cruciate (cross-shaped) ligaments are strong bands of fibers that provide anterior and posterior stability to the knee. The cruciate ligaments are located within the joint capsule but outside the synovial membrane (Figures 10.71 through 10.73). The **anterior cruciate ligament** arises from the medial intercondylar tubercle and extends to attach to the posteromedial surface of the lateral femoral condyle (Figures 10.83, 10.84, 10.88, 10.94, and 10.97). It helps prevent hyperextension and anterior displacement of the tibia. The **posterior cruciate ligament** is the stronger of the two and extends from the posterior aspect of the intercondylar eminence to the anteromedial surface of the medial femoral condyle. It functions to prevent hyperflexion and posterior displacement of the tibia (Figures 10.83, 10.84, 10.88, 10.89, 10.95, and 10.97).

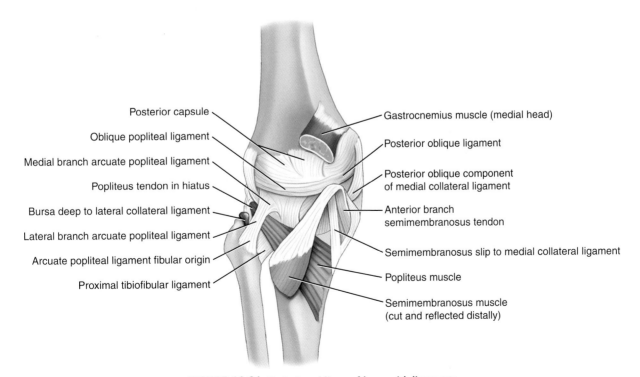

Posterior capsule
Oblique popliteal ligament
Medial branch arcuate popliteal ligament
Popliteus tendon in hiatus
Bursa deep to lateral collateral ligament
Lateral branch arcuate popliteal ligament
Arcuate popliteal ligament fibular origin
Proximal tibiofibular ligament

Gastrocnemius muscle (medial head)
Posterior oblique ligament
Posterior oblique component of medial collateral ligament
Anterior branch semimembranosus tendon
Semimembranosus slip to medial collateral ligament
Popliteus muscle
Semimembranosus muscle (cut and reflected distally)

FIGURE 10.81 Posterior oblique of knee with ligaments.

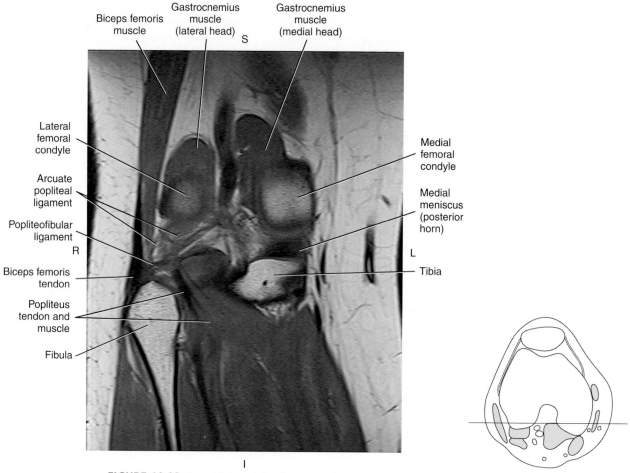

FIGURE 10.82 Coronal, T1-weighted MRI of right knee with arcuate popliteal ligament.

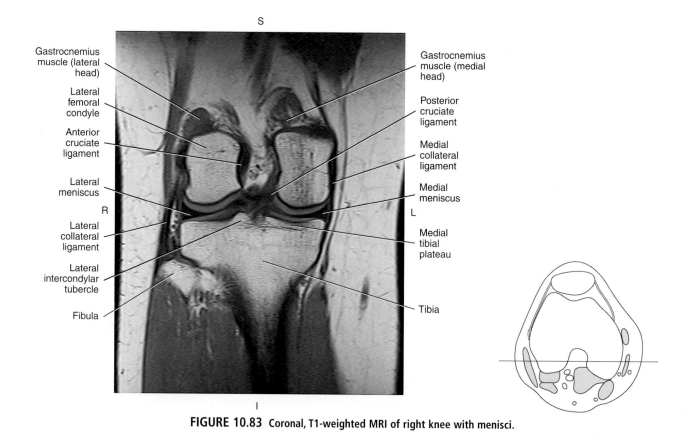

FIGURE 10.83 Coronal, T1-weighted MRI of right knee with menisci.

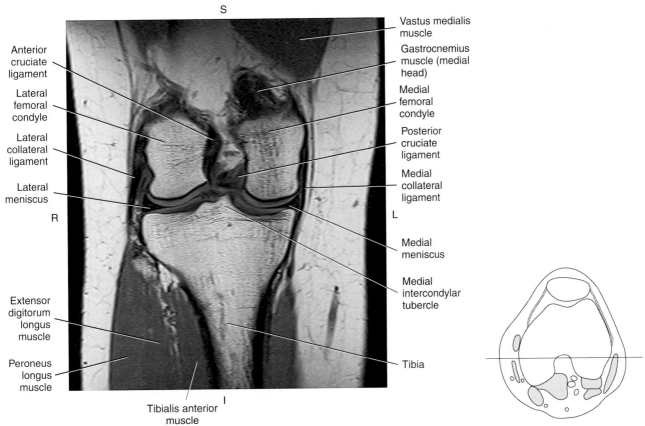

S

Vastus medialis muscle

Anterior cruciate ligament

Gastrocnemius muscle (medial head)

Lateral femoral condyle

Medial femoral condyle

Lateral collateral ligament

Posterior cruciate ligament

Lateral meniscus

Medial collateral ligament

R

L

Medial meniscus

Medial intercondylar tubercle

Extensor digitorum longus muscle

Peroneus longus muscle

Tibia

Tibialis anterior muscle

I

FIGURE 10.84 Coronal, T1-weighted MRI of right knee with collateral ligaments.

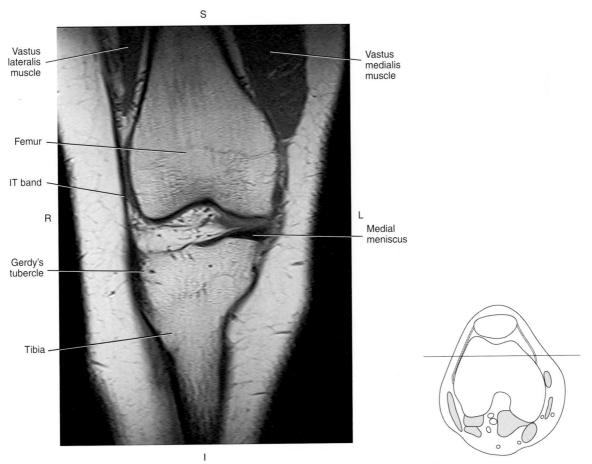

S

Vastus lateralis muscle

Vastus medialis muscle

Femur

IT band

R

L

Medial meniscus

Gerdy's tubercle

Tibia

I

FIGURE 10.85 Coronal, T1-weighted MRI of right knee with IT band.

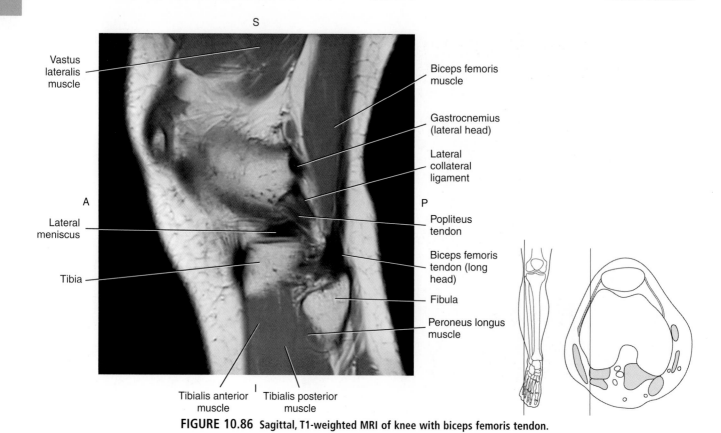

S

| Vastus lateralis muscle | | Biceps femoris muscle |

FIGURE 10.86 Sagittal, T1-weighted MRI of knee with biceps femoris tendon.

FIGURE 10.87 Sagittal, T1-weighted MRI of knee with lateral meniscus.

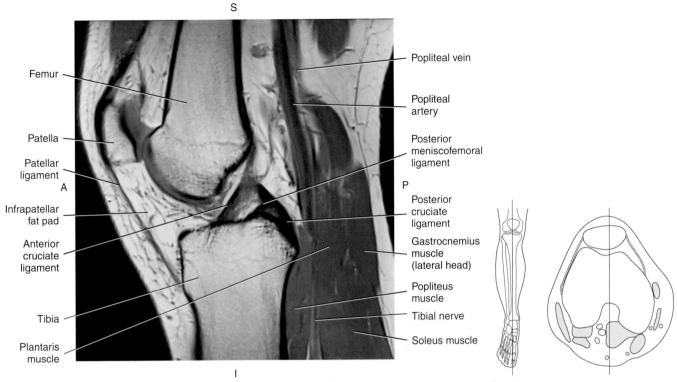

Femur

Patella

Patellar
ligament

A

Infrapatellar
fat pad

Anterior
cruciate
ligament

Tibia

Plantaris
muscle

S

Popliteal vein

Popliteal
artery

Posterior
meniscofemoral
ligament

P

Posterior
cruciate
ligament

Gastrocnemius
muscle
(lateral head)

Popliteus
muscle

Tibial nerve

Soleus muscle

I

FIGURE 10.88 Sagittal, T1-weighted MRI of knee with anterior cruciate ligament.

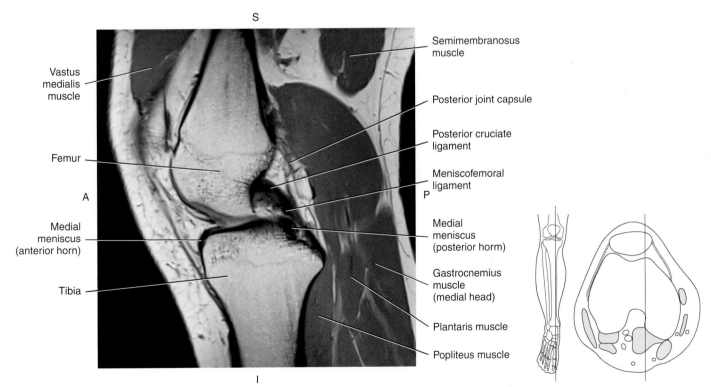

Vastus
medialis
muscle

Femur

A

Medial
meniscus
(anterior horn)

Tibia

S

Semimembranosus
muscle

Posterior joint capsule

Posterior cruciate
ligament

Meniscofemoral
ligament

P

Medial
meniscus
(posterior horn)

Gastrocnemius
muscle
(medial head)

Plantaris muscle

Popliteus muscle

I

FIGURE 10.89 Sagittal, T1-weighted MRI of knee with posterior cruciate ligament.

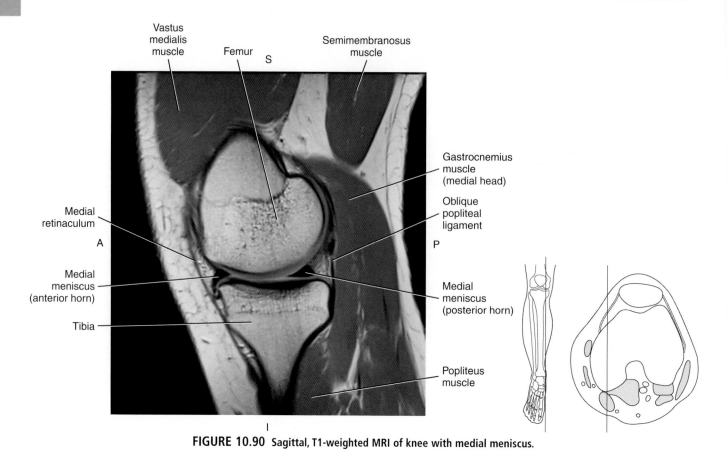

FIGURE 10.90 Sagittal, T1-weighted MRI of knee with medial meniscus.

FIGURE 10.91 Sagittal, T1-weighted MRI of knee with semimembranosus tendon.

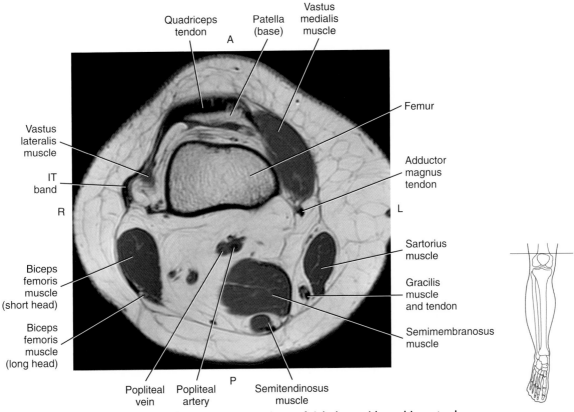

FIGURE 10.92 Axial, T1-weighted MRI of right knee with quadriceps tendon.

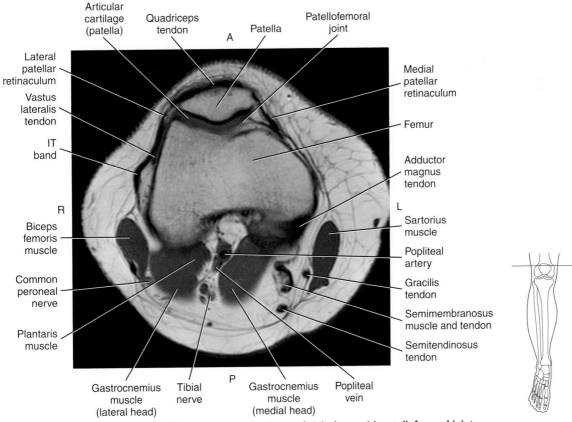

FIGURE 10.93 Axial, T1-weighted MRI of right knee with patellofemoral joint.

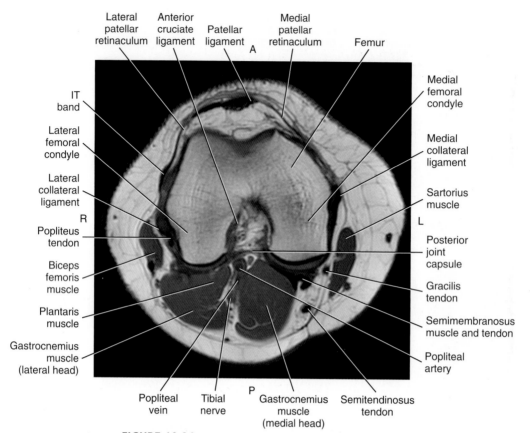

Lateral patellar retinaculum
Anterior cruciate ligament
Patellar ligament
Medial patellar retinaculum
Femur
A

IT band
Lateral femoral condyle
Lateral collateral ligament
R
Popliteus tendon
Biceps femoris muscle
Plantaris muscle
Gastrocnemius muscle (lateral head)

Medial femoral condyle
Medial collateral ligament
Sartorius muscle
L
Posterior joint capsule
Gracilis tendon
Semimembranosus muscle and tendon
Popliteal artery

Popliteal vein
Tibial nerve
P
Gastrocnemius muscle (medial head)
Semitendinosus tendon

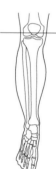

FIGURE 10.94 Axial, T1-weighted MRI of right knee with patellar ligament.

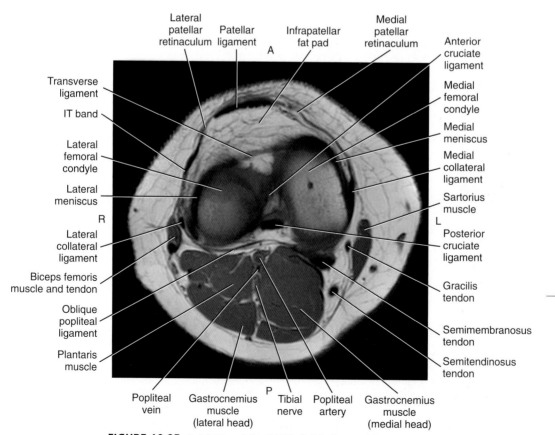

Lateral patellar retinaculum
Patellar ligament
Infrapatellar fat pad
Medial patellar retinaculum
A

Transverse ligament
IT band
Lateral femoral condyle
Lateral meniscus
R
Lateral collateral ligament
Biceps femoris muscle and tendon
Oblique popliteal ligament
Plantaris muscle

Anterior cruciate ligament
Medial femoral condyle
Medial meniscus
Medial collateral ligament
Sartorius muscle
L
Posterior cruciate ligament
Gracilis tendon
Semimembranosus tendon
Semitendinosus tendon

Popliteal vein
Gastrocnemius muscle (lateral head)
P
Tibial nerve
Popliteal artery
Gastrocnemius muscle (medial head)

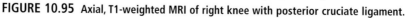

FIGURE 10.95 Axial, T1-weighted MRI of right knee with posterior cruciate ligament.

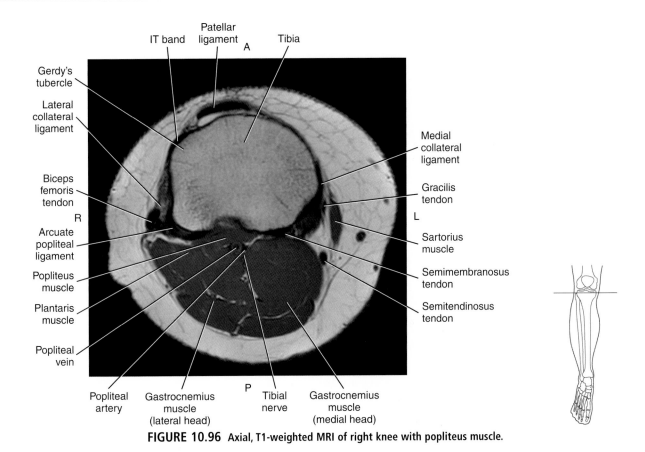

FIGURE 10.96 Axial, T1-weighted MRI of right knee with popliteus muscle.

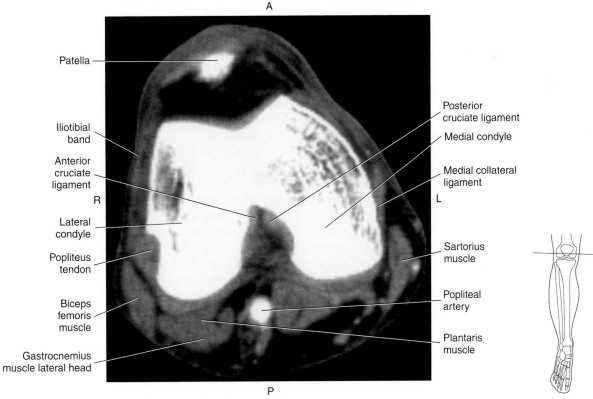

FIGURE 10.97 Axial CT scan of right knee with cruciate and collateral ligaments.

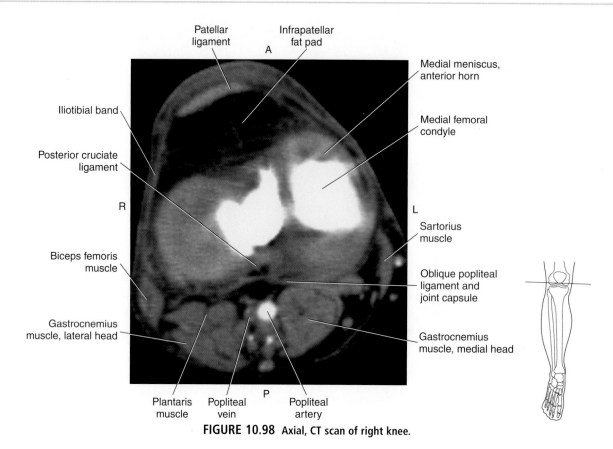

Patellar ligament

Infrapatellar fat pad

A

Medial meniscus, anterior horn

Iliotibial band

Medial femoral condyle

Posterior cruciate ligament

R

L

Sartorius muscle

Biceps femoris muscle

Oblique popliteal ligament and joint capsule

Gastrocnemius muscle, lateral head

Gastrocnemius muscle, medial head

Plantaris muscle

Popliteal vein

P

Popliteal artery

FIGURE 10.98 Axial, CT scan of right knee.

Tendons

The tendons of the sartorius, gracilis, and semitendinosus muscles merge to form a conjoined tendon commonly referred to as the **pes anserinus.** It inserts onto the anteromedial surface of the proximal tibia just superficial to the medial collateral ligament (Figures 10.64, 10.80 A, 10.85, and 10.91 through 10.96).

Bursae

There are more than 10 bursae located around the knee joint owing to the number of muscles associated with the knee. The major bursae include the suprapatellar, prepatellar, infrapatellar (superficial and deep), gastrocnemius (medial and lateral), semimembranosus, and popliteus bursae (Figure 10.99). The **suprapatellar (quadriceps) bursa** is a large extension of the synovial capsule located between the femur and the quadriceps tendon. The **prepatellar bursa** lies between the anterior surface of the patella and the skin, whereas the **superficial infrapatellar bursa** lies over the patellar ligament between the skin and the tibial tuberosity. The **deep infrapatellar bursa** is a small bursa located beneath the patellar ligament and anterior to the tibia just above the tibial tuberosity. Behind each femoral condyle is usually a bursa for the respective head of the gastrocnemius muscle. The **gastrocnemius bursae** are located between each muscle head

and the joint capsule. The **semimembranosus bursa** is located between the medial head of the gastrocnemius and semimembranosus tendon, and the small **popliteus bursa** lies between the lateral tibial condyle and the popliteus tendon. There exists a small bursa adjacent to the tendons of the pes anserinus on the anteromedial surface of the knee called the **pes anserinus bursa.** Bursae are difficult to see in cross-sectional images unless they are abnormal.

Muscles of the Lower Leg

With the exception of the popliteus, all muscles arising from the lower leg are attached to bones of the foot. The muscles of the lower leg can be classified according to their location. They are divided into **anterior** and **posterior groups** by the tibia, fibula, and interosseous membrane. The two main groups are divided again into subgroups or layers. These muscles are demonstrated in Figures 10.100 through 10.116 and described in Table 10.3.

Anterior group.   The anterior muscle group can be subdivided into the extensor group located anteriorly and the peroneus group located laterally. The **extensor group** consists of the tibialis anterior, extensor digitorum longus, extensor hallucis longus, and peroneus tertius muscles, and the **peroneus group** includes the peroneus longus and brevis muscles.

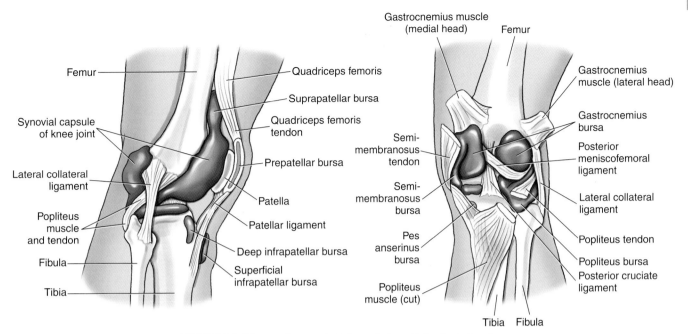

FIGURE 10.99 **Knee bursae.** *Left,* Lateral view. *Right,* Posterior view.

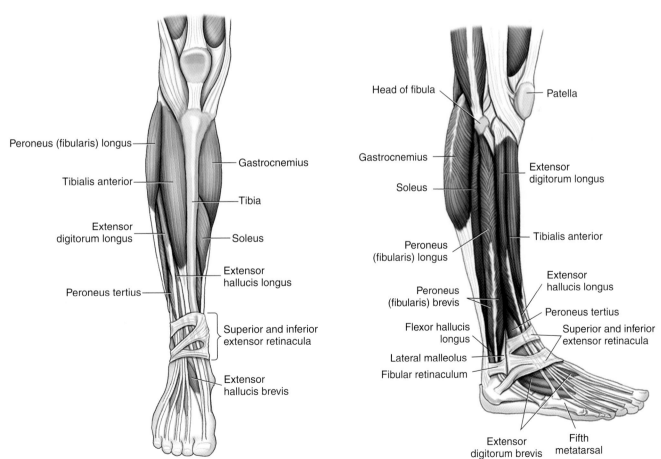

FIGURE 10.100 **Anterior view of muscles and retinacula of right lower leg.**

FIGURE 10.101 **Lateral view of superficial muscles of the right lower leg.**

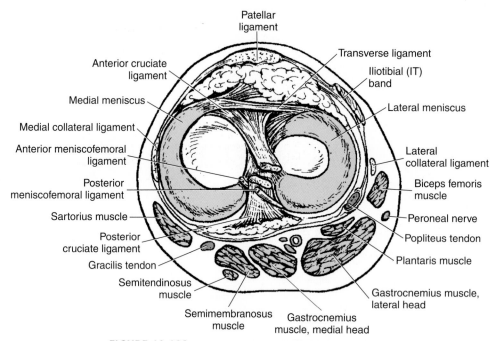

FIGURE 10.102 Axial view of knee with femoral condyles.

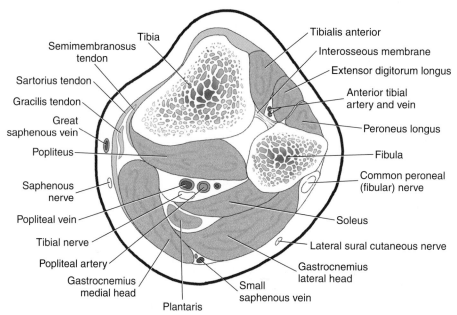

FIGURE 10.103 Axial view proximal portion of left lower leg.

Extensor group. The **tibialis anterior muscle** is a long spindle-shaped muscle located just lateral to the anterior surface of the tibia. It arises from the upper two-thirds of the lateral surface of the tibia and adjoining interosseous membrane, becoming tendinous over the lower third. The tibialis anterior runs distally and medially over the tibia to insert on the plantar surface of the medial cuneiform and first metatarsal. Its actions include dorsiflexion of the foot at the ankle joint, and together

with the tibialis posterior muscle it inverts the foot (Figures 10.100 through 10.109).

The **extensor digitorum longus muscle** is located lateral to the tibialis anterior muscle in the anterior aspect of the leg. It arises from the upper two-thirds of the fibula and adjoining interosseous membrane and the lateral condyle of the tibia. The tendon of the extensor digitorum longus passes over the front of the ankle joint and gives rise to four separate tendons at the level of the

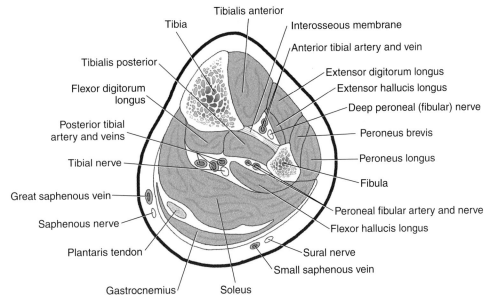

FIGURE 10.104 Axial view middle portion of left lower leg.

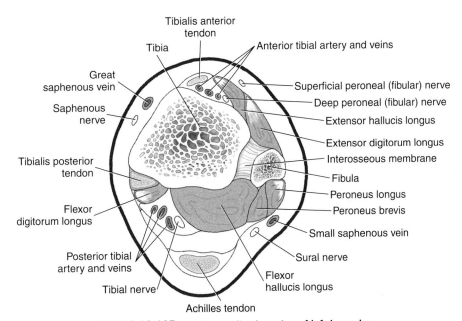

FIGURE 10.105 Axial view distal portion of left lower leg.

inferior extensor retinaculum that run to the dorsal surface of the second through fifth digits. The extensor digitorum longus muscle is an extensor of the lateral four digits at the metatarsophalangeal joints (Figures 10.100, 10.101, 10.103 through 10.109, and 10.112).

The **extensor hallucis longus muscle** lies posterior to and between the tibialis anterior and extensor digitorum longus muscles. It arises from the middle half of the anterior fibula and interosseous membrane. The tendon of

the extensor hallucis longus passes through the inferior extensor retinaculum to the base of the great toe and inserts into the distal phalanx. The extensor hallucis longus muscle extends the joints of the great toe and provides dorsiflexion of the foot at the ankle joint (Figures 10.100, 10.101, 10.104 through 10.109, and 10.112).

The **peroneus tertius muscle** is considered by some to be a distal extension of the extensor digitorum longus

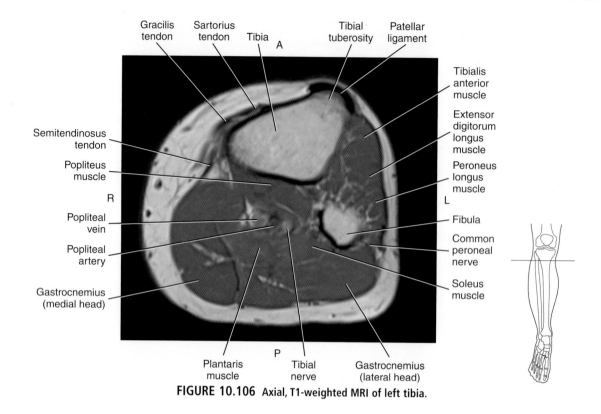

FIGURE 10.106 Axial, T1-weighted MRI of left tibia.

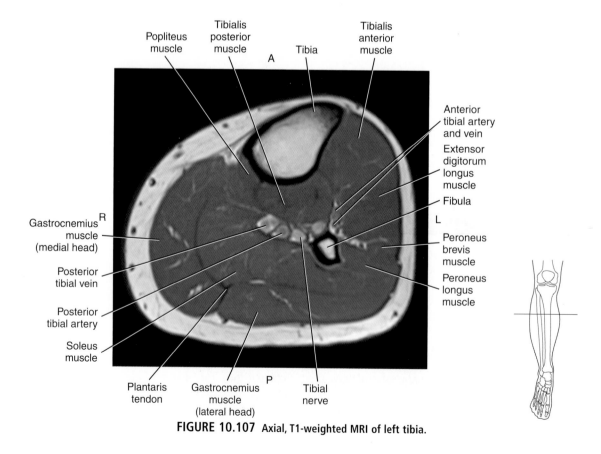

FIGURE 10.107 Axial, T1-weighted MRI of left tibia.

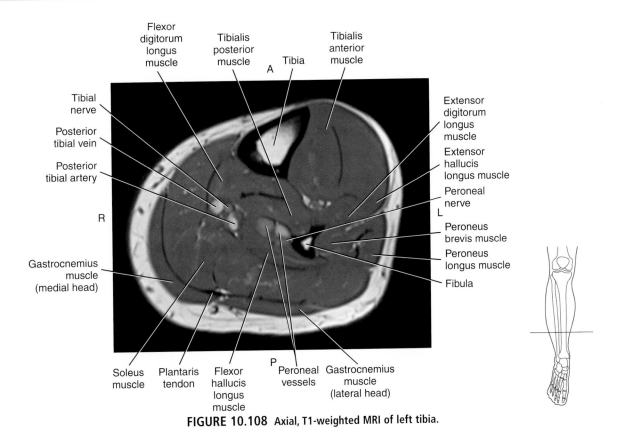

Flexor digitorum longus muscle
Tibialis posterior muscle
A
Tibia
Tibialis anterior muscle
Tibial nerve
Posterior tibial vein
Posterior tibial artery
R
Extensor digitorum longus muscle
Extensor hallucis longus muscle
Peroneal nerve
L
Peroneus brevis muscle
Peroneus longus muscle
Gastrocnemius muscle (medial head)
Fibula
Soleus muscle
Plantaris tendon
Flexor hallucis longus muscle
P
Peroneal vessels
Gastrocnemius muscle (lateral head)

FIGURE 10.108 Axial, T1-weighted MRI of left tibia.

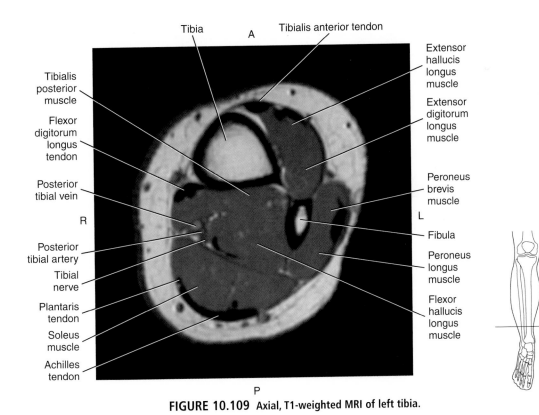

Tibia
A
Tibialis anterior tendon
Tibialis posterior muscle
Flexor digitorum longus tendon
Posterior tibial vein
R
Extensor hallucis longus muscle
Extensor digitorum longus muscle
Peroneus brevis muscle
L
Fibula
Peroneus longus muscle
Posterior tibial artery
Tibial nerve
Plantaris tendon
Soleus muscle
Achilles tendon
Flexor hallucis longus muscle
P

FIGURE 10.109 Axial, T1-weighted MRI of left tibia.

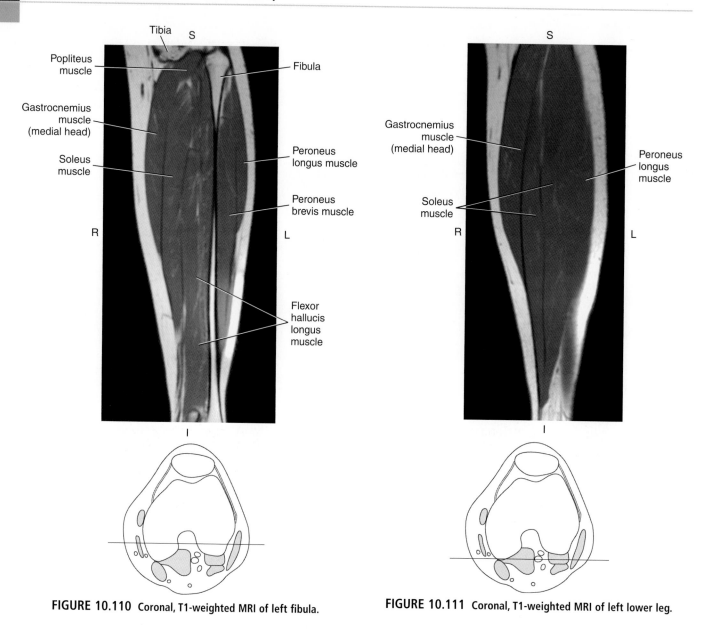

FIGURE 10.110 Coronal, T1-weighted MRI of left fibula.

FIGURE 10.111 Coronal, T1-weighted MRI of left lower leg.

muscle. It arises from the anterior surface of the lower fibula, and its tendon inserts on the dorsal aspect of the base of the fifth metatarsal. This muscle functions as a weak evertor and dorsiflexor of the foot at the ankle joint (Figures 10.100 and 10.101).

Peroneus group. The two peroneus muscles act as plantar flexors but also stabilize the lateral ankle and longitudinal arch of the foot (Figures 10.100 and 10.101). The **peroneus (fibularis) longus muscle** is located on the lateral side of the leg arising from the tibiofibular joint, the head of the fibula, and the lateral condyle of the tibia. The peroneus longus has a long belly and an even longer tendon. The tendon of the peroneus longus runs in a shallow groove behind the lateral malleolus, passing below the peroneal tubercle of the calcaneus and across lower lateral side of the cuboid. It then runs obliquely across the sole of the

foot to insert on the base of the first metatarsal and lateral surface of the medial cuneiform (Figures 10.100, 10.101, 10.103 through 10.111, and 10.114 through 10.116).

The **peroneus (fibularis) brevis muscle** is shorter and smaller than its counterpart. It lies under the peroneus longus, arising from the distal two-thirds of the lateral surface of the fibula. The tendon of the peroneus brevis accompanies the tendon of the peroneus longus in a common synovial sheath behind the lateral malleolus, with the peroneus brevis just anterior to the peroneus longus. At approximately the level of the peroneal tubercle of the calcaneus, the tendons separate into their own synovial sheath, with the peroneus brevis tendon attaching to the base of the fifth metatarsal (Figures 10.100, 10.103 through 10.111, and 10.114 through 10.116).

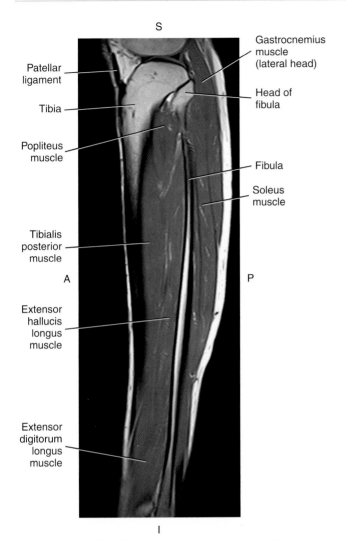

FIGURE 10.112 Sagittal, T1-weighted MRI of fibula.

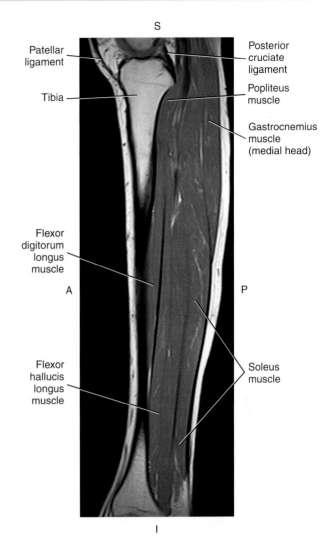

FIGURE 10.113 Sagittal, T1-weighted MRI of tibia.

Posterior group. The posterior group is functionally considered the **flexors,** which are responsible for plantar flexion of the foot. This group is subdivided into the superficial layer consisting of the gastrocnemius, soleus, and plantaris muscles, and the deep layer with the tibialis posterior, flexor hallucis longus, flexor digitorum longus, and popliteus muscles. These muscles are demonstrated in Figures 10.101 through 10.116 and described in Table 10.3.

Superficial layer. The **gastrocnemius muscle** is a prominent flexor of the foot and is responsible for giving the calf its shape on the back of the leg. It consists of two heads arising from the medial and lateral femoral condyles. The medial head arises from the medial supracondylar ridge and adductor tubercle on the popliteal surface of the femur. The lateral head arises just behind the lateral epicondyle on the outer surface of the lateral

femoral condyle. The two heads form the lower boundaries of the popliteal fossa, and their fibers run distally where they join the tendon of the soleus muscle to form the **Achilles tendon,** which inserts on the calcaneal tuberosity (Figures 10.101 through 10.116).

The **soleus muscle** is a broad, flat muscle located beneath the gastrocnemius. It arises from the soleal line on the posterior tibia and the upper third of the fibula. The muscle fibers run distally and merge with the tendon of the gastrocnemius to form the superficial Achilles tendon (Figures 10.101, 10.103, 10.104, and 10.106 through 10.116).

The **plantaris muscle** is a long, thin muscle that arises from the lowest part of the lateral supracondylar ridge, the adjacent popliteal surface, and the joint capsule. The tendon runs inferiorly between the gastrocnemius and soleus muscles, following the medial edge of the Achilles

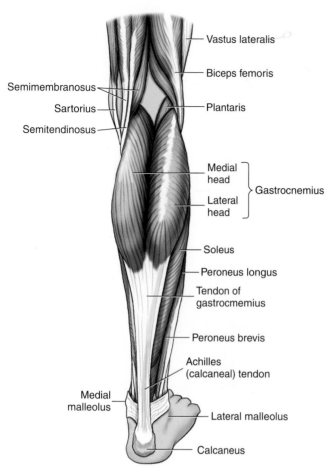

FIGURE 10.114 Posterior view of superficial muscles of leg.

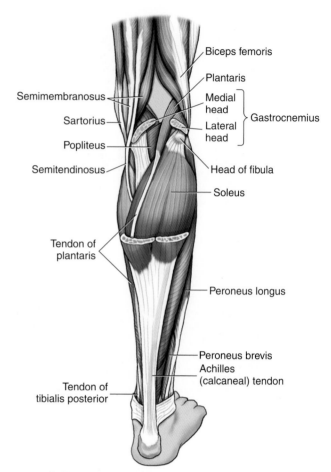

FIGURE 10.115 Posterior view of soleus muscle.

tendon (Figures 10.102 through 10.104, 10.106, and 10.114 through 10.116).

Deep layer. The **tibialis posterior muscle** is the deepest muscle located on the back of the leg. It arises from the superolateral surface of the posterior tibia just below the soleal line, the interosseous membrane, and the posterior surface of the fibula. The tendon of the tibialis posterior passes through the malleolar groove of the tibia behind the medial malleolus to attach to the tuberosity of the navicular and plantar surface of the medial cuneiform bones (Figures 10.104, 10.105, 10.107 through 10.109, 10.112, and 10.116).

The **flexor hallucis longus muscle** is a powerful muscle located beneath the gastrocnemius and soleus muscles. It arises from the distal two-thirds of the posterior fibula, the interosseous membrane, and adjacent fascia. The tendon of the flexor hallucis longus runs distally, crossing over the dorsal aspect of the ankle, through the malleolar groove of the tibia to the sole of the foot, where it inserts into the base of the distal phalanx of the

first toe (Figures 10.104, 10.105, 10.108 through 10.110, and 10.113).

The **flexor digitorum longus muscle** arises from the posterior surface of the body of the tibia immediately below the soleal line. The muscle descends along the tibial side of the leg to become tendinous just above the medial malleolus. The tendon of the flexor digitorum longus passes behind the medial malleolus to the sole of the foot, deep to the flexor hallucis longus, and divides into four individual tendons that insert into the bases of the distal phalanges of the second through fifth digits (Figures 10.104, 10.105, 10.108, 10.109, 10.113, and 10.116).

The **popliteus muscle** is a thin triangular muscle that forms the lower floor of the popliteal fossa. It arises just below the lateral femoral epicondyle and extends obliquely to the triangular surface above the soleal (popliteal) line on the posterior tibia (Figures 10.103, 10.106, 10.107, 10.110, 10.112, 10.113, 10.115, and 10.116).

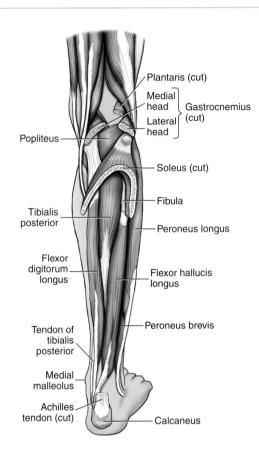

Plantaris (cut)
Medial head ⎤
Lateral head ⎦ Gastrocnemius (cut)
Popliteus
Soleus (cut)
Fibula
Tibialis posterior
Peroneus longus
Flexor digitorum longus
Flexor hallucis longus
Peroneus brevis
Tendon of tibialis posterior
Medial malleolus
Achilles tendon (cut)
Calcaneus

FIGURE 10.116 Posterior view of deep muscles of leg.

TABLE 10.3	Muscles of the Lower Leg		
Muscle	**Proximal Insertion**	**Distal Insertion**	**Action**
Anterior Group *Extensor Group*			
Tibialis anterior	Lateral tibia, upper two-thirds	Medial cuneiform, first metatarsal	Dorsiflexion of foot
Extensor digitorum longus	Proximal fibula	Second-fifth digits of foot	Extensor of lateral four digits at the metatarsophalangeal joints
Extensor hallucis longus	Anterior fibula and interosseous membrane	Distal phalanx of first toe	Extends joints of first toe and dorsiflexion of foot
Peroneus Group			
Peroneus tertius	Distal fibula	Fifth metatarsal	Evertor and dorsiflexion of the foot
Peroneus longus	Tibiofibular joint, head of fibula, and lateral condyle of tibia	First metatarsal and medial cuneiform	Plantar flexion and stabilizer of ankle
Peroneus brevis	Lateral surface of distal fibula	Fifth metatarsal	Plantar flexion and stabilizer of ankle
Posterior Group *Superficial Layer*			
Gastrocnemius		Calcaneal tuberosity	Flexor of the foot
Medial head	Supracondylar ridge and adductor tubercle	Joins soleus tendon at Achilles tendon	
Lateral head	Lateral epicondyle of femur	Joins soleus tendon at Achilles tendon	
Soleus	Soleal line of tibia and proximal fibula	Achilles tendon	Flexor of the foot
Plantaris	Lateral supracondylar ridge	Achilles tendon or calcaneus	Flexor of the foot
Tibialis posterior	Posterior tibia, interosseous membrane, and posterior fibula	Navicular and medial cuneiform	Flexor of the foot
Deep Layer			
Flexor hallucis longus	Posterior fibula, interosseous membrane, and adjacent fascia	Distal phalanx of first toe	Flexor of the foot
Flexor digitorum longus	Body of tibia below soleal line	Distal phalanges of second-fifth toes	Flexor of the foot
Popliteus	Lateral femoral epicondyle	Posterior, proximal tibia	Flexor of the foot

ANKLE AND FOOT

Bony Anatomy

The bony anatomy of the ankle and foot includes the tarsals, metatarsals, and phalanges. The tarsals consist of seven bones: talus, calcaneus, navicular, cuboid, and three cuneiform bones. Five metatarsals and 14 phalanges make up the toes (Figures 10.117 through 10.141).
Tarsals. The **talus** (**astragalus**) is the second largest tarsal bone. Together with the calcaneus, it is responsible for transmitting the entire weight of the body to the foot. The talus consists of a body, head, and neck. The **body** is

wedge-shaped with an upper articular surface (trochlea) that is wider in front than in back (Figures 10.117, 10.118, 10.121, and 10.122). The trochlea provides articulation with the tibia and fibula (Figures 10.121 through 10.128). The **head** faces anteriorly to articulate with the navicular bone (Figure 10.121). The largest tarsal bone is the **calcaneus**, which lies beneath the talus. It has an elongated cuboid shape with a posterior surface comprising the prominence of the heel. On the medial surface of the calcaneus is a shelflike process termed the **sustentaculum tali**, which provides support for the talus (Figures 10.119, 10.120, and 10.124 through 10.126). On the plantar surface of the posterior calcaneus is the

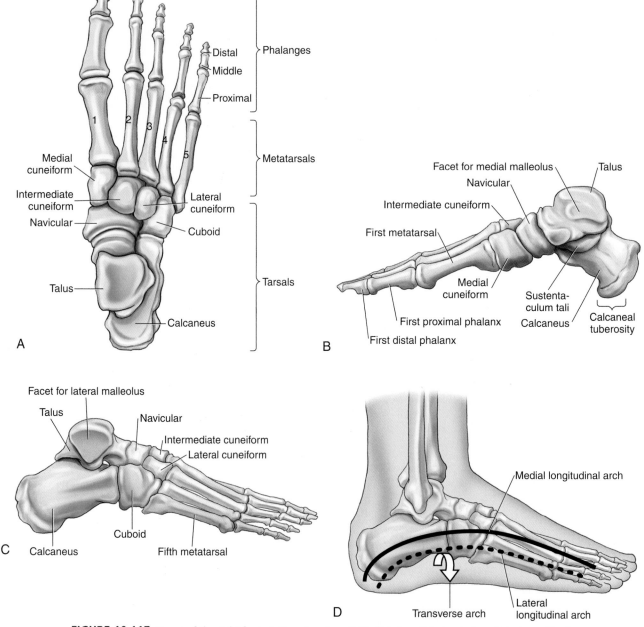

FIGURE 10.117   Bones of the right foot. A, Superior view. B, Medial view. C, Lateral view. D, Arches of foot.

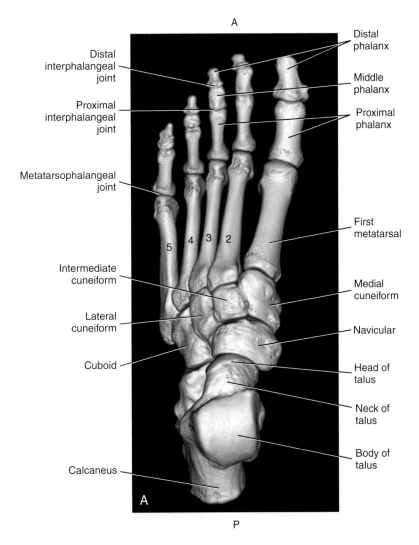

Distal
interphalangeal
joint

Proximal
interphalangeal
joint

Metatarsophalangeal
joint

Intermediate
cuneiform

Lateral
cuneiform

Cuboid

Calcaneus

A

P

Distal
phalanx

Middle
phalanx

Proximal
phalanx

First
metatarsal

Medial
cuneiform

Navicular

Head of
talus

Neck of
talus

Body of
talus

5 4 3 2

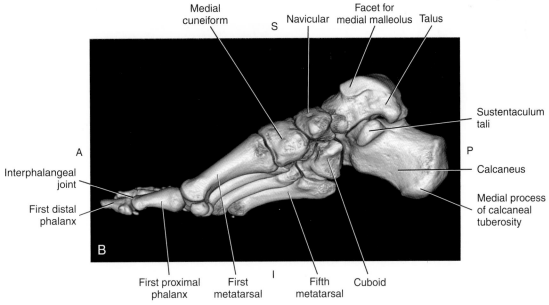

Medial
cuneiform

S

Navicular

Facet for
medial malleolus Talus

Sustentaculum
tali

A

Calcaneus

P

Interphalangeal
joint

First distal
phalanx

B

Medial process
of calcaneal
tuberosity

First proximal
phalanx

First
metatarsal

I

Fifth
metatarsal

Cuboid

FIGURE 10.118 A, 3D CT of foot, superior view. B, 3D CT of foot, medial view.

(Continued)

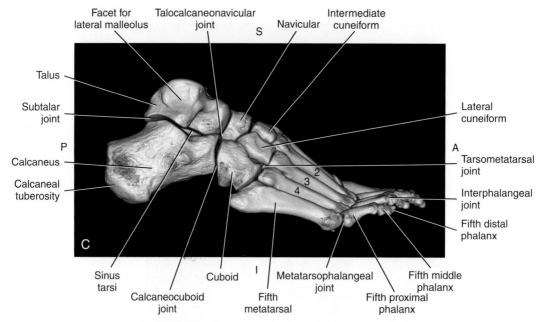

FIGURE 10.118, cont'd   C, 3D CT of foot, lateral view.

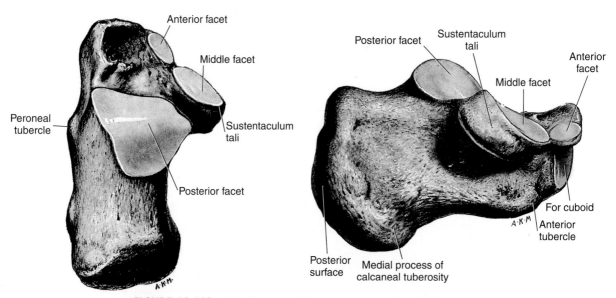

FIGURE 10.119   Left calcaneus. *Left,* Dorsal aspect. *Right,* Medial aspect.

large **calcaneal tuberosity** for insertion of ligaments and tendons, the largest being the Achilles tendon (Figures 10.119 through 10.123). The articulation between the talus and calcaneus is termed the **subtalar joint,** which is composed of three articulations formed by the **anterior, middle,** and **posterior facets** (Figures 10.119 and 10.120). The smallest of the three is the anterior facet, which can be independent of or continuous with the middle facet. The middle facet lies on a ledge of bone projecting off the medial surface of the calcaneus at the sustentaculum tali (Figures 10.119, 10.120, 10.125, and 10.126). This shelf

and the entire middle facet joint provide weight-bearing support to the medial side of the ankle. The posterior facet joint is the largest and provides support for most of the body of the talus (Figures 10.119 through 10.123). Separating this facet from the middle facet is the **tarsal canal.** This canal contains blood vessels, fat, and the interosseous talocalcaneal ligament widens laterally to form the **sinus tarsi,** which contains the cervical ligament (Figures 10.121 through 10.124, 10.139, and 10.140). In addition to the talus and calcaneus, the cuboid, navicular, and three cuneiform bones make up the remaining five

A

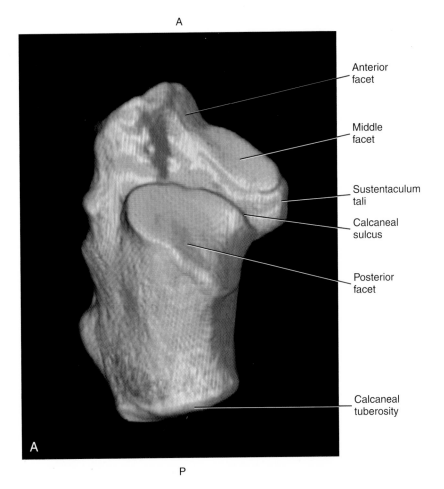

Anterior
facet

Middle
facet

Sustentaculum
tali

Calcaneal
sulcus

Posterior
facet

Calcaneal
tuberosity

A

P

Anterior facet   Middle facet   Posterior facet

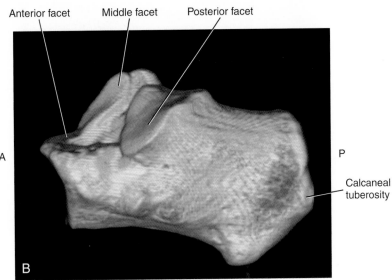

A

P

Calcaneal
tuberosity

B

FIGURE 10-120 A, 3D CT of calcaneus, dorsal view. B, 3D CT of calcaneus, lateral view.

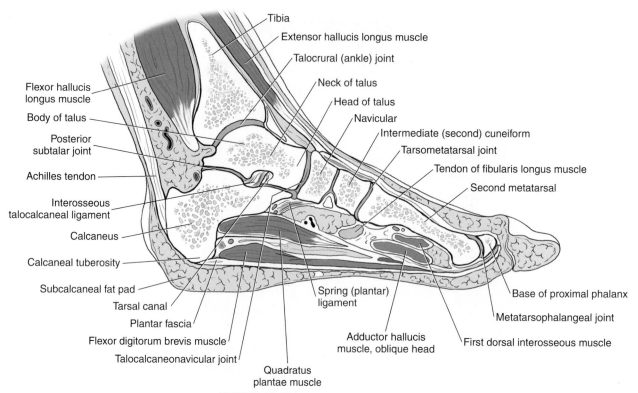

FIGURE 10.121 Sagittal section of foot.

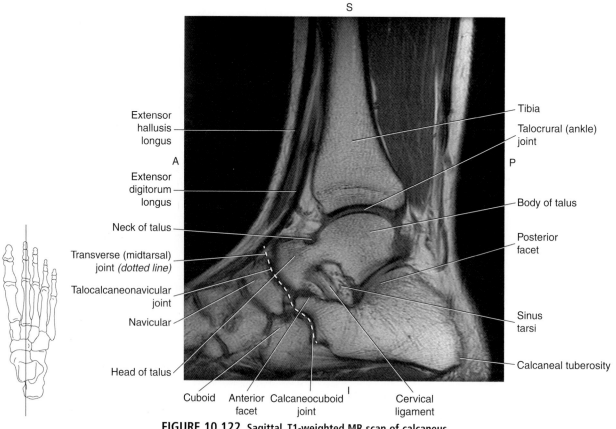

FIGURE 10.122 Sagittal, T1-weighted MR scan of calcaneus.

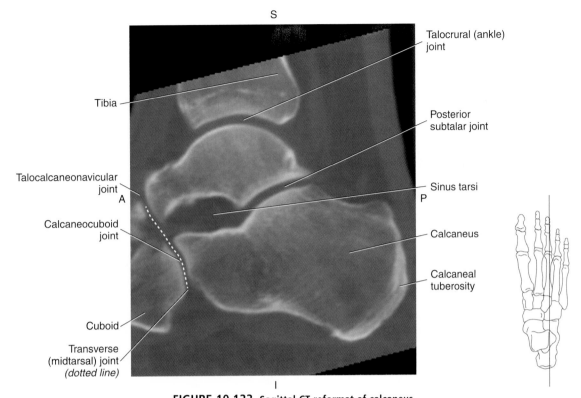

S

Tibia

Talocalcaneonavicular
joint

A

Calcaneocuboid
joint

Cuboid

Transverse
(midtarsal) joint
(dotted line)

I

Talocrural (ankle)
joint

Posterior
subtalar joint

Sinus tarsi

P

Calcaneus

Calcaneal
tuberosity

FIGURE 10.123 Sagittal CT reformat of calcaneus.

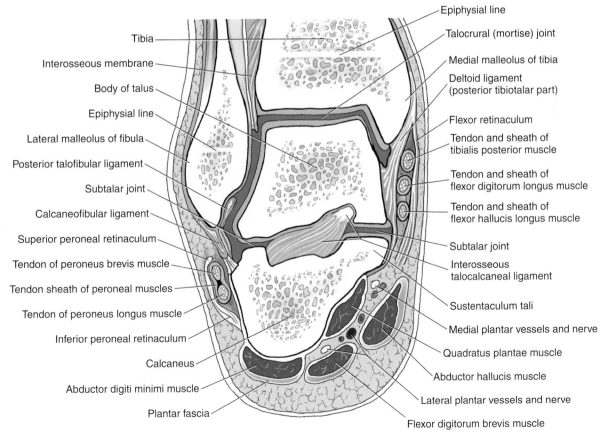

Tibia

Interosseous membrane

Body of talus

Epiphysial line

Lateral malleolus of fibula

Posterior talofibular ligament

Subtalar joint

Calcaneofibular ligament

Superior peroneal retinaculum

Tendon of peroneus brevis muscle

Tendon sheath of peroneal muscles

Tendon of peroneus longus muscle

Inferior peroneal retinaculum

Calcaneus

Abductor digiti minimi muscle

Plantar fascia

Epiphysial line

Talocrural (mortise) joint

Medial malleolus of tibia

Deltoid ligament
(posterior tibiotalar part)

Flexor retinaculum

Tendon and sheath of
tibialis posterior muscle

Tendon and sheath of
flexor digitorum longus muscle

Tendon and sheath of
flexor hallucis longus muscle

Subtalar joint

Interosseous
talocalcaneal ligament

Sustentaculum tali

Medial plantar vessels and nerve

Quadratus plantae muscle

Abductor hallucis muscle

Lateral plantar vessels and nerve

Flexor digitorum brevis muscle

FIGURE 10.124 Coronal view of subtalar joint.

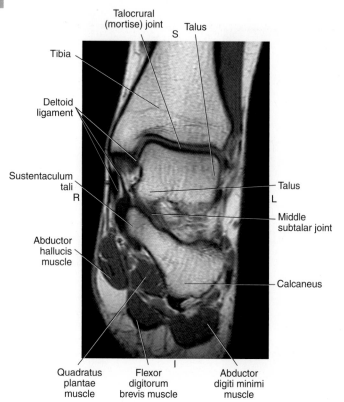

FIGURE 10.125 Coronal, T1-weighted MRI of talocrural joint, left ankle.

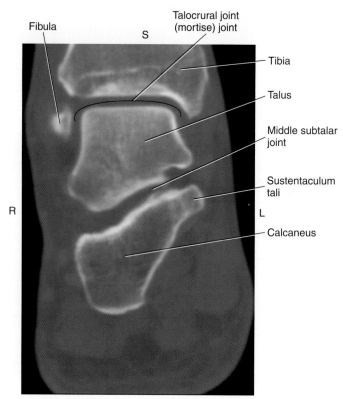

FIGURE 10.126 Coronal CT reformat of subtalar joint, right ankle.

tarsal bones of the foot (Figures 10.117, 10.118, and 10.129 through 10.141). Lateral and anterior to the calcaneus is the **cuboid bone**, which articulates anteriorly with the bases of the fourth and fifth metatarsal bones. The **navicular bone** articulates posteriorly with the talus and anteriorly with the cuneiform bones on the medial side of the foot. The three **cuneiform bones** medial, intermediate, and lateral articulate anteriorly with the first three metatarsal bones.

Sinus Tarsi Syndrome

Sinus tarsi syndrome is a common syndrome associated with post-traumatic lateral hindfoot pain. The interosseous ligament, when injured due to lateral ankle sprains or an inflammatory process, such as arthritis, can lead to characteristic pain. Sinus tarsi syndrome treatment may include anti-inflammatory medication, a period of immobilization, or injection of local anesthetic.

Metatarsals. The metatarsals are long, slender bones. There are five metatarsals in each foot, with each bone having a distal head, proximal base, and body or shaft in between. The heads articulate with the proximal phalanges of the toes and the bases articulate with the tarsals (Figures 10.117, 10.118, 10.129 through 10.132, and 10.136 through 10.141).

Phalanges. Each foot has 14 phalanges—3 phalanges for each toe (proximal, middle, distal), except the great toe, which has just 2 (proximal and distal). The phalanges of the toes are shorter and stouter than their counterparts in the fingers (Figures 10.117, 10.118, 10.131, 10.132, and 10.139).

Joints

The joints of the ankle and foot include the talocrural (ankle) joint, intertarsal, tarsometatarsal and intermetatarsal, metatarsophalangeal, and interphalangeal joints. The joints of the ankle and foot are demonstrated in Figures 10.118 and 10.121 through 10.141.

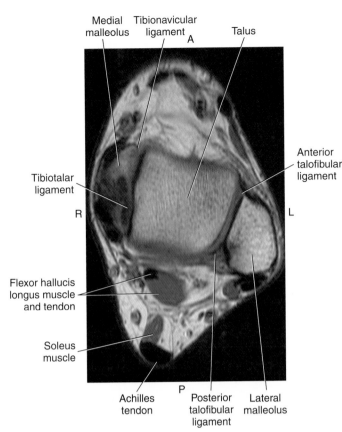

FIGURE 10.127 Axial, T1-weighted MRI of left ankle.

Medial malleolus
Tibionavicular ligament
Talus
Anterior talofibular ligament
Tibiotalar ligament
Flexor hallucis longus muscle and tendon
Soleus muscle
Achilles tendon
Posterior talofibular ligament
Lateral malleolus

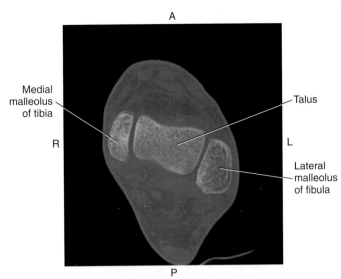

FIGURE 10.128 Axial CT of left ankle.

Medial malleolus of tibia
Talus
Lateral malleolus of fibula

Talocrural. The **talocrural joint (ankle joint)** is created by the articulations between the tibia, fibula, and talus (astragalus). The tibia and fibula rest on the trochlear surface of the talus to form what is commonly termed the **mortise joint**, which allows for dorsal and plantar flexion. Both the tibia and fibula terminate distally in projections termed **malleoli**, which prevent medial and lateral displacement of the talus (Figures 10.121 through 10.126).

Intertarsal. The **intertarsal joints** are created by the articulations between the tarsal bones and include the subtalar, talocalcaneonavicular, calcaneocuboid, transverse (midtarsal), cuneonavicular, intercuneiform, and the cuneocuboid joints. The **subtalar joint** consists of the articulation between the talus and calcaneus and was discussed under bony anatomy (Figures 10.121 through 10.123). The subtalar joint provides the ability to invert and evert the foot. The **talocalcaneonavicular** and **calcaneocuboid** joints combine to form the **transverse** or **midtarsal joint**. This joint provides an irregular plane

across the foot extending from side to side, with the talus and calcaneus located posteriorly and the navicular and cuboid located anteriorly (Figures 10.122 and 10.123). The transverse tarsal joint plays an important part in putting the spring in your step by acting as a shock absorber during the push-off phase of walking or running. The cuneonavicular, intercuneiform, and cuneocuboid joints contribute to the flexibility of the foot by providing a slight gliding movement between bones.

Tarsometatarsal. The **tarsometatarsal joints** exist between the bases of all five metatarsals and the anterior four tarsal bones (cuboid, three cuneiforms). The articulations between the tarsals and metatarsals permit only limited gliding movement between the bones (Figures 10.121 and 10.129 through 10.132). The **intermetatarsal joints** are the articulations between the bases of the lateral four metatarsals. The intermetatarsal joints permit a small degree of gliding between metatarsals and contribute to eversion and inversion of the foot (Figure 10.131).

Metatarsophalangeal joints. The heads of the metatarsals articulate with the bases of the proximal phalanges at the metatarsophalangeal joints (Figures 10.121, 10.131, and 10.140). This articulation provides flexion and extension of the toes.

Interphalangeal joints. The heads of the phalanges articulate with the bases of the more distal phalanges to create the interphalangeal joints. The interphalangeal joints are hinge joints that permit plantar and dorsiflexion of the phalanges (Figure 10.118).

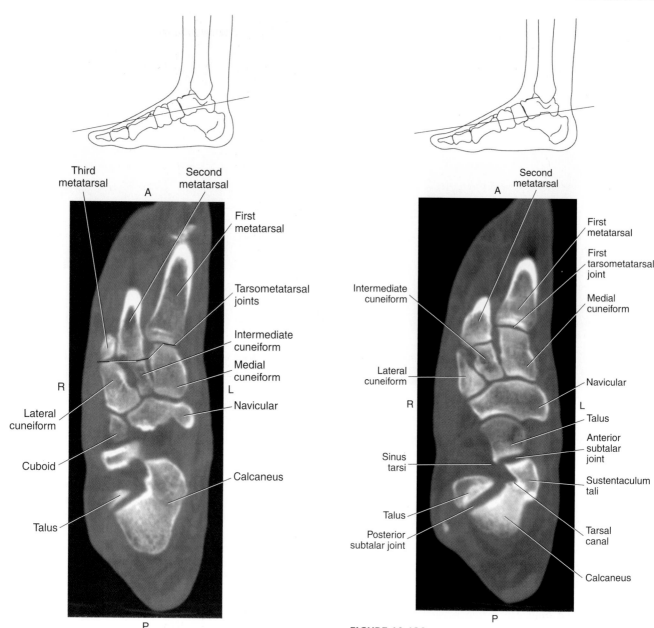

FIGURE 10.129 Axial CT of left ankle and foot with navicular bone.

FIGURE 10.130 Axial CT of left ankle and foot with cuneiform bones.

Arches

The bones of the foot are arranged in transverse and longitudinal arches that provide flexibility and resilience to the foot to support the weight of the body, absorb shocks, and provide spring and lift during activity (Figure 10.117 B through D). The **longitudinal arch** (**plantar arch**) has two parts: one on the lateral side of the foot (**lateral longitudinal arch**) and one on the medial side of the foot (**medial longitudinal arch**). The bony landmarks for the medial longitudinal arch are the head of the first metatarsal anteriorly and the calcaneal tuberosity posteriorly. On the lateral side the bony landmarks include the head of the fifth metatarsal anteriorly and the

calcaneal tuberosity posteriorly. The medial longitudinal arch is more elastic and is associated with greater curvature, whereas the lateral longitudinal arch is flatter and less flexible because it makes contact with the ground. The longitudinal arches provide a firm base for support of the body in the upright position. The **transverse arch** is formed by the distal row of tarsal bones (cuboid, three cuneiforms) and the bases of the metatarsals that create a domed curve across the foot. The transverse arch is the major weight-bearing arch of the foot and helps to distribute body weight over the base of the foot. The integrity of arches is maintained by the tarsal, tarsometatarsal, and intermetatarsal joints and their supporting ligaments (Figure 10.117 D).

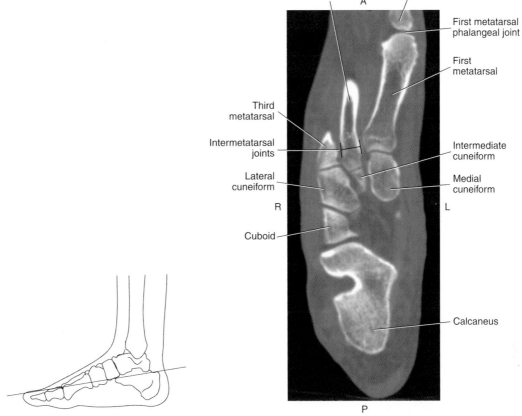

FIGURE 10.131 Axial CT scan of left ankle and foot with cuboid bone.

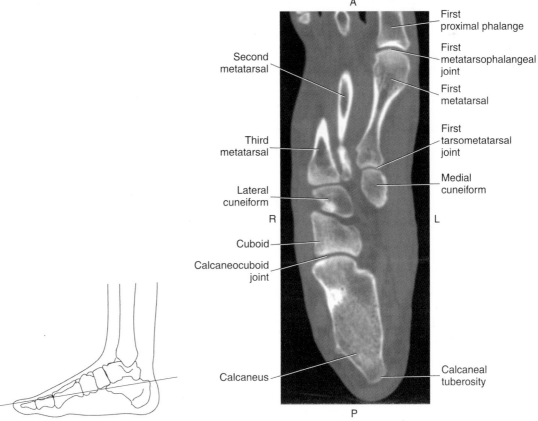

FIGURE 10.132 Axial CT of left ankle and foot with calcaneus.

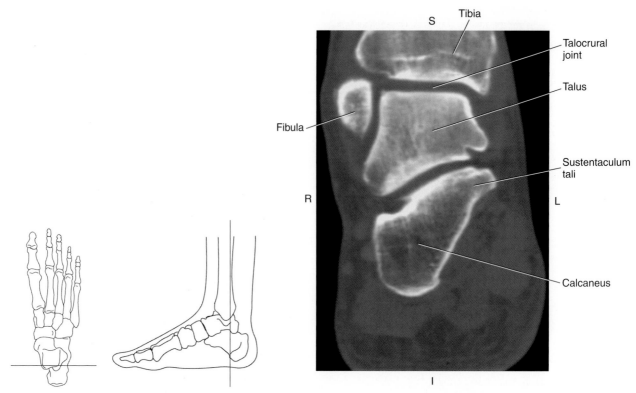

FIGURE 10.133 Coronal CT reformat of right ankle and foot with talus.

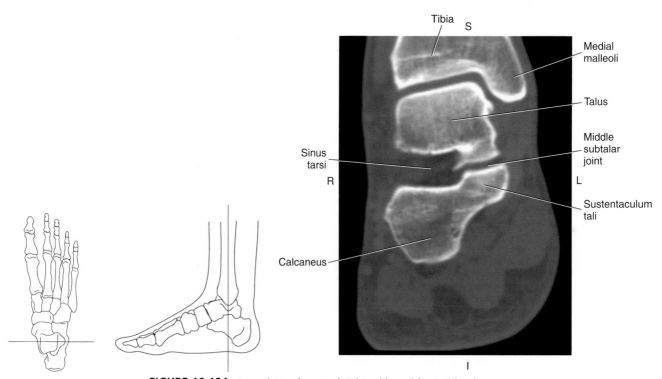

FIGURE 10.134 Coronal CT reformat of right ankle and foot with calcaneus.

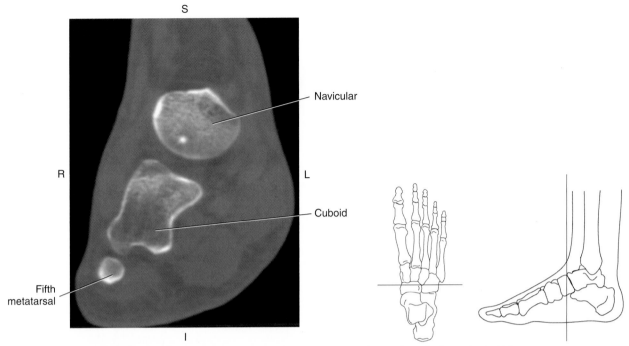

FIGURE 10.135 Coronal CT reformat of right ankle and foot with navicular and cuboid bones.

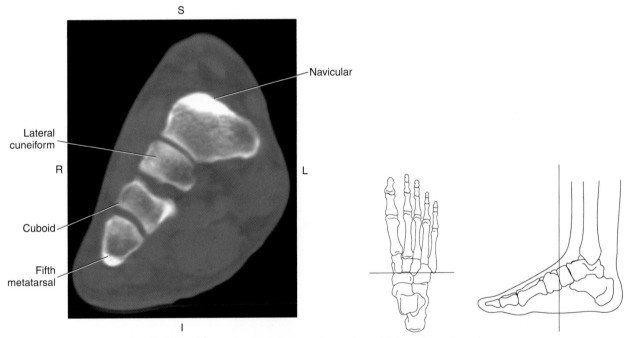

FIGURE 10.136 Coronal CT reformat of right foot with lateral cuneiform bone.

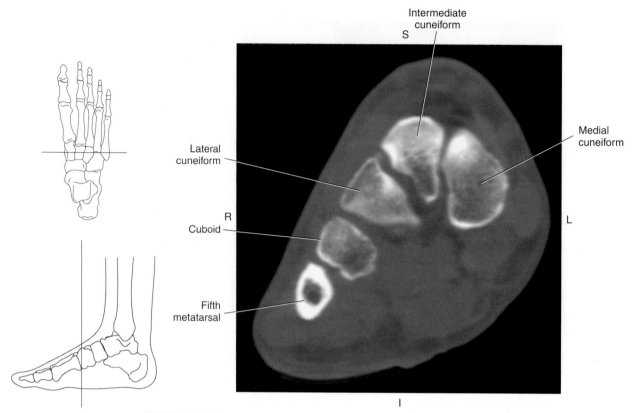

FIGURE 10.137 Coronal CT reformat of right foot with cuneiform bones.

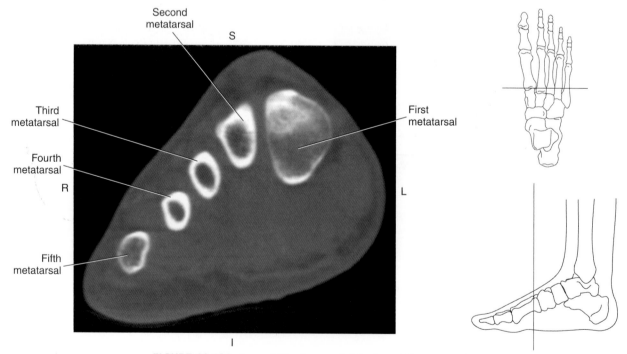

FIGURE 10.138 Coronal CT reformat of right foot with metatarsals.

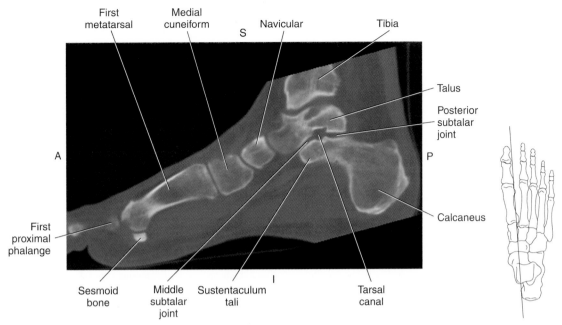

FIGURE 10.139 Sagittal CT reformat of ankle and foot, medial aspect.

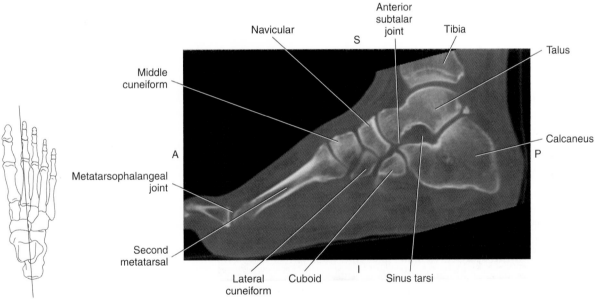

FIGURE 10.140 Sagittal CT reformat of ankle and foot with talus.

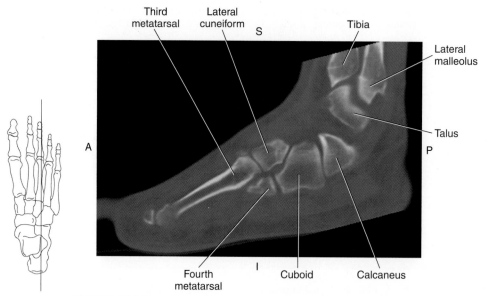

Third metatarsal

Lateral cuneiform

S

Tibia

Lateral malleolus

A

Talus

P

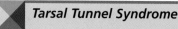

Fourth metatarsal

I

Cuboid

Calcaneus

FIGURE 10.141 Sagittal CT reformat of ankle and foot, lateral aspect.

Retinacula, Fascia, and Ligaments

Retinacula. As in the wrist, fascia in various regions of the ankle will thicken to form retinacula. The retinacula form sheaths for stabilizing tendons crossing over the joints of the ankle. They are called the flexor, extensor, and peroneal retinacula, after the tendons they serve (Figures 10.142, 10.144, and 10.145). The **flexor retinaculum** is located between the medial malleolus and the medial tubercle of the calcaneus. It forms four tunnels, collectively called the **tarsal tunnel,** for the passage of the tendons of the tibialis posterior, flexor digitorum longus, and flexor hallucis longus muscles, as well as the posterior tibial vessels and nerve. The **extensor retinaculum** consists of two portions: an upper portion (superior extensor retinacula) and lower portion (inferior extensor retinacula). The **superior extensor retinaculum** runs horizontally between the tibia and fibula just above the ankle joint. It extends over the tendons of the tibialis anterior and extensor hallucis muscles. The **inferior extensor retinaculum** splits into two bands that extend across the dorsum of the foot, originating from the upper surface of the calcaneus and sinus tarsi. The upper band of the inferior extensor retinaculum attaches to the medial malleolus, whereas the lower band extends to the fascia on the medial side of the foot. The tendons of the extensor digitorum longus and peroneus tertius muscles run deep to the inferior extensor retinaculum. The **peroneal retinacula** split into two bands, forming the superior and inferior peroneal retinaculum. The **superior peroneal retinaculum** extends from the lateral side of the calcaneus to the posterior border of the lateral malleolus. The **inferior peroneal retinaculum** extends from the lateral side of the calcaneus to blend with the fibers of the inferior extensor retinaculum. The superior and inferior peroneal retinacula transmit the tendons for the peroneus brevis and peroneus longus muscles (Figures 10.142, 10.144, and 10.145).

Fascia. In addition to the retinacula, another area of thickened fascia is located on the plantar surface of the foot. The **plantar fascia (aponeurosis)** is approximately 80 layers thick, creating some of the thickest fascia within the human body. It begins at the inferior aspect of the calcaneus and spreads anteriorly into five separate slips that create the fibrous flexor sheaths of the toes (Figures 10.121 and 10.124). The plantar fascia is extremely important for maintaining the longitudinal arch of the foot.

Ligaments. Other support structures of the ankle and foot include a complex architecture of multiple ligaments that provide necessary stability. The ligaments of the ankle and foot can be identified in Figures 10.143 through 10.161. The main support structures of the ankle include the deltoid ligament, lateral ligaments, spring (plantar) ligament, and interosseous ligament. The **deltoid ligament** provides medial support and is the strongest ligament in the ankle joint. It arises from the medial malleolus and fans out into deep and superficial bands that include the **tibiotalar, tibiocalcaneal, tibionavicular,** and **tibiospring ligaments,** which insert on the talus, calcaneus, navicular bones, and spring ligament, respectively (Figures 10.143A, 10.145 through 10.147, 10.156, and 10.157). The lateral border of the ankle joint is strengthened by several ligaments termed the **anterior talofibular, calcaneofibular, posterior talofibular, anterior tibiofibular,** and **posterior tibiofibular ligaments** (Figures 10.143 B and C, 10.144

through 10.147, 10.155, and 10.156). All of these ligaments originate at the fibular malleolus and insert on the adjacent bone structures. The **spring (plantar) ligament** is a triangular band of fibers that arises from the sustentaculum tali and attaches to the posterior surface of the navicular bone (Figures 10.121 and 10.148). It is an important ligament in maintaining the longitudinal arch of the foot. A strong band of tissue binding the talus to the calcaneus is the **interosseous talocalcaneal ligament,** which is obliquely oriented in the tarsal canal and helps limit eversion. The **cervical ligament** located in the sinus tarsi helps to limit inversion of the ankle (Figures 10.121, 10.122, 10.124, 10.152, 10.153, 10.156, and 10.157).

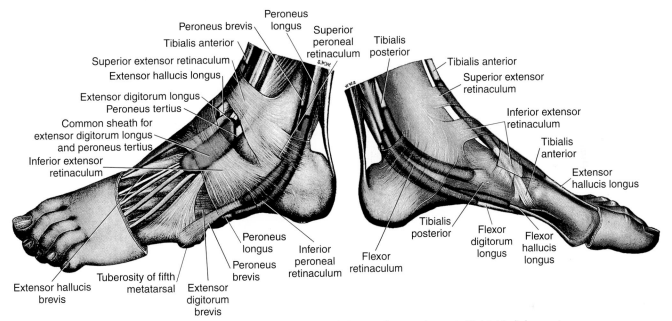

FIGURE 10.142 **Tendons and retinaculum of left foot.** *Left,* Lateral aspect. *Right,* Medial aspect.

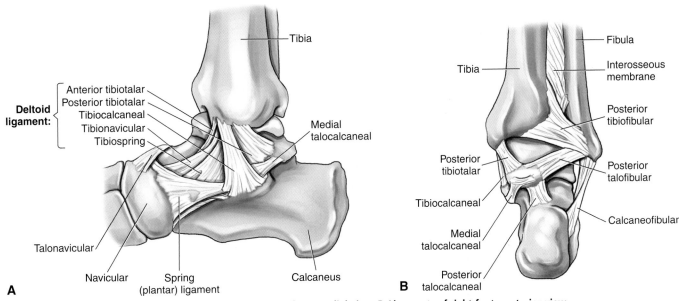

FIGURE 10.143 A, Ligaments of right foot, medial view. B, Ligaments of right foot, posterior view.

(Continued)

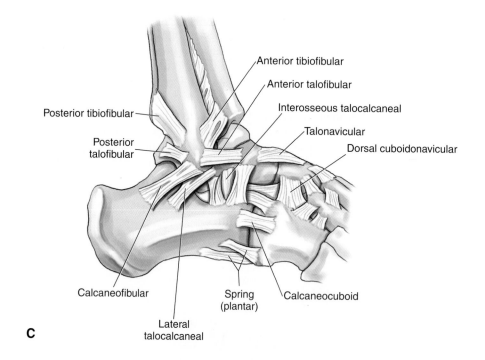

Anterior tibiofibular
Anterior talofibular
Interosseous talocalcaneal
Talonavicular
Dorsal cuboidonavicular
Posterior tibiofibular
Posterior talofibular
Calcaneofibular
Spring (plantar)
Calcaneocuboid
Lateral talocalcaneal

C

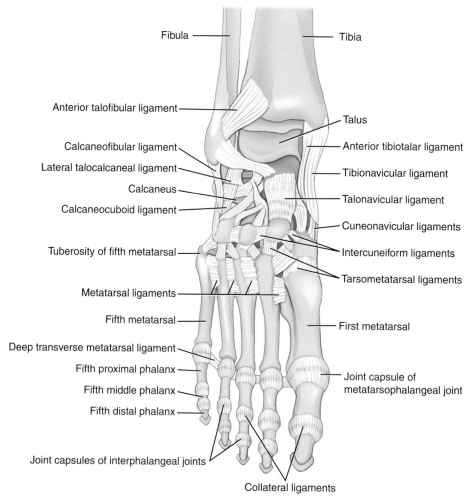

Fibula
Tibia
Anterior talofibular ligament
Talus
Anterior tibiotalar ligament
Calcaneofibular ligament
Tibionavicular ligament
Lateral talocalcaneal ligament
Talonavicular ligament
Calcaneus
Cuneonavicular ligaments
Calcaneocuboid ligament
Intercuneiform ligaments
Tuberosity of fifth metatarsal
Tarsometatarsal ligaments
Metatarsal ligaments
Fifth metatarsal
First metatarsal
Deep transverse metatarsal ligament
Fifth proximal phalanx
Joint capsule of metatarsophalangeal joint
Fifth middle phalanx
Fifth distal phalanx
Joint capsules of interphalangeal joints
Collateral ligaments

D

Anterior view

FIGURE 10.143, cont'd C, Ligaments of right foot, lateral view. D, Collateral ligaments.

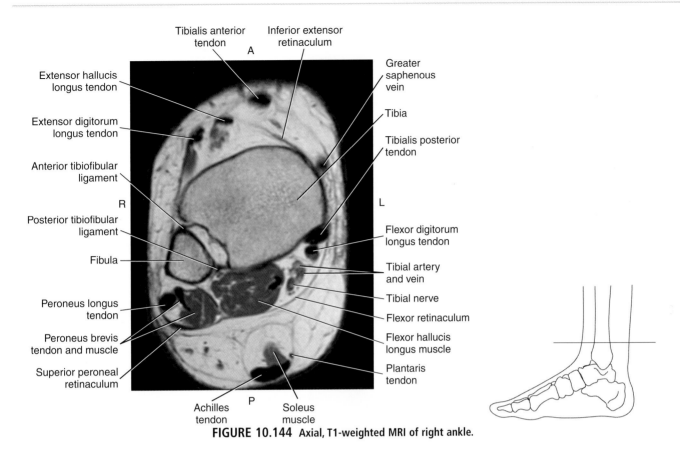

Tibialis anterior tendon

Inferior extensor retinaculum

Extensor hallucis longus tendon

Extensor digitorum longus tendon

Anterior tibiofibular ligament

Posterior tibiofibular ligament

Fibula

Peroneus longus tendon

Peroneus brevis tendon and muscle

Superior peroneal retinaculum

Greater saphenous vein

Tibia

Tibialis posterior tendon

Flexor digitorum longus tendon

Tibial artery and vein

Tibial nerve

Flexor retinaculum

Flexor hallucis longus muscle

Plantaris tendon

Achilles tendon

Soleus muscle

FIGURE 10.144 Axial, T1-weighted MRI of right ankle.

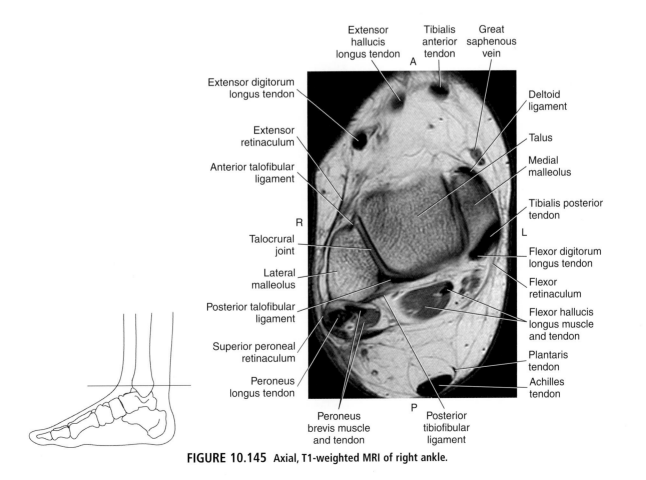

Extensor hallucis longus tendon

Tibialis anterior tendon

Great saphenous vein

Extensor digitorum longus tendon

Extensor retinaculum

Anterior talofibular ligament

Talocrural joint

Lateral malleolus

Posterior talofibular ligament

Superior peroneal retinaculum

Peroneus longus tendon

Deltoid ligament

Talus

Medial malleolus

Tibialis posterior tendon

Flexor digitorum longus tendon

Flexor retinaculum

Flexor hallucis longus muscle and tendon

Plantaris tendon

Achilles tendon

Peroneus brevis muscle and tendon

Posterior tibiofibular ligament

FIGURE 10.145 Axial, T1-weighted MRI of right ankle.

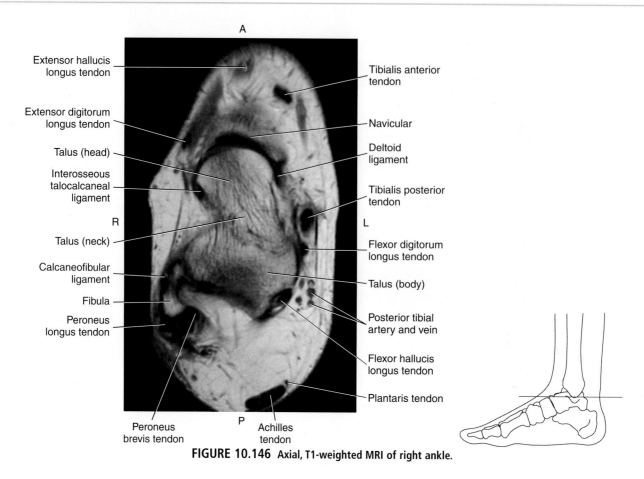

Extensor hallucis longus tendon

Extensor digitorum longus tendon

Talus (head)

Interosseous talocalcaneal ligament

Talus (neck)

Calcaneofibular ligament

Fibula

Peroneus longus tendon

Peroneus brevis tendon

Achilles tendon

Tibialis anterior tendon

Navicular

Deltoid ligament

Tibialis posterior tendon

Flexor digitorum longus tendon

Talus (body)

Posterior tibial artery and vein

Flexor hallucis longus tendon

Plantaris tendon

A

R

L

P

FIGURE 10.146 Axial, T1-weighted MRI of right ankle.

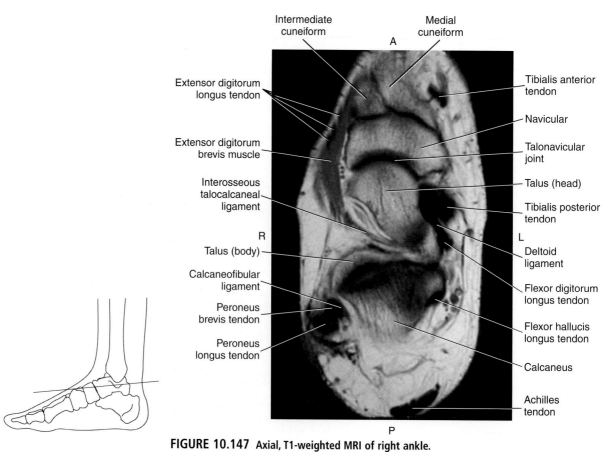

Intermediate cuneiform

Medial cuneiform

Extensor digitorum longus tendon

Extensor digitorum brevis muscle

Interosseous talocalcaneal ligament

Talus (body)

Calcaneofibular ligament

Peroneus brevis tendon

Peroneus longus tendon

Tibialis anterior tendon

Navicular

Talonavicular joint

Talus (head)

Tibialis posterior tendon

Deltoid ligament

Flexor digitorum longus tendon

Flexor hallucis longus tendon

Calcaneus

Achilles tendon

A

R

L

P

FIGURE 10.147 Axial, T1-weighted MRI of right ankle.

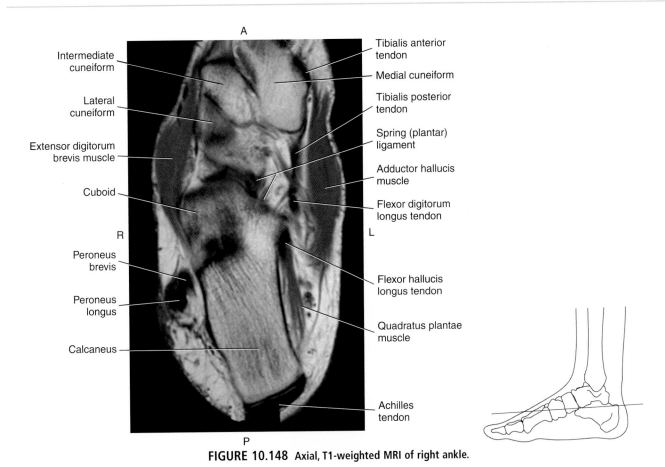

A

Intermediate cuneiform

Lateral cuneiform

Extensor digitorum brevis muscle

Cuboid

R

Peroneus brevis

Peroneus longus

Calcaneus

Tibialis anterior tendon

Medial cuneiform

Tibialis posterior tendon

Spring (plantar) ligament

Adductor hallucis muscle

Flexor digitorum longus tendon

L

Flexor hallucis longus tendon

Quadratus plantae muscle

Achilles tendon

P

FIGURE 10.148 Axial, T1-weighted MRI of right ankle.

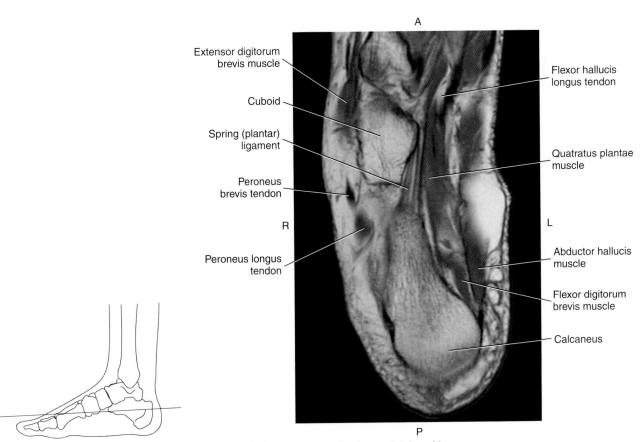

A

Extensor digitorum brevis muscle

Cuboid

Spring (plantar) ligament

Peroneus brevis tendon

R

Peroneus longus tendon

Flexor hallucis longus tendon

Quatratus plantae muscle

L

Abductor hallucis muscle

Flexor digitorum brevis muscle

Calcaneus

P

FIGURE 10.149 Axial, T1-weighted MRI of right ankle.

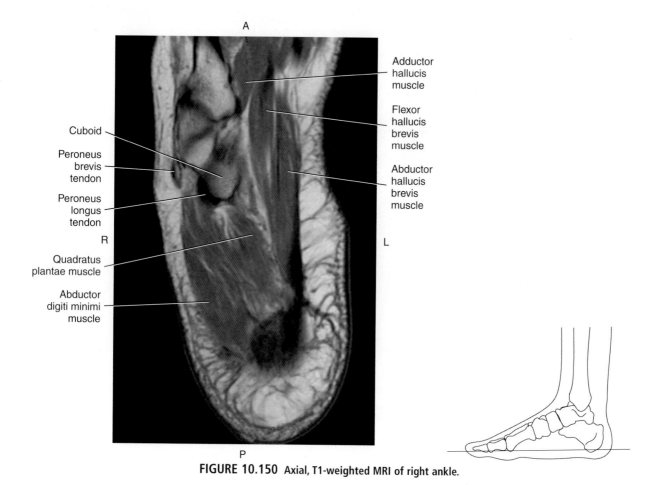

Adductor
hallucis
muscle

Flexor
hallucis
brevis
muscle

Abductor
hallucis
brevis
muscle

Cuboid

Peroneus
brevis
tendon

Peroneus
longus
tendon

Quadratus
plantae muscle

Abductor
digiti minimi
muscle

FIGURE 10.150 Axial, T1-weighted MRI of right ankle.

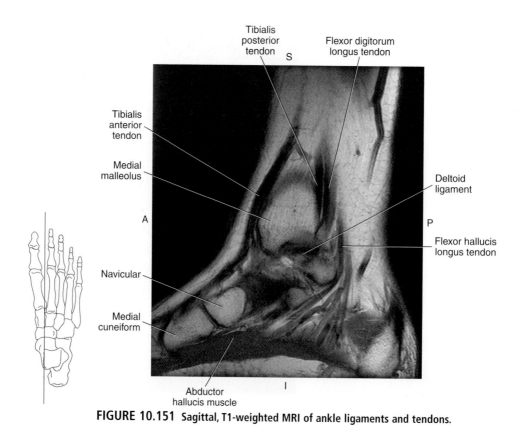

Tibialis
posterior
tendon

Flexor digitorum
longus tendon

Tibialis
anterior
tendon

Medial
malleolus

Deltoid
ligament

Flexor hallucis
longus tendon

Navicular

Medial
cuneiform

Abductor
hallucis muscle

FIGURE 10.151 Sagittal, T1-weighted MRI of ankle ligaments and tendons.

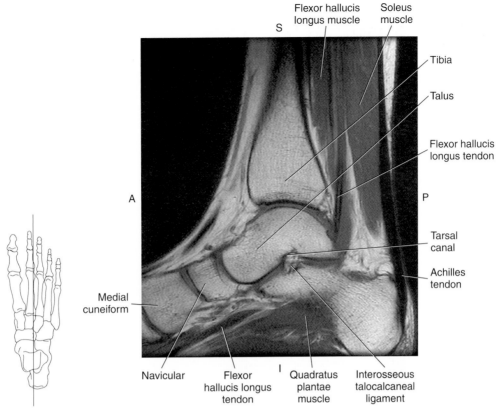

FIGURE 10.152 Sagittal, T1-weighted MRI of ankle ligaments and tendons.

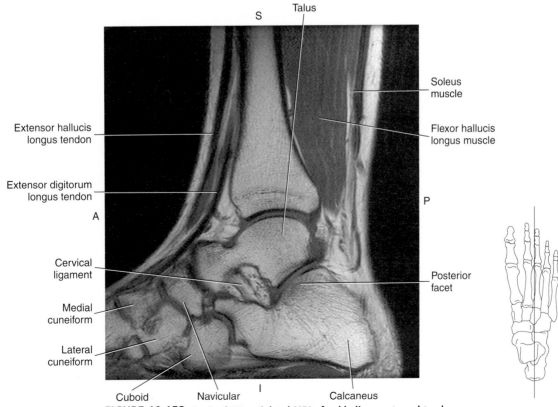

FIGURE 10.153 Sagittal, T1-weighted MRI of ankle ligaments and tendons.

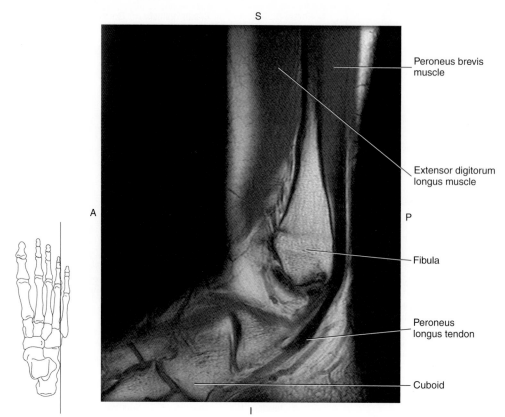

S

Peroneus brevis
muscle

Extensor digitorum
longus muscle

A   P

Fibula

Peroneus
longus tendon

Cuboid

I

FIGURE 10.154 Sagittal, T1-weighted MRI of ankle ligaments and tendons.

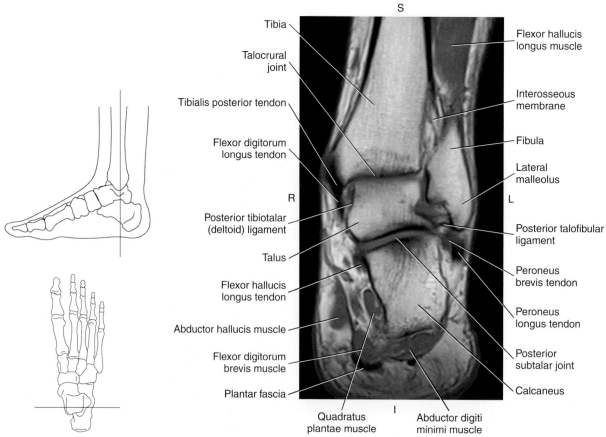

S

Tibia

Talocrural
joint

Tibialis posterior tendon

Flexor digitorum
longus tendon

R

Posterior tibiotalar
(deltoid) ligament

Talus

Flexor hallucis
longus tendon

Abductor hallucis muscle

Flexor digitorum
brevis muscle

Plantar fascia

Flexor hallucis
longus muscle

Interosseous
membrane

Fibula

Lateral
malleolus

L

Posterior talofibular
ligament

Peroneus
brevis tendon

Peroneus
longus tendon

Posterior
subtalar joint

Calcaneus

Quadratus
plantae muscle

I

Abductor digiti
minimi muscle

FIGURE 10.155 Coronal, T1-weighted MRI of left ankle.

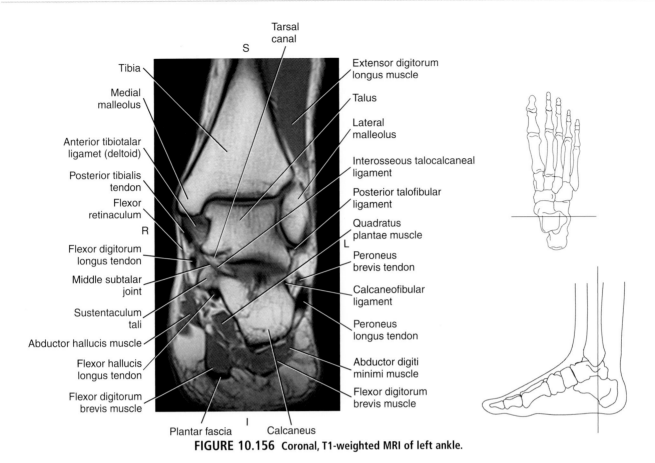

Tarsal canal

S

Tibia

Medial malleolus

Anterior tibiotalar ligamet (deltoid)

Posterior tibialis tendon

Flexor retinaculum

R

Flexor digitorum longus tendon

Middle subtalar joint

Sustentaculum tali

Abductor hallucis muscle

Flexor hallucis longus tendon

Flexor digitorum brevis muscle

Plantar fascia

I

Calcaneus

Extensor digitorum longus muscle

Talus

Lateral malleolus

Interosseous talocalcaneal ligament

Posterior talofibular ligament

Quadratus plantae muscle

L

Peroneus brevis tendon

Calcaneofibular ligament

Peroneus longus tendon

Abductor digiti minimi muscle

Flexor digitorum brevis muscle

FIGURE 10.156 Coronal, T1-weighted MRI of left ankle.

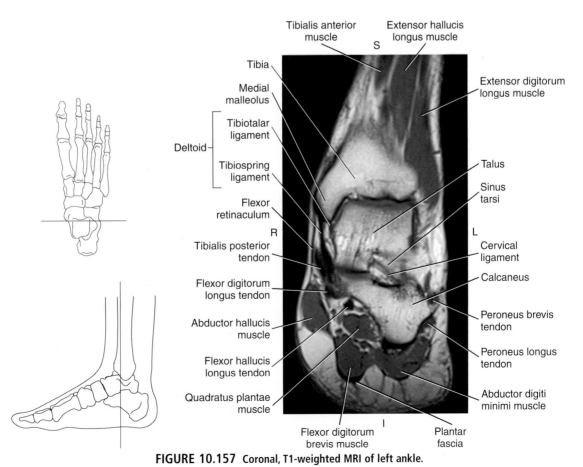

Tibialis anterior muscle

Extensor hallucis longus muscle

S

Tibia

Medial malleolus

Tibiotalar ligament

Deltoid

Tibiospring ligament

Flexor retinaculum

R

Tibialis posterior tendon

Flexor digitorum longus tendon

Abductor hallucis muscle

Flexor hallucis longus tendon

Quadratus plantae muscle

Flexor digitorum brevis muscle

I

Extensor digitorum longus muscle

Talus

Sinus tarsi

L

Cervical ligament

Calcaneus

Peroneus brevis tendon

Peroneus longus tendon

Abductor digiti minimi muscle

Plantar fascia

FIGURE 10.157 Coronal, T1-weighted MRI of left ankle.

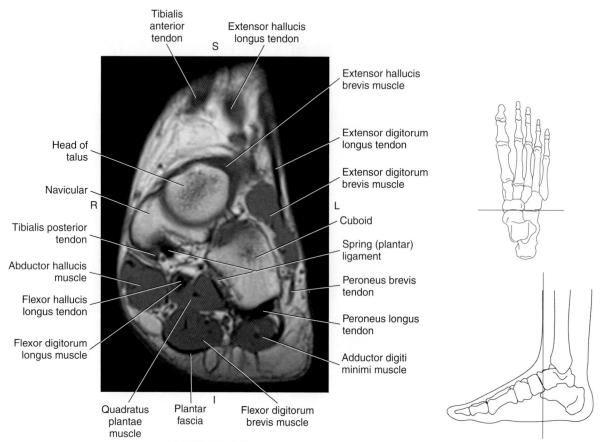

Tibialis anterior tendon

Extensor hallucis longus tendon

S

Extensor hallucis brevis muscle

Extensor digitorum longus tendon

Extensor digitorum brevis muscle

Head of talus

Navicular

R

Tibialis posterior tendon

Abductor hallucis muscle

Flexor hallucis longus tendon

Flexor digitorum longus muscle

L

Cuboid

Spring (plantar) ligament

Peroneus brevis tendon

Peroneus longus tendon

Adductor digiti minimi muscle

Quadratus plantae muscle

Plantar fascia

I

Flexor digitorum brevis muscle

FIGURE 10.158 Coronal, T1-weighted MRI of left foot.

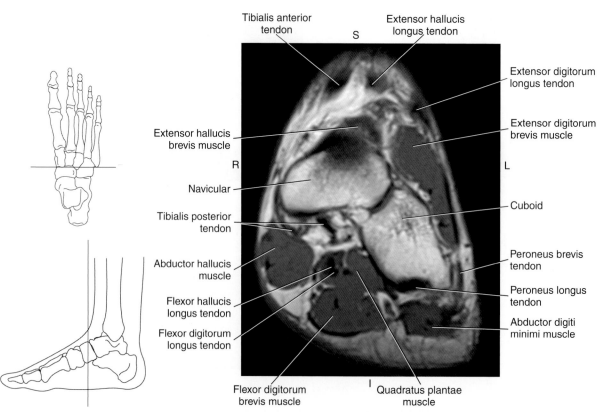

Tibialis anterior tendon

Extensor hallucis longus tendon

S

Extensor digitorum longus tendon

Extensor digitorum brevis muscle

Extensor hallucis brevis muscle

R

Navicular

Tibialis posterior tendon

Abductor hallucis muscle

Flexor hallucis longus tendon

Flexor digitorum longus tendon

L

Cuboid

Peroneus brevis tendon

Peroneus longus tendon

Abductor digiti minimi muscle

Flexor digitorum brevis muscle

I

Quadratus plantae muscle

FIGURE 10.159 Coronal, T1-weighted MRI of left foot.

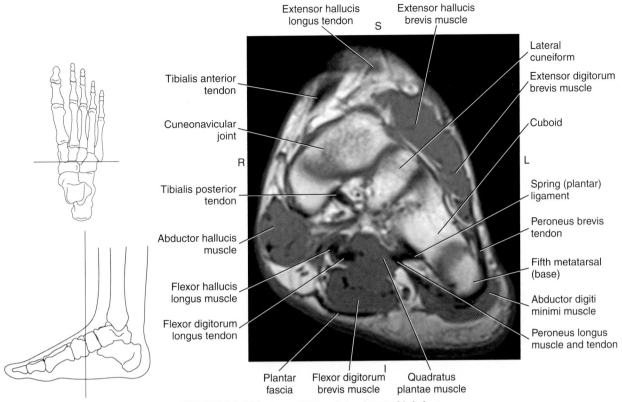

FIGURE 10.160 Coronal, T1-weighted MRI of left foot.

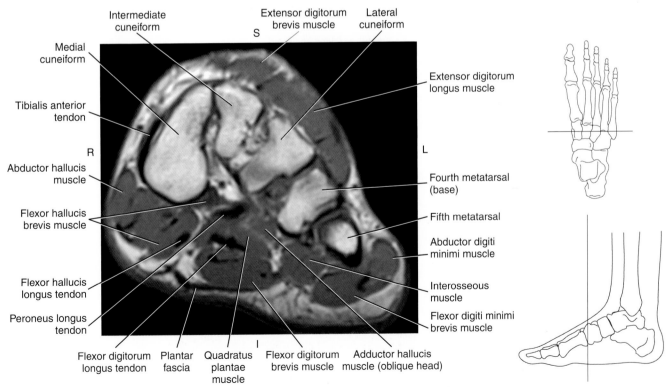

FIGURE 10.161 Coronal, T1-weighted MRI of left foot.

Ligaments of the toes. The metatarsophalangeal joint is strengthened medially and laterally by strong collateral ligaments, dorsally from fibers of the extensor tendons, and underneath by the plantar ligament. The **plantar plate (ligament)** is a thick fibrocartilaginous plate that attaches to the proximal base of the proximal phalanges, the collateral ligaments, and the deep transverse metatarsal ligaments. The **collateral ligaments** extend from the heads of the metatarsal, fanning out to attach to the bases of the proximal phalanges. The heads of the second through fifth metatarsals are interconnected by the **deep transverse metatarsal ligament.** In a similar manner as the metatarsophalangeal joints, the interphalangeal joints are strengthened medially and laterally by collateral ligaments and on the plantar surface by the plantar plate (Figures 10.143 D and 10.162 through 10.164).

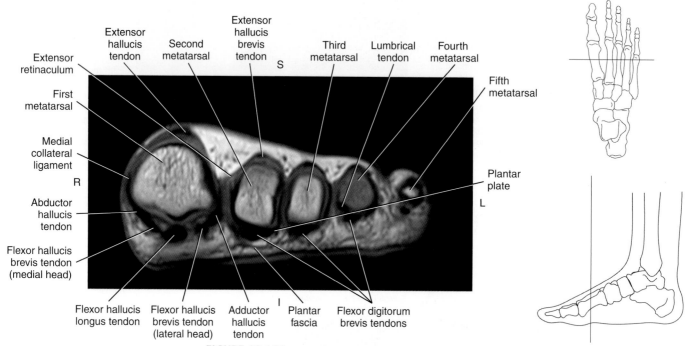

FIGURE 10.162 Coronal, T1-weighted MRI of metatarsals.

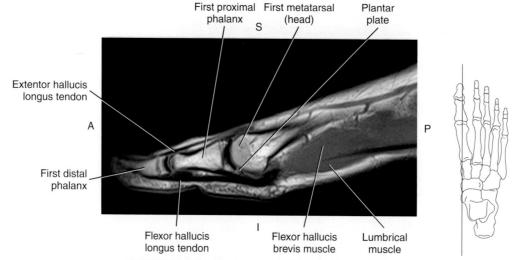

FIGURE 10.163 Sagittal, T1-weighted MRI of great toe.

A

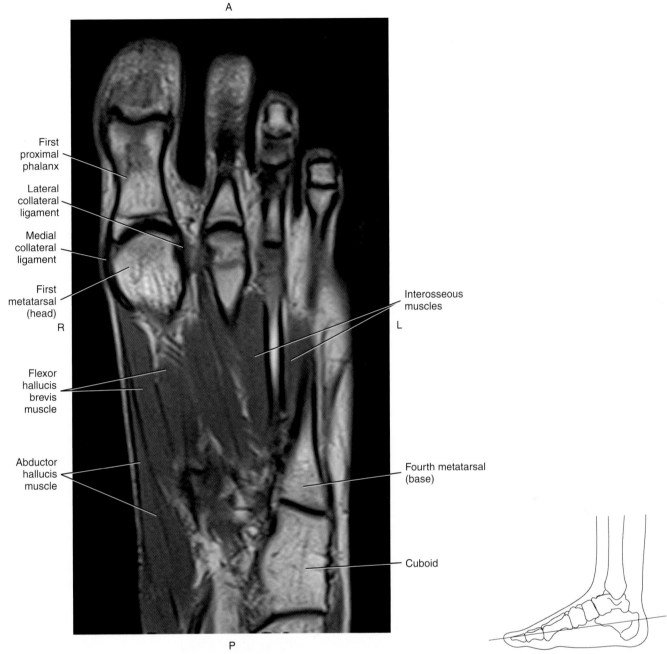

First
proximal
phalanx

Lateral
collateral
ligament

Medial
collateral
ligament

First
metatarsal
(head)

R

Flexor
hallucis
brevis
muscle

Abductor
hallucis
muscle

Interosseous
muscles

L

Fourth metatarsal
(base)

Cuboid

P

FIGURE 10.164 Axial, T1-weighted MRI of foot.

Tendons

The musculotendinous structures of the ankle can be divided into posterior, anterior, medial, and lateral groups.

Posterior group. The posterior group is composed of the single **Achilles tendon,** the largest and most powerful tendon of the body. The Achilles tendon arises from the gastrocnemius and soleus muscles and attaches to the calcaneal tuberosity on the posterior aspect of the calcaneus (Figures 10.115, 10.121, 10.144 through 10.148, 10.152, and 10.153).

Anterior group. The anterior group is made up of the tibialis anterior, extensor hallucis longus, and extensor digitorum longus tendons, which are named medial to lateral and act to extend and dorsiflex the foot. The **tibialis anterior** muscle becomes tendinous at the distal tibia and attaches to the plantar and medial aspects of the first cuneiform and metatarsal bones. The tendon of the **extensor hallucis longus** muscle originates from the anterior fibula and inserts on the great toe. The most lateral of this group is the **extensor digitorum longus tendon,** which originates at the level of the lateral malleolus and inserts on the second through the fifth digits (Figures 10.142, 10.144 through 10.148, 10.151, 10.153, 10.158 through 10.163, and 10.165).

Medial group. The medial group is composed of the posterior tibialis tendons, flexor digitorum longus, and flexor hallucis longus tendons, which as a group act to invert and plantar flex the foot. The **tibialis posterior tendon** fans out in multiple strands that insert on the plantar aspect of the sustentaculum tali, navicular bone, first cuneiform bone, and second through fourth metatarsal bones. Coursing posterior and lateral to the tibialis posterior tendon is the **flexor digitorum longus tendon**, which inserts on the second through fourth phalanges. The tendon of the **flexor hallucis longus** muscle curves under the sustentaculum tali and then courses along the plantar surface of the foot to insert on the great toe (Figures 10.142, 10.144 through 10.148, 10.151, 10.152, 10.155 through 10.163, and 10.165).

Lateral group. The two peroneus tendons, **peroneus longus** and **peroneus brevis**, make up the lateral group and act to evert, weakly plantar flex the foot, and stabilize the ankle joint laterally. These two tendons share a common tendinous sheath behind the lateral malleolus. Below the malleolus they diverge into separate tendon sheaths, with the peroneus brevis tendon inserting on the base of the fifth metatarsal, and the peroneus longus tendon curving beneath the calcaneus to insert on the base of the first metatarsal and medial cuneiform bones (Figures 10.142, 10.144 through 10.149, 10.154 through 10.161, and 10.165.

Muscles of the Foot

The muscles of the foot are divided into the **muscles of the dorsum** and **muscles of the sole of the foot.** These muscles are demonstrated in Figures 10.147 through 10.167 and described in Table 10.4. The dorsal muscles include the extensor digitorum brevis and the extensor hallucis brevis muscles, which form a fleshy mass on the lateral part of the dorsal foot. The **extensor digitorum brevis** muscle arises from the anterior, upper surface of the calcaneus and passes obliquely across the dorsum to end in three tendons that insert onto the dorsal aponeurosis of the second through fourth digits (Figure 10.165). The extensor digitorum brevis muscle is responsible for dorsiflexion of the second through fourth digits. The **extensor hallucis brevis muscle** splits off of the extensor digitorum brevis muscle to insert on the dorsal aponeurosis of the first toe. It acts to dorsiflex the first digit. The muscles of the sole of the foot can be described by four muscular layers.

First layer. The muscles located within the first layer are the most superficial and include the abductor hallucis, flexor digitorum brevis, and abductor digiti minimi muscles (Figures 10.121, 10.124, 10.166 A, and 10.167). The **abductor hallucis muscle** arises from the medial process of the calcaneal tuberosity and lies along the medial border of the foot to insert on the medial base of the proximal phalanx of the first digit. The **flexor digitorum brevis** muscle also arises from the medial process of the calcaneal tuberosity, as well as the plantar aponeurosis, to insert on both sides of the middle phalanges of the lateral four digits. The **abductor digiti minimi muscle** arises from the lateral process of the calcaneal tuberosity, the tuberosity of the fifth metatarsal, and the plantar aponeurosis to form the lateral margin of the foot. It inserts on the lateral side of the base of the proximal phalanx of the fifth digit.

Second layer. This layer is located deep to the first layer and includes the quadratus plantae and lumbrical muscles (Figures 10.121, 10.124, and 10.166 B). The **quadratus plantae muscle** is a small flat muscle that arises as two small slips from the medial and lateral margins of the plantar surface of the calcaneus and joins with the tendon of the flexor digitorum longus that continues to the distal phalanges of the lateral four digits. The four small **lumbrical muscles** arise from the medial surfaces of the individual tendons of the flexor digitorum longus. They insert on the medial margin of the proximal phalanges of

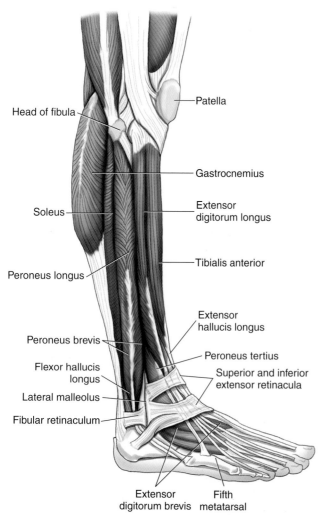

FIGURE 10.165   **Extensor tendons of the lower leg.**

Labels on figure:
- Head of fibula
- Patella
- Gastrocnemius
- Soleus
- Extensor digitorum longus
- Peroneus longus
- Tibialis anterior
- Peroneus brevis
- Extensor hallucis longus
- Flexor hallucis longus
- Peroneus tertius
- Superior and inferior extensor retinacula
- Lateral malleolus
- Fibular retinaculum
- Extensor digitorum brevis
- Fifth metatarsal

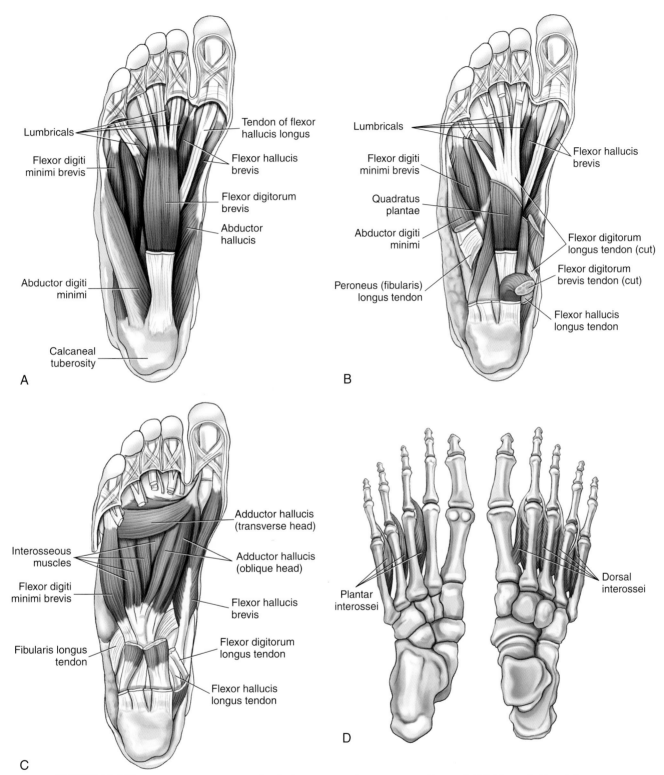

Lumbricals

Tendon of flexor
hallucis longus

Flexor digiti
minimi brevis

Flexor hallucis
brevis

Flexor digitorum
brevis

Abductor
hallucis

Abductor digiti
minimi

Calcaneal
tuberosity

A

Lumbricals

Flexor hallucis
brevis

Flexor digiti
minimi brevis

Quadratus
plantae

Abductor digiti
minimi

Flexor digitorum
longus tendon (cut)

Flexor digitorum
brevis tendon (cut)

Peroneus (fibularis)
longus tendon

Flexor hallucis
longus tendon

B

Interosseous
muscles

Adductor hallucis
(transverse head)

Flexor digiti
minimi brevis

Adductor hallucis
(oblique head)

Fibularis longus
tendon

Flexor hallucis
brevis

Flexor digitorum
longus tendon

Flexor hallucis
longus tendon

C

Plantar
interossei

Dorsal
interossei

D

FIGURE 10.166 Dorsal view of muscles of right foot. A, First layer. **B,** Second layer. **C,** Third layer. **D,** Fourth layer.

the second through fifth digits and extend into the extensor aponeurosis.

Third layer. The third layer consists of three muscles: the flexor hallucis brevis, adductor hallucis, and flexor digiti minimi brevis muscles (Figures 10.121, 10.166 C, and 10.167). The **flexor hallucis brevis muscle** arises from the medial cuneiform bone and the tibialis posterior tendon. It has two heads that cover the plantar surface of the first metatarsal, extending to both sides of the base of the proximal phalanx of the first digit. The **adductor hallucis muscle** has two heads; the oblique head arises from the cuboid and lateral cuneiform bones and the bases of the second and third metatarsals, and the transverse head arises from the deep transverse metatarsal ligament and the metatarsal joint capsule. Both heads insert on the lateral side of the base of the

proximal phalanx of the first digit. The slender **flexor digiti minimi brevis muscle** arises from the base of the fifth metatarsal and inserts on the base of the proximal phalanx of the fifth digit.

Fourth layer. This layer consists of the interosseous muscles (Figures 10.121, 10.166 D, and 10.167). Three plantar and four dorsal interossei muscles are located between the metatarsal bones. The **plantar interosseous muscles** arise from the bases and medial surfaces of the third through fifth metatarsals and insert on the medial sides of the bases of the proximal phalanges of the third through fifth digits. The **dorsal interosseous muscles** are larger than their plantar counterparts, arising from adjacent surfaces of the metatarsal bones and extending to attach to the sides of the proximal phalanx and capsules of the metatarsal phalangeal joints of the second through fourth digits.

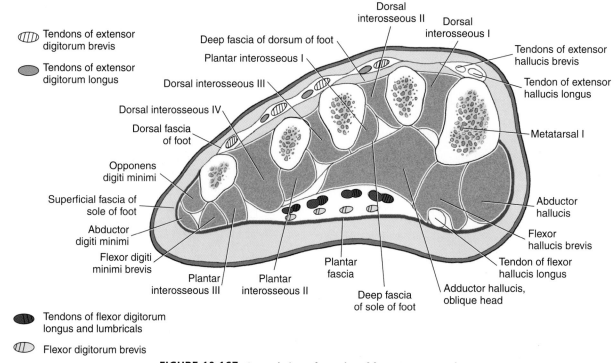

FIGURE 10.167 Coronal view of muscles of foot at metatarsals.

TABLE 10.4	Muscles of the Foot		
Muscle	**Proximal Insertion**	**Distal Insertion**	**Action**
Dorsal Surface			
Extensor digitorum brevis	Calcaneus	Second to fourth digits of the foot	Dorsiflexion of second to fourth digits
Extensor hallucis brevis	Extensor digitorum brevis	First toe	Dorsiflexes the first digit
Sole of Foot			
First Layer			
Abductor hallucis	Calcaneal tuberosity	Proximal phalanx of first digit	Abducts first toe from second, flexes metatarsophalangeal joint
Flexor digitorum brevis	Calcaneal tuberosity and plantar aponeurosis	Middle phalanges of second to fifth digits	Flexes metatarsophalangeal and proximal interphalangeal joints of second to fifth digits
Abductor digiti minimi	Calcaneal tuberosity, fifth metatarsal	Proximal phalanx of fifth digit	Abducts fifth toe and flexes metatarsophalangeal joint
Second Layer			
Quadratus plantae	Calcaneus	Distal phalanges of second to fifth digits	Assists the flexor digitorum longus in flexion of toes
Lumbrical	Flexor digitorum longus tendons	Proximal phalanges of second to fifth digits	Flexes metatarsophalangeal joints, extends proximal and distal interphalangeal joints of second to fifth digits
Third Layer			
Flexor hallucis brevis	Medial cuneiform and tibialis posterior tendon	Proximal phalanx of first digit	Flexes metatarsophalangeal joint of first toe
Adductor hallucis		Proximal phalanx of first digit	Adduct first toe toward second and flexes first toe
Oblique head	Cuboid, lateral cuneiform and second and third metatarsals		
Transverse head	Transverse metatarsal ligament and metatarsal joint capsule		
Flexor digiti minimi	Fifth metatarsal	Proximal phalanx of fifth digit	Flexes metatarsophalangeal joint of fifth digit
Fourth Layer			
Plantar interosseous	Third to fifth metatarsals	Proximal phalanges of third to fifth digits	Adducts third to fifth toes, flexes metatarsophalangeal and extends nterphalangeal joints of third to fifth digits
Dorsal interosseous	Metatarsals	Proximal phalanx and capsules of metatarsal phalangeal joints of second to fourth digits	Abducts second to fourth digits away from midline, flexes metatarsophalangeal joints, and extends interphalangeal joints of second to fourth digits

NEUROVASCULATURE

Arteries

Femoral. Traveling vertically along the anteromedial aspect of the hip is the **femoral artery**. The femoral artery, an extension of the external iliac artery, enters the anterior compartment of the thigh beneath the inguinal ligament, where it is relatively superficial and easily palpable (Figures 10.168 through 10.172). It descends the thigh and continues through the opening in the adductor magnus muscle as the popliteal artery in the knee. The femoral artery and its main branches, superficial and deep, supply all the compartments of the thigh, as well as the skin of the anterior abdominal wall, inguinal region, and external genitalia. The superficial branches of the femoral artery accompany the veins of the hip and include the **inferior epigastric, superficial circumflex iliac,** and the **external pudendal arteries**. The largest deep branch of the femoral artery is the **profunda femoris artery,** which arises from the posterolateral aspect of the femoral artery about 4 cm below the inguinal ligament and runs distally behind the femoral artery (Figures 10.168, 10.169, and 10.171 through 10.174). It passes between the vastus medialis muscle and the muscles of the adductor group. The profundus femoris gives off two large branches: the **medial** and **lateral circumflex femoral arteries** (Figures 10.173 and 10.174). The branches curve around the proximal femur and hip joint to supply the muscles of the adductor group and parts of the gluteal musculature, as well as the extensors and flexors at the thigh. The terminal branches of the profunda femoris artery are the **perforating arteries** (3-5) near the linea aspera that pass through the adductor muscles (Figures 10.173 and 10.174).

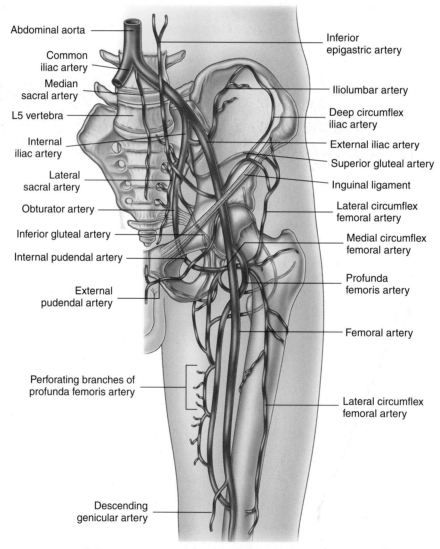

FIGURE 10.168 Anterior view of iliac and femoral arteries.

External
iliac artery

Internal
iliac artery

S

Aorta

Common
iliac artery

Femoral
artery

Profunda
femoris
artery

Lateral
circumflex
artery

Popliteal
artery

R

L

I

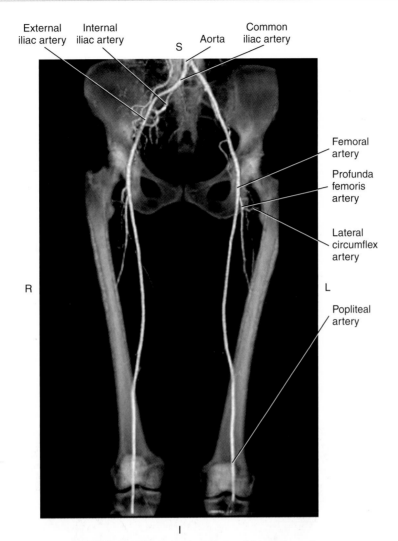

FIGURE 10.169 3D CTA of iliac and femoral arteries.

Popliteal. The popliteal artery is the continuation of the femoral artery. It runs deep near the bones of the knee joint during its course through the popliteal fossa. It passes distally over the popliteus muscle and divides into the **anterior** and **posterior tibial arteries** (Figures 10.173 through 10.176). The popliteal artery accompanies the popliteal vein and tibial nerve. The tibial nerve is the most superficial structure in the popliteal fossa (Figures 10.177 and 10.178). The popliteal artery supplies the surrounding muscles and forms a substantial plexus of articular branches anastomosing around the knee joint. The popliteal artery gives off branches to portions of the thigh muscles near the knee joint, dispatches the **sural arteries** distally to the gastrocnemius muscle, and supplies the knee joint with the anastomosing **genicular arteries** (lateral superior, lateral inferior, medial superior, medial inferior, and descending) (Figures 10.173 and 10.174).

Anterior tibial. The anterior tibial artery courses anteriorly at the level of the fibular head into the anterior compartment of the lower leg. It runs distally as far as the anterior side of the ankle, where it becomes the **dorsalis pedis artery**. The branches of the anterior tibial artery are the posterior tibial recurrent, the anterior tibial recurrent, the medial anterior malleolar, the lateral anterior malleolar, and numerous muscular branches (Figures 10.174, 10.175, and 10.176).

Posterior tibial. The posterior tibial artery is usually larger than the anterior tibial artery. As it passes distally in the posterior compartment, it courses toward the medial side of the leg. The posterior tibial artery terminates by dividing into the **medial** and **lateral plantar arteries** in the foot. The **peroneal (fibular) artery** arises from the posterior tibial artery approximately 2 cm below the distal border of the popliteal muscle. It descends posteriorly along the medial aspect of the fibula and terminates on the lateral surface of the calcaneal tuberosity. Branches of the peroneal artery include the fibular nutrient, communicating, perforating, posterior lateral malleolar, and lateral calcaneal, as well as numerous muscular and cutaneous branches (Figures 10.174, 10.175, and 10.176).

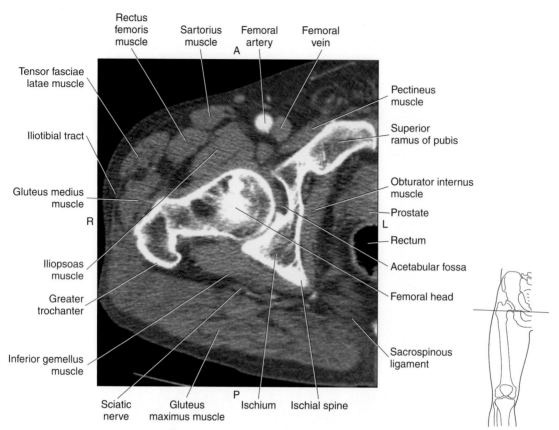

FIGURE 10.170 Axial, contrast-enhanced CT of right hip with femoral artery.

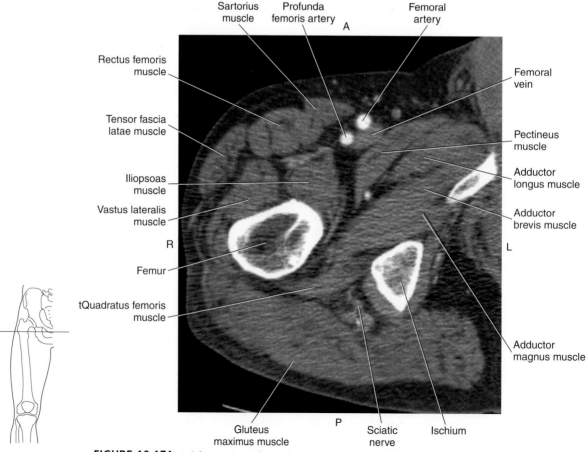

FIGURE 10.171 Axial, contrast-enhanced CT of right hip with femoral artery and vein.

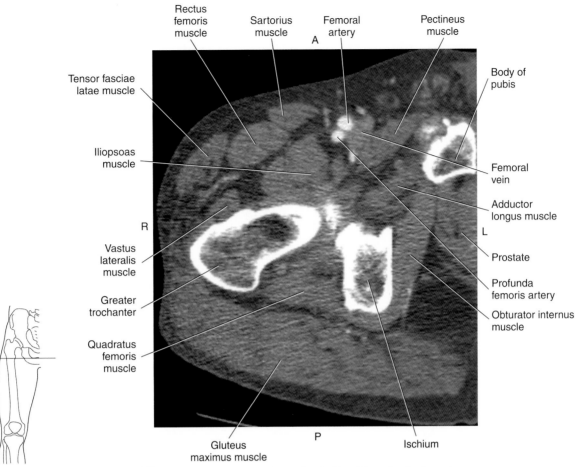

Rectus femoris muscle

Sartorius muscle

Femoral artery

Pectineus muscle

Tensor fasciae latae muscle

Body of pubis

Iliopsoas muscle

Femoral vein

Adductor longus muscle

Vastus lateralis muscle

Prostate

Greater trochanter

Profunda femoris artery

Quadratus femoris muscle

Obturator internus muscle

Gluteus maximus muscle

Ischium

FIGURE 10.172 Axial, contrast-enhanced CT of right hip with profundus femoris artery.

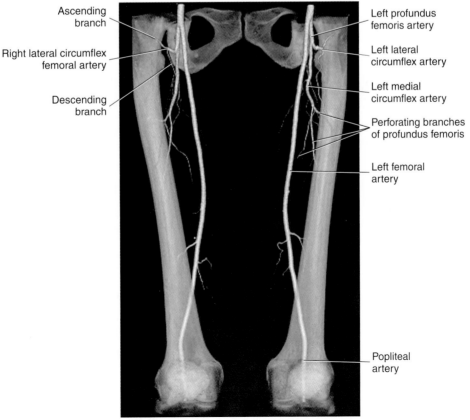

Ascending branch

Left profundus femoris artery

Right lateral circumflex femoral artery

Left lateral circumflex artery

Descending branch

Left medial circumflex artery

Perforating branches of profundus femoris

Left femoral artery

Popliteal artery

FIGURE 10.173 3D CT of femoral artery.

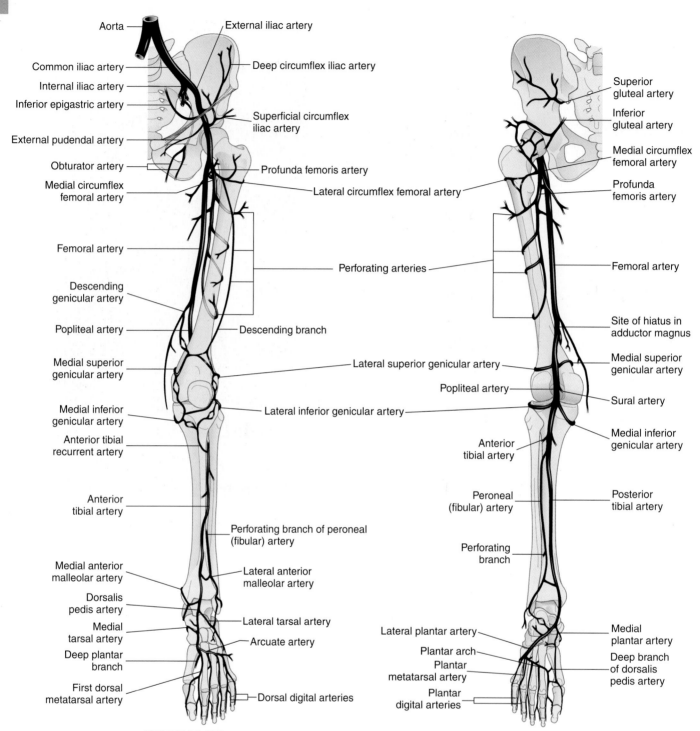

FIGURE 10.174 Arteries of lower extremity. *Left,* Anterior view. *Right,* Posterior view.

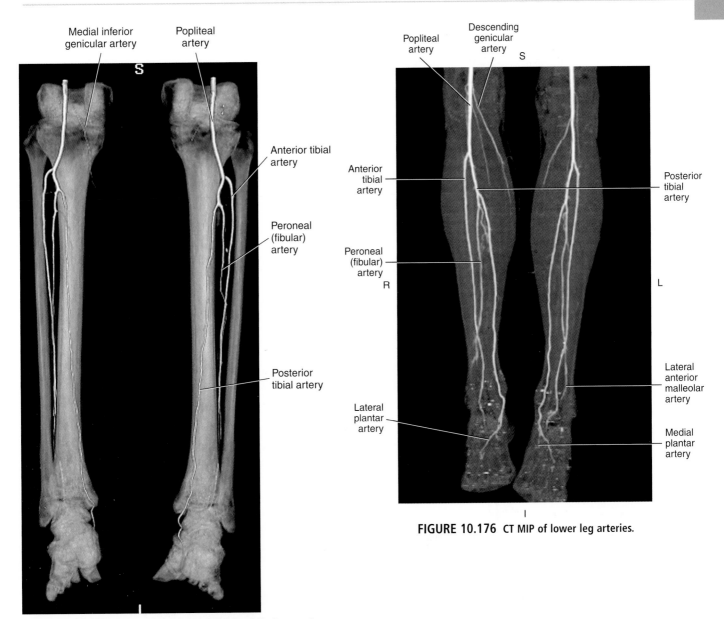

FIGURE 10.175 3D CT angiography of tibial and fibular arteries.

FIGURE 10.176 CT MIP of lower leg arteries.

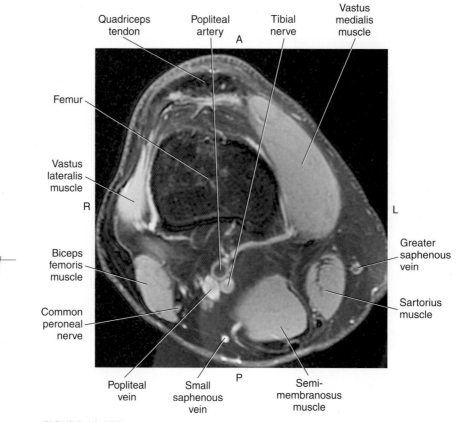

FIGURE 10.177 Axial, T1-weighted MRI of right knee with vessels.

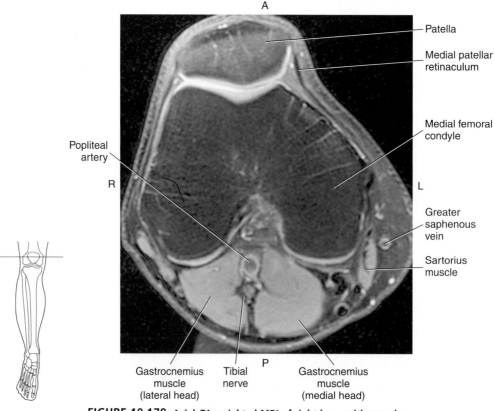

FIGURE 10.178 Axial, T1-weighted MRI of right knee with vessels.

Veins

There are two groups of veins in the lower extremity: superficial and deep. The superficial veins arise in the foot from the dorsal venous arch and merge chiefly into two main trunks, the great saphenous and the small saphenous. The **great saphenous vein** ascends the medial aspect of the leg and thigh to drain into the femoral vein near the hip joint. From the lateral side of the foot, the **small saphenous vein** passes posterolaterally to join the popliteal vein

(Figure 10.179). Between these two superficial veins and the system of the deep veins are numerous deep anastomoses. The deep veins accompany their corresponding arteries and include the **anterior** and **posterior tibial veins**. They unite to form the popliteal vein on the posterior aspect of the knee. The popliteal vein becomes the femoral vein in the thigh, which courses medial to the femoral artery and continues deep to the inguinal ligament as the **external iliac vein** (Figures 10.40 through 10.48, 10.102 through 10.109, 10.170 through 10.172, 10.179, and 10.180).

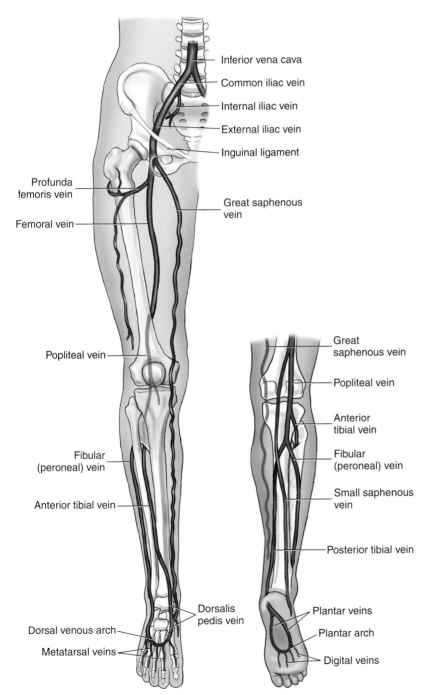

FIGURE 10.179 Anterior view of veins of the lower leg.
Left, Anterior view. *Right,* Posterior view.

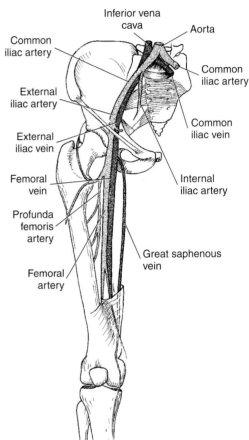

FIGURE 10.180 Anterior view of femoral artery and vein and great saphenous vein.

Nerves

The nerves of the lower extremity are derived from the lumbar and sacral plexuses (see Chapter 4). The **femoral nerve** enters the thigh beneath the inguinal ligament and divides into several superficial and deep branches to supply the anterior compartment of the thigh. The femoral nerve terminates as the **saphenous nerve** to innervate the skin on the medial side of the leg and foot. The **obturator nerve** courses through the obturator canal and immediately

divides into anterior and posterior divisions to supply the medial compartment of the thigh. The **sciatic nerve** is the largest peripheral nerve in the body. Its branches supply the posterior compartment of the thigh and all compartments of the distal leg and foot. The sciatic nerve runs deep to the gluteus maximus muscle and descends in the midline of the thigh, where it usually divides into two terminal branches: the **tibial** and **common peroneal (common fibular) nerves** (Figures 10.40 through 10.45, 10.102 through 10.108, 10.170, 10.177, 10.178, and 10.181).

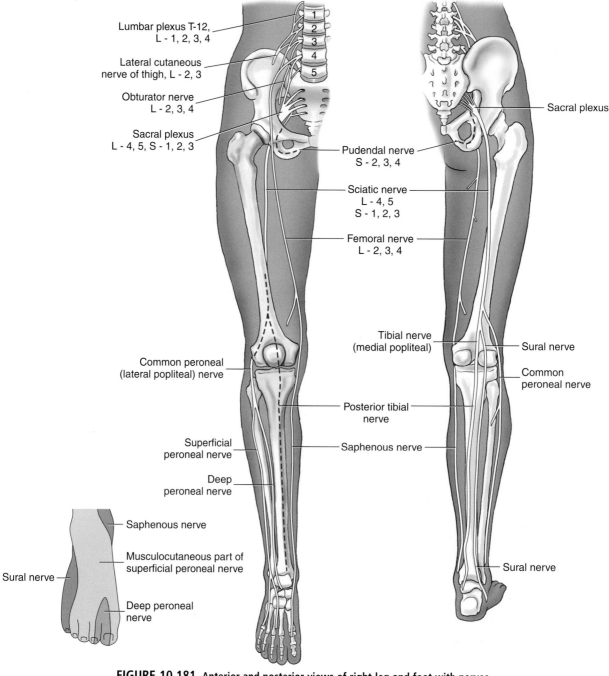

Lumbar plexus T-12,
L - 1, 2, 3, 4

Lateral cutaneous
nerve of thigh, L - 2, 3

Obturator nerve
L - 2, 3, 4

Sacral plexus
L - 4, 5, S - 1, 2, 3

Pudendal nerve
S - 2, 3, 4

Sciatic nerve
L - 4, 5
S - 1, 2, 3

Femoral nerve
L - 2, 3, 4

Sacral plexus

Common peroneal
(lateral popliteal) nerve

Tibial nerve
(medial popliteal)

Sural nerve

Common
peroneal nerve

Posterior tibial
nerve

Superficial
peroneal nerve

Saphenous nerve

Deep
peroneal nerve

Saphenous nerve

Musculocutaneous part of
superficial peroneal nerve

Sural nerve

Sural nerve

Deep peroneal
nerve

FIGURE 10.181 Anterior and posterior views of right leg and foot with nerves.

Illustration Credits

Chapter 1

Figure 1.4 from Applegate E: *The sectional anatomy learning system*, ed 3, St. Louis, 2010, Saunders.

Figures 1.8, 1.9 from Frank: *Merrill's atlas of positioning and radiographic procedures*, ed 12, St. Louis, 2012, Mosby.

Figure 1.7 from Jacob S: *Atlas of human anatomy*, Philadelphia, 2002, Churchill Livingstone.

Figure 1.10 from Seeram E: *Computed tomography: Physical principles, clinical applications, and quality control*, ed 3, St. Louis, 2009, Saunders.

Figure 1.11 from Mitchell DG: *MRI principles*, ed 2, Philadelphia, 2004, Saunders.

Figure 1.14 from Stark DD, Bradley WG: *Magnetic resonance imaging*, ed 3, St. Louis, 1999, Mosby.

Chapter 2

Figures 2.2, 2.3, 2.18, 2.20, 2.27, 2.67, 2.68, 2.81 from Frank: *Merrill's atlas of positioning and radiographic procedures*, ed 12, St. Louis, 2012, Mosby.

Figure 2.24 from *Mosby's dictionary of medical and health professions*, ed 8, St. Louis, 2009, Mosby.

Figures 2.47, 2.70, 2.76, 2.88, 2.80, 2.90, 2.107, 2.108, 2.110 from Som PM, Curtin HD: *Head and neck imaging*, ed 5, St. Louis, 2012, Mosby.

Chapter 3

Figure 3.9 from Frank: *Merrill's atlas of positioning and radiographic procedures*, ed 12, St. Louis, 2012, Mosby.

Figures 3.17, 3.35 from Applegate E: *The sectional anatomy learning system*, ed 3, St. Louis, 2010, Saunders.

Figures 3.45, 3.84, 3.104 from Standring S: *Gray's anatomy*, ed 40, Philadelphia, 2009, Churchill Livingstone.

Figures 3.60, 3.73, 3.112, 3.113, 3.118, 3.119, 3.134 from Fitzgerald MJT: *Clinical neuroanatomy and related neuroscience*, ed 6, Philadelphia, 2012, Saunders.

Figure 3.94 from Noback CR, Demarest RJ: *The nervous system: Introduction and review*, New York, 1972, McGraw-Hill.

Figure 3.103 from Langley LL, et al: *Dynamic anatomy and physiology*, ed 4, New York, 1974, McGraw Hill. Copyright Mosby-Year Book, Inc.

Figure 3.115 from Weir J: *Imaging atlas of human anatomy*, ed 4, Philadelphia, 2011, Mosby.

Figure 3.130 from Jacob S: *Atlas of human anatomy*, Philadelphia, 2002, Churchill Livingstone.

Chapter 4

Figure 4.7 from Frank: *Merrill's atlas of positioning and radiographic procedures*, ed 12, St. Louis, 2012, Mosby.

Figures 4.19, 4.54, 4.55, 4.59, 4.65B from Larsen WL: *Anatomy development, function, clinical correlations*, Philadelphia, 2002, Saunders.

Figures 4.48, 4.65A, 4.88 from Standring S: *Gray's anatomy*, ed 40, Philadelphia, 2009, Churchill Livingstone.

Figure 4.69 from *Mosby's dictionary of medical and health professions*, ed 8, St. Louis, 2009, Mosby.

Figure 4.70 from Jacob S: *Atlas of human anatomy*, Philadelphia, 2002, Churchill Livingstone.

Figure 4.76 from Weir J: *Imaging atlas of human anatomy*, ed 4, Philadelphia, 2011, Mosby.

Figures 4.101, 4.102, 4.106 from Palastanga N, Field D, Soames R, et al: *Anatomy and human movement*, ed 4, Boston, 2002, Butterworth-Heinemann.

Figure 4.116 from Stark DD, Bradley WG: *Magnetic resonance imaging*, ed 3, St. Louis, 1999, Mosby.

Figure 4.125 Netter illustration used with permission from Icon Learning Systems, a division of MediMedia USA, Inc. All rights reserved.

Chapter 5

Figure 5.2 from Applegate E: *The sectional anatomy learning system*, ed 3, St. Louis, 2010, Saunders.

Figures 5.49, 5.51, 5.52, 5.53, 5.54, 5.55 from Som PM, Curtin HD: *Head and neck imaging*, ed 5, St. Louis, 2012, Mosby.

Figure 5.19 from *Mosby's dictionary of medical and health professions*, ed 8, St. Louis, 2009, Mosby.

Figures 5.70, 5.75, 5.77, 5.78 from Standring S: *Gray's anatomy*, ed 40, Philadelphia, 2009, Churchill Livingstone.

Figure 5.81 from Curry RA, Tempkin BB: *Sonography: Introduction to normal structure and function*, ed 3, St. Louis, 2011, Saunders.

Chapter 6

Figure 6.3 courtesy of Anne Marie Sawyer, Radiologic Sciences Laboratory, Stanford University School of Medicine, Stanford, Calif.

Figure 6.7 from Frank: *Merrill's atlas of positioning and radiographic procedures*, ed 12, St. Louis, 2012, Mosby.

Figures 6.15, 6.25, 6.87, 6.90 from Standring S: *Gray's anatomy*, ed 40, Philadelphia, 2009, Churchill Livingstone.

Figures 6.41, 6.48, 6.126, 6.131 from Manning WJ, Pennell DJ: *Cardiovascular magnetic resonance*, Philadelphia, 2011, Churchill Livingstone.

Figures 6.21, 6.148 from Palastanga N, Field D, Soames R, et al: *Anatomy and human movement*, ed 4, Boston, 2002, Butterworth-Heinemann.

Figures 6.27, 6.32 from Haaga JR, Lanzieri CF, Gilkeson RC, et al: *CT and MR imaging of the whole body*, ed 5, Philadelphia, 2009, Mosby.

Figures 6.34, 6.157 from Seidel HM, Ball JW, Dains JE, et al: *Mosby's guide to physical examination*, ed 7, St. Louis, 2011, Mosby.

Figures 6.37, 6-44 from Applegate E: *The sectional anatomy learning system*, ed 3, St. Louis, 2010, Saunders.

Figures 6.39, 6.58, 6.64, 6.65, 6.70, 6.77, 6.83, 6.85, 6.88, 6.91, 6.93, 6.114 from Weir: *Imaging atlas of human anatomy*, ed 4, Philadelphia, 2011, Mosby.

Figure 6.75 from Wilson SF, Thompson JM: *Respiratory disorders*, St. Louis, 1990, Mosby.

Figure 6.140 from Jacob: *Atlas of human anatomy*, Philadelphia, 2002, Churchill Livingstone.

Figures 6.145, 6.146 from Larsen WL: *Anatomy development, function, clinical correlations*, Philadelphia, 2002, Saunders.

Figure 6.158 from *Mosby's dictionary of medical and health professions*, ed 8, St. Louis, 2009, Mosby.

Chapter 7

Figures 7.3, 7.23, 7.27, 7.28, 7.63, 7.70, 7.80, 7.87, 7.151, 7.158, 7.166, 7.169, 7.172, 7.181, 7.185, 7.186 from Hagen-Ansert SL: *Textbook of diagnostic sonography*, ed 7, St. Louis, 2012, Mosby.

Figure 7.6 from Larsen WL: *Anatomy development, function, clinical correlations*, Philadelphia, 2002, Saunders.

Figures 7.8, 7.9, 7.13, 7.16, 7.40, 7.43, 7.46, 7.49 from Haaga JR, Lanzieri CF, Gilkeson RC, et al: *CT and MR imaging of the whole body*, ed 5, Philadelphia, 2009, Mosby.

Figures 7.12, 7.142, 7.167, 7.173 from Standring S: *Gray's anatomy*, ed 40, Philadelphia, 2009, Churchill Livingstone.

Figures 7.29, 7.112, 7.122 from Frank: *Merrill's atlas of positioning and radiographic procedures*, ed 12, St. Louis, 2012, Mosby.

Figures 7.39, 7.42, 7.45, 7.48, 7.102 from Stark DD, Bradley WG: *Magnetic resonance imaging*, ed 3, St. Louis, 1999, Mosby.

Figures 7.179, 7.180 from Webb WR, Brant WE, Major N: *Fundamentals of body CT*, ed 3, Philadelphia, 2006, Saunders.

Chapter 8

Figures 8.9, 8.11 from Frank: *Merrill's atlas of positioning and radiographic procedures*, ed 12, St. Louis, 2012, Mosby.

Figure 8.18 from Larsen WL: *Anatomy development, function, clinical correlations*, Philadelphia, 2002, Saunders.

Figures 8.25, 8.26, 8.31, 8.65, 8.121 from Hagen-Ansert: *Textbook of diagnostic sonography*, ed 7, St. Louis, 2012, Mosby.

Figures 8.43, 8.45, 8.58, 8.79, 8.83, 8.101 from Applegate E: *The sectional anatomy learning system*, ed. 3, St. Louis, 2010, Saunders.

Figures 8.96, 8.100 courtesy of GE Medical Systems, Milwaukee, Wisc.

Figures 8.54, 8.123 from Seidel HM, Ball JW, Dains JE, et al: *Mosby's guide to physical examination*, ed 7, St. Louis, 2011, Mosby.

Figure 8.85 from Haaga JR, Lanzieri CF, Gilkeson RC, et al: *CT and MR imaging of the whole body*, ed 5, Philadelphia, 2009, Mosby.

Figure 8.98 from Standring S: *Gray's anatomy*, ed 40, Philadelphia, 2009, Churchill Livingstone.

Chapter 9

Figures 9.20, 9.21, 9.22, 9.51, 9.52 from Weir J: *Imaging atlas of human anatomy*, ed 4, Philadelphia, 2011, Mosby.

Figure 9.36 from Seidel HM, Ball JW, Dains JE, et al: *Mosby's guide to physical examination*, ed 7, St. Louis, 2011, Mosby.

Figures 9.87, 9.127 from Miller MD, Cooper DE: *Review of sports medicine and arthroscopy*, ed 2, Philadelphia, 2002, Saunders.

Figure 9.111 from Frank: *Merrill's atlas of positioning and radiographic procedures*, ed 12, St. Louis, 2012, Mosby.

Figure 9.124 from Palastanga N, Field D, Soames R, et al: *Anatomy and human movement*, ed 4, Boston, 2002, Butterworth-Heinemann.

Figures 9.126, 9.142 from Kang HS, Ahn JM: *MRI of the extremities*, ed 2, Philadelphia, 2002, Saunders.

Chapter 10

Figure 10.2 from Frank: *Merrill's atlas of positioning and radiographic procedures*, ed 12, St. Louis, 2012, Mosby.

Figure 10.12 from Byrd JWT: Gross anatomy. In Byrd JET (ed): *Operative hip arthroscopy*, New York, 1998, Thieme, pp. 69-82.

Figures 10.40, 10.41, 10.42, 10.119, 10.142, 10.168, 10.174 from Standring S: *Gray's anatomy*, ed 40, Philadelphia, 2009, Churchill Livingstone.

Figure 10.102 from Haaga JR, Lanzieri CF, Gilkeson RC, et al: *CT and MR imaging of the whole body*, ed 5, Philadelphia, 2009, Mosby.

Index

Renal fascia, 410, 410f, 411f, 442f, 446-449, 450f, 451f
Renal hilum, 451f
Renal impression, 412f
Renal medulla, 446, 450f
Renal papilla, 449f
Renal pelvis, 447f, 448f, 450f, 451f, 452f
Renal pyramids, 446, 447f, 448f, 449f, 450f
Renal vein, 6f, 442f, 446f, 487, 487f, 559-560f
Respiratory muscles, 389
Rete testis, 537, 537f
Reticular formation, 121f
Retina, 79
Retromandibular vein, 271f, 284f, 285f, 286f, 305, 305f
Retro-orbital fat, 79f, 80f, 81, 82f, 83f, 84f, 85f
Retroperitoneal space, 409t, 410, 410f
Retroperitoneum, 398f, 399f, 410, 456f
Retropharyngeal nodes, 279t
Retropharyngeal space, 259f, 283f, 287f, 289f
Retropubic space, 512f, 513f, 519f, 522f, 525f, 533, 534f, 543f, 546f, 548f
Rhomboid major muscle, 582f, 584f, 585t
Rhomboid minor muscle, 582f, 584f, 585t
Rhomboid muscle, 298f, 390f
Ribs, 230f, 308, 308f, 310f, 311f
Right adrenal gland, 419f, 442-443, 442f, 443f, 444f, 448f, 479f
Right aortic sinus, 348f, 371f
Right atrial appendage, 359f
Right atrioventricular valve, 346
Right atrium, 309f, 310f, 332f, 337f, 338f, 339f, 340f, 341f, 342f, 344f, 345f, 347f, 348f, 349f, 350f, 354f, 359f, 360f, 362, 362f, 368f, 369f, 370f, 371f, 373f, 375f, 376f, 378f, 379f, 380f, 381f, 382f, 384f, 387f, 425f, 463f
Right auricle, 336-337, 337f, 349f
Right brachiocephalic artery, 365f
Right brachiocephalic trunk, 364f
Right brachiocephalic vein, 300f, 323f, 325f, 349f, 350f, 363f, 365f, 366f, 367f, 368f, 376f
Right bundle branch, 336f
Right cardiac vein, 376
Right colic artery, 477-478, 482f
Right colic flexure, 459f, 462f
Right common carotid artery, 300, 301f, 302f, 303t, 356f, 363, 363f, 364f, 366f, 368f
Right common iliac artery, 472f, 482f, 551f
Right coronary artery, 344f, 349f, 350f, 359f, 368-369, 369f, 370f, 371f, 373f, 374f, 375f, 379f, 381f, 384f
Right coronary sinus, 370f
Right crus of diaphragm, 330f
Right descending pulmonary artery, 356f, 357f
Right external carotid artery, 301f
Right external iliac artery, 520f
Right facial artery, 301f
Right gastric artery, 426f, 477
Right gastric vein, 559-560f
Right gastroduodenal artery, 476f, 477f
Right gastroepiploic artery, 474f, 477
Right gonadal artery, 473f, 476f, 483f
Right gonadal vein, 487

Right hepatic artery, 426-427, 426f, 427f, 428f, 469f, 474f, 477f, 478f
Right hepatic duct, 431f, 433f, 435f
Right hepatic vein, 416f, 417f, 418f, 419f, 422f, 425f, 426-427, 429f, 430f
Right horizontal fissure, 319f
Right inferior lobe, 310f, 314f, 315f, 318f, 319f, 360f
Right inferior lobe bronchus, 319f
Right inferior phrenic artery, 470, 472f
Right inferior phrenic vein, 485, 485f
Right inferior pulmonary vein, 310f, 339f, 340f, 349-358, 356f, 357f, 359f, 360f, 370f
Right inferior thyroid artery, 301f
Right infracolic space, 406f, 408f
Right inguinal ligament, 468f
Right internal carotid artery, 301f
Right internal jugular vein, 329f, 363f, 366f, 367f
Right internal thoracic artery, 301f
Right internal thoracic vein, 376f
Right jugular trunk, 329f
Right kidney, 411f, 434f, 443f, 445f
Right lower quadrant, 7, 8f, 8t
Right lymphatic duct, 329, 329f
Right mainstem artery, 316f
Right mainstem bronchus, 315f, 317f, 318f, 319f, 353f, 355f, 387f
Right marginal artery, 349f
Right mediastinum, 360f
Right middle lobe bronchus, 319f
Right oblique fissure, 314f, 315f, 318f
Right ovary, 402f
Right paracolic gutter, 406f, 408f, 409t
Right perirenal space, 409t, 411f
Right phrenic nerve, 231f
Right pleural cavity, 312f
Right portal vein, 416f, 419f, 420f, 421f, 559-560f
Right principal bronchus, 316f, 360f
Right pulmonary artery, 309f, 315f, 317f, 344f, 345f, 346, 350f, 353f, 354f, 355f, 356f, 357f, 358f, 360f, 362f, 366f, 376f, 383f
Right pulmonary vein, 338f, 376f
Right pulmonary venous recess, 335f
Right pulmonic recess, 335f, 335t
Right renal artery, 468f, 469f, 471f, 472f, 476f, 482f, 483f, 550f, 556f
Right renal vein, 485f, 487, 487f, 558f
Right subclavian artery, 301f, 363, 363f, 364f, 366f, 368f
Right subclavian trunk, 329f
Right subclavian vein, 233f, 329f, 363f, 367f
Right subhepatic space, 401f, 405f, 406f, 407f, 408f, 409t
Right subphrenic space, 406f, 407f, 408f, 409t
Right superior lobe, 314f, 315f, 318f, 319f, 360f
Right superior lobe bronchus, 319f, 358f
Right superior pulmonary vein, 349-358, 356f, 358f, 360f, 370f, 372f
Right suprarenal artery, 468f
Right triangular ligament, 412, 412f
Right upper quadrant, 7, 8f, 8t
Right ureter, 452f

Right vagus nerve, 231f
Right ventricle, 309f, 310f, 334f, 336-337, 336f, 337f, 338f, 339f, 340f, 341f, 342f, 343f, 345f, 347f, 349f, 350f, 351f, 353f, 360f, 361f, 362, 362f, 368f, 369f, 370f, 371f, 373f, 374f, 375f, 378f, 379f, 380f, 381f, 382f, 383f, 384f, 385f, 418f, 463f
Right ventricular outflow tract, 344f, 377-379, 380f, 383f, 384f, 463f
Right vertebral artery, 233f, 284f, 285f, 301f
Rivinus's ducts, 270
Rostral, 4t
Rotator cuff, 590
Rotator cuff muscles, 592f
Rotatores muscle, 201t, 205f, 207f
Round ligament of uterus, 402, 406f, 412f, 413, 436f, 527f, 528, 528f, 531f, 534f
Round window, 37f, 39f, 40, 44f, 166f
Rugae, 453f, 455f

S
Saccular duct, 39f
Sacral ala, 452f
Sacral flexure, 518f, 523
Sacral foramina, 187f, 191-193, 191f, 192f, 495, 496f, 497f, 659f
Sacral ligament, 191f
Sacral nerve root sleeve, 225f, 239f
Sacral nerves, 210f, 225f, 239f
Sacral promontory, 187f, 188-189f, 192f, 193f, 216f, 398f, 495, 497f, 498f, 504f, 659f
Sacroiliac joint, 191-193, 192f, 193f, 208f, 225f, 238f, 239f, 495, 496f, 497f, 498f, 503f, 508f, 552f, 553f, 659f
Sacrospinous ligament, 542f, 748f
Sacrotuberous ligament, 511f, 515f
Sacrum, 187f, 188-189f, 191-193, 191f, 192f, 204f, 223f, 225f, 238f, 239f, 242f, 495-497, 496f, 497f, 498f, 499f, 504f, 514f, 519f
Sagittal plane, 2, 2f
Sagittal suture, 46, 49f
Salivary glands, 270, 270f, 271f, 272f, 273f, 274f, 275f
    parotid gland, 233f, 252f, 254f, 258f, 270, 270f, 271f, 272f, 285f, 286f, 293f
    sublingual glands, 270, 270f, 275f, 294f, 295f
    submandibular glands, 252f, 255f, 256f, 257f, 264f, 270, 270f, 273f, 274f, 278f, 287f, 288f
Salpingopharyngeus muscle, 291, 292t
Saphenous nerve, 237, 237f, 674f, 754f
Saphenous vein, 6f, 685f
Sartorius muscle, 507f, 509f, 538f, 540f, 541f, 554f, 561f, 562f, 656f, 661f, 670f, 671f, 672-677, 672f, 677f, 678f, 681t, 683f, 685f, 691f, 701f, 702f, 712f, 748f, 752f
Scala tympani, 39f
Scala vestibuli, 39f
Scaphoid bone, 621, 622f, 623f, 624f, 625f, 626f, 628f, 629f, 634f, 635f, 644f
Scapholunate ligament, 629f, 634f
Scapula, 298f, 365f, 565-567, 566f, 582f, 590
Scapular notch, 564-565, 564f, 567f

Scapular spine, 575f, 577f, 583f, 585f
Sciatic nerve, 237f, 239, 240f, 241f, 562f, 656f, 661f, 676f, 748f, 754
Scrotal septum, 536f
Scrotum, 519f, 535-536, 536f, 538f, 540f
Secondary pulmonary lobule, 318, 321f
Segmental artery, 238f, 241, 244f
Segmental bronchi, 318, 321f
Segmental pulmonary veins, 321f
Sella turcica, 18f, 19f, 25-27, 25f, 26f, 31f, 53f, 72, 77f
Semicircular canals, 33f, 36f, 37f, 38f, 40, 40f, 43f, 166f, 167f
Semicircular duct, 33f
Semilunar hiatus, 74-75, 74f, 75f
Semilunar valves, 346
Semimembranosus bursae, 704
Semimembranosus muscle, 668f, 674f, 676f, 678-681, 679f, 680f, 681t, 691f, 692f, 699f, 700f, 701f, 712f
Semimembranosus tendon, 549f, 676f, 683f, 693f, 700f, 701f, 703f, 705f
Seminal vesicle, 513f, 519f, 523f, 535f, 542, 542f, 543f, 546f
Seminiferous tubules, 537f
Semispinalis capitis muscle, 202f, 203f, 204f, 205f, 207, 207f, 234f, 255f, 256f, 259f, 262f, 274f, 281f, 282f, 284f, 285f, 286f, 287f, 288f, 289f
Semispinalis cervicis muscle, 203f, 205f, 207, 256f, 259f, 282f, 283f, 286f, 287f, 288f
Semispinalis thoracis muscle, 206f, 207
Semitendinosus muscle, 239f, 538f, 549f, 668f, 674f, 676f, 678-681, 679f, 680f, 681t, 712f
Semitendinosus tendon, 683f, 700f, 701f, 703f, 708f
Septal pulmonary vein, 321f
Septal vein, 156f
Septum pellucidum, 93, 93b, 95f, 99f, 106f, 112f, 117f
Serous pericardium, 333
Serratus anterior muscle, 236f, 298f, 390f, 392f, 394, 395t, 492f, 593-594, 593f, 594t, 597f
Serratus posterior inferior muscle, 389, 389t, 390f, 391f
Serratus posterior superior muscle, 389, 389t, 390f, 391f
Shaded surface display, 12, 13f
Shingles, 211b
Short axis view, 377-379, 377f, 380f, 381f, 382f
Shoulder, 564-600
    arterial supply of, 646-650
    articular joint capsule of, 580-581, 580f
    bony anatomy of, 564-568, 564f, 565f, 566f, 567f, 568f
    bursae of, 581, 581f
    clavicle, 236f, 273f, 310f, 326f, 328f, 332f, 348f, 366f, 564-565, 564f, 573f
    humerus, 568, 568f, 569f, 570f, 595f, 596f, 597f, 598f, 599f, 601f
    labrum of, 569f, 571-572, 571f, 573f, 574f, 576f, 577f, 580f
    ligaments of, 571-572, 571f, 572f, 573f, 574f, 575f, 576f, 577f, 578f, 579f, 580f
    muscles of, 582-595, 582f, 583f, 584f, 585f, 586f, 587f, 588f, 589f, 591f, 592f, 593f, 594f, 595f, 596f, 597f, 598f, 599f, 600, 600f